Bayesian Biostatistics

Statistics in Practice

Series Advisors

Human and Biological Sciences
Stephen Senn
CRP-Santé, Luxembourg

Earth and Environmental Sciences
Marian Scott
University of Glasgow, UK

Industry, Commerce and Finance
Wolfgang Jank
University of Maryland, USA

Statistics in Practice is an important international series of texts which provide detailed coverage of statistical concepts, methods and worked case studies in specific fields of investigation and study.

With sound motivation and many worked practical examples, the books show in down-to-earth terms how to select and use an appropriate range of statistical techniques in a particular practical field within each title's special topic area.

The books provide statistical support for professionals and research workers across a range of employment fields and research environments. Subject areas covered include medicine and pharmaceutics; industry, finance and commerce; public services; the earth and environmental sciences, and so on.

The books also provide support to students studying statistical courses applied to the above areas. The demand for graduates to be equipped for the work environment has led to such courses becoming increasingly prevalent at universities and colleges.

It is our aim to present judiciously chosen and well-written workbooks to meet everyday practical needs. Feedback of views from readers will be most valuable to monitor the success of this aim.

A complete list of titles in this series can be found at
www.wiley.com/go/statisticsinpractice

Bayesian Biostatistics

Emmanuel Lesaffre

Erasmus MC, Rotterdam, The Netherlands and K.U. Leuven, Belgium

Andrew B. Lawson

Medical University of South Carolina, Charleston, USA

WILEY

A John Wiley & Sons, Ltd., Publication

This edition first published 2012

Registered of ce
John Wiley & Sons Ltd, The Atrium, Southern Gate, Chichester, West Sussex, PO19 8SQ, United Kingdom

For details of our global editorial offices, for customer services and for information about how to apply for permission to reuse the copyright material in this book please see our website at www.wiley.com.

Library of Congress Cataloging-in-Publication Data

Lesaffre, Emmanuel.
Bayesian biostatistics / Emmanuel Lesaffre, Andrew Lawson.
p. ; cm.
Includes bibliographical references and index.
ISBN 978-0-470-01823-1 (cloth)
1. Biometry–Methodology. 2. Bayesian statistical decision theory. I. Lawson, Andrew (Andrew B.) II. Title.
[DNLM: 1. Biostatistics–methods. 2. Bayes Theorem. QH 323.5]
QH323.5.L45 2012
570.1′5195–dc23

2012004237

A catalogue record for this book is available from the British Library.

ISBN: 978-0-470-01823-1

Typeset in 10/12pt Times by Aptara Inc., New Delhi, India

Contents

Part II BAYESIAN TOOLS FOR STATISTICAL MODELING

Preface

The growth of biostatistics as a subject has been phenomenal in recent years and has been marked by a considerable technical innovation in methodology and computational practicality. One area that has a significant growth is the class of Bayesian methods. This growth has taken place partly because a growing number of practitioners value the Bayesian paradigm as matching that of scientific discovery. But the computational advances in the last decade that have allowed for more complex models to be fitted routinely to realistic data sets have also led to this growth.

In this book, we explore the Bayesian approach via a great variety of medical application areas. In effect, from the elementary concepts to the more advanced modeling exercises, the Bayesian tools will be exemplified using a diversity of applications taken from epidemiology, exploratory clinical studies, health promotion studies and clinical trials.

This book grew out of a course that the first author has taught for many years (especially) in the Master programs in (bio)statistics at the universities of Hasselt and Leuven, both in Belgium. The course material was the inspiration for two out of three parts in the book. Therefore, the intended readership of this book are Master program students in (bio)statistics, but we hope that applied researchers with a good statistical background will also find the book useful. The structure of the book allows it to be used as course material for a course in Bayesian methods at an undergraduate or early stage postgraduate level. The aim of the book is to introduce the reader smoothly into Bayesian statistical methods with chapters that gradually increase in the level of complexity. The book consists of three parts. The first two parts of this work were the chapters primarily covered by the first author, while the last five chapters were primarily covered by the second author.

In Part I, we first review the fundamental concepts of the significance test and the associated P-value and note that frequentist methods, although proved to be quite useful over many years, are not without conceptual flaws. We also note that there are other methods on the market, such as the likelihood approach, but more importantly, the Bayesian approach. In addition, we introduce (an embryonic version of) the Bayes theorem. In Chapter 2, we derive the general expression of Bayes theorem and illustrate extensively the analytical computations to arrive at the posterior distribution on the binomial, the Gaussian and the Poisson case. For this, simple textbook examples are used. In Chapter 3, the reader is introduced to various posterior summary measures and the predictive distributions. Since sampling is fundamental to contemporary Bayesian approaches, sampling algorithms are introduced and exemplified in this chapter. While these sampling procedures will not yet prove their usefulness in practice, we believe that the early introduction of relatively simple sampling techniques will prepare the reader better for the advanced algorithms seen in later chapters. In this chapter, approaches to Bayesian hypothesis testing are treated and we introduce the Bayes factor. In Chapter 4, we extend all the concepts and computations seen in the first three chapters for univariate problems to the multivariate case, introducing also Bayesian regression models. It is then seen that, in general, no analytical methods to derive the posterior distribution are available, neither are the classical numerical approaches to integration sufficient. A new approach is then needed. Before addressing the solution to the problem, we treat in Chapter 5 the choice of the prior distribution. The prior distribution is the keystone to the Bayesian methodology. Yet, the appropriate choice of the prior distribution has been the topic of extensive discussions between non-Bayesians and Bayesians, but also among Bayesians. In this chapter, we extensively treat the various ways of specifying prior knowledge. In Chapters 6 and 7, we treat the basics of the Markov chain Monte Carlo methodologies. In Chapter 6, the Gibbs and the Metropolis–Hastings samplers are introduced again illustrated using a variety of medical examples. Chapter 7 is devoted to assessing and accelerating the convergence of the Markov chains. In addition, we cover the extension of the EM-algorithm to the Bayesian context, i.e. the data augmentation approach is exemplified. It is then time to see how Bayesian analyses can be done in practice. For this reason, we review in Chapter 8 the Bayesian software. We focus on two software packages: the most popular WinBUGS and the recently released Bayesian SAS® procedures. In both cases, a simple regression analysis serves as a guiding example helping the readers in their first analyzes with these packages. We end this chapter with a review of other Bayesian software, such as the packages OpenBUGS and JAGS, and also various R packages written to perform specific analyses.

In Part II, we develop Bayesian tools for statistical modeling. We start in Chapter 9 with reviewing hierarchical models. To fix ideas, we focus first on two simple two-level hierarchical models. The first is the Poisson-gamma model applied to a spatial data set on lip cancer cases in former East Germany. This example serves to introduce the concepts of hierarchical modeling. Then, we turn to the Gaussian hierarchical model as an introduction to the more general mixed models. A variety of mixed models are explored and amply exemplified. Also in this chapter comparisons between frequentist and Bayesian solutions aim to help the reader to see the differences between the two approaches. Model building and assessment are the topics of Chapter 10. The aim of this chapter is to see how statistical modeling could be performed entirely within the Bayesian framework. To this end, we reintroduce the Bayes factor (and its variants) to select between two statistical models. The Bayes factor is an important tool in model selection but is also fraught with serious computational difficulties. We then move to the Deviance Information Criterion (DIC). For a better understanding of this popular model selection criterion, we introduce at length the classical model selection criteria, i.e. AIC and BIC and relate them to DIC. The part on model checking describes all classical actions one would take to construct and evaluate a model, such as checking the residuals for outliers and influential observations, finding the correct scale of the response and the covariates, choosing the correct link function, etc. In this chapter, we also elaborate on the posterior predictive check as a general tool for goodness-of-fit testing. The final chapter, Chapter 11, in Part II handles Bayesian variable selection. This is a rapidly evolving topic that received a great impetus from the developments in bioinformatics. A broad overview of possible variable and model selection approaches and the associated software is given. While in the previous two chapters, the WinBUGS software and to a lesser extent the Bayesian SAS procedures were dominant, in this chapter we focus on software packages in R.

In Part III, we address particular application areas for Bayesian modeling. We include the most important areas from a practical biostatistical standpoint. In Chapter 12, we examine bioassay, where we consider preclinical testing methods: both Ames and Mouse Lymphoma *in vitro* assays and the famous Beetles LD50 toxicity assay are considered. In Chapter 13, we consider the important and pervasive problem of measurement error and also the misclassification in biostatistical studies. We discuss Berkson and classical joint models, bias such as attenuation and the problem of discrete error in the form of misclassification. In Chapter 14, we examine survival analysis from a Bayesian perspective. In this chapter, we cover basic survival time models and risk-set-based approaches and extend models to consider contextual effects within hazards. In Chapter 15, longitudinal analysis is considered in greater depth. Correlated prior distributions for parameters and also temporally correlated errors are considered. Missingness mechanisms are discussed and a nonrandom missingness example is explored. In Chapter 16, two important spatial biostatistical application areas are then considered: disease mapping and image analysis. In disease mapping, basic Poisson convolution models that include spatially structured random effects are examined for risk estimation, while in image analysis a focus on Bayesian fMRI analysis with correlated prior distributions is presented.

In Chapter 17, we end the book with a brief review of the topics that we did not cover in this book and give some key references for further reading. Finally, in the appendix, we provide an overview of the characteristics of most popular distributions used in Bayesian analyses.

Throughout the book there are numerous examples. In Parts I and II, explicit reference is made to the programs associated with the examples. These programs can be found at the website `www.wiley.com/go/bayesian_methods_biostatistics`. The programs used in Part III can also be found at this website.

Acknowledgments

When writing the early chapters, the first author benefitted from discussions with master students at Leuven, Hasselt and Leiden who pointed out various typos and ambiguities in earlier versions of the book. In addition, thanks go to the colleagues and former/current PhD students at L-Biostat at KU Leuven and at the Department of Biostatistics, Erasmus MC, Rotterdam, for illustrative discussions, critical remarks and help with software. In this respect, special thanks go to Susan Bryan, Silvia Cecere, Luwis Diya, Alejandro Jara, Arnošt Komárek, Marek Molas, Mukendi Mbuyi, Timothy Mutsvari, Veronika Rockova, Robin Van Oirbeek and Sten Willemsen. Software support was received from Sabanés Bové on the R package `glmBfp`, Fang Chen on the Bayesian SAS programs, Robert Gramacy on the R program `monomvn`, David Hastie and Peter Green on an R program for RJMCMC, David Lunn on the Jump interface in WinBUGS, Elizabeth Slate and Karen Vines. Thanks also go to those who provided data for the book or who gave permission to use their data, i.e. Steven Boonen, Elly Den Hondt, Jolanda Luime, the Signal-Tandmobiel® team, Bako Topal and Vincent van Weel. The authors also wish to thank, for interesting discussions, their colleagues in Leuven, Rotterdam and Charleston especially Dipankar Bandyopadhyay, Paul Eilers, Steffen Fieuws, Mulugeta Gebregziabher, Dimitris Rizopoulos and Elizabeth Slate. Finally, insightful conversations with George Casella, James Hodges, Helmut Küchenhoff and Paul Schmitt were much appreciated.

Last, the first author especially wishes to thank his wife Lieve Sels for her patience not only during the preparation of the 'book' but also during his whole professional career. To his children, Annemie and Kristof, he apologizes for the many times that their father was present but 'absent'.

Emmanuel Lesaffre (Rotterdam and Leuven)
Andrew B. Lawson (Charleston)

December 2011

Notation, terminology and some guidance for reading the book

Notation and terminology

In this section, we review some notation used in the book. We limit ourselves to outline some general principles; for precise definitions, we refer to the text.

First, both the random variable and its realization are denoted in this book as y. The vector of covariates is most often denoted as $\boldsymbol{x}$. The distribution of a discrete y as well as the density of a continuous variable will be denoted as $p(y)$, unless otherwise stated. In the text, we make clear which of the two meanings applies. A sample of observations $y_1, \ldots, y_n$ is denoted as $\boldsymbol{y}$, but also, a d-dimensional vector will be denoted in bold, i.e. $\boldsymbol{y}$. We make it clear from the context what is implied. Further, independent, identically distributed random variables are indicated as i.i.d. A distribution (density) depending on a parameter vector $\boldsymbol{\theta}$ is denoted as $p(y \mid \boldsymbol{\theta})$. The joint distribution of y and z is denoted as $p(y, z \mid \boldsymbol{\theta})$ and the conditional distribution of y, given z will be denoted as $y \mid z, \boldsymbol{\theta} \sim p(y \mid z, \boldsymbol{\theta})$. Alternatively, we use the notation $p(y \mid z, \boldsymbol{\theta})$. The probability that an event happens will occasionally be denoted as P for reasons of clarity.

A particular distribution will be addressed in two ways. For example, $y \sim \text{Gamma}(\alpha, \beta)$ indicates that the random variable y has a gamma distribution with parameters α and β, but to indicate that the distribution is evaluated in y we will use the notation $\text{Gamma}(y \mid \alpha, \beta)$. When parameters have been given almost the same notation, say $\beta_0, \beta_1, \beta_3$, then the notation β_* is used where * is a place holder for 1, 2, 3.

In the normal case, some Bayesian textbooks use the *precision* notation while others use the *variance* notation. More specifically, if y has a normal distribution with mean μ and variance σ^2, then instead of $y \sim \text{N}(\mu, \sigma^2)$ (classical notation) the alternative notation $y \sim \text{N}(\mu, \tau^{-1})$ (or even $y \sim \text{N}(\mu, \tau)$) with the precision $\tau = \sigma^{-2}$ is used by some. This alternative notation is inspired by the fact that in Bayesian statistics some key results are better expressed in terms of the precision rather than the variance. This is also the notation used by WinBUGS. In this book, we frequently refer to classical, frequentist statistics. The use of precision would then be more confusing, rather than illuminating. In addition, when it comes to summarizing the results of a statistical analysis, the standard deviation is a better tool than the precision. For these reasons, we primarily used in this book the variance notation. But, throughout the book (especially in the later chapters) we regularly make the transition from one notation to the other.

Finally, we use some generally accepted standard notations, such as $\boldsymbol{x}$ always denotes a column vector, $|A|$ denotes the determinant of a matrix A, tr(A) is the trace of a matrix and A^T denotes the transpose of a matrix A. The sample mean of $\{y_1, y_2, \ldots, y_n\}$ is denoted as $\overline{y}$ and their standard deviation as s, s_y or simply SD.

Guidance for reading the book

No particular guidance is needed to read this book. The flow in the book is natural: starting from elementary Bayesian concepts we gradually introduce the more complex topics. This book deals, basically, only with parametric Bayesian methods. This means that all our random variables are assumed to have a particular distribution with a finite number of parameters. In the Bayesian world, many more distributions are used than in classical statistics. So for the classical reader (whatever meaning this may have), many of the distributions that pop-up in the book will be new. A brief characterization of these distributions, together with a graphical display, can be found in the appendix of the book.

Finally, some of the sections indicated by '*' are technical and may be skipped at first reading.

Part I

BASIC CONCEPTS IN BAYESIAN METHODS

1

Modes of statistical inference

The central activity in statistics is inference. Statistical inference is a procedure or a collection of activities with the aim to extract information from (gathered) data and to generalize the observed results beyond the data at hand, say to a population or to the future. In this way, statistical inference may help the researchers in suggesting or verifying scientific hypotheses, or decision makers in improving their decisions. Inference obviously depends on the collected data and on the assumed underlying probabilistic model that generated these data, but it also depends on the approach to generalize from the known (data) to the unknown (population). We distinguish two mainstream views/paradigms to draw statistical inference, i.e. the frequentist approach and the Bayesian approach. In-between these two paradigms is the (pure) likelihood approach.

In most of the empirical research, but definitely in medical research, scientific conclusions need to be supported by a 'significant result' using the classical P-value. Significance testing belongs to the frequentist paradigm. However, the frequentist approach does not consist of one unifying theory but is rather the combination of two approaches, i.e. the inductive approach of Fisher who introduced the null-hypothesis, the P-value and the significance level and the deductive procedure of Neyman and Pearson who introduced the alternative hypothesis and the notion of power. First, we review the practice of frequentist significance testing and focus on the popular P-value. More specifically we look at the value of the P-value in practice. Second, we treat an approach that is purely based on the likelihood function not involving any classical significance testing. This approach is based on two fundamental likelihood principles that are also essential for the Bayesian philosophy. Finally, we end this chapter by introducing the principles of the Bayesian approach and we give an outlook of what the Bayesian approach can bring to the statistician. However, at least three more chapters will be needed to fully develop the Bayesian theory.

Bayesian Biostatistics, First Edition. Emmanuel Lesaffre and Andrew B. Lawson.

1.1 The frequentist approach: A critical reflection

1.1.1 The classical statistical approach

It is perhaps an oversimplification to speak of a classical statistical approach. Nevertheless, we mean by this the ensemble of methods that provides statistical inference based on the classical P-value, the significance level, the power and the confidence interval (CI). To fix ideas, we now exemplify current statistical practice with a *randomized controlled clinical trial* (*RCT*). In fact, the RCT is the study design that, by excellence, is based on the classical statistical tool box of inferential procedures. We assume that the reader is familiar with the classical concepts in inferential statistics.

For those who have never experienced a RCT, here is a brief description. A clinical trial is an experimental study comparing two (or more) medical treatments on human subjects, most often patients. When a control group is involved, the trial is called *controlled*. For a *parallel* group design, one group of patients receives one treatment and the other group(s) receive(s) the other treatment and all groups are followed up in time to measure the effect of the treatments. In a *randomized study*, patients are assigned to the treatments in a random manner. To minimize bias in evaluating the effect of the treatments, patients and/or care givers are blinded. When only patients are blinded one speaks of a *single-blinded* study, but when both patients and care givers are blinded (and everyone involved in running the trial) one speaks of a *double-blinded* trial. Finally, when more than one center (e.g. hospital) is involved one deals with a multicenter study.

Example I.1: Toenail RCT: Evaluation of two oral treatments for toenail infection using the frequentist approach

A randomized, double-blind, parallel group, multicenter study was set up to compare the efficacy of two oral treatments for toenail infection (De Backer *et al.* 1996). In this study, two groups of 189 patients were recruited, and each received 12 weeks of treatment (Lamisil: treatment A and Itraconazol: treatment B), with 48 weeks of follow-up (FU). The significance level was set at $\alpha = 0.05$. The *primary endpoint* (upon which the sample size was based) in the original study was negative mycology, i.e. a negative microscopy and a negative culture. Here, we look at another endpoint, i.e. *unaffected nail length at week 48* on a subset of patients for whom the big toenail was the target nail. One hundred and thirty-one patients treated with A and 133 treated with B were included in this comparison. Note that we only included those patients present at the end of the study. The observed mean (SD) lengths in millimeter at week 48 were 9.07 (4.92) and 7.70 (5.33), for treatments A and B, respectively. Suppose the (population) average for treatment A is μ_1 while for treatment B it is μ_2. Therefore, the null-hypothesis is $H_0 : \Delta = \mu_1 - \mu_2 = 0$ and can be evaluated with an unpaired t-test at a two-sided significance level of $\alpha = 0.05$. Upon completion of the study, the treatment estimate was $\widehat{\Delta} = 1.38$ with an observed value of the t-statistic equal to $t_{obs} = 2.19$. This result lies in the rejection region corresponding to $\alpha = 0.05$ yielding a statistically significant result (at 0.05). Thus, according to the Neyman–Pearson (NP) approach we (can) reject that A and B are equally effective.

It is common to report also the P-value of the result to indicate the strength of evidence against the hypothesis of two equally effective treatments. Here, we obtained a two-sided P-value equal to 0.030, which is a measure of evidence against H_0 in a Fisherian sense. □

In Section 1.1.2, we reflect on what message the P-value can bring to the researcher. We will also indicate what properties the P-value does not have (but assumed to have).

1.1.2 The *P*-value as a measure of evidence

Fisher developed the P-value in the context of well-planned limited agricultural experiments in a time when computations had to be done by hand. Nowadays, a great variety of studies are undertaken in the medical research usually of an exploratory nature and often evaluating hundreds to thousands of P-values. The P-value is an intuitively appealing measure against the null-hypothesis, but that it is not always perceived in the correct manner. Here, we will further elaborate on the use and misuse of the P-value in practice.

The *P*-value is not the probability that H_0 is (not) true A common error is to interpret the P-value as a probability that H_0 is (not) true. However, the P-value only measures the extremeness of the observed result under H_0. The probability that H_0 is true is formally $p(H_0 \mid \text{data})$, which we shall call the posterior probability of the null-hypothesis in the following text, given the observed data. This probability is based on Bayes theorem and depends on the prevalence of H_0 (see also Example I.11).

The *P*-value depends on fictive data The P-value does not express the probability that the observed result occurred under H_0, but is rather the probability of observing this or a more extreme result under H_0. This implies that the calculation of the P-value is based not only on the observed result but also on fictive (never observed) data.

Example I.2: Toenail RCT: Meaning of *P*-value
The P-value is equal to the probability that the test statistic exceeds the observed value if the null-hypothesis were true. The computation of the P-value is done using probability laws, but could also be represented by a simulation experiment. For instance, in the toenail infection study the P-value is approximately equal to the proportion of studies, out of (say) 10 000 imaginary studies done under H_0 (two identical treatments), that yield a t-value more extreme than $t_{\text{obs}} = 2.19$. In Figure 1.1, the histogram of imaginary results is displayed together with the observed result. □

The *P*-value depends on the sample space The above simulation exercise shows that the P-value is computed as a probability using the *long-run frequency definition*, which means that a probability for an event A is defined as the ultimate proportion of experiments that generated that event to the total number of experiments. For a P-value, the event A corresponds to a t-value located in the rejection region. This makes it clear that the P-value depends on the choice of the fictive studies and, hence, also on the sample space. The particular choice can have surprising effects, as illustrated in Example I.3.

Example I.3: Accounting for interim analyses in a RCT
Suppose that a randomized controlled trial has been set up to compare two treatments and that four *interim analyses for efficacy* were planned. An interim analysis for efficacy is a statistical comparison between the treatment groups prior to the end of the study to see

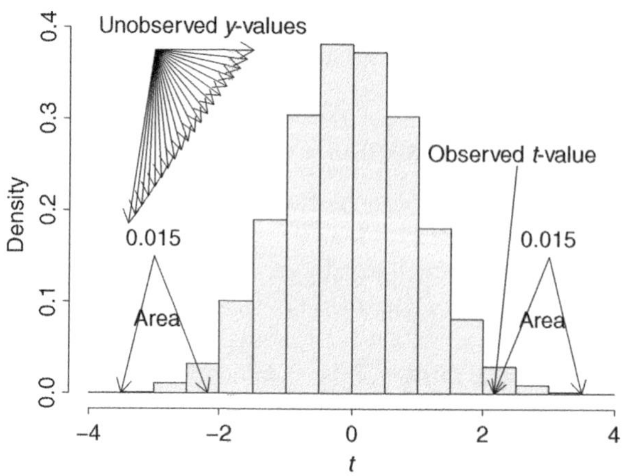

Figure 1.1 Graphical representation of the P-value by means of a simulation study under H_0.

whether the experimental treatment is better than the control treatment. The purpose is to stop the trial earlier if possible. When more than one comparison is planned, one needs to correct in a frequentist approach for *multiple testing*. A classical correction for multiple testing is *Bonferroni's rule* which dictates that the significance level at each comparison (*nominal significance level*) needs to be made more stringent, i.e. α/k where k is the total number of tests applied, to arrive at an overall (across all comparisons) type I error rate less or equal to α. Bonferroni's procedure is approximate; an exact control of the type I error rate is obtained with a *group sequential design* (Jennison and Turnbull 2000). With Pocock's group sequential method and 5 analyses (4 interim + 1 final analyses), a significance level of 0.016 is handled at each analysis to achieve a global significance level of 0.05. Thus, when the study ran until the end and at the last analysis a P-value of 0.02 was obtained, then the result cannot be claimed significant with Pocock's rule. However, if the same result had been obtained without planning interim analyses, then this trial produced a significant result! Thus, in the presence of two identical results, one cannot claim evidence against the null-hypothesis in one case, while in the other case we would conclude that the two treatments have a different effect. □

In statistical terminology, the different evidence for the treatment effect in the two RCTs of Example I.3 (with an identical P-value) is due to a different sample space (see below) in the two scenarios. This is further illustrated in Example I.4.

Example I.4: Kaldor' *et al.* case-control study: Illustration of sample space

In the (matched) case-control study (Kaldor *et al.* 1990) involving 149 cases (leukaemia patients) and 411 controls, the purpose was to examine the impact of chemotherapy on leukaemia in Hodgkin's survivors (Ashby *et al.* 1993). The 5-year survival of Hodgkin's disease (cancer of the lymph nodes) is about 80%, but the survivors have an excess risk of developing solid tumors, leukaemia and/or lymphomas. In Table 1.1, the cases and controls are subdivided according to exposure to chemotherapy or not.

Table 1.1 Kaldor' *et al.* case-control study (Kaldor *et al.* 1990): frequency table of cases and controls subdivided according to their exposure to chemotherapy.

Treatment	Controls	Cases
No chemo	160	11
Chemo	251	138
Total	411	149

Ignoring the matched character of the data, the analysis of the 2×2-contingency table by a Pearson chi-squared test results in $P = 7.8959 \times 10^{-13}$ with a chi-squared value of 51.3. With the Fisher's exact test, a P-value of 1.487×10^{-14} was obtained. Finally, the estimated odds ratio is equal to 7.9971 with a 95% CI of [4.19, 15.25]. □

The chi-squared test and the Fisher's exact test have a different *sample space*, which is the space of possible samples considered to calculate the null distribution of the test statistic. The sample space for the chi-squared test consists of the 2×2-contingency tables with the same total sample size (n), while for Fisher's exact test the sample space consists of the subset of 2×2-contingency tables with the same row and column marginal totals. The difference between the two sample spaces explains here partly the difference in the two test results. In Example I.3, it is the sole reason for the different evidence from the two RCTs. The conclusion of a scientific experiment, hence, not only depends on the results of that experiment but also on the results of experiments that did not and will never happen. This finding has triggered a lot of debate among statisticians (see Royall 1997).

The *P*-value is not an absolute measure A small P-value does not necessarily imply a large difference between two treatments or a strong association among variables. Indeed, as a measure of evidence the P-value does not take the size of the study into account. There have been vivid discussions on how a small P-value should be interpreted as a function of the size of the study (see Royall 1997).

The *P*-value does not take all evidence into account Let us take the following example also discussed by Ashby *et al.* (1993).

Example I.5: Merseyside registry results

Ashby *et al.* (1993) reported on data obtained from a subsequent registry study in UK (after Kaldor *et al.*'s case-control study) to check the relationship between chemotherapy and leukemia among Hodgkin's survivors. Preliminary results of the Merseyside registry were reported in Ashby *et al.* (1993) and are reproduced in Table 1.2. The P-value obtained from the chi-squared test with continuity correction equals 0.67. Thus, formally there is no reason to worry that chemotherapy may cause leukemia among Hodgkin's survivors. Of course, every epidemiologist would recognize that this study has no chance of finding a relationship between chemotherapy and leukemia because of the small study size. By simply analyzing the data of the Merseyside registry, no evidence of a relationship can be established. □

Table 1.2 Merseyside registry: frequency table of cases and controls subdivided according to their exposure to chemotherapy.

Treatment	Controls	Cases
No chemo	3	0
Chemo	3	2
Total	6	2

Is it reasonable to analyze the results of the Merseyside registry in isolation, not referring to the previous study of Kaldor *et al.* (1990)? In other words, should one forget about the historical data and assume that one cannot learn anything from the past? The answer will depend on the particular circumstances, but it is not obvious that the past should never play a role in the analysis of data.

1.1.3 The confidence interval as a measure of evidence

While the P-value has been criticized by many statisticians, it is more the (mis)use of the P-value that is under fire. Nevertheless, there is a growing preference to replace the P-value by the (95%) CI.

Example I.6: Toenail RCT: Illustration of 95% confidence interval
The 95% CI for Δ is equal to [0.14, 2.62]. Technically speaking we can only say that in the long run 95% of those intervals will contain the true parameter (the 95% CI is based on the long-run frequency definition of probability). But for our RCT, the 95% CI will either contain the true parameter or not (with probability 1)! In our communication to nonstatisticians, we never use the technical definition of the CI. Rather, we say that the 95% CI [0.14, 2.62] expresses that we are uncertain about the true value of Δ and that it most likely lies between 0.14 and 2.62 (with 0.95 probability). □

The 95% CI expresses our uncertainty about the parameter of interest and as such is considered to give better insight into the relevance of the obtained results than the P-value. However, the adjective '95%' refers to the procedure of constructing the interval and not to the interval itself. The interpretation that we give to nonstatisticians has a Bayesian flavor as will be seen in Chapter 2.

1.1.4 An historical note on the two frequentist paradigms*

In this section, we expand on the difference between the two frequentist paradigms and how they have been integrated in practice into an apparently one unifying approach. This section is not essential for the remainder of the book and can be skipped. A more in-depth treatment of this topic can be found in Hubbard and Bayarri (2003) and the papers of Goodman (1993, 1999a, 1999b) and Royall (1997).

The Fisherian and the NP approach are different in nature but are integrated in current statistical practice. Fisher's views on statistical inference are elaborated in two of his books: *Statistical Methods for Research Workers* (Fisher 1925) and *The Design of Experiments* (Fisher 1935). He strongly advocated the inductive reasoning to generate new hypotheses. Fisher's approach to inductive inference goes via the rejection of the *null-hypothesis*, say $H_0 : \Delta = 0$. His *significance test* constitutes of a statistical procedure based on a test statistic for which the sampling distribution, given that $\Delta = 0$ holds, is determined. He called the probability under H_0 of obtaining the observed value of that test statistic or a more extreme one, the P-value. To Fisher, the P-value was just a practical tool for inductive inference whereby the smaller the P-value implies a greater evidence against $\Delta = 0$. Further, according to Fisher the null-hypothesis should be 'rejected' when the P-value is small, say less than a prespecified threshold $\alpha = 0.05$ called the *level of significance*. Fisher's rule for rejecting H_0 is, therefore, when $P \leq 0.05$, but he recognized (Fisher 1959) that rejection may have two meanings: either that an exceptionally rare chance has occurred or the theory (according to the null-hypothesis) is not true.

In their approach to statistical testing, Neyman and Pearson (1928a, 1928b, 1933) needed an *alternative hypothesis* (H_a), say $\Delta \neq 0$. Once the data have been observed, the investigator needs to decide between two actions: reject H_0 (and accept H_a) or accept H_0 (and reject H_a). NP called their procedure an *hypothesis test*. Their approach to research has a decision theoretic flavor, i.e. decision makers can commit two errors: (1) type I error with probability P(type I error) $= \alpha$ (*type I error rate*) when H_0 is rejected while in fact true and (2) type II error with probability P(type II error) $= \beta$ (*type II error rate*) when H_a is rejected while in fact true. In this respect they introduced the *power* of a test, equal to $1 - \beta$ for an alternative hypothesis $H_a : \Delta = \Delta_a$. NP argued that a statistical test must minimize the probability of making the wrong decision and demonstrated (Neyman and Pearson 1933) that the well-known *likelihood-ratio test* minimizes β for given a value for α. The NP approach is in fact deductive and reasons from the general to the particular and thereby makes claims from the particular to the general only in the long run. NP strived that one shall not be wrong too often. In other words, they rather advocated 'inductive behavior'. Fisher strongly disliked this viewpoint and both parties ended up in a never-ending debate.

Despite the strong historical disagreement between the proponents of the two approaches, nowadays the two philosophies are mixed up and presented as a unifying methodology. Hubbard and Bayarri (2003) (see also references therein) warned for the confusion this unification might imply, especially for the danger that the P-value is wrongly interpreted as a type I error rate. Indeed, the P-value was introduced by Fisher as a surprise index vis-à-vis the null-hypothesis and in the light of the data. It is an a posteriori determined probability. A problem occurs when the P-value is given the status of an a priori determined error rate. For example, suppose the significance level is $\alpha = 0.05$, chosen in advance. Thus, if upon completion of the study, we obtain $P = 0.023$ we say that H_0 is rejected at 0.05. However, we cannot say that H_0 is rejected at the 0.025 level, because in this sense α is chosen after the facts and P obtains the status of a prespecified level. In medical papers, the P-value is often given the nature of a prespecified value. For instance when significant results are indicated by asterisks, e.g. '*' for $P < 0.05$, '**' for $P < 0.01$ and '***' for $P < 0.001$, then the impression is created that for a '**' result significance at 0.01 can be claimed. Following Carl Popper (Popper 1959), Fisher claimed that one can never accept the null-hypothesis, only disprove it. In contrast, according to the NP approach subsequent to the hypothesis test there are two possible actions: one 'rejects' the null-hypothesis (and accepts the alternative hypothesis) or vice versa. This creates another clash of the two approaches. Namely, if the NP approach is the basis for statistical inference, then there is in principle no problem in accepting the null-hypothesis. However, one of the basic principles in classical statistical practice is never to accept H_0 in case of a nonsignificant result that is in the spirit of Fisher's significance testing. Note that in clinical trials the standard approach is the NP approach, but accepting the null-hypothesis would be a major flaw.

Because of the above difficulties with the P-value and that classical statistical inference is claimed to be not coherent, Goodman (1993, 1999a, 1999b) and others advocated to use Bayesian inference tools such as the Bayes factor. Having said this, others still regard it as a useful tool in some circumstances. For instance, Hill (1996) writes: 'Like many others, I have come to regard the classical P-value as a useful diagnostic device, particularly in screening large numbers of possibly meaningful treatment comparisons.' Further, in some cases (one-sided hypothesis testing) the P-value and Bayesian inference come close (see Section 3.8.3). Finally, Weinberg (2001) argues that 'It is time to stop blaming the tools, and turn our attention to the investigators who misuse them.'

1.2 Statistical inference based on the likelihood function

1.2.1 The likelihood function

The concept of *likelihood* was introduced by Fisher (1922). It expresses the plausibility of the observed data as a function of the parameters of a stochastic model. As a function of the parameters the likelihood is called the *likelihood function*. Statistical inference based on the likelihood function differs fundamentally from inference based on the P-value, although both approaches were promoted by Fisher as a tool for inductive inference. To fix ideas, let us look at the likelihood function of a binomial sample. The following example dates back to Cornfield (1966) but is rephrased in terms of a surgery experiment.

Example I.7: A surgery experiment

Assume that a new but rather complicated surgical technique was developed in a hospital with a nonnegligible risk for failure. To evaluate the feasibility of the technique the chief surgeon decides to operate on $n = 12$ patients with this new procedure. Upon completion of the 12 operations, he reports $s = 9$ successes. Let the outcome of the ith operation be denoted as $y_i = 1$ for a success and $y_i = 0$ for a failure. The total experiment yields a sample of n independent binary observations $\{y_1, \ldots, y_n\} \equiv \mathbf{y}$ with s successes. Assume that the probability of success remains constant over the experiment, i.e. $p(y_i) = \theta$, $(i = 1, \ldots, n)$. Then the probability of the observed number of successes is expressed by the *binomial distribution*, i.e. the probability that s successes out of n experiments occur when the probability of success in a single experiment is equal to θ, is given by

$$f_\theta(s) = \binom{n}{s} \theta^s (1-\theta)^{n-s} \text{ with } s = \sum_{i=1}^{n} y_i, \tag{1.1}$$

where $f_\theta(s)$ is a discrete distribution (as a function of s) with the property that $\sum_{s=0}^{n} f_\theta(s) = 1$. When s is kept fixed and θ is varying, $f_\theta(s)$ becomes a continuous function of θ, called the *binomial likelihood function*. The likelihood function could be viewed as expressing the plausibility of θ in the light of the data and is therefore denoted as $L(\theta \mid s)$. The graphical representation of the binomial likelihood function is shown in Figure 1.2(a) for $s = 9$ and

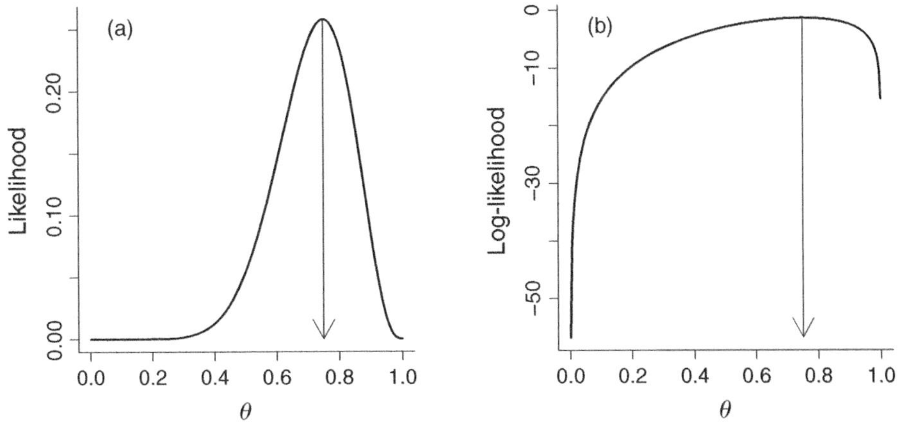

Figure 1.2 Surgery experiment: likelihood (a) and log-likelihood function (b) corresponding to $s = 9$ successes out of $n = 12$ operations from Example I.7.

$n = 12$. The figure shows that values of θ close to zero and close to one are not supported by the observed result of 9 successes out of 12 operations. On the other hand, values above 0.5 and below 0.9 are relatively well supported by the data with the value $\theta = 9/12 = 0.75$ best supported. □

The value of θ that maximizes $L(\theta \mid s)$ is called the *maximum likelihood estimate* (*MLE*) and is denoted as $\widehat{\theta}$. To determine $\widehat{\theta}$, we maximize $L(\theta \mid s)$ with respect to θ. It is equivalent and easier to maximize the logarithm of $L(\theta \mid s)$, called the *log-likelihood*, and denoted as $\ell(\theta \mid s)$.

Example I.7: (continued)
The log-likelihood for the surgery experiment is given by

$$\ell(\theta \mid s) = c + [s \log \theta + (n - s) \log(1 - \theta)], \tag{1.2}$$

where c is a constant. The first derivative with respect to θ gives the expression $\frac{s}{\theta} - \frac{(n-s)}{(1-\theta)}$. Equating this expression to zero gives the MLE equal to s/n, and thus, $\widehat{\theta} = 0.75$ (for $s = 9$ and $n = 12$), which is the sample proportion. Figure 1.2(b) shows $\ell(\theta \mid s)$ as a function of θ. □

1.2.2 The likelihood principles

Inference based on the likelihood function naturally adheres to two *likelihood principles* (*LP*) (Berger and Wolpert 1984):

1. *Likelihood principle 1*: All evidence, which is obtained from an experiment, about an unknown quantity θ is contained in the likelihood function of θ for the given data.

2. *Likelihood principle 2*: Two likelihood functions for θ contain the same information about θ if they are proportional to each other.

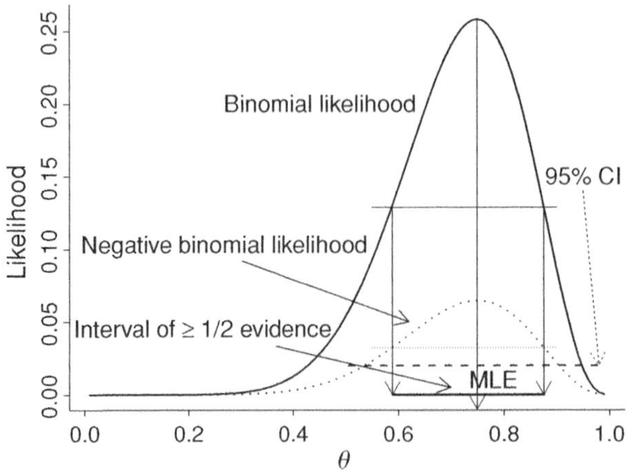

Figure 1.3 Surgery experiments: binomial and negative binomial (Pascal) likelihood functions together with MLE and interval of at least 0.5 maximal evidence and the classical two-sided 95% CI.

The first LP implies that the choice between two values of an unknown parameter is made via the likelihood function evaluated at those values. This leads to the *standardized likelihood* and the *interval of evidence*, which will be introduced in Example I.7 (continued) below.

Example I.7: (continued)
The binomial likelihood for $s = 9$ and $n = 12$ is maximal at $\widehat{\theta} = 0.75$. In a frequentist context, we could test the observed proportion against an a priori chosen value for θ, say 0.5 and we calculate a 95% CI for θ.

According to the likelihood function, there is maximal evidence for $\theta = 0.75$. The ratio of the likelihood functions at $\theta = 0.5$ and at $\theta = 0.75$ can be used as a measure of the relative evidential support given by the data for the two hypotheses. This ratio is called the *likelihood ratio* and is here equal to 0.21. The function $L(\theta \mid s)/L(\widehat{\theta} \mid s)$ (here $L(\theta \mid s)/L(0.75 \mid s)$) is called the *standardized likelihood*. On the standardized likelihood scale, one can read off that the evidence for $\theta = 0.5$ is about 1/5 the maximal evidence. Note that this comparison does not involve any fictive data, only the observed data play a role.

One can also construct an interval of parameter values that show at least a fraction of the maximal evidence. For instance, the *interval of (at least half of the maximal) evidence* consists of those θ-values that correspond to at least half of $L(\widehat{\theta} \mid s)$, i.e. with a standardized likelihood of at least 0.5 (see Figure 1.3). This interval provides direct evidence on the parameter of interest and is related to the highest posterior density interval introduced in Section 3.3.2. On the same figure, the classical 95% CI [0.505, 0.995] is indicated. In general, the 95% CI only represents an interval of evidence when the likelihood function is symmetric. □

The second LP states that two likelihood functions for θ contain the same information about that parameter if they are proportional to each other. This is called the *relative likelihood principle*. Thus, when the likelihood is proportional under two experimental conditions, irrespective of the way the results were obtained, the information about the unknown parameter must be the same. Example I.8 contrasts in this respect the difference between the frequentist and the likelihood viewpoints.

Example I.8: Another surgery experiment

Assume that the chief surgeon of another hospital wished to test the same surgical technique introduced in Example I.7 but decided to operate until k failures occur. The probability of the observed number of successes is now expressed by the *negative binomial (Pascal) distribution*. With θ again the probability of success in a single experiment, the negative binomial distribution is given by

$$g_\theta(s) = \binom{s+k-1}{s} \theta^s (1-\theta)^k. \tag{1.3}$$

Since $s + k = n$ represents the total sample size, $g_\theta(s)$ differs from $f_\theta(s)$ only in the binomial coefficient. The chief surgeon fixed k to 3. Suppose that again 9 successes were realized. As a result, for both chief surgeons 9 successes and 3 failures were observed but the mechanism for stopping the experiment (stopping rule) was different. We now show that the stopping rule does not affect likelihood inference, in contrast to the frequentist approach (see Example I.8 (continued)).

For the first surgeon, the sum $s = \sum_{i=1}^{n} y_i$ has a binomial distribution. Therefore, the likelihood function given that s is observed is given by

$$L_1(\theta \mid s) = \tbinom{n}{s}\theta^s(1-\theta)^{(n-s)}. \tag{1.4}$$

On the other hand, for the second surgeon the likelihood is

$$L_2(\theta \mid s) = \tbinom{n-1}{s}\theta^s(1-\theta)^{(n-s)}. \tag{1.5}$$

Since for the two surgery experiments $s = 9$ and $k = 3$, $L_1(\theta \mid 9) = \tbinom{12}{9}\theta^9(1-\theta)^3$ differs from $L_2(\theta \mid 9) = \tbinom{11}{9}\theta^9(1-\theta)^3$ only in a factor. According to the second likelihood principle, the two experiments must, therefore, give us the same information about θ. This can be seen in Figure 1.3, which shows that the binomial and the negative binomial likelihood result in the same MLE and in the same intervals of evidence. □

The stopping rule affects, though, frequentist inference as seen in the following text.

Example I.8: (continued)

Suppose that we wish to test null-hypothesis $H_0 : \theta = 0.5$ versus the alternative hypothesis $H_a : \theta > 0.5$ in a frequentist way. The significance test depends on the null distribution of the test statistic, which is here the number of successes. For the binomial experiment, we obtain under H_0:

$$p(s \geq 9 \mid \theta = 0.5) = \sum_{s=9}^{12} \binom{12}{s} 0.5^s (1-0.5)^{12-s}. \tag{1.6}$$

This gives an exact one-sided P-value of 0.0730. On the other hand, for the negative binomial experiment we obtain under H_0:

$$p(s \geq 9 \mid \theta = 0.5) = \sum_{s=9}^{\infty} \binom{s+2}{s} 0.5^s (1-0.5)^3, \tag{1.7}$$

giving $P = 0.0337$. Thus, the significance of the test $\theta = 0.5$ depends on what other results could have been achieved besides 9 successes and 3 failures. □

The example shows the fundamental difference between the likelihood and frequentist approaches when dealing with stopping rules. The likelihood function is a central concept in the two paradigms. But in the likelihood approach only the likelihood function is used, while in the frequentist approach the likelihood function is used to construct significance tests. Finally, note that the classical likelihood ratio test for the binomial experiment coincides with that of the negative binomial experiment (see Exercise 1.1).

1.3 The Bayesian approach: Some basic ideas

1.3.1 Introduction

In Examples I.7 and I.8, the surgeons were interested in estimating the true proportion of successful operations, i.e. θ, in order to decide upon the usefulness of the newly developed surgical technique. Suppose that in the past the first surgeon experienced another technique with similar difficulties and recollects that the first 20 operations were the most difficult (learning curve). In that case, it is conceivable to think that he will implicitly or explicitly combine this prior information with the outcome of the current experiment to draw his final conclusions. In other words, he will adjust the obtained proportion of 9/12 in view of the past experience, a process that is an example of a Bayesian exercise.

Research is not done in isolation. When planning a phase III RCT, comparing a new treatment for treating breast cancer with a standard treatment, a lot of background information has already been collected on the two treatments. This information has been incorporated in the protocol of the trial, but is not explicitly used in the classical statistical analysis of the trial results afterward. For example, when a small-scale clinical trial shows an unexpectedly positive result, e.g. $P < 0.01$ in favor of the new treatment, the first reaction (certainly of the drug company) might be 'great'! However, if in the past none of such drugs had a large effect and the new drug is biologically similar to the standard drug one would probably be cautious in claiming strong effects. With the Bayesian approach, one can formally incorporate such prior skepticism as will be seen in Chapter 5.

Take another example. A new mouthwash is introduced into the market and a study is set up to show its efficacy. The study must evaluate whether daily use of the new mouthwash before tooth brushing reduces plaque when compared to using tap water alone. The results were that the new mouthwash reduced 25% of the plaque with a 95% CI = [10%, 40%]. This seems to be a great result. However, previous trials on similar products showed that the overall reduction in plaque lies between 5% to 15%, and experts argue that plaque reduction from a mouthwash will probably not exceed 30%. What to conclude then?

An approach is needed that combines in a natural manner the past experience (call it prior knowledge) with the results of the current experiment. This can be accomplished with the Bayesian approach, which is based on *Bayes theorem*. In this chapter, we introduce the basic (discrete) version of the theorem. General Bayesian statistical inference as well as its connection with the likelihood approach will be treated in next chapters.

The central idea of the Bayesian approach is to combine the likelihood (data) with *Your* prior knowledge (*prior probability*) to result in a revised probability (*posterior probability*). The adjective 'Your' indicates that the prior knowledge can differ from individual to individual and thus might have a subjective flavor. It will imply that probability statements will not necessarily have a long run frequency interpretation anymore as in the frequentist approach.

Before stating the fundamental theorem of Bayes, we illustrate that the Bayesian way of thinking is naturally incorporated in our daily life.

Example I.9: Examples of Bayesian reasoning in daily life

In everyday life, but also in our professional activities, we often reason and act according to the Bayesian principle.

As a first example, assume that you visit Belgium for the first time. Belgium is a small country located in Western Europe. It may well be that you never met a Belgian in the past. Hence, prior to your visit your information (prior knowledge) about Belgians could range from no information to some information that you gathered from travel books, e.g. that Belgians produce excellent beers and chocolate. During your visit, you meet Belgians (data) so that upon your return you have a revised impression (posterior knowledge) of how Belgian people are. Consequently, your personal impression of Belgians will probably have changed.

Suppose that a company wishes to launch for the first time an 'energy' drink. The marketing director responsible for launching the product has many years of experience with energy drinks from his previous job in another company. He believes that the drink will be a success (prior belief). But, to strengthen his prior belief he conducts a small-field experiment (data), say by setting up a booth in a shopping area delivering free samples of the drink to the target group and eliciting their first reactions. After this limited experiment his prior faith in the product will be reinforced or weakened (posterior belief) depending on the outcome of the experiment.

A cerebral vascular accident (CVA) is a life-threatening event. One of the causes of a CVA is a blocked brain artery induced by a blood clot. This event is called an ischemic stroke. Adequate treatment of a patient with an ischemic stroke to prevent lifelong disability is a difficult task. One possibility is to dissolve the clot by a thrombolytic. However, choosing the right dose of the drug is not easy. The higher the dose the higher the potency of dissolving the clot but also the higher the risk of suffering from bleeding accidents. In the worst case, the ischemic stroke is converted into a hemorrhagic stroke causing a severe bleeding in the brain. Suppose that a new thrombolytic agent was developed and that there is some evidence from animal models and experience with other thrombolytic agents that about 20% of the patients (prior knowledge) might suffer from a severe bleeding accident (SBA) with this new drug. A small pilot trial resulted in 10% of patients with a SBA (data). What can we conclude for the true percentage of SBA (posterior knowledge) when combining the current evidence with the past evidence? Bayes theorem allows us to tackle such prior–posterior questions. □

1.3.2 Bayes theorem – discrete version for simple events

The simplest case of Bayes theorem occurs when there are only two possible events, say A and B, which may or may not occur. A typical example is that A represents a positive diagnostic test and B a diseased patient. When the event does not occur it is denoted as B^C (patient is not diseased) or A^C (diagnostic test is negative). Bayes theorem describes the relation between the probability that A occurs (or not) given that B has occurred and the probability that B occurs (or not) given that A has occurred.

Bayes theorem is based on the following elementary property in probability theory: $p(A, B) = p(A) \cdot p(B \mid A) = p(B) \cdot p(A \mid B)$, where $p(A)$, $p(B)$ are marginal probabilities and $p(A \mid B)$, $p(B \mid A)$ are conditional probabilities. This leads to the basic form of the Bayes theorem (also called *Bayes rule*), given by

$$p(B \mid A) = \frac{p(A \mid B) \cdot p(B)}{p(A)}. \tag{1.8}$$

Because of the Law of Total Probability

$$p(A) = p(A \mid B) \cdot p(B) + p(A \mid B^C) \cdot p(B^C), \tag{1.9}$$

we can elaborate Bayes theorem in the following way:

$$p(B \mid A) = \frac{p(A \mid B) \cdot p(B)}{p(A \mid B) \cdot p(B) + p(A \mid B^C) \cdot p(B^C)}. \tag{1.10}$$

Expressions (1.8) and (1.10) can be read also as $p(B \mid A) \propto p(A \mid B)$, where $\propto$ means 'proportional to'. Thus, Bayes theorem allows us to calculate the inverse probability $p(B \mid A)$ from $p(A \mid B)$ and is, therefore, also called the *Theorem on Inverse Probability*.

In Example I.10, we show that expression (1.10) has some advantages over expression (1.8). In the example, we derive the *positive* and *negative predictive value* of a diagnostic test from its *sensitivity* and *specificity*. Sensitivity (S_e) is the probability of a positive diagnostic test when the patient is indeed diseased. Specificity (S_p) is the probability of a negative diagnostic test when the patient is indeed not-diseased. When the event 'diseased' is represented by B, then the event 'nondiseased' is B^C. Likewise, the event 'positive diagnostic test' can be represented by A and the event 'negative diagnostic test' by A^C. Thus, the sensitivity (specificity) is equal to the probability $p(A \mid B)$ ($p(A^C \mid B^C)$). The positive (negative) predictive value, on the other hand, is the probability that the person is (not) diseased given a positive (negative) test. So, in probability terms, the positive (negative) predictive value is equal to $p(B \mid A)$ ($p(B^C \mid A^C)$) and is denoted as pred+ (pred−). In practice, the predictive values of a diagnostic are needed, because they express the probability that a patient is (not) diseased given a positive (or a negative test). When a 2×2 table of results is provided, pred+ and pred− can be readily computed. However, often the predictive values are needed in a new population and then we need Bayes theorem. Indeed, Bayes rule expresses the positive (negative) predictive value as a function of the sensitivity and the specificity, and the marginal probability that B happens ($p(B)$). This marginal probability is known as the *prevalence* of the disease and is abbreviated as *prev*. Hence, Bayes rule offers us a tool to compute the predictive values in each population once the prevalence in that population is available. The computation assumes that the sensitivity and specificity are intrinsic qualities of the diagnostic test and do not vary with the population (see also Example V.6). Example I.10 is an illustration of the mechanics of calculating the probability $p(B \mid A)$ from $p(A \mid B)$.

Example I.10: Sensitivity, specificity, prevalence, and their relation to predictive values
Fisher and van Belle (1993) described the results of the Folin-Wu blood test, a screening test for diabetes, on patients seen in the Boston City hospital. A group of medical consultants established criteria for the gold standard, so that the true disease status is known. In Table 1.3, the results on 580 patients are given. From this table, we determine $S_e = 56/70 = 0.80$ and $S_p = 461/510 = 0.90$. The prevalence of the disease, as recorded in the Boston City hospital, is equal to $prev = 70/580 = 0.12$. But we need the predictive values for different populations. The world prevalence of diabetes is about 3%. Expression (1.10) can easily be transformed

Table 1.3 Folin-Wu blood test: diagnostic test to detect diabetes applied to 580 patients seen in the Boston City Hospital (Fisher and van Belle 1993) split up according to true disease status and outcome of diagnostic test.

Test	Diabetic	Nondiabetic	Total
+	56	49	105
−	14	461	475
Total	70	510	580

to an expression relating the predictive values to the intrinsic characteristics of the test and the prevalence of diabetes. When suffering from diabetes is denoted as D^+, diabetes-free as D^-, a positive screening test as T^+ and a negative screening test as T^-, then Bayes theorem translates into

$$p(D^+ \mid T^+) = \frac{p(T^+ \mid D^+) \cdot p(D^+)}{p(T^+ \mid D^+) \cdot p(D^+) + p(T^+ \mid D^-) \cdot p(D^-)}. \tag{1.11}$$

In terms of sensitivity, specificity and prevalence, Bayes theorem reads as

$$\text{pred+} = \frac{S_e \cdot \text{prev}}{S_e \cdot \text{prev} + (1 - S_p) \cdot (1 - \text{prev})}. \tag{1.12}$$

The predictive values for a population are obtained by plugging-in the prevalence for that population in expression (1.12). For $p(B) = 0.03$, the positive (negative) predictive value is equal to 0.20 (0.99). □

The above calculations merely show the mechanics of Bayes theorem. We now show how Bayes theorem could work in the office of a general practitioner (GP). Suppose an elderly patient visits his GP for a check-up. The GP wishes to check whether his patient suffers from diabetes or not. He knows that in his elderly population the prevalence of diabetes is around 10%. The prior probability for that patient to suffer from diabetes is thus 0.10. The GP takes a Folin-Wu blood test and a positive result appears. The outcome of this diagnostic test represents the data. With Bayes theorem the physician can then formally combine his prior belief with the data obtained from the diagnostic test to arrive at a positive predictive value of 0.47 (posterior probability). The conclusion is that the patient has a reasonable chance of suffering from diabetes and it is likely that more tests are needed to give assurance to the patient. Note that in the above example, the prior probability was based on observed data, but this is not a must. Indeed, the prior probability could originate from a guess, a hunch, a belief, etc., from the treating GP. In that case, the prior and posterior probabilities will not have a long-run frequency interpretation anymore.

We end this section with another illustration of Bayes theorem. In this case, we evaluate the quality of published research findings in medicine. This example also highlights the difference between the message a P-value brings us and the probability $p(H_a \mid \text{data})$ (or the probability of a positive result for the experimental treatment).

Example I.11: The Bayesian interpretation of published research findings
Many medical research findings prove afterwards to be false and there is a growing concern about such misreporting. Ioannidus (2005) examined the publishing behavior in current medical research. More specifically, he calculated the probability of a falsely reported positive result using Bayes theorem.

Suppose that classical significance tests are employed at significance level α (= P(type I error)) and with the probability of a type II error equal to β. Suppose also that the purpose is to find true relationships between, say, risk indicators (life style, genetic disposition, etc.) and a particular disease. If there are G (possibly very large) likely relationships to examine with only one true relationship, then $1/G$ could be viewed as the prior probability of a true research finding. Let $R = 1/(G-1)$ be the prior odds, then for c relationships examined in an independent manner on average $c(1-\beta)R/(R+1)$ are truly positive. On the other hand, the average number of false positive findings is equal to $c\alpha/(R+1)$. Using Bayes theorem, this results in a positive predictive value for a positive finding equal to

$$\frac{(1-\beta)R}{(1-\beta)R+\alpha}. \tag{1.13}$$

When $(1-\beta)R > \alpha$, the posterior probability of finding a true relationship is higher than 0.5. Thus, the power to find a positive result needs to be higher than $0.05/R$ for the probability of finding a true relationship is relatively high, which is impossible for G large. Ioannidus (2005) then continues to quantify the effect of biased reporting on the probability of a true scientific result and highlighted the dangers of the current reporting practice in medical research. □

1.4 Outlook

Bayes theorem will be further developed in Chapter 2 in such a way that it can be used in statistical practice. A first step will be to reanalyze examples such as those seen in this chapter, whereby inference will be done without the help of fictive data and whereby prior information on parameters may be incorporated if we feel the need to do so. But this is just a first step. From an applied point of view, it is reasonable to ask what more a Bayesian analysis can do than a classical frequentist analysis. However, to show what extra tools the Bayesian approach can offer to the practitioner we will need at least six additional chapters. That the Bayesian methodology has become popular only in the last decades is not without a reason. In the first 230 years, Bayesians were basically only selling their ideas, but could not offer a practical tool. This situation has changed now. The Bayesian methods can handle far more complex problems than classical approaches.

To let the reader taste already a bit of the possibilities of Bayesian methods, we now reanalyze the toenail data of Example I.1. How the analysis was done will become clear later.

Example I.12: Toenail RCT: A Bayesian analysis
We reanalyzed the toenail data using the popular package WinBUGS. The aim is to show a few of the possibilities of Bayesian methods without going into details on how the results were obtained. The program can be found in 'chapter 1 toenail.odc'. In the first analysis, we simply replayed the original analysis. A typical output of WinBUGS is shown in Figure 1.4(a). The (posterior) density represents what evidence we have on Δ after having seen the data. For

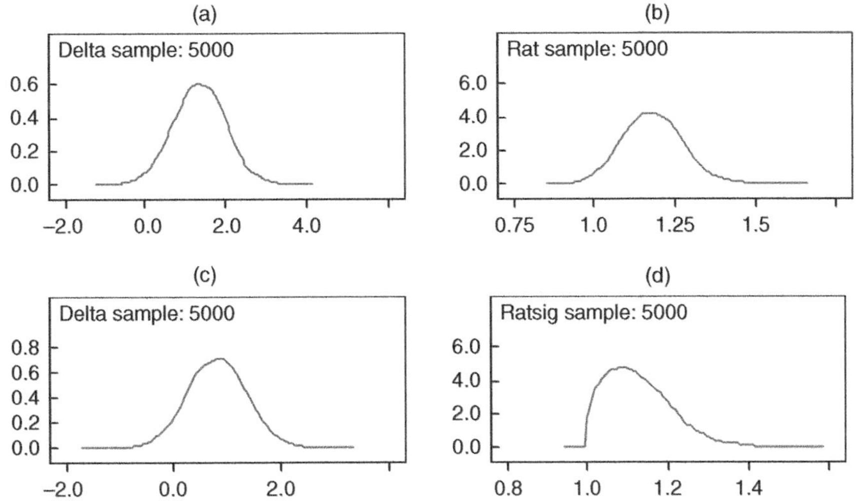

Figure 1.4 Toenail RCT: (a) posterior distribution of Δ, (b) posterior distribution of μ_1/μ_2, (c) posterior distribution of Δ, and (d) posterior distribution of σ_2/σ_1 both when taking prior information into account.

instance, the area under the curve (AUC) on the positive x-axis represents our belief that Δ is positive. This was here 0.98. In a classical analysis it would be more difficult to perform a test on the ratio μ_1/μ_2. In a Bayesian analysis, this is just as easy as looking at the difference. The posterior density on that ratio is shown in Figure 1.4(b) and the area under the curve (AUC) for the interval $[1, \infty)$ can be easily determined. In a Bayesian analysis, one can also bring in prior information on the parameters of the model. Suppose we were skeptical about Δ being positive and that we rather believed a priori that its value is around -0.5 (with of course some uncertainty), then this information can be incorporated into our analysis. In the same way, we can include information about the variance parameters. For instance, suppose that in all past studies σ_2^2 was greater than σ_1^2 and that the ratio varied around 2. Then that finding can be incorporated in the Bayesian estimation procedure. In Figure 1.4(c), we show the evidence that Δ is positive taking into account the above-described prior information, which is now 0.95. Figure 1.4(d) shows the ratio of σ_2/σ_1 when the prior information on the variances was taken into account. □

This example just shows a small portion of what nowadays can be done with Bayesian methodology. In later chapters, we demonstrate the flexibility of the Bayesian methods and software.

Exercises

Exercise 1.1 Show that the likelihood ratio test for the binomial distribution coincides with the corresponding likelihood ratio test for the negative binomial distribution.

Exercise 1.2 Prove expression (1.13) based on A = "test is significant at α" and B = "relationship is true".

2

Bayes theorem: Computing the posterior distribution

2.1 Introduction

In this chapter, we derive the general Bayes theorem and illustrate it with a variety of examples. Comparisons of the Bayesian solution with the frequentist and the likelihood solution will be made for a better understanding of the Bayesian concepts. In fact, inference will turn out to be quite different from the classical case, even probability will get a different flavor in the Bayesian paradigm.

2.2 Bayes theorem – the binary version

The Bayes theorem will now be applied to statistical models. The first step is to change the notation in expression (1.11). Let us replace D^+ and D^- by a parameter θ assuming two values, i.e. $\theta = 1$ for D^+ and $\theta = 0$ for D^-. The results of the diagnostic test represent *data*, and hence, T^+ is recoded as $y = 1$ and T^- as $y = 0$, then expression (1.11) can be reformulated as

$$p(\theta = 1 \mid y = 1) = \frac{p(y = 1 \mid \theta = 1) \cdot p(\theta = 1)}{p(y = 1 \mid \theta = 1) \cdot p(\theta = 1) + p(y = 1 \mid \theta = 0) \cdot p(\theta = 0)}. \quad (2.1)$$

In expression (2.1), $p(\theta = 1)$ ($p(\theta = 0)$) represents the prevalence (1-prevalence) of a disease in the context of Example I.10, but in general it is called the *prior* probability that $\theta = 1$ ($\theta = 0$). The probability $p(y = 1 \mid \theta = 1)$ describes the probability that a positive test is obtained, given that $\theta = 1$. As a function of θ, it is the likelihood for $\theta = 1$ with a positive test. Likewise, $p(y = 1 \mid \theta = 0)$ describes the likelihood for $\theta = 0$ for a positive test. Here, the terms $p(y = 1 \mid \theta = 1)$ and $p(y = 1 \mid \theta = 0)$ define completely the *likelihood* for θ. Finally, $p(\theta = 1 \mid y = 1)$ is the probability that an individual is diseased upon observing a positive

Bayesian Biostatistics, First Edition. Emmanuel Lesaffre and Andrew B. Lawson.

test. This probability is called the *posterior* probability and is derived from combining the prior information with the observed data.

By classical probability rules, the denominator of expression (2.1) is $p(y)$, so that a shorthand notation of expression (2.1) is

$$p(\theta \mid y) = \frac{p(y \mid \theta)p(\theta)}{p(y)}, \tag{2.2}$$

where θ can stand for $\theta = 0$ or $\theta = 1$. Note also that the rule immediately applies to random variables y that are categorical or continuous. In the latter case then $p(y \mid \theta)$ represents a density.

Since Bayes theorem follows immediately from probability rules, Cornfield (1967) noted 'Actually Bayes result follows so directly from the formal definitions of probability and related concepts that it is perhaps overly solemn to call it a theorem at all.' However, this should not be interpreted as a criticism to this ingenious result, on the contrary. The ingenious idea Bayes had 250 years ago is to give parameters a stochastic nature as can be seen from expressions (2.1) and (2.2). At first sight, this may look bizarre since in classical statistics a parameter is assumed to be fixed. In the Bayesian paradigm, however, a parameter is stochastic but the term *stochastic* does not necessarily imply a classical meaning, as will be seen in Section 2.3.

2.3 Probability in a Bayesian context

When tossing a (honest) coin, two types of probabilities come into play. First, there is the classical probability that a coin will show heads when tossed up. For an 'honest' coin, this probability is 0.50 since the proportion of times that heads will show converges to 0.50 as the tossing experiment proceeds. In this case, the probability has a *long-run frequency meaning*. Now suppose that a coin is tossed only once but the result is hidden and you are asked about the probability that it is heads. Suppose you do not believe that there exist honest coins then you might give it a probability of 0.6. This kind of probability expresses your personal belief on the outcome of the experiment and is typically an example of a *Bayesian probability*.

For a medical example, assume that patients are screened for diabetes. The probability that a patient suffers from diabetes is equal to the prevalence of diabetes in the population. Conditional on a positive screening test, the probability that a patient suffers from diabetes is then equal to the prevalence of diabetes patients in the subpopulation of positively tested patients. Both probabilities have a long-run frequency interpretation. Now suppose that a physician examines a patient for diabetes, then prior to the screening test the patient's probability for diabetes is equal to the prevalence of diabetes in the whole population but after the positive result it changes to the prevalence of diabetes in the subpopulation. Applied to the individual patient, these probabilities become expressions of the physician's belief in the patient's health status. This is again an example of a Bayesian probability.

Hence when we speak of probabilities they can have two meanings. They might express a limiting proportion that an event happens in a true or fictive experiment or they might express a personal belief that this event will happen or has happened. The first type of probability is called *objective*, while the second type is called *subjective*. Subjective probabilities express our uncertainties in life in a probabilistic language. We can be uncertain about basically all things in life, but typically these uncertainties exhibit a great range, may change in time and vary with the individual. For instance, there is always a lot of speculation of the future winner of the Tour de France. The prior opinion of the fans of a specific cyclist that he will win the Tour certainly differs from that of sports journalists and bookmakers and probably also from the prior opinion of the cyclist himself. In addition, these opinions will change when the Tour unfolds and definitely become clearer when the mountains stage has been taken. Another example is the speculation in the past about whether global warming is taking place. Nowadays there is little doubt about this, but the speculation is now about how fast global warming will take place and to what extent, and even more importantly how it will affect our lives. These speculations varied and still vary considerably across individuals and in time.

Hence, subjective probabilities are probabilistic reformulations of our uncertainty. In order for them to be used in computations, they should have the same properties as classical probabilities, i.e. those that have the long-run frequency nature. This means that they need to satisfy the axioms of a probability system. In particular for mutually exclusive events $A_1, A_2, \ldots, A_K$ with the total event S (A_1 or A_2 or ... or A_K), a (subjective) probability p should have the following properties:

- For each event A (from $A_1, A_2, \ldots, A_K$): $0 \leq p(A) \leq 1$.
- The sum of all probabilities should be one: $p(S) = p(A_1 \text{ or } A_2 \text{ or} \ldots \text{or } A_K) = 1$, and also $p(A_i \text{ or } A_j \text{ or} \ldots \text{or } A_k) = p(A_i) + p(A_j) + \ldots + p(A_k)$.
- The probability that event A will not happen (event A^C) is 1 − the probability that A will happen: $p(A^C) = 1 - p(A)$.
- Suppose $B_1, B_2, \ldots, B_L$ represent another subdivision of S, then

$$p(A_i \mid B_j) = \frac{p(A_i, B_j)}{p(B_j)},$$

  with $p(A_i, B_j)$ the probability that A_i and B_j happen together and $p(A_i \mid B_j)$ the conditional probability that A_i happens given that B_j has already happened.

In short, subjective probabilities should constitute a coherent system of probabilities. Surely for pure mathematicians this description of a probability system is too naive. For a more mathematical description of a probability system and different axiom systems, they could consult Press (2003).

In his book on understanding uncertainty, Lindley (2006) argues that probability is a totally different concept from, say, distance. The distance between two points is the same for all of us, but that is the not case with probability of events since it depends on the person looking at the world. Therefore, he prefers to talk about *your* probability instead of *the* probability.

2.4 Bayes theorem – the categorical version

Suppose a subject can belong to $K > 2$ diagnostic classes corresponding to K values for θ: $\theta_1, \theta_2, \ldots, \theta_K$. Assuming that y can take on L different values: $y_1, \ldots, y_L$, then Bayes theorem generalizes to

$$p(\theta_k \mid y) = \frac{p(y \mid \theta_k)\, p(\theta_k)}{\sum_{m=1}^{K} p(y \mid \theta_m)\, p(\theta_m)}, \tag{2.3}$$

where y stands for one of the possible values in $\{y_1, \ldots, y_L\}$.

In expression (2.3), the parameter is discrete but the data y can be discrete or continuous. When the observed data are multidimensional, the random variable y is turned into a random vector $\mathbf{y}$. Expression (2.3) shows that Bayes theorem provides a rule to classify individuals into one of K diagnostic classes based on the prior belief that they belong to that class and the observed data. Developing classification models is a broad research area in statistics covering a great range of applications. Many of the classification techniques are based on Bayes theorem. For instance, Lesaffre and Willems (1988) examined the ability to predict a heart-related disease using electrocardiogram measurements and used thereby basically expression (2.3). The prior probabilities were obtained from the relative proportions of the diagnostic classes in the population.

2.5 Bayes theorem – the continuous version

Let us now look at how we can learn about a (one-dimensional) continuous parameter θ based on collected data and given prior information on θ. The data y can again be discrete or continuous such that $p(y \mid \theta)$ represents a distribution function or a density function. Because in a Bayesian context, parameters are assumed to be stochastic, we assume here that θ is a continuous random variable. Let $\mathbf{y}$ represent a sample of n i.i.d. observations. The joint distribution of the sample is given by $p(\mathbf{y} \mid \theta) = \prod_{i=1}^{n} p(y_i \mid \theta)$, which we also denote as $L(\theta \mid \mathbf{y})$.

For a discrete parameter, the prior information was expressed as a discrete probability distribution, but for a continuous parameter, our prior information needs to be specified differently. Only prior statements that θ lies in a particular interval make sense. This leads to a probability density function for θ, which we again denote as $p(\theta)$.

Bayes theorem or rule can be derived in a similar manner as before. Namely, when the data and the parameter are stochastic, the joint distribution $p(\mathbf{y}, \theta)$ can be split up into either $p(\mathbf{y} \mid \theta)p(\theta)$ or $p(\theta \mid \mathbf{y})p(\mathbf{y})$. This yields Bayes rule for continuous parameters, i.e.

$$p(\theta \mid \mathbf{y}) = \frac{L(\theta \mid \mathbf{y})p(\theta)}{p(\mathbf{y})} = \frac{L(\theta \mid \mathbf{y})p(\theta)}{\int L(\theta \mid \mathbf{y})p(\theta)\,\mathrm{d}\theta}. \tag{2.4}$$

The interpretation of expression (2.4) is as follows: when the prior opinion about the parameter expressed as a distribution $p(\theta)$ is combined with the observed data, the opinion will be updated and is expressed by the posterior distribution $p(\theta \mid \mathbf{y})$. Figure 2.3 shows a prior distribution that is transformed into a posterior distribution after having observed data $\mathbf{y}$. Expression (2.4) also tells us that when both the prior and the likelihood support a particular θ, then this θ is also supported a posteriori. But, if θ is not supported by either the prior distribution or the likelihood or both, then neither θ is supported a posteriori. Finally, the denominator of Bayes theorem ensures that $p(\theta \mid \mathbf{y})$ is indeed a distribution. Expression (2.4) shows that the posterior distribution is proportional to the product of the likelihood with the prior distribution, i.e.

$$p(\theta \mid \mathbf{y}) \propto L(\theta \mid \mathbf{y})p(\theta),$$

since the denominator is depending only on the observed data which is assumed to be fixed in a Bayesian context.

The denominator in expression (2.4) is called the *averaged likelihood* because it is the weighted average of $L(\theta \mid \mathbf{y})$ over the possible values of θ with a weight function given by the prior distribution $p(\theta)$. Note that expression (2.4) could be viewed as a limiting form of expression (2.3) when the number of possible parameter values increases to infinity.

Finally, let there be no misunderstanding: it can also be assumed in the Bayesian paradigm that there is a true parameter value θ_0. Indeed, we regard θ as stochastic because we do not know its true value and, therefore, express our belief on θ_0. The ultimate purpose of a Bayesian analysis is to get a good idea of this true value θ_0 by combining data and prior information.

It is now time to show the mechanics of Bayes theorem in more detail. Three cases are exemplified: the binomial, the normal and the Poisson case. For each of the cases, a medical example is used as guidance: (a) a stroke clinical trial for the binomial case, (b) a dietary cross-sectional study for the normal case, and (c) a dental study on caries experience for the Poisson case. In the remainder of the book, *prior* and *posterior* are shorthand notations for prior and posterior distributions, respectively. For each of the cases, the prior will be specified on the basis of historical studies possibly combined with 'expert' knowledge.

2.6 The binomial case

The following example in stroke research illustrates the mechanism of Bayes theorem when the data are discrete and the parameter is continuous.

Example II.1: Stroke study: Monitoring safety of a thrombolytic drug administered for ischemic stroke

Patients suffer from a *stroke* or cerebrovascular accident (CVA), when brain cells die or are seriously damaged due to ischemia (ischemic stroke) or bleeding (hemorrhagic stroke) impairing the local brain function. About 70% of strokes are ischemic, resulting from blockage of a blood vessel as a result of atherosclerotic plaques or an embolus from another vessel. An ischemic stroke is treated with a thrombolytic drug that reperfuses the blocked blood vessel as quickly as possible. Early attempts with streptokinase given within 6 hours of stroke onset were terminated prematurely because they resulted in more deaths and bleeding complications (Donnan *et al.* 1996). Administration of recombinant tissue plasminogen activator (rt-PA), a more recent type of thrombolytic, gave more promising results (placebo-controlled RCTs (randomized controlled clinical trials) ECASS 1 (Hacke *et al.* 1995) and ECASS 2 (Hacke *et al.* 1998)). However, for all thrombolytic drugs, an important bleeding complication is symptomatic intercerebral hemorrhage (SICH) defined as an intracerebral hemorrhage associated with neurological deterioration. A third ECASS study, the ECASS 3 study, was set up and finalized in 2008 (Hacke *et al.* 2008) to further document the outcome (efficacy and safety) of patients with acute ischaemic hemispheric stroke in whom rt-PA can be initiated between 3 and 4.5 hours after onset of symptoms. The trial ended after 821 patients were enrolled in the study (418 to rt-PA and 403 to placebo). The result was that significantly ($P = 0.04$) more patients had a favorable outcome (absence of disability at 90 days) with rt-PA than with placebo (52.4% vs. 45.2%). Here, we focus on statistical aspects during the conduct of the trial, but the data are fictive. Indeed, the study only serves as a motivation for the statistical developments.

Clinical trials on life-threatening diseases most often have a committee of clinicians and statisticians, called the Data and Safety Monitoring Board (DSMB), which monitors the study at regular time intervals. In this respect, interim analyses reporting on the safety of the administered treatments are evaluated by the DSMB. In the ECASS 3 study, there was a need to monitor the incidence of SICH. There existed prior data from ECASS 1 and ECASS 2 and from a meta-analysis of other trials on SICH. For instance, in the ECASS 2 study SICH occurred in 8.8% in the 409 rt-PA treated patients.

Suppose now that the ECASS 3 DSMB is asked to examine the interim results of rt-PA treated stroke patients with an emphasis on SICH and in the light of the results of the ECASS 2 study. For ease of exposition, we assume that in the ECASS 2 study 100 patients were treated with rt-PA and 8 patients suffered from SICH. Assume also that at the first interim analysis of the ECASS 3 study, 50 patients were treated with rt-PA and that SICH occurred in 10 patients. The DSMB wishes to obtain an accurate picture of the risk for SICH. The results of the first interim analysis could be viewed in separation of the ECASS 2 data, but it seems reasonable to informally or formally combine the two sources of information. The decision to continue or to stop the trial (stopping rule) will then involve the combined ECASS 2 and ECASS 3 results.

We now (a) compare the different approaches (frequentist, likelihood and Bayesian) to estimate the incidence of SICH in the first interim analysis of the ECASS 3 study; (b) exemplify the mechanics of calculating the posterior distribution using Bayes theorem, and (c) compare various Bayesian analyses differing by the prior distribution.

Let the probability of showing SICH (SICH incidence) under rt-PA be θ and $y_1, \ldots, y_n$ a sample of n i.i.d. Bernoulli random variables with $y_i = 1$ if the ith patient suffered from SICH and 0 otherwise. Then the random variable $y = \sum_1^n y_i$ has a binomial distribution Bin(n, θ), given by $p(y \mid \theta) = \binom{n}{y}\theta^y(1-\theta)^{(n-y)}$.

Likelihood and frequentist approach

The information that the data provide on θ is expressed by the likelihood function. In the likelihood approach, preference for certain θ-values is given via inspecting the likelihood function at these values. The MLE of the incidence of SICH in the first interim analysis of the (fictive) ECASS 3 study, i.e. $\widehat{\theta}$, is equal to $y/n = 10/50 = 0.20$. The binomial likelihood function and the MLE are shown in Figure 2.1. The '0.05 interval of evidence', i.e. the interval that contains θs with a standardized likelihood of at least 0.05 (Section 1.2.2), is equal to [0.09, 0.36].

In the frequentist approach, one could test the hypothesis whether $\theta = 0.08$, which is the result obtained from the ECASS 2 study, with a binomial test or a Z-test. The classical 95% confidence interval (CI) based on the asymptotic normal distribution of $\widehat{\theta}$ is equal to [0.089, 0.31].

Bayesian approach: Prior obtained from ECASS 2 study

1. Specifying the (ECASS 2) prior distribution

The data collected in the ECASS 2 study provide valuable information, and it would be a flaw to ignore them. As mentioned above, in the rt-PA arm of our (fictive) ECASS 2 study 8 ($= y_0$) patients out of 100 ($= n_0$) suffered from SICH. The corresponding likelihood is $L(\theta \mid y_0) = \binom{n_0}{y_0}\theta^{y_0}(1-\theta)^{(n_0-y_0)}$ and yields the most likely value for θ, i.e. $\widehat{\theta}_0 = y_0/n_0 = 0.08$. Figure 2.2 shows that the ECASS 2 data do not support much a proportion (of patients suffering from SICH) outside the interval [0.02, 0.18]. In fact, the ECASS 2 likelihood expresses our opinion about θ based on a study conducted prior to the ECASS 3 study. Thus, the ECASS 2 likelihood may be used to express our prior belief on θ for the ECASS 3 study. As a function of θ, the

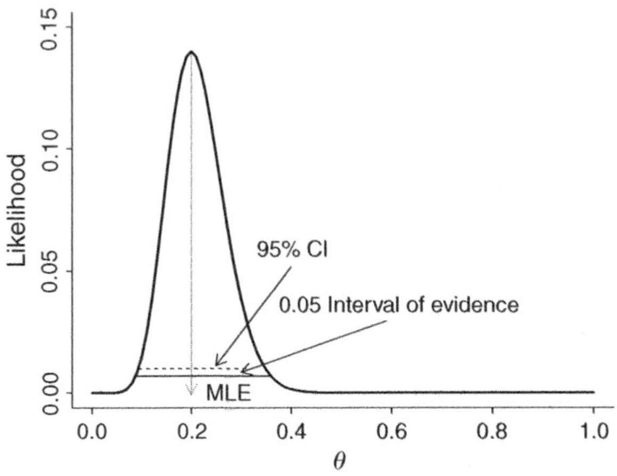

Figure 2.1 Stroke study: binomial likelihood for first interim analysis in the (fictive) ECASS 3 study.

likelihood function is not a distribution since the area under $L(\theta \mid y_0)$ is not equal to 1. But the area under the curve (AUC) can easily be turned to 1. For instance, when $\int L(\theta \mid y_0)\,d\theta = a$, then $p(\theta) \equiv L(\theta \mid y_0)/a$ ('proportional to likelihood' in Figure 2.2) satisfies the requirements of a prior distribution. The calculation of the AUC involves in general a numerical procedure, but here analytical calculations are possible which we will now show.

The kernel of the binomial likelihood of the ECASS 2 study, $\theta^{y_0}(1-\theta)^{(n_0-y_0)}$, is up to a constant value, the expression of a *beta density*, i.e.

$$p(\theta) = \frac{1}{B(\alpha_0, \beta_0)}\,\theta^{\alpha_0-1}(1-\theta)^{\beta_0-1}, \tag{2.5}$$

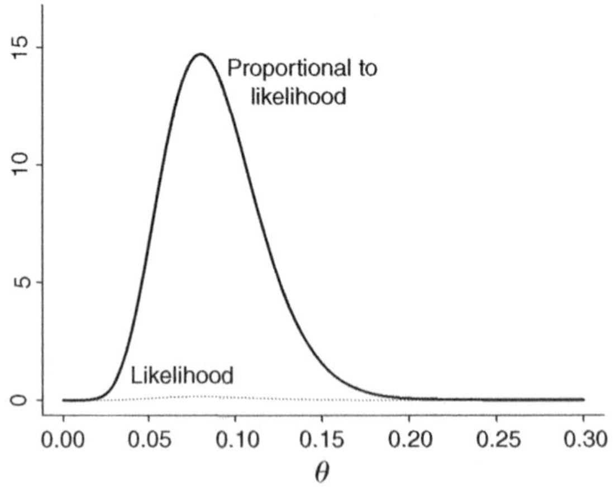

Figure 2.2 Stroke study: binomial likelihood obtained from ECASS 2 study and the rescaled likelihood (proportional to likelihood) equal to Beta(θ | 9, 93).

with

$$B(\alpha, \beta) = \frac{\Gamma(\alpha)\Gamma(\beta)}{\Gamma(\alpha + \beta)} = \int \theta^{\alpha-1}(1-\theta)^{\beta-1}\, d\theta,$$

and $\Gamma(\cdot)$ the gamma function. When α_0 is replaced by $y_0 + 1$ and β_0 by $n_0 - y_0 + 1$ in expression (2.5), the ECASS 2 likelihood is obtained up to a constant. In other words, to turn the prior likelihood into a distribution of θ we need to replace the binomial coefficient by $1/B(\alpha_0, \beta_0)$. Figure 2.2 shows the beta density with $\alpha_0 = 9$ and $\beta_0 = 100 - 8 + 1 = 93$.

The beta distribution with parameters α and β is denoted as Beta(α, β) and represents a flexible family of distributions defined on the unit interval.

2. Constructing the posterior distribution

The task of the DSMB is to protect the safety of the patients enrolled in the ECASS 3 trial, and therefore, all the existing evidence about the safety of the drug needs to be taken into consideration. On the other hand, the DSMB should also be aware of the natural variability of the statistical information collected in an interim analysis. Especially in an early interim analysis, the gathered information is limited and prone to high variability. Prior information obtained from the ECASS 2 study could, therefore, be useful for the first ECASS 3 interim analysis to yield, when combined with the data obtained from the interim analysis, an updated estimate of the safety.

The ingredients of expression (2.4) applied to this setting are (a) the prior $p(\theta)$, here obtained from the ECASS 2 study; (b) the likelihood $L(\theta \mid y)$, here obtained from the rt-PA treated patients from the first ECASS 3 interim analysis (remember that $y = 10$ and $n = 50$); and (c) the averaged likelihood $\int L(\theta \mid y)p(\theta)\, d\theta$. The numerator of Bayes theorem is the product of the prior and the likelihood and is equal to

$$L(\theta \mid y)\, p(\theta) = \binom{n}{y} \frac{1}{B(\alpha_0, \beta_0)}\, \theta^{\alpha_0+y-1}(1-\theta)^{\beta_0+n-y-1}.$$

The averaged likelihood $p(y) = \int L(\theta \mid y)\, p(\theta)\, d\theta$ is readily obtained when one realizes that $\theta^{\alpha_0+y-1}(1-\theta)^{\beta_0+n-y-1}$ is the kernel of a beta density with parameters $\alpha_0 + y$ and $\beta_0 + n - y$. Hence,

$$p(y) = \binom{n}{y} \frac{B(\alpha_0 + y, \beta_0 + n - y)}{B(\alpha_0, \beta_0)}.$$

Combining the numerator and the denominator, results in the posterior distribution for θ and is given by

$$p(\theta \mid y) = \frac{1}{B(\overline{\alpha}, \overline{\beta})}\, \theta^{\overline{\alpha}-1}(1-\theta)^{\overline{\beta}-1}, \tag{2.6}$$

where $\overline{\alpha} = \alpha_0 + y$ and $\overline{\beta} = \beta_0 + n - y$. Then the posterior (2.6) corresponds again to a beta distribution, i.e. Beta($\overline{\alpha}, \overline{\beta}$) with $\overline{\alpha} = 19$ and $\overline{\beta} = 133$. For the first interim analysis of the ECASS 3 study, the beta prior, the binomial likelihood (scaled to have AUC=1), and the beta posterior are graphically displayed in Figure 2.3.

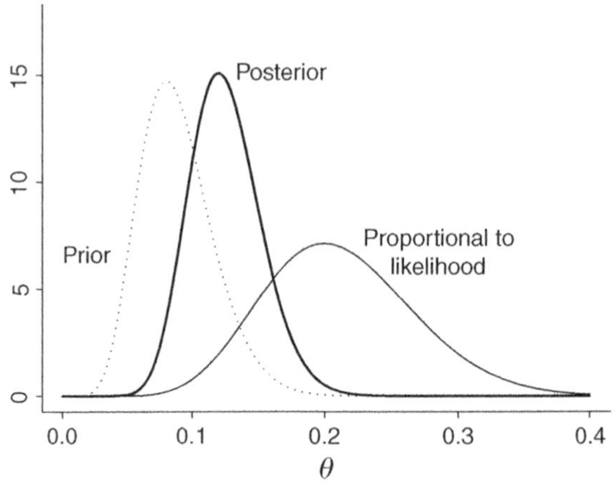

Figure 2.3 Stroke study: beta prior density, binomial likelihood, and beta posterior density.

3. Characteristics of the posterior distribution

Our computations and Figure 2.3 illustrate the following properties of the posterior distribution:

- The posterior is a compromise of the prior and the likelihood function since the posterior lies midway between the prior and the likelihood function (Figure 2.3). This can also be seen numerically as follows: let the prior be obtained from a binomial experiment with y_0 successes in n_0 experiments. The value that maximizes the prior distribution, i.e. the 'most plausible' a priori value of θ is $\theta_0 = y_0/n_0$, while for the likelihood it is the MLE $\widehat{\theta} = y/n$. The value that maximizes the posterior distribution $p(\theta \mid y)$ is $\widehat{\theta}_M = (\overline{\alpha} - 1)/(\overline{\alpha} + \overline{\beta} - 2) = (y + y_0)/n + n_0)$, then

$$\widehat{\theta}_M = \frac{n_0}{n_0 + n}\,\theta_0 + \frac{n}{n_0 + n}\,\widehat{\theta}. \tag{2.7}$$

  This shows that the most plausible value a posteriori is a weighted average of the most plausible value a priori and the most plausible value calculated from the data. It also shows that there is *shrinkage* toward θ_0, i.e. $\theta_0 \leq \widehat{\theta}_M \leq \widehat{\theta}$, when $y_0/n_0 \leq y/n$. The reverse inequality holds when $y/n \leq y_0/n_0$.

- The posterior contains more information about the parameter of interest than the prior and the likelihood function separately since the posterior is more concentrated than the prior and the likelihood function. Consequently, an a posteriori statement about the parameter θ will be more precise than the prior statement and the information represented by the likelihood function. However, when the prior distribution is 'in conflict' with the likelihood, the beta posterior might be less concentrated than that of the beta prior (Exercise 2.1). Note that the prior and the likelihood are in conflict when they support largely different values for θ.

- From the expressions of $\overline{\alpha}$ and $\overline{\beta}$, we conclude that when the study size increases (y and n increase) the impact of the prior parameters (α_0 and β_0) on the posterior decreases. This result is classically coined as 'the likelihood dominates the prior for large sample sizes'.

- The posterior is of the same type (beta) as the prior. This property is called *conjugacy* and will be treated in more generality in Chapter 5.

Finally, since the prior distribution in the stroke example is based on prior data, the maximum posterior value for θ, $(y + y_0)/(n + n_0)$, is in fact the MLE of the combined experiment (data from ECASS 2 and interim analysis data from ECASS 3). This is a reflection of the implicit assumption that the conditions under which the ECASS 2 and ECASS 3 studies were conducted are identical, and hence, we in fact assumed that the past data are *exchangeable* with the present data. More on exchangeability can be found in Chapter 3.

4. Equivalence of prior information and extra data
The aforementioned reasoning shows that a Beta(α, β) prior is equivalent to a binomial experiment with $(\alpha - 1)$ successes in $(\alpha + \beta - 2)$ experiments. Further, the scaled likelihood is equal to a Beta($y + 1, n - y + 1$)-distribution and adding the Beta(α_0, β_0) prior to the data yields the Beta($\alpha_0 + y$, $\beta_0 + n - y$)-distribution. Summarized, the prior corresponds to adding extra data to the observed data set, $(\alpha_0 - 1)$ successes and $(\beta_0 - 1)$ failures. This equivalence of prior information and 'imaginary' data can be used to construct prior distributions that combine elegantly with the likelihood allowing even to use frequentist software for estimation purposes (see Chapter 3 and subsequent chapters).

Bayesian approach: Using a subjective prior
Suppose that at the start of the ECASS 3 study, the DSMB neurologists believed that the incidence of SICH lies probably between 5% and 20%. If their prior belief coincides with the prior density $p(\theta)$ as obtained from the ECASS 2 study data, then all posterior inference would be the same as before. Indeed, nowhere in Bayes theorem is it specified how the prior information should be collected.

The neurologists could also combine their qualitative prior belief with the data collected in the ECASS 2 study in order to construct a prior distribution. For instance, suppose that the patient population in the ECASS 3 study is on average 5 years older than in the ECASS 2 study. In that case, the neurologists might adjust the prior distribution obtained from the ECASS 2 study toward higher incidences, as done in Figure 2.4.

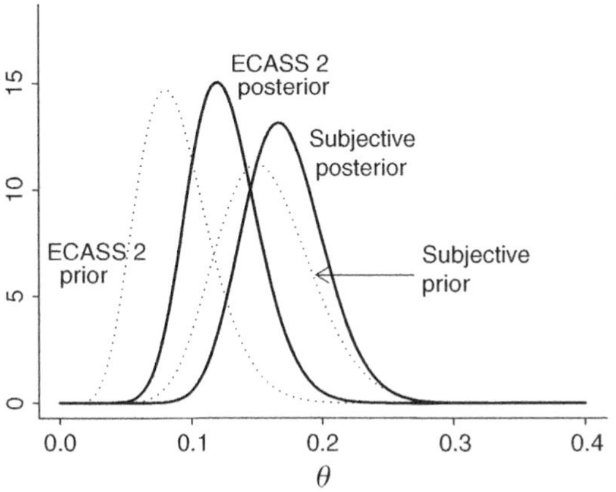

Figure 2.4 Stroke study: prior and posterior based on the ECASS 2 study data or based on a subjective prior belief.

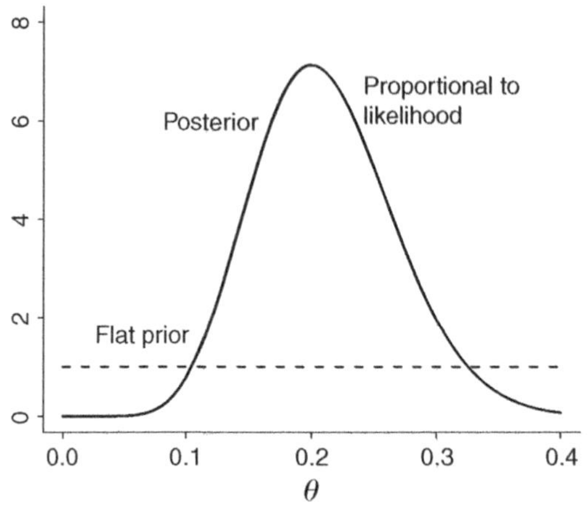

Figure 2.5 Stroke study: prior, likelihood, and posterior based on flat prior.

Bayesian approach: No prior information is available
When there is little prior information available or when one is reluctant to use the available prior knowledge, a prior distribution is needed that expresses our lack of information. Such a prior is called a *noninformative* (*NI*) prior. Other terms used in the literature are *weakly informative, vague, diffuse*, etc.

A popular NI prior for θ is a uniform distribution, also called a *flat prior*. Since θ has support [0, 1], we take the uniform distribution on the unit interval, i.e. U(0, 1), to express that we have no preference for any particular value for θ. Why this flat prior may be a good choice is seen from combining the prior with the data collected in the ECASS 3 study. Using expression (2.4), we immediately see that this yields a posterior that is equal to the scaled likelihood (see Figure 2.5). Hence, it appears that the flat prior has done a good job in expressing our lack of knowledge since the posterior distribution depends only on the likelihood. We also see that the posterior only depends on the data and not on the prior distribution. Note that a uniform prior is a beta distribution with parameters $\alpha = \beta = 1$. □

2.7 The Gaussian case

The binomial likelihood combined with a beta prior produces a beta posterior. A similar conjugacy property holds in the Gaussian case, since a normal likelihood combined with a normal prior gives a normal posterior. As in Section 2.6 the results will be derived by making use of a motivating example which is now a dietary survey conducted in Belgium about two decades ago.

Example II.2: Dietary study: Monitoring dietary behavior in Belgium
There is an increasing awareness that we should improve our life style. In Western Europe, a variety of campaigns have been set up in the last decades to give up smoking and to render our diet more healthy, say by lowering our daily consumption of saturated fat. As a consequence, there is a tendency to lowering the intake of dietary cholesterol in order to lower the serum cholesterol. Around 1990 a dietary survey, the Inter-regional Belgian Bank

Employee Nutrition Study (IBBENS) (Den Hond *et al.* 1994), was set up to compare the dietary intake in different geographical areas in Belgium, especially in Flanders.

The IBBENS study was performed in eight subsidiaries of one bank situated in seven Dutch-speaking cities in the north and in one French-speaking city in the south of Belgium. The food habits of 371 (66%) male and 192 female healthy employees with average age 38.3 years were examined by a 3-day food record with an additional interview. The results showed regional differences in fat consumption.

Here, we look at the intake of cholesterol. First, we describe the results obtained in the IBBENS study. These data will then be used to create a prior density for the IBBENS-2 study, a fictive dietary survey organized 1 year after the IBBENS study to monitor the evolution in dietary behavior of the Belgian population.

Bayesian approach: Prior obtained from the IBBENS study

1. Specifying the (IBBENS) prior distribution

Figure 2.6(a) shows the histogram of the dietary cholesterol in mg/day (*chol*) of the 563 bank employees. The approximating Gaussian distribution pinpoints that *chol* has a slightly positively skewed distribution. To simplify matters, we will assume that *chol* has a Gaussian distribution, but as shown below, this assumption is not crucial for a large sample. The observed mean *chol* is 328 mg/day with a standard deviation equal to 120.3 mg/day.

Let the random variable y has a normal distribution with mean μ and standard deviation σ, then its density is

$$\frac{1}{\sqrt{2\pi}\,\sigma}\exp\left[-(y-\mu)^2/2\sigma^2\right]. \tag{2.8}$$

We denote this as $y \sim \mathrm{N}(\mu, \sigma^2)$ or $\mathrm{N}(y \mid \mu, \sigma^2)$. To simplify matters, we assume in this chapter that σ is known. For a sample $\boldsymbol{y} \equiv \{y_1, \ldots, y_n\}$ of i.i.d. Gaussian random variables,

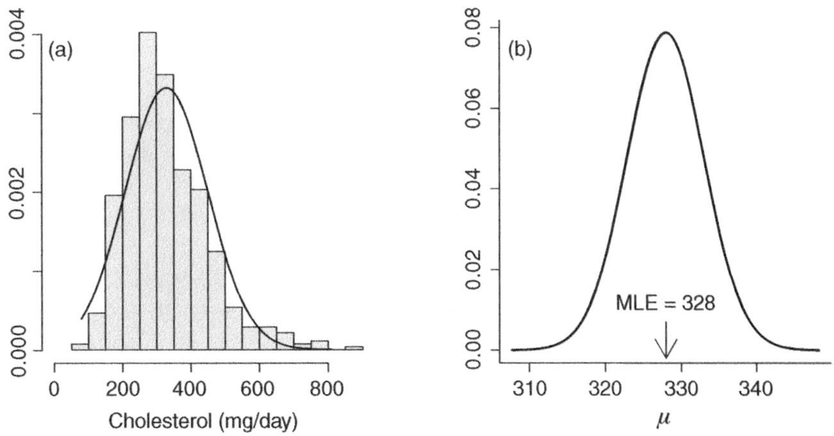

Figure 2.6 Dietary study: (a) histogram of dietary cholesterol obtained from the IBBENS study and approximating normal distribution, and (b) normal likelihood for unknown population mean μ.

the likelihood is

$$L(\mu \mid \mathbf{y}) = \frac{1}{(2\pi)^{n/2}\sigma^n} \exp\left[-\frac{1}{2\sigma^2}\sum_{i=1}^{n}(y_i - \mu)^2\right]. \tag{2.9}$$

Because $\sum(y_i - \mu)^2 = \sum(y_i - \overline{y})^2 + \sum(\overline{y} - \mu)^2$, with $\overline{y}$ the sample average of the y_i, we can rewrite expression (2.9) as

$$L(\mu \mid \mathbf{y}) \propto L(\mu \mid \overline{y}) \propto \exp\left[-\frac{1}{2}\left(\frac{\mu - \overline{y}}{\sigma/\sqrt{n}}\right)^2\right]. \tag{2.10}$$

Expression (2.10) is the kernel of a Gaussian distribution with mean $\overline{y}$ and variance σ^2/n. But, even when y does not have a Gaussian distribution, the likelihood will still have an (approximately) normal shape for a large sample size according to the classical Central Limit Theorem (CLT).

In order to use the IBBENS data as prior information for the IBBENS-2 study, we need to change the notation slightly. Namely, the random variable that expresses the dietary intake of cholesterol in the IBBENS study will now be denoted as y_0, the sample of observations of size n_0 as $\mathbf{y}_0 \equiv \{y_{0,1}, \ldots, y_{0,n_0}\}$ and the sample mean as $\overline{y}_0$.

From expression (2.10) and using the above change in notation, it is immediately seen that, up to a factor, the likelihood is given by the normal curve $\mathrm{N}(\mu \mid \mu_0, \sigma_0^2)$ (see Figure 2.6(b)), where $\mu_0 = \overline{y}_0$ and $\sigma_0 = \sigma/\sqrt{n_0}$ is the standard error of the mean. For the IBBENS, $\sigma_0 = 120.3/\sqrt{563} = 5.072$. Thus, the IBBENS prior distribution is

$$p(\mu) = \frac{1}{\sqrt{2\pi}\,\sigma_0} \exp\left[-\frac{1}{2}\left(\frac{\mu - \mu_0}{\sigma_0}\right)^2\right], \tag{2.11}$$

with $\mu_0 = \overline{y}_0$ and has the same shape as that of Figure 2.6(b).

2. Constructing the posterior distribution

Suppose that, to monitor dietary behavior in Belgium, and more specifically cholesterol intake, a new dietary survey was set up and finished one year after the IBBENS ended. Because of budget limitations, the new study was much smaller ($n = 50$). The average intake of cholesterol in this IBBENS-2 study was 318 mg/day with SD = 119.5 mg/day with 95% CI = [284.3, 351.9] mg/day.

The 95% CI is wide because the IBBENS-2 study is small sized. The CI is based on only the IBBENS-2 data, but is this reasonable? Do we believe that the IBBENS cannot learn us anything about the mean dietary intake in Belgium? This is, though, the consequence of using a frequentist/likelihood approach. In the Bayesian approach, we believe that information from the past can be used as prior for the current data.

To obtain the IBBENS-2 posterior, we combine the IBBENS normal prior (2.11) with the IBBENS-2 normal likelihood. Let $\mathbf{y}$ represent the n cholesterol intake values in the IBBENS-2 study with sample average as $\overline{y}$ producing the IBBENS-2 likelihood $L(\mu \mid \overline{y})$. Further, suppose that we tentatively 'forget' how the prior density was constructed and only use the fact that it is a $\mathrm{N}(\mu \mid \mu_0, \sigma_0^2)$ density. The posterior distribution is then proportional to $p(\mu)L(\mu \mid \overline{y})$, and therefore,

$$p(\mu \mid \mathbf{y}) \propto p(\mu \mid \overline{y}) \propto \exp\left\{-\frac{1}{2}\left[\left(\frac{\mu-\mu_0}{\sigma_0}\right)^2+\left(\frac{\mu-\overline{y}}{\sigma/\sqrt{n}}\right)^2\right]\right\}. \tag{2.12}$$

In the next step, we look for the constant such that expression (2.12) becomes a density. Instead of tackling this problem directly, we may have a closer look at expression (2.12) to possibly simplify it. Indeed, the expression behind the exponent is a quadratic function of μ which, up to a constant (function of $\overline{y}$ and σ_0 only), can be turned into $[(\mu-\overline{\mu})/\overline{\sigma}]^2$ with $\overline{\mu}$ and $\overline{\sigma}$ defined below (see also Exercise 2.6). Thus, the posterior distribution for μ after having observed the IBBENS-2 data and using the IBBENS as prior is given by the Gaussian density

$$p(\mu \mid \mathbf{y}) = \mathrm{N}(\mu \mid \overline{\mu}, \overline{\sigma}^2),$$

with

$$\overline{\mu} = \frac{\frac{1}{\sigma_0^2}\mu_0 + \frac{n}{\sigma^2}\overline{y}}{\frac{1}{\sigma_0^2}+\frac{n}{\sigma^2}} \quad \text{and} \quad \overline{\sigma}^2 = \frac{1}{\frac{1}{\sigma_0^2}+\frac{n}{\sigma^2}}. \tag{2.13}$$

In Figure 2.7, the IBBENS normal prior distribution, the IBBENS-2 normal (scaled) likelihood and the IBBENS-2 normal posterior distribution are shown. The latter distribution has mean $\overline{\mu} = 327.2$ and standard deviation $\overline{\sigma} = 4.79$.

3. Characteristics of the posterior distribution

We note the following properties of the posterior distribution:

- The posterior distribution is a 'compromise' between the prior distribution and the likelihood function (see Figure 2.7). As for the binomial case, there is shrinkage toward

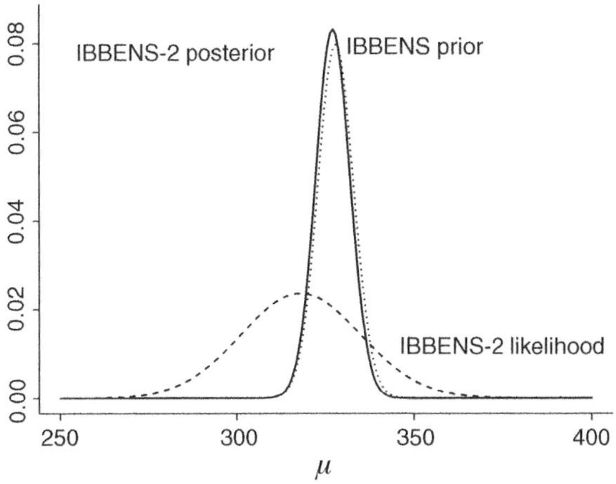

Figure 2.7 Dietary study: IBBENS normal prior density, IBBENS-2 normal likelihood (scaled) and IBBENS-2 normal posterior density.

the prior mean: $\overline{\mu}$, the mean of the posterior distribution is a weighted average of the prior and the sample mean, i.e.

$$\overline{\mu} = \frac{w_0}{w_0 + w_1}\,\mu_0 + \frac{w_1}{w_0 + w_1}\,\overline{y}, \tag{2.14}$$

with

$$w_0 = \frac{1}{\sigma_0^2},\; w_1 = \frac{1}{\sigma^2/n}. \tag{2.15}$$

In Bayesian statistics, it has been customary to work with the inverse of the variance, called the *precision*, rather than with the variance. Therefore, the weight w_0 is called the *prior precision* and the weight w_1 the *sample precision*.

- The *posterior precision* is the sum of the prior and the sample precision, i.e.

$$\frac{1}{\overline{\sigma}^2} = w_0 + w_1. \tag{2.16}$$

This shows that the posterior is more peaked than the prior and the likelihood function which means that the posterior contains more information about μ than the prior and the likelihood function. The property holds even when prior and likelihood are in conflict (in contrast to the binomial-beta case). This may look counterintuitive since in the presence of conflicting information, there is more uncertainty a posteriori rather than less uncertainty. Note that this result only holds for the special, and unrealistic, case of a known σ (see Example IV.2).

- Expression (2.13) clearly shows that for n large, $p(\mu \mid \mathbf{y}) \approx \mathrm{N}(\mu \mid \overline{y}, \sigma^2/n)$. This demonstrates that with the increasing sample size the likelihood dominates the prior. The same result is obtained under a fixed sample size when $\sigma_0 \to \infty$.

- The posterior is of the same type (normal density) as the prior (normal density). In other words, the conjugacy property also holds here.

As in the stroke example, the posterior estimate of μ is equal to the MLE of the combined experiment (data from IBBENS and IBBENS-2 studies). This reflects that, as before, we have assumed that the conditions under which the two studies were done are identical.

Note that in the Bayesian literature, the Gaussian distribution $\mathrm{N}(\mu, \sigma^2)$ is often denoted as $\mathrm{N}(\mu, 1/\sigma^2)$. This notation is also used by WinBUGS, the most popular Bayesian software on the market. It reflects that in the Bayesian world precision is more popular than variance, at least in the past. However, we continue using the classical notation to avoid confusion when making comparisons with frequentist results.

4. Equivalence of prior information and extra data

Suppose that the prior variance σ_0^2 is taken equal to the variance of the data, i.e. equal to σ^2 yielding the *unit-information* prior. Then the posterior variance is equal to $\overline{\sigma}^2 = \sigma^2/(n+1)$ and the prior distribution corresponds to adding one extra observation to the sample. This finding can be generalized since the prior variance σ_0^2 can always be reexpressed as σ^2/n_0, where n_0 is not necessarily an integer. Hence, any prior density with variance σ_0^2 corresponds to adding n_0 extra data points to the data set. This allows us to reexpress the posterior mean and variance as

$$\overline{\mu} = \frac{n_0}{n_0 + n}\,\mu_0 + \frac{n}{n_0 + n}\,\overline{y}, \tag{2.17}$$

and

$$\overline{\sigma}^2 = \frac{\sigma^2}{n_0 + n}. \tag{2.18}$$

Again we can use this result to base our prior distribution on imaginary data and even use standard frequentist software for the Bayesian estimation of parameters.

Bayesian approach: Using a subjective prior

The IBBENS prior has a large impact on the posterior distribution. We may wish to downplay this impact by increasing σ_0^2 from 25 (IBBENS prior variance) to say 100. The resulting prior is called *discounted* since the information from the IBBENS is discounted (see Figure 2.8(a)).

Further, suppose the IBBENS prior is not entirely appropriate for the study at hand, e.g. when the IBBENS-2 study was performed only in the south of Belgium. A further modification of the prior can reflect this prior knowledge better. In Figure 2.8(b), the mean of the prior was changed to $\mu_0 = 340$ mg/day mimicking the prior belief that in the south of Belgium there is somewhat more saturated fat intake and hence also more cholesterol intake.

When a 'wrong' choice for the subjective prior is made, e.g. when it is not supported by evidence, the validity of the Bayesian analysis is low. Luckily, as for the binomial-beta case, the impact of the prior decreases when the study size increases.

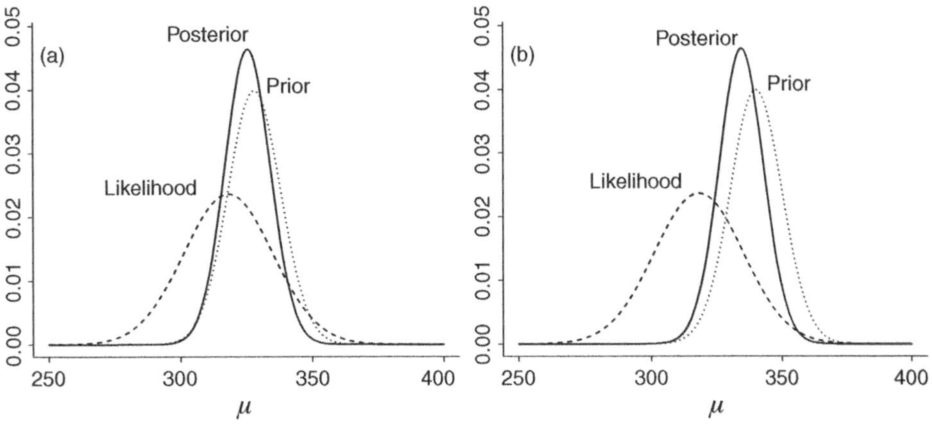

Figure 2.8 Dietary study: (a) discounted IBBENS normal prior density (variance = 100), and (b) adapted IBBENS normal prior distribution (variance = 100) both in combination with IBBENS-2 normal likelihood (scaled).

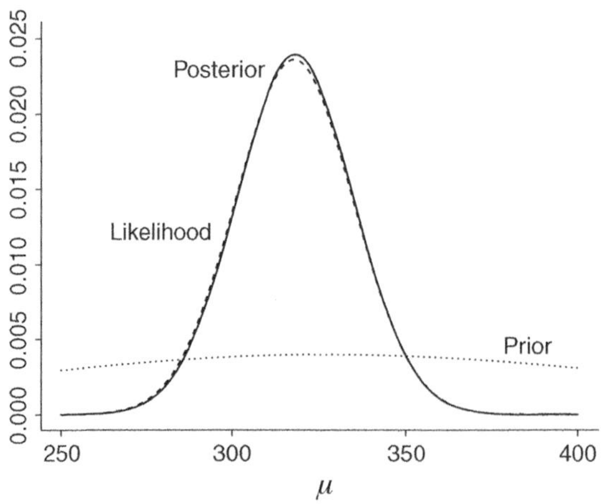

Figure 2.9 Dietary study: noninformative normal prior (variance = 10 000) in combination with IBBENS-2 normal likelihood (scaled).

Bayesian approach: No prior information is available

Had IBBENS-2 study been organized in Asia, the IBBENS prior would be inappropriate, even a discounted version of it. In that case, one must admit that there is not much prior information. But, how do we specify our lack of knowledge? In other words, what is the NI or vague prior here? The answer to this question can be found in expression (2.13). Indeed, as seen above, when $\sigma_0^2 \to \infty$, the posterior becomes

$$\mathrm{N}(\mu \mid \overline{y}, \sigma^2/n), \tag{2.19}$$

which appears to be independent of prior information. Thus, putting it loosely, the NI prior in the normal case is a normal distribution with a very large variance. In the binomial case, we have chosen the flat prior to express no prior knowledge. Here, a flat prior is obtained as the limit.

In Figure 2.9, the normal prior with mean 328 and variance 10 000 is combined with the likelihood. The prior is relatively flat in the interval of plausible μ-values and the posterior is only slightly more peaked than the scaled likelihood. The posterior mean is equal to 318.3, close to the observed mean of 318 and the posterior variance is equal to 277.6 a bit lower than the observed SEM^2 of 285.6. If the prior has to have a lower impact on the posterior estimates, then the prior variance should be further increased. □

2.8 The Poisson case

Assume that y_i $(i = 1, \ldots, n)$ are independent counts. Examples are the number of epileptic seizures in a month of epilepsy patients, the number of medical errors in hospitals in a year, the counts of a disease in census tracts, etc. The *Poisson distribution* is the most popular model to describe the distribution of counts. The random variable y is said to have a Poisson distribution with parameter θ, denoted as Poisson(θ), when

$$p(y \mid \theta) = \frac{\theta^y \, \mathrm{e}^{-\theta}}{y!}. \tag{2.20}$$

It is well-known that the mean and variance of the Poisson distribution are equal to θ. Note that in the above examples the y_i are the counts observed in a unit of time, e.g. year, month, etc. When the time periods differ between the subjects, say the count y_i is observed in a time period of length t_i, then the Poisson model is extended to

$$p(y_i \mid \theta) = \frac{(\theta\, t_i)^{y_i}\, \mathrm{e}^{-\theta\, t_i}}{y_i!}. \tag{2.21}$$

A Bayesian Poisson analysis of the number of deciduous teeth with caries is shown in Example II.3.

Example II.3: Caries study: Describing caries experience in Flanders
The Signal-Tandmobiel® (ST) study is a longitudinal oral health intervention study involving a sample of 4468 children. A stratified cluster random sample was taken by selecting primary schools at random and therein all children from the first class. Hereby, a sample was established representative of the 7% of children born in 1989 in Flanders. The children were examined in 1996 by 16 trained dentists (examiners) and annually thereafter for 6 years. Data on caries experience (current or past caries) status, oral hygiene and dietary habits were obtained at yearly intervals, through structured questionnaires. Here, we look at the caries experience on primary teeth of the first year of the study; hence, the data of 7-year old children are evaluated here. Caries experience on primary teeth is classically measured by the dmft-index. This score represents the number of primary teeth that are decayed (d), missing due to extraction for caries reasons (m) or filled (f) because of caries. It varies from 0 (no caries experience) to 20 (all primary teeth affected). The dmft-index was available on 4351 children (see Figure 2.10). Apart from the oral health information, dietary habits and oral hygiene behavior was also recorded. For a more detailed description of the ST study, we refer to Vanobbergen *et al.* (2000).

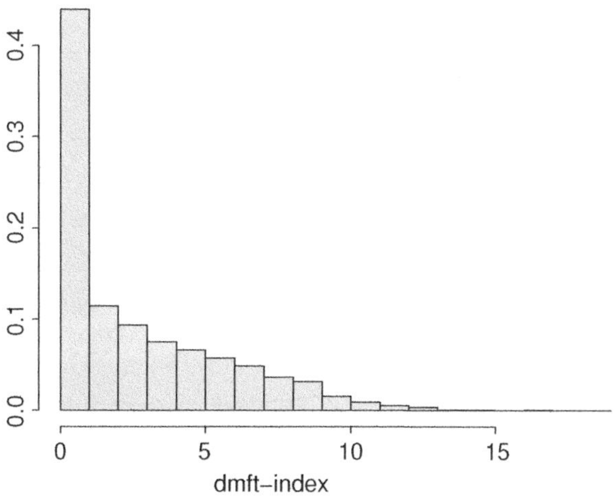

Figure 2.10 Caries study: histogram of dmft-index.

The Poisson likelihood of the dmft-index is the product of terms $p(y_i \mid \theta)$ given by expression (2.20) resulting in

$$L(\theta \mid \mathbf{y}) \equiv \prod_{i=1}^{n} p(y_i \mid \theta) = \prod_{i=1}^{n} (\theta^{y_i}/y_i!)\ \mathrm{e}^{-n\theta}. \tag{2.22}$$

Maximizing expression (2.22) with respect to θ yields the MLE of θ, i.e. $\widehat{\theta} = \overline{y}$ which is equal to 2.24 for the ST study. A likelihood-based frequentist 95% CI for θ is equal to [2.1984, 2.2875].

Bayesian approach: Prior distribution based on historical data

1. Specifying the prior distribution for the ST study

We wish to combine the Poisson likelihood with any available prior information. However, prior to the ST study there was only limited information available on the degree of caries experience among 7-year-old children in Flanders. The review paper of Vanobbergen *et al.* (2001) reported an average dmft-index of 4.1 obtained in a study based on 109 seven-year-old children and conducted in Liège in 1983, while an average of 1.39 was obtained around Ghent on 200 five-year-old children examined in 1994. Further, it is known that oral hygiene had improved considerably in Flanders in the recent years. Thus, we do not materially restrict the mean dmft-index when we bound it above by a value around 10. An appropriate prior distribution for θ should reflect all of the above available knowledge. While in principle any distribution expressing the prior knowledge in a probabilistic way could do the job, we look here for a distribution (as for the binomial and normal likelihood) that allows us to determine the posterior distribution in a relatively easy manner. For a Poisson likelihood, this is the *gamma density*, denoted as Gamma(α,β) where α is a shape parameter and β is the inverse of a scale parameter.

Thus, we assumed here that $\theta \sim \text{Gamma}(\alpha_0, \beta_0)$ a priori, implying that $E(\theta) = \alpha_0/\beta_0$ and $var(\theta) = \alpha_0/\beta_0^2$. When $\alpha_0 = 3$ and $\beta_0 = 1$, the knowledge prior to the ST seems adequately represented (see Figure 2.11).

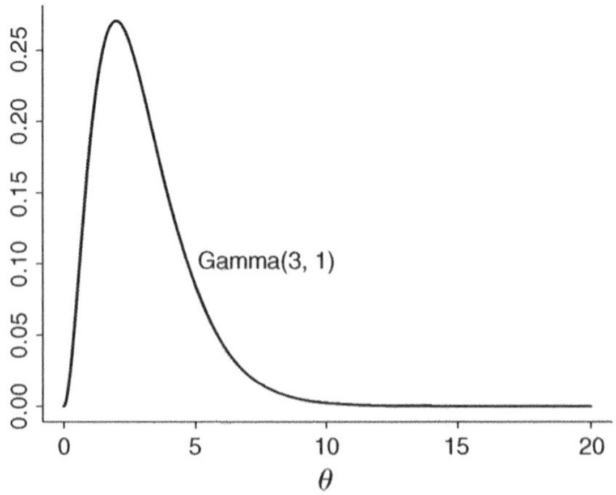

Figure 2.11 Caries study: Gamma(3, 1) prior density.

2. Constructing the posterior distribution
The Gamma(α_0, β_0) prior distribution as a function of θ is given by

$$p(\theta) = \frac{\beta_0^{\alpha_0}}{\Gamma(\alpha_0)} \theta^{\alpha_0 - 1} \, \mathrm{e}^{-\beta_0 \theta}. \tag{2.23}$$

The posterior density is proportional to $L(\theta \mid \boldsymbol{y})p(\theta)$, which leads to

$$\begin{aligned} p(\theta \mid \boldsymbol{y}) &\propto \mathrm{e}^{-n\theta} \prod_{i=1}^{n} (\theta^{y_i}/y_i!) \frac{\beta_0^{\alpha_0}}{\Gamma(\alpha_0)} \theta^{\alpha_0 - 1} \mathrm{e}^{-\beta_0 \theta} \\ &\propto \theta^{(\sum y_i + \alpha_0) - 1} \mathrm{e}^{-(n+\beta_0)\theta}. \end{aligned} \tag{2.24}$$

Expression (2.24) is the kernel of a Gamma($\sum y_i + \alpha_0, n + \beta_0$) distribution; hence,

$$p(\theta \mid \boldsymbol{y}) \equiv p(\theta \mid \overline{y}) = \frac{\overline{\beta}^{\overline{\alpha}}}{\Gamma(\overline{\alpha})} \theta^{\overline{\alpha} - 1} \, \mathrm{e}^{-\overline{\beta} \theta}, \tag{2.25}$$

where $\overline{\alpha} = \sum y_i + \alpha_0$ and $\overline{\beta} = n + \beta_0$. For the ST study, we obtained $\overline{\alpha} = 9758 + 3 = 9761$ and $\overline{\beta} = 4351 + 1 = 4352$. Clearly, the effect of the prior on the posterior is minimal here.

3. Characteristics of the posterior distribution
We note the following properties of the posterior distribution:

- The posterior distribution is again a compromise between the prior distribution and the likelihood function (see Exercise 3.6).
- In the ST study, the posterior distribution is more peaked than the prior distribution and the likelihood function. However, as in the binomial case, the prior gamma distribution might sometimes be more concentrated than the posterior gamma distribution (see Exercise 3.7).
- It can easily be verified that the prior is again dominated by the likelihood when the sample size is large.
- The posterior distribution belongs to the same class (gamma) as the prior distribution, providing another example of conjugacy.

4. Equivalence of prior information and extra data
Since the scaled Poisson likelihood (such that AUC $= 1$) as a function of θ is equal to a Gamma($\sum y_i + 1, n$)-distribution, the Gamma(α_0, β_0) prior can be viewed as equivalent to imaginary data corresponding to an experiment of size β_0 and where the counts sum up to $(\alpha_0 - 1)$. Applied to the ST study, the prior corresponds to an experiment of size 1 with count equal to 2.

Bayesian approach: No prior information is available
When there is no prior information available on the mean parameter of the Poisson distribution, the absence of knowledge should be reflected in the prior distribution. Comparing the expression of the (scaled) Poisson likelihood and that of the posterior distribution, informs us that $\alpha_0 \approx 1$ and $\beta_0 \approx 0$ correspond to almost no extra (prior) information added to the likelihood. □

While the Poisson distribution is usually the first choice to describe the distribution of counts, in medical applications it is often not the best choice. For the Poisson distribution, the counts represent the sum of independent events that happen with a constant average. The dmft-index is the sum of binary responses expressing the caries experience in each of the 20 primary teeth. However, cavities in the same mouth are correlated. This leads to (Poisson-) overdispersion, which means that the variance is (much) larger than the mean. Here, we obtained $var(\text{dmft})/mean(\text{dmft}) = 3.53$. In Chapter 10, we will look for more appropriate distributions to model the dmft-index.

2.9 The prior and posterior distribution of $h(\theta)$

Suppose that h defines a monotone transformation of the parameter θ, i.e. $h(\theta) \equiv \psi$ defines a new parameter. Since θ is stochastic, also ψ is stochastic and has a prior and a posterior distribution. By the standard transformation rule for random variables (also called change-of-variables rule), the (prior or posterior) distribution of ψ is

$$p(h^{-1}(\psi)) \left(\left| \frac{\mathrm{d}\psi}{\mathrm{d}\theta} \right| \right)^{-1}, \tag{2.26}$$

when $p(\theta) = p(h^{-1}(\psi))$ is the (prior or posterior) distribution of θ. Expression (2.26) involves the Jacobian when changing from θ to ψ.

Example II.4: Stroke study: Posterior distribution of $\log(\theta)$
The probability of developing SICH could be modeled on the log-scale (or logit-scale). Transformation rule (2.26) yields the posterior distribution of $\psi = \log(\theta)$, i.e.

$$p(\psi \mid \mathbf{y}) = \frac{1}{B(\overline{\alpha}, \overline{\beta})} \exp \psi^{\overline{\alpha}} (1 - \exp \psi)^{\overline{\beta}-1},$$

where $\overline{\alpha} = 19$ and $\overline{\beta} = 133$. In Figure 3.3, the posterior distribution of ψ is shown. □

2.10 Bayesian versus likelihood approach

The Bayesian approach satisfies the relative likelihood principle (second LP). Indeed, take two proportional likelihoods, i.e. $L_2(\theta \mid \mathbf{y}) = c L_1(\theta \mid \mathbf{y})$, then

$$\begin{aligned} p_2(\theta \mid \mathbf{y}) &= L_2(\theta \mid \mathbf{y}) p(\theta) \Big/ \int L_2(\theta \mid \mathbf{y}) p(\theta) \mathrm{d}\theta, \\ &= c L_1(\theta \mid \mathbf{y}) p(\theta) \Big/ \int c L_1(\theta \mid \mathbf{y}) p(\theta) \mathrm{d}\theta, \\ &= p_1(\theta \mid \mathbf{y}). \end{aligned}$$

The Bayesian approach also satisfies the first likelihood principle in the sense that it does not need to generate artificial data (under H_0) to make conclusions about the outcome of the experiment. However, in the Bayesian approach the parameter is stochastic, in contrast to the likelihood approach. Indeed, the likelihood approach is invariant to a change from θ to $h(\theta)$

(for a strict monotone function h), but from expression (2.26) we know that with a parameter change the prior and the posterior also change. A consequence of this is that the outcome from a Bayesian analysis will change when a flat prior is put on $h(\theta)$ instead of θ (see also Chapter 5).

2.11 Bayesian versus frequentist approach

In the frequentist approach, inference about a parameter is based on the repeated sampling behavior of a summary measure while hypothesis testing relies on the repeated sampling behavior of a test statistic under H_0. In Bayesian inference, probability enters via the uncertainty that one has about the parameter conditioned on the observed data. Thus, in frequentist statistics the parameter is considered fixed and inference is based on repeated sampling, while in Bayesian statistics the parameter is stochastic and inference is done given the observed data. Both approaches aim to discover the 'true' parameter value of the parameter but take a different route to achieve this goal. The consequence of this difference is that the computations for statistical inference differ in important ways. Indeed, many frequentist approaches rely on asymptotic theory. For example, in logistic regression models the importance of a regressor is assessed via the Wald, score or likelihood-ratio statistic, all based on their asymptotic distribution. In contrast, Bayesian inference only relies on the posterior distribution that provides inference for any sample size. A striking illustration of the difference in inferential procedures is the lack of importance of the CLT in the Bayesian paradigm (see Section 3.6.2). Also, in a computational sense the two approaches are markedly different. Namely, in frequentist statistics maximization is the key for drawing statistical inference (see likelihood-ratio test statistic), while in the Bayesian approach integration is central.

While the Bayesian and frequentist approach differ in their fundament and in computational aspects, we will illustrate in the book that the approaches can lead to (about) the same numerical output. For instance, in Section 4.3.1, we show that for the Gaussian distribution the classical CI coincides with the Bayesian counterpart for a particular choice of the prior. However, in some cases the two approaches will lead to drastically different conclusions. For example, when stopping rules are involved the Bayesian approach acts like the likelihood approach and may, therefore, give drastically different conclusions.

Despite all differences between the two approaches, the Bayesian approach makes use of frequentist ideas at several places. For instance, the techniques to evaluate the Markov chain Monte Carlo runs are based on frequentist approaches. In addition, increasingly more Bayesians believe that their solutions should be evaluated on their long-run frequency properties. As seen in Chapter 1, there is even a reconciliation possible between the P-value and Bayesian inference.

2.12 The different modes of the Bayesian approach

The Bayesian approach is often criticized for introducing subjectivism into (medical) research by allowing probabilities to be subjective. However, the concept that research is objective is a myth. Those who claim objectivity sweep a lot of their subjective decisions under the carpet (see Good (1978) and references therein). Indeed, researchers are driven by previous scientific findings, background knowledge, intuition, etc. When combined in an intelligent manner, it can lead to great scientific discoveries. Press and Tanur (2001) describe the discoveries of great scientists such as Newton, Kepler, Mendel, etc., and how their findings and theories were lead by subjective decisions. Of course, subjectivity should be not confused with manipulation of results and cheating. The aim of research is to go for the truth, but the way to the truth runs over subjective paths. Subjectivity enters research also in a completely other manner. Medical (and other ...) research findings are always disseminated to a mix of consumers: medical colleagues, policy makers, patients, etc., each with their own belief in the result. Therefore, the appreciation of a research finding will differ between individuals. By combining prior beliefs (and past results) with results from the present experiment and producing a posterior belief, the Bayesian approach mimics this behavior. Spiegelhalter *et al.* (2004) state that 'Bayesian methods explicitly allow for the possibility that the conclusions of an analysis may depend on who is conducting it and their available evidence and opinion'. If little or no information is available, then a Bayesian analysis may yield similar results as the frequentist procedure.

Bayesians differ in opinion in how to deal with prior information. For a *subjective Bayesian*, the prior information always reflects a personal opinion. This opinion may express the belief of one individual or of a group. The appropriateness of the posterior, and thus the trustworthiness of the conclusions, depends much on the appropriateness of the prior. For an *objective Bayesian*, the prior is chosen by a formal rule expressing lack of knowledge on the subject. Such a prior is also called a *default prior*. This approach keeps the appearance of objectivity, which is necessary, e.g. for phase III controlled trials. But Bayesians may disagree with each other on many other fundamentals. Good (1982) sees at least 46 656 varieties of Bayesians. Nowadays, many Bayesians may be classified as *pragmatic Bayesians*. Their aim is to solve a scientific question and they are willing to combine subjective and objective Bayesian approaches with frequentist ideas. Another class, perhaps the biggest group, consists of those who just use Bayesian statistical software to crack their problems, but it is not clear whether all of them should be called Bayesians.

2.13 An historical note on the Bayesian approach

The cornerstone of the Bayesian approach is *Bayes theorem* named after its originator, Thomas Bayes born around 1701 (not exactly known) and died in 1761. He was a Presbyterian minister, studied logic and theology at Edinburgh University, and had strong mathematical interests. Immediately after his death, Richard Price, a friend of Thomas Bayes, was asked to look into Bayes mathematical papers. As a result he submitted the paper *An Essay toward a Problem in the Doctrine of Chances* in 1763 to *Philosophical Transactions of the Royal Society* after having added personal comments and extensions of his own. Note that a copy of the original paper can be found in Press (2003).

Bayes appears to be the first to formulate the problem of Inverse Probability. Indeed, while in the eighteen century great developments in mathematics (the term statistics was not used then) were seen, e.g. De Moivre (1667–1754) derived the normal approximation to the binomial in 1733, mathematicians had developed methods only to compute the (direct) probability. Namely, they could predict that, say, 7 people aged 50 die in a given year out of a sample of 100 if the probability of any one of them dying was known, but they were not able to find the (inverse) probability of one 50-year-old dying based on the observation that 7 had died out of 100. Bayes made a start to derive this inverse probability. He also derived the distribution of the binomial parameter in a two-stage sampling experiment and thereby discovered the beta distribution.

Up to 1950, Bayes theorem was called *The Theorem of Inverse Probability*. However, attributing this fundamental theorem to Bayes alone is not justified. The fundament of Bayesian theory is actually due to Laplace (1749–1827). Laplace is also responsible for many other achievements. In his time, mathematicians used both inverse and direct probability arguments and chose whatever was more convenient. There was no clear split between the Bayesian and frequentist approaches. Therefore, results developed in what we now call frequentist statistics were later picked up to be used in a Bayesian context, and vice versa. For example, Laplace first proved the asymptotic normality of posterior distributions (see Theorem 3.6.1), which is called the CLT for inverse probability. From this result, the classical CLT was derived.

At first, Laplace assumed that prior probabilities are uniform that is referred to as the *principle of insufficient reason* or the *principle of indifference*. Later on, he relaxed this assumption by allowing the prior distribution to be nonuniform and he derived the general expression (2.3) of Bayes theorem. Hereby, Laplace assigned hypotheses and parameters a stochastic behavior and, therefore, put them on an equal footing with observations (as of course Bayes did but in a less formal manner). The fact that with the inverse probability principle parameters were given a distribution was a thorn in the flesh of many influential statisticians such as Poisson in the nineteenth century (see especially Chapter 11 in Hald (2007)). However, the strongest opposition came from Fisher and Jerzy Neyman.

Fisher laid down the fundamentals of current (classical) statistical theory and is probably the most influential statistician. However, Fisher was also one of the most fervent opposers to Bayesian theory. His (but also others) main objection was the use of the flat prior to express ignorance. He argued that the flat prior was not appropriate to express ignorance in most practical cases, but there was another annoying problem with the flat prior. Namely, Fisher showed that the inverse probability estimate depends on the chosen parameterization of the model. Indeed, as seen in Section 2.9, when a flat prior is put on $h(\theta)$ rather than on θ, the posterior distribution for θ changes and also inference on θ changes. Since it is not clear on which scale the uniform prior should be specified, Fisher concluded that the Bayesian approach leads to arbitrary conclusions and, therefore, must be rejected completely. Fisher's tool for inductive inference was the likelihood function although he did attempt to mimic the Bayesian approach with his theory on *fiducial inference*, without much success though; see also Edwards (1997) for a historical note on how and when Fisher moved from inverse probability to likelihood.

Both Fisher, Neyman, and Pearson strongly rejected the Bayesian paradigm, but as seen above they were also strongly opposed to one another's viewpoints. Their impact on the practice of statistical inference is immense and led most applied statisticians to ignore the Bayesian approach for a long period. Concurrent to the developments of Fisher, Neyman and Pearson, important theoretical advances in Bayesian theory were made by de Finetti, Jeffreys, Savage and Lindley. For example, the *Representation Theorem* proved by Bruno de Finetti (1906–1985) in 1931 is seen by many Bayesians as one of the most fundamental results in Bayesian theory (see Section 3.5). Other examples are the developments of Harold Jeffreys (1891–1989), who suggested a system to define noninformative priors (see Section 5.4.3) and the Bayes factor, which is a fundamental tool for Bayesian hypothesis testing and model selection (see Section 3.8.2). Unfortunately, initially the impact of these developments on applied statistics was limited since the Bayesian approach suffered from serious computational limitations, making it impossible to provide answers to practical problems. The main obstacle for the Bayesian approach was the calculation of the denominator in Bayes theorem. It was only after the introduction of fast computational methods (such as Markov chain Monte Carlo) into the statistical world in the late 1980s and the implementation of the BUGS package in

1989) and its Windows version WinBUGS that the Bayesian approach became accessible to practitioners.

The enthusiasm for the Bayesian paradigm may not be shared by all statisticians, not even today. But the days are over when frequentists and Bayesians were raging against each other (especially the frequentists against the Bayesians). To get an idea of this hostility, look at the discussion part of the seminal paper of Lindley and Smith (1972), but especially at the comments of Kempthorne and the replies from the authors. Nowadays many Bayesians would classify themselves merely as pragmatic and dedicated to find solutions to practical problems.

To end this historical note, we strongly encourage the reader to read the book '*The theory that would not die. How Bayes rule cracked the enigma code, hunted down Russian submarines & emerged triumphant from two centuries of controversy*' by Mc Grayne (2011). It is an amazing and most entertaining story of the 'life of the Bayesian paradigm' and reads almost as a detective romance novel.

2.14 Closing remarks

In this chapter, we have introduced the reader to the general expression of Bayes theorem. We have also shown how, in elementary cases, the posterior distribution can be computed. Further, we have illustrated the impact of choosing different priors on the posterior distribution and indicated that the prior is the cause of much of the controversy around the Bayesian paradigm. In Chapter 3, we continue with introducing the fundamental Bayesian concepts, but it will take until Chapter 6 before practical problems can be tackled.

Exercises

Exercise 2.1 Show by a practical example that when the binomial likelihood is in conflict with the beta prior, the variance of the posterior may be larger than that of the prior.

Exercise 2.2 Write a program in R, which reproduces Figure 2.1 and calculate the 95% interval of evidence.

Exercise 2.3 Write a program in R, which reproduces Figure 2.3. Analyze this example also with FirstBayes (can be downloaded from http://tonyohagan.co.uk/1b/).

Exercise 2.4 Write a program in R, which reproduces Figure 2.7. Analyze this example also with FirstBayes.

Exercise 2.5 Calculate the posterior distribution for $1/\theta$, θ^2, etc., for the ECASS 3 study. Show the posterior distributions graphically.

Exercise 2.6 Prove expression (2.13). This is done by observing that the expression behind the exponent is in fact quadratic in μ and by searching for the extra terms to make the expression a square. This is called 'completing the square'.

Exercise 2.7 Suggest for the Signal-Tandmobiel® study a gamma prior distribution, which has a substantial impact on the posterior distribution. Derive the result using an R program or FirstBayes.

Exercise 2.8 The negative binomial distribution

$$p(y \mid \theta, r) = \binom{y+r-1}{r-1} \theta^r (1-\theta)^y, \; y = 0, 1, \ldots, \quad (0 < \theta < 1)$$

expresses the distribution of the number of failures until r successes have been observed. Show that a beta prior distribution combined with a negative binomial likelihood, results in a beta posterior distribution.

Exercise 2.9 The exponential distribution is a candidate distribution for a positive random variable y. Show that a gamma prior distribution combined with an exponential likelihood, results in a gamma posterior distribution.

Exercise 2.10 Show that for the gamma-Poisson case

$$\frac{\overline{\alpha}}{\overline{\beta}} = \frac{w_0}{w_0 + w_1} \frac{\alpha_0}{\beta_0} + \frac{w_1}{w_0 + w_1} \frac{\sum y_i}{n},$$

with $w_0 > 0$ and $w_1 > 0$.

3

Introduction to Bayesian inference

3.1 Introduction

In this chapter, we introduce the Bayesian tools for statistical inference. To focus on concepts and to minimize computational issues, we treat here only one-parameter models. The extension of the concepts to multiparameter models is the subject of Chapter 4, but is in fact the topic of the remainder of the book.

The posterior distribution contains all information of the parameter of interest. Nevertheless, it is desirable to summarize the posterior information in a concise manner. In this chapter, we derive (a) summary measures for location and variability of the posterior distribution; (b) an interval estimator for the parameter of interest, and (c) the posterior predictive distribution (PPD) to predict future observations.

We also introduce the concept of exchangeability which is fundamental in the Bayesian paradigm and extends the notion of independence. Further, we elaborate on the conditions when the posterior distribution can be approximated well by a normal distribution. This brings us to the Bayesian version of the Central Limit Theorem (CLT). Sampling techniques are introduced in this chapter. They illustrate that sampling can replace analytical procedures to explore the posterior distribution. Hereby, we prepare the reader for more complex sampling procedures such as the Method of Composition in Chapter 4 and the Markov chain Monte Carlo (MCMC) procedures treated in the subsequent chapters. At the end of this chapter, we return to the topic that we started in Chapter 1, i.e. hypothesis testing. In this respect, we treat a Bayesian version of a P-value and the Bayes factor which is the key tool for Bayesian hypothesis testing.

3.2 Summarizing the posterior by probabilities

A simple way to characterize the posterior information is by calculating probabilities $P(a < \theta < b \mid \mathbf{y})$ for various values of a and b. This is illustrated later, on the stroke study of Example II.1.

Example III.1: Stroke study: SICH incidence
The posterior distribution of θ (probability of suffering from symptomatic intercerebral hemorrhage (SICH)) after observing the data from the first ECASS 3 interim analysis is a Beta(19, 133)-distribution. This enables one to compute the posterior probability $P(a < \theta < b \mid \mathbf{y})$, for any two values of a and b. For instance, one could compute the probability that the incidence is greater than 0.20, which is the incidence observed in the first interim analysis. The area under the curve (AUC) of the interval [0.2, 1] can be readily computed using standard software and is equal to 0.0062. Thus, we doubt that the incidence is greater than 0.20. It is also unlikely that θ is smaller than 0.088, which is the value observed in the ECASS 2 study, since $P(\theta < 0.088 \mid \mathbf{y}) = 0.072$. □

Summarizing the posterior information in probabilities $P(a < \theta < b \mid \mathbf{y})$ is useful, but more is needed. In the frequentist approach, the results of most statistical analyses consist of a parameter estimate together with its standard error or 95% confidence interval (CI). Similar reporting is also useful in a Bayesian context.

3.3 Posterior summary measures

In this section, we review the most frequently used summary measures of the posterior distribution. It goes without saying that these measures can also be computed for the prior distribution. In that case, they receive the adjective 'prior'.

3.3.1 Characterizing the location and variability of the posterior distribution

The aim is to summarize the posterior distribution by representative values of location and variability. Three measures for location of the posterior $p(\theta \mid \mathbf{y})$ are in use: (a) the posterior mode; (b) the posterior mean, and (c) the posterior median.

The *posterior mode* is defined as

$$\widehat{\theta}_M = \arg\max_\theta p(\theta \mid \mathbf{y}), \tag{3.1}$$

i.e. it is the value of θ for which $p(\theta \mid \mathbf{y})$ is maximal. The posterior mode has the following properties:

- The posterior mode only involves maximization and hence to compute $\widehat{\theta}_M$ only $L(\theta \mid \mathbf{y})p(\theta)$ is involved.
- For a flat prior distribution, i.e. $p(\theta) \propto c$, the posterior mode is equal to the MLE of the likelihood function since then $p(\theta \mid \mathbf{y}) \propto L(\theta \mid \mathbf{y})$.
- The image of the posterior mode under a monotone transformation h is in general not a posterior mode anymore. In other words, $\widehat{\psi}_M \neq h(\widehat{\theta}_M)$ for $\psi = h(\theta)$.

The second measure of location is the *posterior mean*, also referred to as *Bayesian estimate*, defined as

$$\overline{\theta} = \int \theta p(\theta \mid \mathbf{y})\, d\theta, \tag{3.2}$$

with the following properties:

- The posterior mean minimizes the squared loss, i.e. it minimizes

$$\int (\theta - \widehat{\theta})^2 p(\theta \mid \mathbf{y})\, d\theta \tag{3.3}$$

over all estimators $\widehat{\theta}$. It means that $\overline{\theta}$ is closest to all θ as measured by the quadratic loss function, $L(\theta, \phi) = (\theta - \phi)^2$ weighted by the posterior distribution.

- To calculate the posterior mean, integration is needed twice: (a) for the posterior distribution and (b) for expression (3.2).

- The image of the posterior mean under a monotone transformation h is in general not a posterior mean anymore, i.e. $\overline{\psi} \neq h(\overline{\theta})$.

The third posterior measure of location is the *posterior median* $\overline{\theta}_M$ defined by the equation

$$0.5 = \int_{\overline{\theta}_M} p(\theta \mid \mathbf{y})\, d\theta. \tag{3.4}$$

The posterior median has the following properties:

- If the quadratic loss function in expression (3.3) is replaced by $a\,|\theta - \widehat{\theta}|$ with $a > 0$, the posterior median is obtained.

- The calculation of the posterior median involves one integration and solving an integral equation.

- The image of a posterior median under a monotone transformation h is again a posterior median, i.e. $\overline{\psi}_M = h(\overline{\theta}_M)$.

- For a unimodal symmetric posterior distribution, the posterior median is equal to the posterior mean and equal to the posterior mode.

The three posterior measures may be useful to characterize what we know a posteriori about the parameter of interest. The choice between the measures depends, among other things, on computational considerations and on the shape of the posterior distribution.

The most common posterior measure of variability is the *posterior variance:*

$$\overline{\sigma}^2 = \int (\theta - \overline{\theta})^2 p(\theta \mid \mathbf{y})\, d\theta. \tag{3.5}$$

The square root $\overline{\sigma}$, the *posterior standard deviation* is a common measure to indicate the posterior uncertainty about the parameter of interest. To calculate the posterior variance (and standard deviation), three integrals need to be evaluated.

Example III.2: Stroke study: Posterior summary measures
The posterior distribution of θ (probability of suffering from SICH), based on the data from the first interim analysis in ECASS 3, i.e. 10 ($=y$) patients with SICH out of 50 ($=n$) patients and using the prior observation obtained from a pilot study is Beta($\theta \mid \overline{\alpha}, \overline{\beta}$), with $\overline{\alpha}(= \alpha_0 + y) = 19$ and $\overline{\beta}(= \beta_0 + n - y) = 133$ (see Example II.1).

The posterior mode is obtained by maximizing $(\overline{\alpha} - 1)\log(\theta) + (\overline{\beta} - 1)\log(1 - \theta)$ with respect to θ yielding $\widehat{\theta}_M = (\overline{\alpha} - 1)/(\overline{\alpha} + \overline{\beta} - 2)$. Here, $\widehat{\theta}_M$ is equal to $18/150 = 0.12$.

The posterior mean involves the integral $\frac{1}{B(\overline{\alpha},\overline{\beta})}\int_0^1 \theta\theta^{\overline{\alpha}-1}(1-\theta)^{\overline{\beta}-1}\mathrm{d}\theta = B(\overline{\alpha}+1,\overline{\beta})/B(\overline{\alpha},\overline{\beta}) = \overline{\alpha}/(\overline{\alpha}+\overline{\beta})$. For the stroke example $\overline{\theta} = 19/152 = 0.125$.

To compute the posterior median, $0.5 = \frac{1}{B(\overline{\alpha},\overline{\beta})}\int_{\overline{\theta}_M}^1 \theta^{\overline{\alpha}-1}(1-\theta)^{\overline{\beta}-1}\mathrm{d}\theta$ needs to be solved for θ. With the R function *qbeta*, we obtained 0.122 as posterior median for the stroke example.

The variance of the Beta($\overline{\alpha}, \overline{\beta}$)-distribution is equal to $\overline{\alpha}\overline{\beta}/\left[(\overline{\alpha}+\overline{\beta})^2(\overline{\alpha}+\overline{\beta}+1)\right]$. For $\overline{\alpha} = 19$ and $\overline{\beta} = 133$, the posterior standard deviation is, therefore, equal to $\overline{\sigma} = 0.0267$.

If no pilot study had been executed prior to the first interim analysis, then no hard facts would have been available on the binomial parameter θ and one might prefer to express ignorance. With the uniform prior on [0, 1] as NI prior, the posterior mode is equal to $y/n = 0.20$. The posterior mean is $(y+1)/(n+2) = 0.211$ and the posterior median 0.208. Note that when the posterior mode is chosen as the summary measure for θ the result from a classical frequentist analysis is reproduced since in that case the posterior measure is equal to the MLE. □

Example III.3: Dietary study: Posterior summary measures

In Chapter 2, we have seen that the posterior distribution for the mean parameter is normal when a normal prior is combined with a normal likelihood. In this case, $\widehat{\mu}_M \equiv \overline{\mu} \equiv \overline{\mu}_M$. For the Inter-regional Belgian Bank Employee Nutrition Study (IBBENS)-prior combined with the IBBENS-2 data, the posterior mean for cholesterol-intake is $\overline{\mu} = 327.2$ mg/day. The posterior variance is also readily obtained as it is the variance of the normal distribution. For the IBBENS-2, we obtained $\overline{\sigma}^2 = 22.99$ and hence $\overline{\sigma} = 4.79$. □

3.3.2 Posterior interval estimation

From the posterior distribution, one can determine the range (most often the interval) of parameter values θ that are a posteriori most plausible with probability $(1-\alpha)$, with α usually taken equal to 0.05. Such an interval is called a *95% credible (or credibility) interval*, abbreviated as 95% CI. Formally, $[a, b]$ is a $100(1-\alpha)\%$ credible interval for θ if $P(a \leq \theta \leq b \mid \mathbf{y}) = 1 - \alpha$. Denoting the posterior cumulative distribution function (cdf) as $F(\theta)$, the $100(1-\alpha)$ credible interval $[a, b]$ satisfies

$$P(a \leq \theta \leq b \mid \mathbf{y}) = 1 - \alpha = F(b) - F(a). \tag{3.6}$$

Expression (3.6) does not define uniquely a credible interval. Two special cases of a credible interval are most popular: (a) the equal tail CI and (b) the highest (posterior) density interval.

The $100(1-\alpha)\%$ *equal tail* credible interval $[a, b]$ satisfies the following two properties: $P(\theta \leq a \mid \mathbf{y}) \equiv F(a) = \alpha/2$ and $P(\theta \geq b \mid \mathbf{y}) \equiv 1 - F(b) = \alpha/2$. In the equal tail CI, some values of θ have a lower value of $p(\theta \mid \mathbf{y})$ than some values outside that interval. Therefore, a second CI has been defined.

The $100(1-\alpha)\%$ *highest posterior density (HPD)* interval $[a, b]$ is a $100(1-\alpha)\%$ credible interval with

$$\text{for all } \theta_1 \in [a, b] \text{ and for all } \theta_2 \notin [a, b] \;:\; p(\theta_1 \mid \mathbf{y}) \geq p(\theta_2 \mid \mathbf{y}). \tag{3.7}$$

Thus, the HPD interval contains the values of θ that are a posteriori most plausible, i.e. $p(\theta \mid \mathbf{y})$ is higher for all θs inside the HPD interval than for values outside the interval. Graphically, the HPD interval is constructed by determining the intersection of a horizontal line with the posterior density. The x-coordinates of the two intersection points define the HPD interval. The HPD interval obtains the correct size by adjusting the height of the horizontal line until the AUC is equal to $(1-\alpha)$. This is the basis for determining the HPD interval numerically (see Exercise 3.8). It is clear that the HPD interval is a kind of interval of evidence but now determined on the posterior distribution rather than on the likelihood. Note that the HPD interval explicitly needs a density, while the equal tail interval only needs the cdf. The following properties are useful:

- The $100(1-\alpha)\%$ HPD interval is the shortest interval such that $P(a \le \theta \le b \mid \mathbf{y}) = 1-\alpha$; see Press (2003, p. 211) for a proof.
- Some speak of the highest density interval, e.g. in the software *FirstBayes*, when referring to the HPD interval computed either for the prior or the posterior distribution.
- The image of an equal tail CI under a monotone transformation h is again an equal tail CI, but this property does not hold in general for an HPD interval; see Example III.5 and Exercise 3.9 for an illustration.
- For a unimodal symmetric posterior distribution, the equal tail credible interval equals the corresponding HPD interval.
- For common cdfs (beta, gamma, etc.) software (e.g. in R) is available to readily compute the equal tail CI. However, to determine the HPD interval numerical optimization is required. For an illustration of the numerical procedure, we refer to Example III.5.

A 95% credible interval has a natural interpretation not shared by the classical CI in frequentist statistics. In fact, a 95% credible interval contains the 95% most plausible parameter values a posteriori, while the 95% CI does or does not contain the true value for a particular data set $\mathbf{y}$. In the frequentist paradigm, the adjective 95% gets its meaning only in the long run. Having said this, in practice the classical CI is often interpreted in a Bayesian manner, especially by clinicians. Historically, the credible and CI were developed in about the same period. Already in 1812 Laplace derived that the large sample credible interval and CI for the binomial parameter coincide (Hald 2007).

We now illustrate Bayesian interval estimation using the examples introduced in Chapter 2.

Example III.4: Dietary study: Interval estimation of dietary intake

The posterior distribution of the mean cholesterol intake is given by $N(\overline{\mu}, \overline{\sigma}^2)$, with $\overline{\mu}$ and $\overline{\sigma}$ defined by expression (2.13). An obvious choice for a 95% CI is

$$[\overline{\mu} - 1.96\,\overline{\sigma}, \overline{\mu} + 1.96\,\overline{\sigma}]. \tag{3.8}$$

The 95% CI defined in expression (3.8) is both an equal tail CI as well as a HPD interval because the normal distribution is symmetric. On the basis of the IBBENS prior distribution, expression (3.8) yields for the IBBENS-2 a 95% CI for μ equal to [317.8, 336.6] mg/day.

For a normal prior with mean 328 and variance 10 000, the 95% CI for μ becomes [285.6, 351.0] mg/day. On the other hand, the classical 95% CI $[\overline{y} - 1.96\ \text{SD}, \overline{y} + 1.96\ \text{SD}]$ is here

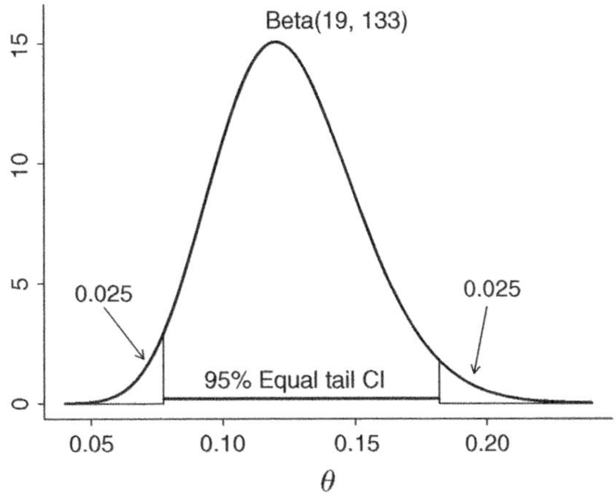

Figure 3.1 Stroke study: 95% equal tail credible interval.

equal to [284.9, 351.1] mg/day. Hence, the CI is practically equal to the credible interval and they will become virtually indistinguishable when the prior variance would be increased further. However, we must realize that the interpretation of the two intervals is drastically different. □

Example III.5: Stroke study: Interval estimation of probability of SICH

The 95% equal tail CI for θ (probability of suffering from SICH due to recombinant tissue plasminogen activator (rt-PA)) is calculated from the Beta(19, 133)-distribution. This can be readily done using the R function *qbeta* and yields here a 95% equal tail CI equal to [0.077, 0.18]; see Figure 3.1 for a graphical presentation.

For the 95% HPD interval, a numerical optimization algorithm is needed. In fact, the 95% HPD interval is the interval $[a, a+h]$, such that $F(a+h) - F(a) = 0.95$ and $f(a+h) = f(a)$, with f the posterior density and F the posterior cdf. The R function *optimize* yields both a and h. The result [0.075, 0.18] is shown in Figure 3.2. It is shown that the θ-values inside the 95% HPD interval have a higher posterior likelihood than those outside that interval.

The HPD interval is not invariant to (monotone) transformations. As an illustration, suppose interest lies in $\log(\theta)$. The 95% HPD interval of $\log(\theta) \equiv \psi$ is not equal to $[\log(a), \log(b)]$ when $[a, b]$ is the 95% HPD interval of θ. This is graphically depicted in Figure 3.2. In other words, the 95% most plausible values of ψ a posteriori do not correspond to the 95% most plausible values of θ. This is due to the introduction of the Jacobian when the posterior of ψ is determined from the posterior of θ (see Section 2.26). □

3.4 Predictive distributions

Let $p(y \mid \theta)$ be the distribution of y and an i.i.d. sample $\boldsymbol{y} \equiv \{y_1, \ldots, y_n\}$ be available. Suppose we wish to predict future observations $\widetilde{y}$ or sets of observations $\widetilde{\boldsymbol{y}}$. More formally, we wish to know the distribution of $\widetilde{y}$ that belongs to the same population as the observed sample, i.e. $\widetilde{y} \sim p(y \mid \theta)$ and assume that it is independent of $\boldsymbol{y}$, given θ. The distribution of $\widetilde{y}$ is called

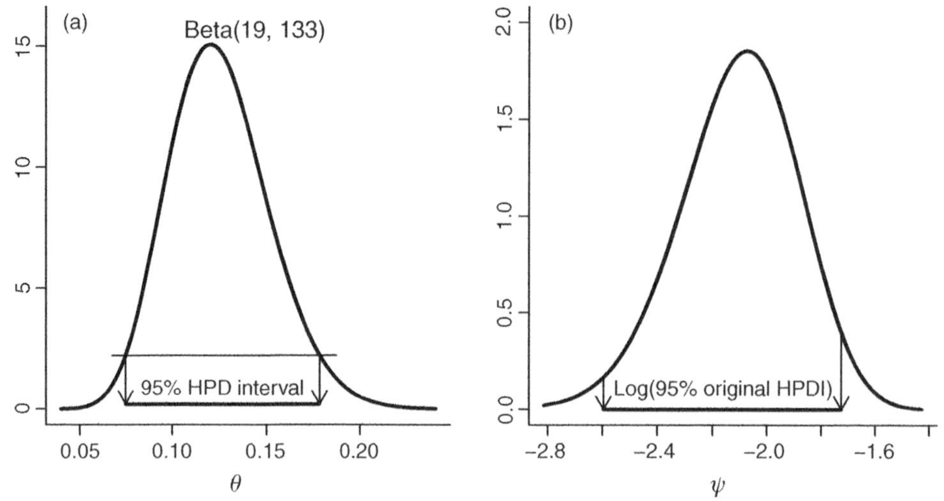

Figure 3.2 Stroke study: (a) 95% HPD interval of θ, and (b) log(95% HPD interval of θ) on ψ scale.

a *predictive distribution*. Since the true value of θ is not known, the aim is to predict the distribution of $\widetilde{y}$, given $\mathbf{y}$ and taking into account the uncertainty about θ.

Prediction is an important issue in all application areas but especially in medicine, since we hope that our models (most often regression models) are able to deliver an accurate prognosis of the patient's status. In addition, comparing predicted to observed responses is the default approach to model checking. In this section, we introduce the Bayesian approach of deriving the predictive distribution. In Chapter 4, the ideas are further developed on multiparameter models, and in Chapter 10, the usefulness of the predictive distribution in a MCMC setting will be shown.

It is illustrative to contrast the Bayesian approach to prediction with the frequentist approach. This will be done for three classical cases: (a) Gaussian, (b) binomial, and (c) Poisson.

3.4.1 The frequentist approach to prediction

On the basis of an estimate of θ, say the MLE $\widehat{\theta}$, the predictive distribution of a new observation $\widetilde{y}$ is taken as $p(\widetilde{y} \mid \widehat{\theta})$. From that distribution one can determine the mean, variance, etc., all characterizing the behavior of $\widetilde{y}$. The behavior of $\widetilde{y}$ can also be represented by a $100(1-\alpha)\%$-*predictive interval* (*PI*), which is an interval that contains $100(1-\alpha)\%$ of the future observations. A more popular term is $100(1-\alpha)\%$-*tolerance interval*, extensively treated in Krishnamoorthy and Mathew (2009). In frequentist statistics, one rarely looks at the whole predictive distribution but rather focuses on the predicted mean and the 95% PI. This is in contrast to the Bayesian approach.

The above approach is naive since it does not take into account the sampling variability of $\widehat{\theta}$. Thus, the 95% PI based on $p(\widetilde{y} \mid \widehat{\theta})$ will be too short. A more realistic approach allows for the sampling distribution of $\widehat{\theta}$. But, apart from the normal case, it is complicated to derive the predictive distribution that takes the sampling distribution of $\widehat{\theta}$ into account.

3.4.2 The Bayesian approach to prediction

Prediction of future observations in a Bayesian context takes the parameter uncertainty directly into account. The predictive distribution dates back to Laplace when he was establishing the probability of a future series of events in the binomial case.

We first give an intuitive derivation of the predictive distribution, then a more formal argument follows. The posterior distribution $p(\theta \mid \mathbf{y})$ weights the evidence of each θ after having observed $\mathbf{y}$. When all mass of $p(\theta \mid \mathbf{y})$ is concentrated at the posterior mode $\widehat{\theta}_M$, then the distribution of $\widetilde{y}$ is in fact $p(\widetilde{y} \mid \widehat{\theta}_M)$. In the case that the posterior mass is concentrated on a finite number of values of θ, say $\theta^1, \ldots, \theta^K$, then a reasonable approach is to take a weighted sum of the possible distributions for the predictive distribution, i.e. to take $\sum_{k=1}^{K} p(\widetilde{y} \mid \theta^k)p(\theta^k \mid \mathbf{y})$ as an estimate for the distribution of $\widetilde{y}$. In the continuous case, summation is replaced by integration. Therefore, the distribution of $\widetilde{y}$ is, given the observed data $\mathbf{y}$, equal to

$$p(\widetilde{y} \mid \mathbf{y}) = \int p(\widetilde{y} \mid \theta)p(\theta \mid \mathbf{y})\, \mathrm{d}\theta \tag{3.9}$$

and is called the *posterior predictive distribution*. The notation '$p(\widetilde{y} \mid \mathbf{y})$' reflects that the unknown parameter θ has been integrated out. Indeed, once the uncertainty regarding θ has been taken into account the resulting expression does not depend on θ anymore. Note that the PPD expresses what we know about the distribution of the (future) ys.

Expression (3.9) can be derived formally using elementary integration rules. To see this, write $p(\widetilde{y} \mid \mathbf{y})$ as a marginal density of the density of the future observation given a particular value of the parameter and then integrate out the parameter according to its posterior, given the data, i.e.

$$p(\widetilde{y} \mid \mathbf{y}) = \int p(\widetilde{y}, \theta \mid \mathbf{y})\, \mathrm{d}\theta = \int p(\widetilde{y} \mid \theta, \mathbf{y})p(\theta \mid \mathbf{y})\, \mathrm{d}\theta. \tag{3.10}$$

Expression (3.10) leads to (3.9) by using a property that often holds in practice and is called *hierarchical independence*, i.e.

$$p(\widetilde{y} \mid \theta, \mathbf{y}) = p(\widetilde{y} \mid \theta). \tag{3.11}$$

Hierarchical independence implies that, given the true parameter of the model, the past data cannot teach us anything about the distribution of the future data. In other words, it is assumed that the future data are independent of the past data, given θ.

Similarly, as for parameters, one could define a credible interval for future observations $\widetilde{y}$. More specifically, an interval $[a, b]$ is a $100(1-\alpha)\%$-*posterior predictive interval* (*PPI*) when $P(a \leq \widetilde{y} \leq b \mid \mathbf{y}) = 1 - \alpha$, but a more popular term for this is a *Bayesian tolerance interval*. Two special cases of a PPI are worth mentioning: (a) equal tail PPI and (b) highest PPI; both are defined in a similar way as for a parameter. For a discrete PPD, we need to replace the PPI by a *posterior predictive set* (*PPS*).

Finally, suppose that the data come to us in a sequential manner. At the start no data are available, only prior information. Given only prior information, we replace $p(\theta \mid \mathbf{y})$ by $p(\theta)$ in expression (3.10). This yields the *prior predictive distribution* $p(\widetilde{y}) = \int p(\widetilde{y} \mid \theta)\, p(\theta)\, \mathrm{d}\theta$. Clearly, the prior predictive distribution is the averaged likelihood for observation $\widetilde{y}$ and it is the denominator in expression (2.4) in Bayes theorem. Since the averaged likelihood involves integration, $p(\widetilde{y})$ is also called the *integrated or marginal likelihood*.

3.4.3 Applications

We illustrate prediction for three special cases: (a) the Gaussian distribution, still assuming that σ^2 is known, (b) the binomial distribution, and (c) the Poisson distribution. In the first two examples, we start with the frequentist approach to prediction and show that, apart from the normal case, taking into account the sampling variability of the parameter is not trivial.

3.4.3.1 The Gaussian case

Diagnostic screening tests aim to distinguish healthy from diseased individuals based on a medical/laboratory test often measured on the blood or urine. Most medical tests yield continuous measurements. To have an idea which values of the medical test are indicative for the disease, we need to know the natural variability of that measurement for a 'healthy' population. For this purpose, one uses a 95% reference interval that contains 95% of the central measurements of the values measured in 'healthy' individuals. This interval can indicate whether a future individual is diseased or not. The 95% reference interval is often referred to as the *(95%) normal range*. The adjective 'normal' does not refer to the Gaussian distribution but rather to the belief that 'normal' individuals have been included in the sample. In the case that the lab tests are not normally distributed, often a transformation to normality can be found.

Example III.6: Serum alkaline phosphatase study: 95% reference interval
After having conducted a retrospective study predicting the incidence of common bile duct stones in patients with gallstone disease, Topal *et al.* (2003) measured serum alkaline phosphatase (*alp*) on a prospective set of 250 'healthy' patients.

(a) The frequentist approach
Figure 3.3 shows the histogram of the 250 *alp* measurements. It was found that $y_i = 100/\sqrt{alp_i}$ $(i = 1, \ldots, 250)$ has approximately a Gaussian distribution. For a known Gaussian distribution, $\mathrm{N}(\mu, \sigma^2)$, the 95% reference interval for future observations on the transformed scale, i.e. $\widetilde{y}$, is given by $[\mu - 1.96\,\sigma,\ \mu + 1.96\,\sigma]$. The naive approach in determining the 95% reference interval is to replace μ by $\overline{y}$ and σ by s in the previous expression. Since $\overline{y} = 7.11$ and $s = 1.4$, the 95% reference interval on the *alp* scale is [104.45, 508.95]. However, this interval ignores the sampling variability with which μ is estimated. Note that we assumed in the above calculations that $\sigma = 1.4$.

A more realistic approach acknowledges the sampling distribution of $\overline{y}$. This can be done relatively easy for the Gaussian distribution because $(\widetilde{y} - \overline{y})/\sqrt{\sigma^2(1 + 1/n)}$ is a pivotal statistic (random variable that does not depend on parameters). Namely, $\widetilde{y} - \overline{y} \sim \mathrm{N}[0, \sigma^2(1 + 1/n)]$. Hence, a 95% reference interval that takes into account the estimation of μ is

$$[\overline{y} - 1.96\,\sigma\sqrt{1 + 1/n},\ \overline{y} + 1.96\,\sigma\sqrt{1 + 1/n}].$$

This approach yields on the y scale a 95% reference range equal to $[4.43, 9.79]$. Back-transformed to the *alp* scale, this gives [104.33, 510.18] as 95% reference interval; see Figure 3.3 for the graphical representation of the interval.

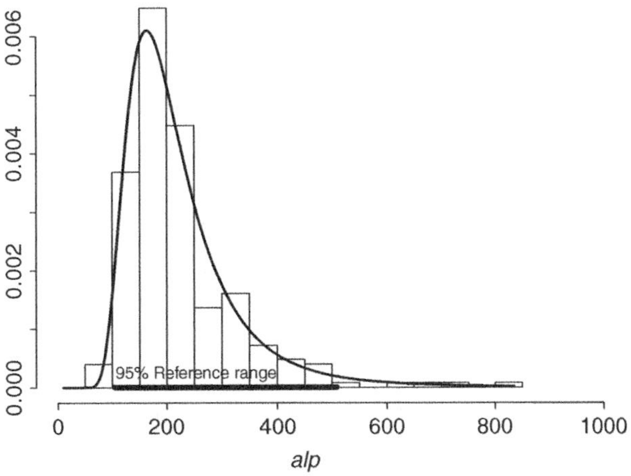

Figure 3.3 Serum alkaline phosphatase study: histogram of serum alkaline phosphatase (*alp*) measurements overlaid with fitted distribution assuming normality of $100/\sqrt{alp}$ and together with 95% reference interval.

(b) The Bayesian approach

We work again with the transformed *alp* measurements (y scale), which are assumed to have a normal distribution $\mathrm{N}(\mu, \sigma^2)$. For a normal prior for μ, expression (2.13) shows that the posterior must be normal too. By a technique similar to that used to derive the normal posterior, we can show that the PPD is again normal, i.e.

$$\widetilde{y} \mid \boldsymbol{y} \sim \mathrm{N}(\overline{\mu}, \sigma^2 + \overline{\sigma}^2). \tag{3.12}$$

In a similar way, the prior predictive distribution is equal to $\mathrm{N}(\mu_0, \sigma^2 + \sigma_0^2)$.

The PPD leads to a 95% PPI

$$[\overline{\mu} - 1.96\sqrt{\sigma^2 + \overline{\sigma}^2}, \overline{\mu} + 1.96\sqrt{\sigma^2 + \overline{\sigma}^2}], \tag{3.13}$$

which is automatically also an equal tail PPI and a highest PPI. When the prior variance σ_0^2 is large, $\overline{\mu} \approx \overline{y}$ and $\overline{\sigma}^2 \approx \sigma^2/n$ and expression (3.12) becomes approximately $\widetilde{y} \mid \boldsymbol{y} \sim \mathrm{N}\left[\overline{y}, \sigma^2(1 + 1/n)\right]$. Consequently, the 95% Bayesian reference interval becomes numerically equal to the frequentist 95% reference interval in the case of no prior information, but of course its interpretation is different. □

Bayesian tolerance intervals were first derived by Aitchison (1964, 1966) for the univariate normal distribution. However, they seem to be rarely used in medical practice. There are essentially only a few contributions, with the most important published in 1975 (Krause *et al.* 1975). In addition, the recent book Krishnamoorthy and Mathew (2009) devotes only 16 pages to the topic of Bayesian tolerance intervals.

3.4.3.2 The binomial case

Prior to setting up a new randomized controlled clinical trial (RCT) it is customary to reflect on a variety of scenarios. For instance, a lot of thinking goes into choosing the inclusion and exclusion criteria of the new RCT. Therefore, The choice of the most promising scenarios might involve predictive calculations. For example, prior to the ECASS 3 study, one might be interested in obtaining an idea of the number of rt-PA treated patients who will suffer from SICH. More specifically, one might be interested in predicting the number of rt-PA patients in the first interim analysis if the same type of patients would be recruited as in the ECASS 2 study.

Example III.7: Stroke study: Predicting SICH incidence in interim analysis

(a) The frequentist approach

The MLE of θ (incidence of suffering from SICH) is equal to $8/100 = 0.08$ for the (fictive) ECASS 2 study. In the naive approach, we assume that the binomial distribution Bin(50, 0.08) represents the predictive distribution of $\widetilde{y}$ well, which is the number of patients with SICH in a future sample of size 50. Because of the discrete nature of the binomial distribution, one cannot take an exact 95% predictive set. The set $\{0, 1, \ldots, 7\}$ contains 94% of the future counts, assuming $\theta = 0.8$. So we should be somewhat worried about the observed (fictive) result of 10 SICH patients out of 50. However, this approach is too simplistic since it does not take into account the sampling variability of $\widehat{\theta}$.

The incorporation of the sampling variability of $\widehat{\theta}$ is a very old problem already formulated in 1920 by Karl Pearson. The problem boils down to: Suppose that, given θ, y and $\widetilde{y}$ are independently distributed according to Bin(n, θ) and Bin(m, θ), respectively, what is then the conditional distribution of $\widetilde{y}$ given y? This is more difficult to solve for the binomial than for a Gaussian distribution, since there is no pivotal statistic now. Pawitan (2001, pp. 430–433) suggested to take the profile likelihood of $\widetilde{y}$, i.e. $L(\widetilde{y}) = \max_\theta L(\theta, \widetilde{y})$ with $L(\theta, \widetilde{y})$ the joint likelihood of the future observation and the parameter based on the observed $\mathbf{y}$. The result gives a distribution for $\widetilde{y}$ very similar to the Bayesian solution described below. For large n, another possibility is to use the asymptotic normal distribution of $\widehat{\theta}$ resulting in a predictive normal distribution (if $\widehat{\theta}$ in the expression of the standard error is assumed fixed), which allows to take into account the sampling variability of $\widehat{\theta}$ in an approximate manner.

(b) The Bayesian approach

The posterior distribution of θ based on the ECASS 2 study data is the Beta(9, 93)-distribution. The PPD describes the distribution of $\widetilde{y}$, the number of future rt-PA treated patients with SICH, in a sample of size $m = 50$. Expression (3.9) with $p(\widetilde{y} \mid \theta)$ replaced by a Bin(m, θ)-distribution and $p(\theta \mid \mathbf{y})$ by a Beta(α, β)-distribution leads to

$$
\begin{aligned}
p(\widetilde{y} \mid \mathbf{y}) &= \int_0^1 \binom{m}{\widetilde{y}} \theta^{\widetilde{y}} (1-\theta)^{(m-\widetilde{y})} \frac{\theta^{\alpha-1}(1-\theta)^{\beta-1}}{B(\alpha, \beta)} \, d\theta \\
&= \binom{m}{\widetilde{y}} \frac{B(\widetilde{y}+\alpha, m-\widetilde{y}+\beta)}{B(\alpha, \beta)},
\end{aligned}
\tag{3.14}
$$

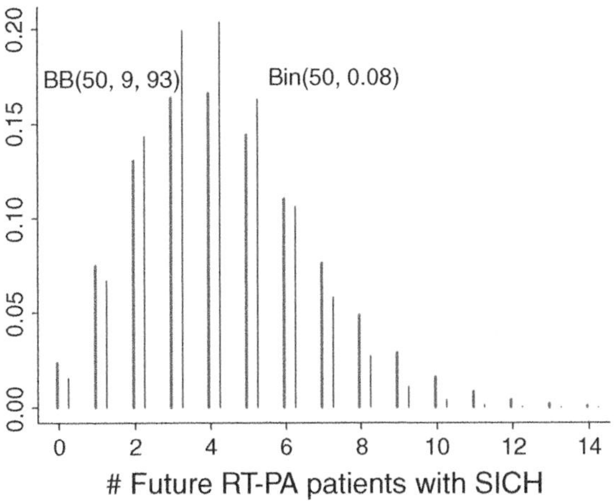

Figure 3.4 Stroke study: binomial (Bin(50, 0.08)) and beta-binomial distribution (BB(50, 9, 93)) predicting the number of patients with SICH in the first interim analysis based on 50 rt-PA treated patients.

which defines a *beta-binomial distribution* $BB(m, \alpha, \beta)$, first derived by Laplace. In Figure 3.4, we show that $BB(m, \overline{\alpha}, \overline{\beta})$ exhibits more variability than the binomial distribution $Bin(m, \widehat{\theta})$, obtained by the frequentist approach. The 94.4% highest PPS is $\{0, 1, \ldots, 9\}$, rendering the observed result of 10 SICH patients out of 50 somewhat less extreme.

Note that the prior predictive distribution is also a beta-binomial distribution, now with parameters α_0 and β_0. □

3.4.3.3 The Poisson case

Only the Bayesian approach is considered now. Recall that a Poisson likelihood combined with a gamma prior distribution results in a gamma posterior. Thus, the PPD is a weighted combination of Poisson distributions, Poisson$(\widetilde{y} \mid \theta)$, with a Gamma$(\alpha,\beta)$-distribution as weight function for θ. Applying expression (3.9) using $p(\widetilde{y} \mid \theta) \equiv \theta^{\widetilde{y}} e^{-\theta}/\widetilde{y}!$ and $p(\theta \mid \mathbf{y}) \equiv \frac{\beta^{\alpha}}{\Gamma(\alpha)}\theta^{\alpha-1}e^{-\beta\theta}$ yields

$$p(\widetilde{y} \mid \mathbf{y}) \equiv \frac{\Gamma(\alpha + \widetilde{y})}{\Gamma(\alpha)\, \widetilde{y}!} \left(\frac{\beta}{\beta + 1}\right)^{\alpha} \left(\frac{1}{\beta + 1}\right)^{\widetilde{y}}, \tag{3.15}$$

which is the expression of a *negative binomial distribution*, denoted as NB(α,β). This distribution is also referred to as the *Pólya distribution*. It generalizes the negative binomial distribution given by expression (1.3) where $\widetilde{y}$ plays the role of s and by allowing k in expression (1.3) to be a real value α. The probability of success in a single experiment is $\theta = 1/(\beta + 1)$.

Example III.8: Caries study: PPD for caries experience

With a Gamma(9761, 4352) posterior distribution, the PPD of a single future count $\widetilde{y}$ is given by a NB(9761, 4352) distribution. In Figure 3.5, we have shown the PPD together with the observed distribution of the dmft-index. Comparing the two distributions, clearly reveals the inadequacy of the Poisson assumption for the dmft-index. □

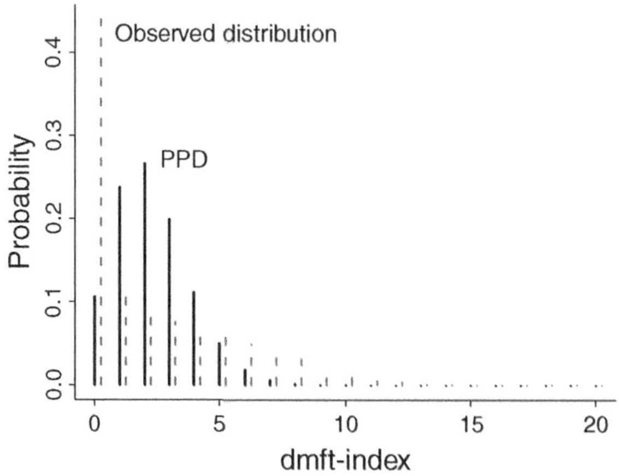

Figure 3.5 Caries study: observed distribution of dmft-index and PPD-distribution (NB(9761, 4352)-distribution).

In Chapter 10, we will see that the comparison of the observed distribution to the PPD is the basis of a goodness-of-fit test.

3.5 Exchangeability

The classical assumption of the independence in a sample $\{y_1, y_2, \ldots, y_n\}$ is expressed as $p(y_1, y_2, \ldots, y_n \mid \theta) = \prod_{i=1}^{n} p(y_i \mid \theta)$. Thus, independence is defined conditional on θ and in the case of independence, the joint distribution of $y_1, y_2, \ldots, y_n$ splits up in a product of marginal distributions.

In practice, we never know θ, but we give it a prior distribution $p(\theta)$ in a Bayesian context. Averaging over the uncertainty of θ, the marginal or unconditional joint distribution of $\{y_1, y_2, \ldots, y_n\}$ is obtained, given by

$$\begin{aligned} p(y_1, y_2, \ldots, y_n) &= \int_\theta p(y_1, y_2, \ldots, y_n \mid \theta) p(\theta)\, d\theta, \\ &= \int_\theta \prod_{i=1}^{n} p(y_i \mid \theta) p(\theta)\, d\theta. \end{aligned} \tag{3.16}$$

From expression (3.16),

$$p(y_1, y_2, \ldots, y_n) = p(y_{\pi(1)}, y_{\pi(2)}, \ldots, y_{\pi(n)}), \tag{3.17}$$

with π any permutation on the set $\{1, 2, \ldots, n\}$. When the above equality holds, we say that the random variables $y_1, y_2, \ldots, y_n$ are *exchangeable*. Note that exchangeability does not imply independence since the product and the integral in expression (3.16) cannot be exchanged, but independence of random variables having the same marginal distribution does imply exchangeability. In a frequentist context, the same phenomenon occurs when θ is not constant but has a random distribution. An example of exchangeable but not independent random variables is the random vector $(y_1, y_2, \ldots, y_n)$, which has a multivariate normal distribution with mean zero and all correlations equal to ρ (for the covariance matrix to be positive definite $\rho \geq -1/(n-1)$). In the case where $(y_1, y_2, \ldots, y_n) \sim \mathrm{N}_n(\boldsymbol{\mu}, \Sigma)$, with $\boldsymbol{\mu}$ and/or Σ general, then $y_1, y_2, \ldots, y_n$ are not exchangeable; see Exercise 3.16 for a more basic probabilistic example that differentiates exchangeability from independence.

Exchangeability is about 'similar' random variables. However, it is an assumption that must follow from the context of the experiment. Suppose that subjects are enrolled in a clinical trial in a sequential manner. Then the (measurements on the) subjects could be judged exchangeable if there is no reason to believe that there is a time trend in the type of patients that are recruited. In practice, one may come up with many reasons why subjects may be considered nonexchangeable, e.g. patients differ in gender, age, etc. Deciding that subjects are 'similar' depends on the goal of the research. For some research questions, say, gender might be irrelevant but in others men and women may correspond to different distributions. Further, exchangeability clearly also depends on how much the researcher is acquainted with the problem. He will be less inclined to declare subjects exchangeable when he is quite knowledgeable in the topic; see Draper *et al.* (1993) for an elaboration on this topic.

Exchangeability is central in prediction. In Section 3.4, we looked for the distribution of a future observation $\widetilde{y}$ assumed to be similar to the past data $\{y_1, \ldots, y_n\}$. We assumed conditional independence of $\widetilde{y}$ and $\{y_1, \ldots, y_n\}$, but since we did not know the true value of θ, the unconditional distribution of $\{\widetilde{y}, y_1, \ldots, y_n\}$ is exchangeable but dependent. It is this kind of dependence that allowed us to learn from the past data. If we knew θ then past data would not help us in determining the distribution of $\widetilde{y}$ because of the conditional independence.

Exchangeability was introduced by de Finetti (1937, 1974) in a more formal manner. de Finetti called condition expression (3.17) *nite exchangeability*. He defined *in nite exchangeability* for an infinite sequence of random variables when each finite subsequence is exchangeable. From above, we know that when we start with conditional independent random variables, then unconditionally we obtain exchangeable random variables satisfying expression (3.16). de Finetti also proved the reverse result stated in Theorem 3.5.1.

Theorem 3.5.1 *(Representation theorem) Let $y_1, y_2, \ldots, y_n$ be an in nitely exchangeable sequence of binary random variables with (unconditional) cdf F and density p, then there exists a cdf Q such that*

$$p(y_1, y_2, \ldots, y_n) = \int_0^1 \prod_{i=1}^{n} \theta^{y_i}(1-\theta)^{1-y_i}\, \mathrm{d}Q(\theta),$$

where $Q(\theta) = \lim_{n\to\infty} F(s_n/n \leq \theta)$, with $s_n = y_1 + y_2 + \ldots + y_n$ and $\theta = \lim_{n\to\infty} s_n/n$.

For a proof, see Bernardo and Smith (1994, pp. 172–173). The above theorem says that when $y_1, \ldots, y_n$ are exchangeable, this is functionally equivalent to assuming that y_i are independent Bern(θ) (Bernoulli) random variables with θ, given a prior distribution $Q(\theta)$. It also implies that $p(y_1, \ldots, y_n \mid \theta) = \prod_{i=1}^{n} \theta^{y_i}(1-\theta)^{1-y_i}$. In other words, exchangeability is equivalent to a simple hierarchical model where the hyperparameter is given a prior (see Chapter 9). Therefore, the representation theorem is seen by Bayesians as a plea for the Bayesian approach in the sense that a natural assumption for random variables immediately leads to a Bayesian model combining a likelihood with a prior.

The representation theorem has been extended to multinomial and real-valued random variables. The theorems and their proofs can be found in Chapter 4 in Bernardo and Smith (1994).

If considered nonexchangeable, subjects can still be exchangeable within a subpopulation. For instance, women and men might be separately exchangeable. Another example is that the effect of an antihypertensive treatment might depend on age and gender, but within each age-gender class patients are considered to be exchangeable. When this happens, then one speaks of *partial* or *conditional exchangeability*. In general, we speak of conditional exchangeability given a covariate x when two subjects i and j with response y_i and y_j are exchangeable conditional on x_i and x_j, respectively. In Chapter 9, we further extend exchangeability to hierarchical models.

3.6 A normal approximation to the posterior

In all of the above examples, the choice of the prior allowed the posterior as well as the posterior summary measures to be derived analytically. If other priors had been chosen, then numerical procedures would have been needed to compute the necessary posterior information. This can become quickly involved especially for the multiparameter case because the integral in the denominator of Bayes theorem needs to be computed numerically.

But even when the problem is numerically complex, the Bayesian analysis can be simplified considerably by using a normal approximation to the posterior distribution for a large sample size.

3.6.1 A Bayesian analysis based on a normal approximation to the likelihood

The ML estimator of θ has (approximately) a normal distribution for a large sample size. Since the MLE is asymptotically sufficient, the likelihood of the data is well approximated by the normal likelihood of the MLE. When this normal likelihood is combined with a normal prior, we know that a normal posterior is the result.

In Example III.9, we analyze the case-control study introduced in Example I.3 in a similar way as in Ashby *et al.* (1993). In the spirit of the previous examples, we start with the frequentist approach.

Example III.9: Kaldor's *et al.* (1990) case-control study: Posterior inference using normal approximations

In Table 1.1, the results of the case-control study conducted by Kaldor *et al.* (1990) were summarized. As in Ashby *et al.* (1993), the matched nature of the case-control design is neglected here.

Let the probability of having the risk factor in the controls (cases) be θ_0 (θ_1), the total number of controls (cases) be n_0 (n_1) and the number of controls (cases) with the risk factor (chemotherapy) be r_0 (r_1). The odds ratio expresses the association between the risk factor and the disease, but for estimation purposes one usually works with the logarithm of the odds ratio, i.e.

$$\gamma = \log\left[\frac{\theta_1/(1-\theta_1)}{\theta_0/(1-\theta_0)}\right].$$

The MLE of γ is equal to

$$\hat{\gamma} = \log\left[\frac{r_1\ (n_0 - r_0)}{r_0\ (n_1 - r_1)}\right],$$

and has approximately a normal distribution with mean γ and variance

$$\text{var}(\hat{\gamma}) \equiv \sigma_{\hat{\gamma}}^2 = \frac{1}{r_0} + \frac{1}{n_0 - r_0} + \frac{1}{r_1} + \frac{1}{n_1 - r_1}.$$

For small numbers of events, augmenting the cell frequencies with 0.5 improves the normal approximation (Agresti 1990).

(a) The frequentist approach

Based on $\hat{\gamma} \sim \text{N}(\gamma, \sigma_{\hat{\gamma}}^2)$ an asymptotic significance test and a 95% CI for γ can be obtained. This also gives a significance test and a CI for the odds ratio e^{γ}. Here, we obtained $\hat{\gamma} = 2.08$ and $e^{\hat{\gamma}} = 8.0$ ($P < 0.0001$). The 95% CI for γ is [1.43, 2.72] and for the odds ratio e^{γ}, it is [4.2, 15.2].

(b) The Bayesian approach

The Bayesian approach does not need a large sample for inference about γ, but the large sample result for $\hat{\gamma}$ simplifies the computations. From Section 2.7, we know that a normal prior $\text{N}(\gamma_0, \sigma_0^2)$ for γ, combined with the normal likelihood of $\hat{\gamma}$, yields a normal posterior $\text{N}(\overline{\gamma}, \overline{\sigma}^2)$ for γ with

$$\overline{\gamma} = \left(\frac{\hat{\gamma}}{\sigma_{\hat{\gamma}}^2} + \frac{\gamma_0}{\sigma_0^2}\right) \times \overline{\sigma}^2,$$

$$\overline{\sigma}^2 = \left(\frac{1}{\sigma_{\hat{\gamma}}^2} + \frac{1}{\sigma_0^2}\right)^{-1}.$$

Figure 3.6(a) shows the prior and posterior distributions of the odds ratio when a weakly informative normal prior ($\gamma_0 = \log(5)$, $\sigma_0 = 10\ 000$) is chosen. The posterior summary measures were computed on the log odds ratio scale (assuming a normal distribution) and then back-transformed to the odds ratio scale. We found that the posterior summary measures for γ are (practically) identical to those obtained from the above frequentist analysis, i.e. the posterior mode/median/mean are equal to the MLE of γ and the 95% CI is equal to the corresponding CI. On the odds ratio scale, the posterior median is equal to the MLE of e^{γ}, but it differs from the posterior mean and mode. Figure 3.6(a) illustrates that the transformed 95% HPD interval on the log odds ratio scale is not an HPD interval anymore on the odds ratio scale (see Section 3.3.2).

The clinicians (Ashby *et al.* 1993) assumed that chemotherapy always induces an increase in risk. Their 'best guess' (median) for e^{γ} was 5 with a 95% prior credible interval on the

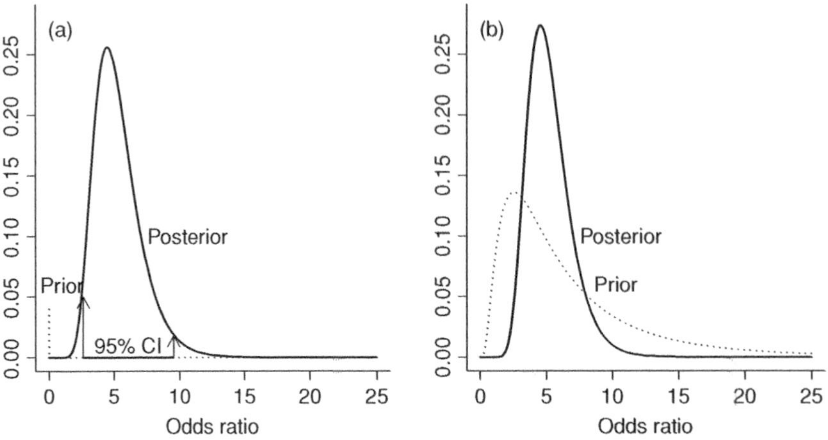

Figure 3.6 Kaldor's *et al.* case-control study: (a) posterior of e^{γ} based on N(1.6, 10 000^2)-prior for γ and (b) posterior of e^{γ} based on N(1.6, 0.82^2)-prior for γ.

odds ratio scale of [1, 25]. Thus, loosely speaking, the experts put their 95% belief in a N(1.6, 0.82^2)-distribution for γ. The prior and posterior distribution for the odds ratio are shown in Figure 3.6(b). The posterior median for γ is now slightly lower, i.e. 7.5, reflecting the belief of the experts that the risk is somewhat lower than that obtained in the data. The 95% CI is [4.1, 13.6]. □

3.6.2 Asymptotic properties of the posterior distribution

The use of a normal posterior is justified even when the likelihood is combined with a non-normal prior as long as the sample size is large. In 1785, Laplace proved the CLT for the inverse probability, i.e. the asymptotic normality of the posterior distribution even before the classical CLT was proven! However, because the posterior is up to a constant equal to the likelihood for a uniform prior, the two results are intimately related to each other. In modern terms, we could say that the asymptotic normality of the posterior follows from the classical result in likelihood theory together with the fact that 'the likelihood dominates the prior for a large sample size'. Only, ... historically seen the reverse happened (Hald 2007). We state below the one-parameter version of *Bayesian CLT;* the multiparameter version is a straightforward generalization.

Theorem 3.6.1 *Let* $\mathbf{y}$ *represent a sample of* n *i.i.d. observations with joint density* $p(\mathbf{y} \mid \theta) \equiv L(\theta \mid \mathbf{y})$ *and* $p(\theta) > 0$ *a prior density for* θ. *Under suitable regularity conditions, the posterior distribution* $p(\theta \mid \mathbf{y})$ *converges to the normal distribution* $N(\widehat{\theta}, \sigma^2_{\widehat{\theta}})$ *when* $n \to \infty$, *where* $\widehat{\theta}$ *is the MLE of* θ *and* $\sigma^2_{\widehat{\theta}} = -\left(\frac{d^2 \log L(\theta|\mathbf{y})}{d\theta^2}\Big|_{\theta=\widehat{\theta}}\right)^{-1}$.

In practice, the regularity conditions are usually met. For instance, one of the regularity conditions is that the support of the prior distribution should contain the MLE. Gelman *et al.* (2004, pp. 108–111) elaborate on the impact of the regularity conditions.

In the frequentist paradigm, the CLT occupies a central role. Indeed, many frequentist tests have intractable small sample properties so that one needs to rely on asymptotic theory. This is not the case in the Bayesian approach since exact Bayesian inference can always be obtained simply by exploring the posterior distribution. Theorem 3.6.1 only states that this exploration becomes simple when n is large.

Example III.10: Caries study: Posterior of mean (dmft-index)
To show that the normal approximation to the posterior can be reasonable even for small sample sizes, we have selected the dmft-index of the first 10 children. Combining the Gamma(3, 1) prior with the likelihood ($\sum_i^{10} y_i = 26$) gives a Gamma(29, 11) distribution as posterior for θ. The normal approximation (computed as in Theorem 3.6.1) to the posterior has, in general, mean $\widehat{\theta} = \overline{y}$ and variance $\sigma^2_{\widehat{\theta}} = \overline{y}/n$. Here, we obtained $\overline{y} = 2.6$ and $\sigma^2_{\widehat{\theta}} = 0.26$, respectively. The normal approximation is remarkably good (not shown). When applied to the whole study, the normal approximation simply overlays the true posterior distribution (not shown). □

Theorem 3.6.1 also implies that for a large sample the choice of the prior is not important and that the posterior is completely determined by the likelihood. However, for a small to moderate sample size one cannot rely, in general, on this result and the posterior needs to be computed explicitly. Analytical determination of the posterior can only be done for a well-chosen prior, called the conjugate prior. For another choice of the prior, numerical procedures are necessary. In Section 3.7, we review some (relative simple) numerical techniques to compute the posterior for any chosen prior.

3.7 Numerical techniques to determine the posterior

In this section, we briefly review two classes of numerical techniques to determine the posterior distribution and posterior summary measures. The first class consists of numerical integration techniques to approximate the involved integrals directly. In the second approach, integration is replaced by sampling from the posterior. We show that sampling has a lot to offer. Moreover, from Chapter 6 on all posterior computations will be done via sampling although using more complicated algorithms. In this chapter we focus on one-dimensional problems, but in principle all techniques can be applied to multidimensional problems in which case the one-dimensional parameter θ becomes a vector $\boldsymbol{\theta}$.

3.7.1 Numerical integration

There are numerous techniques to approximate integrals in a numerical manner. We start with some elementary techniques and end with methods that are nowadays intensively used in random effects models (see also Verbeke and Molenberghs 2000). Let $f(\theta)$ denote a smooth function that we wish to integrate over a possibly infinite interval $[a, b]$ (when infinite, the closed interval is replaced by a half-open or open interval). This function represents $t(\theta)p(\theta \mid \mathbf{y})$ or $t(\theta)p(\mathbf{y} \mid \theta)p(\theta)$ with $t(\theta)$ a summary measure. When $t(\theta) = 1$ in the latter expression, we are interested in determining the denominator of Bayes theorem.

The simplest integration techniques involve a grid $a \equiv \theta_0 < \theta_1 < \ldots < \theta_{(M+1)} \equiv b$ of equidistant grid points with $\delta = \theta_m - \theta_{m-1}$, $(m = 1, \ldots, M + 1)$. A first and simple technique to compute the integral $\int_{\theta_{m-1}}^{\theta_m} f(\theta)\,\mathrm{d}\theta$ is to approximate the function $f(\theta)$ in the mth subinterval by the rectangle with base δ and height $f(\theta_m^*)$, $\theta_m^* = (\theta_{m-1} + \theta_m)/2$ the midpoint of the mth subinterval. This yields $\int_{\theta_{m-1}}^{\theta_m} f(\theta)\,\mathrm{d}\theta \approx \delta\, f(\theta_m^*)$. The total integral is then obtained by summing up all contributions from the subintervals, and hence,

$$\int_a^b f(\theta)\,\mathrm{d}\theta \approx \sum_{m=1}^{M+1} w_m f(\theta_m^*), \tag{3.18}$$

with $w_m = \delta$. For the *trapezoidal rule,* the piecewise constant function is replaced by a piecewise linear function passing through $f(\theta_{m-1})$ and $f(\theta_m)$. The well-known *Simpson's rule* is a further improvement involving piecewise quadratic polynomials. When $f(\theta)$ is well approximated by the product of a normal density and a polynomial in θ, efficient computation of the integral can be done via *Gaussian quadrature*. Naylor and Smith (1982) introduced this technique for Bayesian computations. For the Gaussian quadrature rule, the M grid points, called *quadrature points* (on the infinite interval $(-\infty, \infty)$), are not equidistant anymore, but are the roots of Mth-degree *Hermite polynomials*. The weight w_m is a function of the $(M-1)$th-degree Hermite polynomial evaluated in the mth grid point. An important property of the Gaussian quadrature rule is that the integral is exactly reproduced when the above polynomial is of degree $2M-1$. There are two versions of Gaussian quadrature: *nonadaptive* and *adaptive*. In the nonadaptive case, the grid points do not depend on $f(\theta)$. For the adaptive case, the grid points are centered around the posterior mode, and the curvature of the posterior density at the posterior mode determines the distance between the grid points. Typically, adaptive Gaussian quadrature needs less quadrature points than the nonadaptive version to achieve the same accuracy. This is shown by Lesaffre and Spiessens (2001) in the context of a logistic random-effects model.

For one quadrature point, the adaptive Gaussian quadrature reduces to the *Laplace method for integration* or *Laplace approximation*, an important technique both for numerical approximations and for analytical derivations. To perform the Laplace approximation, the integral in expression (3.18) is rewritten as

$$\int \exp[h(\theta)]\,\mathrm{d}\theta,$$

with $h(\theta) = \log f(\theta)$ a smooth, bounded unimodal function. Often $h(\theta)$ is the log-likelihood function of a sample or the product of the log-likelihood with the prior (see Section 11.4.2 for more details). The method is based on a Taylor series expansion of $h(\theta)$ and yields the approximation

$$\int \exp[h(\theta)]\,\mathrm{d}\theta \approx (2\pi)^{d/2}|A|^{1/2}\exp[h(\widehat{\theta}_M)], \tag{3.19}$$

with $\widehat{\theta}_M$ the value at which $h(\cdot)$ (or $f(\cdot)$) attains its maximum and A is minus the inverse Hessian of h evaluated at $\widehat{\theta}_M$. For alternative formulations of the Laplace method and improvements; see Tanner (1996, pp. 44–47).

In Example III.11, we replace the gamma prior for the dmft-index in the Signal-Tandmobiel® study by a lognormal prior. This increases the complexity of the problem drastically in the sense that the posterior distribution cannot be computed analytically anymore, i.e. the denominator $\int p(\mathbf{y} \mid \theta)p(\theta)\,\mathrm{d}\theta$ of Bayes theorem needs to be evaluated numerically as well as all posterior summary measures.

Example III.11: Caries study: Posterior distribution for a lognormal prior
When the gamma prior in Example III.10 is replaced by a lognormal prior, the posterior becomes a complicated function and the posterior summary measures are not easily calculated. More specifically, suppose the prior distribution for θ is

$$p(\theta) = \frac{1}{\theta\sigma_0\sqrt{2\pi}} e^{-\left(\frac{\log(\theta)-\mu_0}{2\sigma_0}\right)^2}, \ (\theta > 0), \tag{3.20}$$

then the posterior distribution is proportional to

$$\theta^{\sum_{i=1}^{n} y_i - 1} e^{-n\theta - \left(\frac{\log(\theta)-\mu_0}{2\sigma_0}\right)^2}, \ (\theta > 0). \tag{3.21}$$

The above posterior distribution is quite complicated. Press (2003, p. 175) showed that the AUC is not known and that no analytical expressions are available for the posterior. Thus, we need to rely on a numerical technique.

With parameters for the lognormal prior equal to $\mu_0 = \log(2)$ and $\sigma_0 = 0.5$, we have taken the midpoint approach with 10 000 equidistant grid points to produce the solid line in Figure 3.9. Clearly, this is a grossly inefficient method, but it served our purposes here. From the grid approach, we also obtained the posterior summary measures, with 2.52 for the posterior mean and 0.22 for the posterior variance. □

3.7.2 Sampling from the posterior

The Monte Carlo method has taken a prominent position in Bayesian statistics nowadays which will become clear in the following chapters. In the Monte Carlo approach, the expected value is approximated by the sample mean of simulated random variables.

We first treat *Monte Carlo integration* which replaces the integral by the average obtained from sampled values. To sample from standard posterior distributions such as a normal, beta, and gamma, standard software (S+, R, SAS®, STATA®, etc.) can be employed. For other posteriors general purpose samplers might be needed, as seen below. We review general sampling techniques: the *inverse cumulative distribution function (ICDF) method*, the *acceptance–rejection algorithm* and *importance sampling*. But the great potential value of sampling will only become clear in Chapter 6.

3.7.2.1 Monte Carlo integration

The posterior summary $\int t(\theta)\, p(\theta \mid \mathbf{y})\, d\theta$ is the expected value $E\left[t(\theta) \mid \mathbf{y}\right]$ of $t(\theta)$ under the distribution $p(\theta \mid \mathbf{y})$. Assume that we have K independently sampled values $\{\theta^1, \ldots, \theta^K\}$ from $p(\theta \mid \mathbf{y})$, then for K large

$$\int t(\theta)\, p(\theta \mid \mathbf{y})\, d\theta \approx \bar{t}_K = \frac{1}{K}\sum_{k=1}^{K} t(\theta^k),$$

according to the classical Strong Law of Large Numbers. The unbiased estimator $\bar{t}_K$ is called the *Monte Carlo estimator* of $E\left[t(\theta) \mid \mathbf{y}\right]$. For a discrete θ, the integral is replaced by a sum. The consequence of the above result is that probabilities, summations and integrals can be approximated by the Monte Carlo method. Furthermore, the empirical distribution function and, hence, the histogram of the sampled values converges to the true posterior as $K \to \infty$.

According to the classical CLT, the precision with which the true summary measure is estimated may be quantified by the (classical) 95% CI

$$[\bar{t}_K - 1.96\, s_t/\sqrt{K}, \bar{t}_K + 1.96\, s_t/\sqrt{K}], \tag{3.22}$$

with s_t the standard deviation of the sampled $t(\theta^k)$-values and $s_t/\sqrt{K}$ is called the *Monte Carlo error*. The first standard deviation is an approximation of the posterior standard deviation, while the second is an estimate of the uncertainty of the estimated posterior mean. This interval in expression (3.22) indicates the precision with which the sampling procedure has determined the true posterior mean.

The 95% equal tail CI can be approximated with a sample from the posterior distribution simply by determining the 2.5% and 97.5% quantile from that sample. For the HPD interval based on sampled values, we used the procedure by Tanner (1993, pp. 70–71) that is implemented in the R program to analyze Example III.12 ('chapter 3 sample from beta distribution stroke study. R').

Example III.12: Stroke study: Sampling from the posterior distribution
The posterior information on the probability of developing SICH for rt-PA treated patients was summarized by a Beta(19, 133)-distribution (see Example II.1). Using the R function *rbeta* we sampled 5 000 values of θ from the Beta(19, 133)-distribution. From Figure 3.7(a), it is clear that the sample histogram and the true posterior are quite close.

Determining the posterior of $\log(\theta)$ involves the calculation of the Jacobian, which is easy here. But it is even quicker to add one extra line to the R program to get the sample histogram of $\log(\theta)$. Figure 3.7(b) illustrates that the sample histogram of $\log(\theta)$ is close to the true posterior. In addition, the sample summary measures of the beta distribution were practically identical to the true summary measures.

The R function *quantile* was used to construct an 95% equal tail CI for θ, equal to [0.0780, 0.181], which is virtually identical to that obtained from the true posterior. The 95% equal tail CI for $\log(\theta)$ is $[-2.55, -1.71]$. On the basis of the algorithm suggested by Tanner (1993,

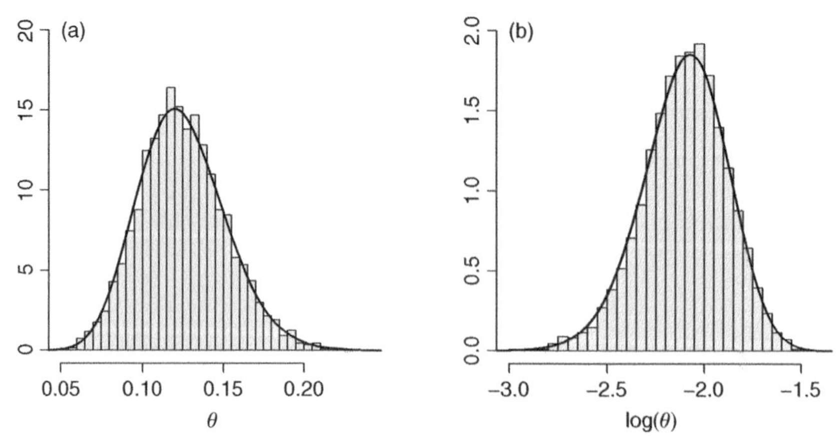

Figure 3.7 Stroke study: true and sampled posterior for (a) θ and (b) $\log(\theta)$.

pp. 70–71), an approximate 95% HPD interval for θ is [0.0747, 0.178]. Chen and Shao (1999) suggested an improvement over the approach of Tanner (1993), which is implemented in the CODA (and BOA) R packages. □

The advantage of sampling is that with a little extra effort the summary measures can be obtained for $\log(\theta)$, $\theta/(1-\theta)$, etc. More (and sometimes laborious) work is needed to derive the analytical expression of the corresponding posterior distributions.

3.7.2.2 General purpose sampling algorithms

For many classical distributions specific algorithms have been suggested to generate random variables (see Ripley 1987; Gentle 1998). If no specific sampling technique exists for the (posterior) distribution at hand, then either a dedicated procedure needs to be developed or one could make use of a general purpose algorithm. The first general approach is the ICDF method. Then we introduce two sampling techniques which make use of an instrumental distribution.

(a) The inverse ICDF method

If the random variable x has a continuous cdf F, then $F(x) \sim \mathrm{U}(0, 1)$. Provided that F^{-1} exists, this suggests sampling from F by $x = F^{-1}(u)$ with $u \sim \mathrm{U}(0, 1)$. This is denoted as the ICDF method. There is also a discrete version of the ICDF method which is used by WinBUGS for discrete parameters.

(b) The accept–reject algorithm

In the accept–reject (AR) algorithm, one first samples from an instrumental distribution $q(\theta)$. In a second step some of the sampled values are rejected to end up with a sample from $p(\theta \mid \mathbf{y})$. The distribution $q(\theta)$ is called the *proposal distribution* and $p(\theta \mid \mathbf{y})$, in this context, the *target distribution*. The AR algorithm assumes that $p(\theta \mid \mathbf{y})$ is bounded above by a multiple of $q(\theta)$, i.e. there is a constant $A < \infty$ such that $p(\theta \mid \mathbf{y}) < A\,q(\theta)$ for all θ. Therefore, the distribution q is also called the *envelope distribution*, A is the *envelope constant* and Aq is the *envelope function*. Sampling proceeds in two stages. In the first stage, $\widetilde{\theta}$ is drawn from $q(\theta)$ independently from u that is drawn from U(0, 1). In the second stage, $\widetilde{\theta}$ is either accepted or rejected according to the following rule:

- *Accept*: When $u \le p(\widetilde{\theta} \mid \mathbf{y})/A\,q(\widetilde{\theta})$, $\widetilde{\theta}$ is accepted as a value from $p(\theta \mid \mathbf{y})$.
- *Reject*: When $u > p(\widetilde{\theta} \mid \mathbf{y})/A\,q(\widetilde{\theta})$, $\widetilde{\theta}$ is rejected.

We now show that, when this sampling algorithm is repeated J times, a sample $\{\theta^1, \ldots, \theta^K\}$ $(K \le J)$ from $p(\theta \mid \mathbf{y})$ is generated. To prove this, we need to show that

$$P(\widetilde{\theta} \le \theta \mid \widetilde{\theta} \text{ is accepted}) = P(\widetilde{\theta} \le \theta \mid \mathbf{y}).$$

This follows from

$$\begin{aligned} P(\widetilde{\theta} \le \theta \;\&\; \widetilde{\theta} \text{ is accepted}) &= \int_{-\infty}^{\theta} P(\widetilde{\theta} \mid \widetilde{\theta} \text{ is accepted})\, P(\widetilde{\theta} \text{ is accepted})\, \mathrm{d}\widetilde{\theta} \\ &= \int_{-\infty}^{\theta} q(\widetilde{\theta})\, \frac{p(\widetilde{\theta} \mid \mathbf{y})}{A\,q(\widetilde{\theta})}\, \mathrm{d}\widetilde{\theta} = \int_{-\infty}^{\theta} \frac{p(\widetilde{\theta} \mid \mathbf{y})}{A}\, \mathrm{d}\widetilde{\theta} \end{aligned}$$

and

$$P(\widetilde{\theta} \text{ is accepted}) = \int_{-\infty}^{\infty} \frac{p(\widetilde{\theta} \mid \mathbf{y})}{A} \, \mathrm{d}\widetilde{\theta} = \frac{1}{A}.$$

From the proof, it follows that the AR algorithm produces a sample from the posterior distribution even if only the product $p(\theta)p(\mathbf{y} \mid \theta)$ is available. This property is extremely useful (see Chapter 6). However, the ARS algorithm will only work properly when the support of $p(\theta \mid \mathbf{y})$ is contained in the support of $q(\theta)$, i.e. $q(\theta) > 0$ if $p(\theta \mid \mathbf{y}) > 0$. The efficiency of the AR algorithm can be measured by the probability that $\widetilde{\theta}$ is accepted, which is equal to $1/A$. Hence, the closer A is to 1 the greater the efficiency of the AR algorithm.

In general, it is not easy to find the envelope function. For log-concave distributions, Gilks and Wild (1992) proposed the *Adaptive Rejection Sampling (ARS) algorithm* that aims to produce a piecewise linear envelope function in an adaptive manner. In addition, a piecewise lower bound to $p(\theta \mid \mathbf{y})$, called the *squeezing function*, is constructed in an adaptive manner. There are two popular versions of the ARS algorithm: the *tangent method of ARS* and the *derivative-free method of ARS*. We focus here on the first approach. A sketch of the sampling algorithm goes as follows. Take the logarithm of the posterior, $\log p(\theta \mid \mathbf{y}) \equiv lp(\theta)$. It is assumed that $lp(\theta)$ is concave and differentiable on its support. Suppose that $lp(\theta)$ has been evaluated already at θ_1, θ_2 and θ_3. The envelope function is determined on these three points by connecting the tangent lines as in Figure 3.8(a). The squeezing function is determined by connecting the points $(\theta_1, lp(\theta_1))$, $(\theta_2, lp(\theta_2))$, $(\theta_3, lp(\theta_3))$, and the boundary points as in Figure 3.8(a). Exponentiate and standardize the envelope and squeezing function such that they have AUC=1 and call these distributions q_U and q_L, respectively. Then draw $\widetilde{\theta}$ from q_U and an independent u from U(0, 1). If $u \leq q_L(\widetilde{\theta})$, then accept $\widetilde{\theta}$. Thus, the squeezing function can prevent the evaluation of the log-likelihood. If $u > q_L(\widetilde{\theta})$, then evaluate $lp(\widetilde{\theta})$ and accept $\widetilde{\theta}$ as done above in the general AR algorithm. If $\widetilde{\theta}$ is rejected in the first step, add $\widetilde{\theta}$ to the grid, compute the tangent at that point and update q_U and q_L. The advantage of this AR algorithm is that much less evaluations of $lp(\theta)$ are needed than the sampled values. Namely, for K sampled points around $K^{1/3}$ evaluations are needed. Usually between 5 and 10 grid points are necessary to have a good performance of the ARS algorithm. In Figure 3.8(b), we can see the envelope and squeezing function of the derivative-free ARS, which differs from the tangent ARS in the envelope function. The derivative-free ARS is implemented in WinBUGS

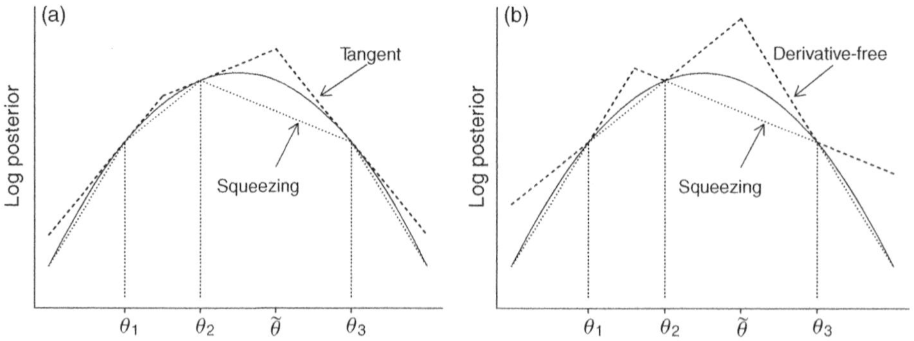

Figure 3.8 ARS algorithm: envelope and squeezing function for (a) tangent ARS, and (b) derivative-free ARS.

and is also the most important sampler of the package. Finally, the ARS approach has also been combined with a Metropolis sampling algorithm (see Chapter 6) to accommodate for nonlog-concave posteriors (Gilks and Tan 1995). This is called the *ARMS algorithm* and is implemented in some of the Bayesian SAS® procedures.

Importance sampling and the SIR algorithm

Now we introduce two sampling procedures which involve sampling from an instrumental distribution in combination with a corrective action, but without needing to find an envelope function. For both methods, the posterior distribution needs to be known only up to a constant.

Importance sampling was first suggested by Kahn and Marshall (1953) as a variance reduction technique to estimate a summary measure of a distribution by sampling from an instrumental distribution $q(\theta)$. Kloek and van Dijk (1978) introduced the approach into the Bayesian world. Let the support of $p(\theta \mid \mathbf{y})$ be part of the support of $q(\theta)$. Suppose that we are interested in the posterior mean of the summary measure $t(\theta)$, then

$$\begin{aligned} E\left[t(\theta) \mid \mathbf{y}\right] &= \int t(\theta) p(\theta \mid \mathbf{y})\,\mathrm{d}\theta \\ &= \int \left[t(\theta)\frac{p(\theta \mid \mathbf{y})}{q(\theta)}\right] q(\theta)\,\mathrm{d}\theta \\ &= E_q\left[t(\theta)\frac{p(\theta \mid \mathbf{y})}{q(\theta)}\right]. \end{aligned} \tag{3.23}$$

Expression (3.23) provides the following sampling algorithm. Given a sample $\theta^1, \ldots, \theta^K$ from $q(\theta)$, then an estimator of $E\left[t(\theta) \mid \mathbf{y}\right]$ is

$$\frac{1}{K}\sum_{k=1}^{K}\frac{t(\theta^k)p(\theta^k \mid \mathbf{y})}{q(\theta^k)} \equiv \frac{1}{K}\sum_{k=1}^{K} t(\theta^k)w(\theta^k), \tag{3.24}$$

with *importance weights* $w(\theta^k) = p(\theta^k \mid \mathbf{y})/q(\theta^k)$. The expected value of the importance weights is equal to 1. But this is not the case for the realized weights. Therefore, an alternative expression based on normalized weights is given by

$$\widehat{t}_{I,K} = \frac{\sum_{k=1}^{K} t(\theta^k)w(\theta^k)}{\sum_{k=1}^{K} w(\theta^k)}. \tag{3.25}$$

The normalized estimator $\widehat{t}_{I,K}$ has the advantage that it can be used when the posterior distribution is only known up to a constant. $\widehat{t}_{I,K}$ converges to $E\left[t(\theta) \mid \mathbf{y}\right]$ for basically any $q(\theta)$ (Geweke 1989), but it can suffer from wild fluctuations unless

$$\int \left[t^2(\theta)\frac{p^2(\theta \mid \mathbf{y})}{q^2(\theta)}\right] q(\theta)\,\mathrm{d}\theta = \int \left[t^2(\theta)\frac{p^2(\theta \mid \mathbf{y})}{q(\theta)}\right] \mathrm{d}\theta < \infty.$$

This condition implies that the tails of $q(\theta)$ must be heavier than those of $p(\theta \mid \mathbf{y})$.

Clearly, importance sampling does not generate a sample from the posterior distribution but makes use of the sample generated from $q(\theta)$ to estimate summary measures from the true posterior. In contrast, the *weighted sampling–resampling method*, called *SIR (sampling/importance resampling)* by Rubin (1988), does produce samples from the posterior. The algorithm goes as follows:

- *First stage*: Draw J (with J large) independent values $\boldsymbol{\theta} \equiv \{\theta^1, \ldots, \theta^J\}$ from $q(\theta)$ and calculate weights $w_j \equiv w(\theta^j)(j = 1, \ldots, J)$ as above. This defines a multinomial distribution, with categories defined by the sampled θ values and associated probabilities $\boldsymbol{w} = (w_1, w_2, \ldots, w_J)$.
- *Second stage*: Take a sample of size $K \ll J$, from $\boldsymbol{\vartheta}$ i.e. draw from Mult(K, $\boldsymbol{w}$).

Here is a sketch of the proof that the SIR algorithm ultimately samples from the correct posterior. The probability that the sampled $\widetilde{\theta}$ is less or equal to θ is equal to

$$\sum_{j:\,\theta^j \leq \theta}^{J} w_j = \frac{\sum_j [p(\theta^j \mid \boldsymbol{y})/q(\theta^j)]\, \mathrm{I}(\theta^j \leq \theta)}{\sum_j p(\theta^j \mid \boldsymbol{y})/q(\theta^j)}.$$

With $J \to \infty$ and a suitable limit operation whereby the θ-range is split up into small intervals with probability $q(\widetilde{\theta})\, d\widetilde{\theta}$ the summation is turned into the integral

$$\frac{\int_{-\infty}^{\theta} [p(\widetilde{\theta} \mid \boldsymbol{y})/q(\widetilde{\theta})] \mathrm{I}(\widetilde{\theta} \leq \theta) q(\widetilde{\theta})\, d\widetilde{\theta}}{\int_{-\infty}^{\infty} [p(\widetilde{\theta} \mid \boldsymbol{y})/q(\widetilde{\theta})] q(\widetilde{\theta})\, d\widetilde{\theta}} = \frac{\int_{-\infty}^{\theta} p(\widetilde{\theta} \mid \boldsymbol{y})\, d\widetilde{\theta}}{\int_{-\infty}^{\infty} p(\widetilde{\theta} \mid \boldsymbol{y})\, d\widetilde{\theta}} = P(\widetilde{\theta} \leq \theta \mid \boldsymbol{y}).$$

Both importance sampling approaches have shown to be quite useful in a great variety of applications. For instance, in Chapter 10 we illustrate their usefulness for detecting influential observations. We now illustrate the AR algorithm and the SIR algorithm on the posterior of Example III.11.

Example III.13: Caries study: Sampling from the posterior distribution with a lognormal prior

Despite the analytical difficulties when replacing the gamma distribution by the lognormal distribution, the posterior and the summary measures can easily be determined via sampling.

(a) The accept–reject algorithm

The lognormal distribution is maximized when $\log(\theta)$ is equal to μ_0. This yields

$$Aq(\theta) = \theta^{\sum_{i=1}^{n} y_i - 1} e^{-n\theta}.$$

The expression of $Aq(\theta)$ is up to a constant that of a Gamma($\sum_i y_i$, n)-distribution. Thus, to apply the AR algorithm we simply generated a random variable $\widetilde{\theta}$ from a gamma distribution, an independent uniform random variable u and evaluated whether $u \leq p(\widetilde{\theta} \mid \boldsymbol{y})/A\, q(\widetilde{\theta})$.

With the same settings as in Example III.11 we applied the AR algorithm and produced the histogram in Figure 3.9. We sampled 1 000 θ-values, but the algorithm rejected 160 values. Thus the histogram is based on 840-sampled θ-values. From the sampled values, we easily derived posterior summary measures. We obtained 2.50 (2.48) as posterior mean (median), 0.21 as posterior variance and [1.66, 3.44] as 95% equal tail CI.

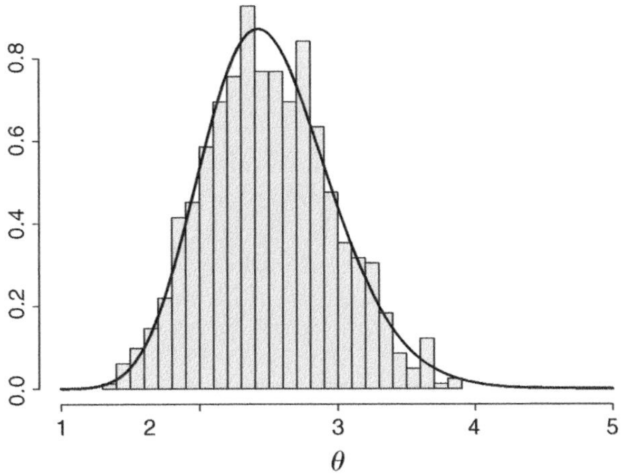

Figure 3.9 Caries study (subsample of the first 10 children): histogram of random sample obtained by AR algorithm (size = 840) from the posterior distribution (lognormal prior-Poisson likelihood). Solid curve is a numerical approximation to the posterior distribution.

(b) The weighted sampling–resampling algorithm

Another approach is to sample first from a posterior gamma distribution obtained by combining a gamma prior with the Poisson likelihood. In a second step, one (re)samples from these sampled values with appropriate weights. In this case, the instrumental distribution q is the posterior based on another prior. This approach was suggested by Smith and Gelfand (1992). However, q could differ also in the likelihood part. More specifically, if the first posterior distribution is

$$p_1(\theta \mid \mathbf{y}) = \frac{L_1(\theta \mid \mathbf{y})\, p_1(\theta)}{p_1(\mathbf{y})}$$

and the second posterior distribution is

$$p_2(\theta \mid \mathbf{y}) = \frac{L_2(\theta \mid \mathbf{y})\, p_2(\theta)}{p_2(\mathbf{y})},$$

then

$$p_2(\theta \mid \mathbf{y}) \propto \frac{L_2(\theta \mid \mathbf{y})\, p_2(\theta)}{L_1(\theta \mid \mathbf{y})\, p_1(\theta)} p_1(\theta \mid \mathbf{y}) = v(\theta) p_1(\theta \mid \mathbf{y}).$$

Here, the SIR method consists in taking first a (large) sample $\theta^1, \ldots, \theta^J$ from $p_1(\theta \mid \mathbf{y})$. In the second stage, one resamples K ($\ll J$) θ-values with weights $w_j = v(\theta^j)/\sum_{i=1}^{J} v(\theta^i)$, ($j = 1, \ldots, J$) resulting in a random sample from $p_2(\theta \mid \mathbf{y})$. First, we have taken a random sample of size $J = 10\,000$ from the Gamma(29, 11) distribution, which was obtained by combining the Gamma(3, 1) distribution as prior $p_1(\theta)$ with the Poisson likelihood. Second, we have taken a random sample from this sample of size $K = 1\,000$ with weights specified as above and $p_2(\theta)$ the above-defined lognormal prior distribution. The histogram of the sampled values is not shown, because it is quite similar to the one in

Figure 3.9. The posterior summary measures are also quite similar to those obtained with the AR algorithm. □

The second application in the previous example is attractive for a Bayesian sensitivity analysis, whereby one can evaluate the effect of omitting an observation from the analysis by simply resampling with weights $w_j = L(\theta^j \mid \mathbf{y}_{(i)})/L(\theta^j \mid \mathbf{y})$ whereby $L(\theta \mid \mathbf{y}_{(i)})$ is the likelihood based on all observations except the ith. If the effect of the ith observation on the summary measure $t(\theta)$ is of interest, then the estimator $\widehat{t_{I,J}}$ with the above defined weights w_j can be computed for each observation $i(= 1, \ldots, n)$ in turn.

3.7.3 Choice of posterior summary measures

Nowadays virtually all Bayesian analyses are based on sampling techniques. In this chapter, we have reviewed sampling techniques that yield independent samples from a distribution, while in Chapter 6 we treat sampling techniques that produce dependent samples. However, the way the posterior summary measures are computed is to a large extent independent of the sampling technique. The posterior summary measures that are most reported in the literature are the mean, median and standard deviation. This is because these measures are easily obtained from a sampling exercise and are the standard output of WinBUGS, which is the most popular Bayesian software. The mode cannot be directly obtained from WinBUGS and is, therefore, rarely reported. However, in Chapter 9 we see that the posterior mode might also be useful, e.g. to compare the Bayesian with the frequentist output (since the MLE is equal to the posterior mode for a flat prior) for reporting the posterior variance. For interval estimation, the equal tail CI is most popular again because it is part of the standard output from WinBUGS. The HPD interval is, though, computed by the R packages CODA and BOA.

3.8 Bayesian hypothesis testing

In this section, we treat two Bayesian tools for hypothesis testing. Recall that, while in the Bayesian approach the parameter θ is a random variable, a true value of the parameter is assumed. This justifies the use of a formal hypothesis test also in a Bayesian context.

3.8.1 Inference based on credible intervals

Let the null-hypothesis be $H_0 : \theta = \theta_0$. This hypothesis can be immediately verified with the help of credible intervals. There are two popular and related ways to do this. In the first approach, one computes the 95% CI of θ. When θ_0 is not included in the interval, then this is seen as a rejection of the null-hypothesis in a Bayesian way. This approach is popular, e.g. when evaluating regression coefficients in Bayesian regression models.

Posterior evidence against the null-hypothesis can also be expressed via the *contour probability* p_B. This probability is calculated from the smallest HPD interval containing θ_0, i.e. the posterior probability that θ lies outside this interval expresses our posterior belief of how extreme the value θ_0 is in the light of the data. Formally, the contour probability p_B is defined as

$$P\left(p(\theta \mid \mathbf{y}) > p(\theta_0 \mid \mathbf{y})\right) \equiv 1 - p_B.$$

Graphically, p_B is the complement of the AUC that is entertained by the smallest HPD interval including the null-hypothesis value. If p_B is small, then the hypothesis $\theta = \theta_0$ is not well-supported a posteriori.

The contour probability was first suggested by Box and Tiao (1973, p. 125) and can be viewed as the Bayesian counterpart of the two-sided P-value in frequentist statistics. Thus, one might refer p_B to a Bayesian P-value keeping in mind that it is based on only the observed data and the prior. However, in the literature, the Bayesian P-value refers to a probability obtained from a posterior predictive check (see Chapter 10).

Example III.14: Cross-over study: Use of credible intervals in Bayesian hypothesis testing
Thirty ($= n$) patients with systolic hypertension were randomized to two antihypertensive treatments A and B. The patients were treated for 1 month and then the reduction in their systolic blood pressure was measured. After a period of no medication (washout period), patients treated with A (B) in the first period were treated with B (A) for 1 month in the second period. At the end of the treatment, $y = 21$ patients treated under A showed a greater systolic blood pressure reduction than under B. Let θ represent the probability that A is better than B in lowering systolic blood pressure. In the case that there is no period effect, one may test $H_0 : \theta = \theta_0 (= 0.5)$ with a two-sided binomial test. It was found that there were significantly more patients better off with A than with B ($P = 0.043$).

In a Bayesian context, one combines a prior (here uniform) with the binomial likelihood. Since 21 successes (A better than B) out of 30 patients were obtained, a Beta(22, 10) posterior is the result.

The 95% HPD interval for θ is given by [0.53, 0.84] excluding the value 0.5. Hence, there is evidence against the null-hypothesis. In Figure 3.10, the smallest HPD interval containing $\theta = 0.5$ is shown corresponding to $p_B = 0.0232$. Thus, also from a Bayesian viewpoint there is serious doubt on the null-hypothesis. □

When the posterior distribution is established by a sampling technique, p_B cannot be determined exactly. However, the contour probability can be approximated using a posterior

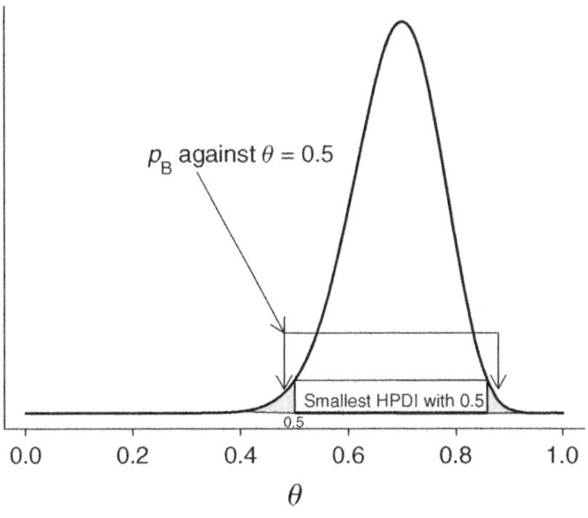

Figure 3.10 Cross-over study: contour probability for null-hypothesis $\theta = 0.5$.

sample $\{\theta^1, \ldots, \theta^K\}$ by $1 - \widehat{p}_B$, with $\widehat{p}_B$ the observed proportion of times that $p(\theta^k \mid \boldsymbol{y}) \geq p(\theta_0 \mid \boldsymbol{y})$, $(k = 1, \ldots, K)$.

3.8.2 The Bayes factor

The *Bayes factor*, one of the major contributions of Jeffreys to Bayesian statistics, measures the change from prior to posterior odds in favor of the null-hypothesis and it is the Bayesian equivalent of the likelihood ratio test.

We are now interested in the posterior probability that a particular hypothesis H is true given the observed data $\boldsymbol{y}$. This probability is denoted as $p(H \mid \boldsymbol{y})$. To compute this probability using Bayes theorem, we need the averaged likelihood under the hypothesis, i.e. $p(\boldsymbol{y} \mid H) = \int p(\boldsymbol{y} \mid \theta)\, p(\theta|H)\, d\theta$ with $p(\theta|H)$ the prior for θ under the hypothesis H. Then, under the settings of Section 3.8.1, we can calculate the posterior probability that H_0 is true, i.e.

$$p(H_0 \mid \boldsymbol{y}) = \frac{p(\boldsymbol{y} \mid H_0)\, p(H_0)}{p(\boldsymbol{y} \mid H_0)\, p(H_0) + p(\boldsymbol{y} \mid H_a)\, p(H_a)}, \tag{3.26}$$

which follows directly from Bayes theorem. The above expression shows that if $p(H_0 \mid \boldsymbol{y}) > 0.5$, the null hypothesis is given greater posterior belief and might be opted for. In that case, the null-hypothesis will be considered more plausible than the alternative hypothesis. However, such a conclusion is not accepted in a frequentist context.

Since H_a is the complement of H_0, $p(H_a) = 1 - p(H_0)$ and $p(H_a \mid \boldsymbol{y}) = 1 - p(H_0 \mid \boldsymbol{y})$, we obtain

$$\frac{p(H_0 \mid \boldsymbol{y})}{1 - p(H_0 \mid \boldsymbol{y})} = \frac{p(\boldsymbol{y} \mid H_0)}{p(\boldsymbol{y} \mid H_a)} \times \frac{p(H_0)}{1 - p(H_0)}. \tag{3.27}$$

Expression (3.27) states that the prior odds for hypothesis H_0 is transformed into a posterior odds by multiplication with $p(\boldsymbol{y} \mid H_0)/p(\boldsymbol{y} \mid H_a)$. The latter term is called the Bayes factor and is denoted as $BF(\boldsymbol{y})$. The Bayes factor is the ratio of the likelihoods under hypotheses H_0 & H_a and varies between 0 and ∞. For $BF(\boldsymbol{y})$ greater than 1 (smaller than 1), the posterior odds for H_0 is greater (smaller) than the prior odds and the posterior probability of H_0 is greater (smaller) than its prior probability. So, the Bayes factor expresses the impact of the data on the odds for H_0. Traditionally, the numerator in the Bayes factor pertains to the null-hypothesis, such that, when small, there is preference for H_a which is in the spirit of a small classical P-value. Jeffreys (1961, p. 432) classified the Bayes factor (favoring H_0 against H_a) into: 'decisive' ($BF(\boldsymbol{y}) > 100$), 'very strong' ($32 < BF(\boldsymbol{y}) \leq 100$), 'strong' ($10 < BF(\boldsymbol{y}) \leq 32$), 'substantial' ($3.2 < BF(\boldsymbol{y}) \leq 10$) and 'not worth more than a bare mention' ($1 < BF(\boldsymbol{y}) \leq 3.2$). As with the frequentist significance level of 0.05, this classification of the Bayes factor is to some extent arbitrary. To give an idea of the impact of a particular $BF(\boldsymbol{y})$, suppose that the prior probability for H_0 is equal to 0.10, then for $BF(\boldsymbol{y}) = 3.2$ the posterior probability for H_0 becomes 0.26, which represents a relatively small change. On the other hand, when $BF(\boldsymbol{y}) = 100$, this posterior probability increases to 0.92 that represents a dramatic change.

We now discuss the use of the Bayes factor on three classical hypothesis testing scenarios in Example III.15.

Example III.15: Cross-over study: Use of the Bayes factor
Consider the following three scenarios for a parameter θ:

- $H_0 : \theta = 0.5$ versus $H_a : \theta = 0.8$ (only 0.5 and 0.8 are possible),
- $H_0 : \theta \leq 0.5$ versus $H_a : \theta > 0.5$,
- $H_0 : \theta = 0.5$ versus $H_a : \theta \neq 0.5$,

where as before, H_0 and H_a represent the null- and alternative hypothesis, respectively. For each of the three scenarios, the Bayes factor will be derived.

Scenario 1: $H_0 : \theta = 0.5$ **versus** $H_a : \theta = 0.8$
In this scenario θ is discrete assuming only two possible values. Suppose that there is a priori no preference of either hypothesis so that we are prepared to give them equal prior weight: $p(H_0) = p(H_a) = 0.5$. The likelihoods under H_0 and H_a are

- $p(y = 21|H_0) = \binom{30}{21} 0.5^{21}\, 0.5^9 = 0.0133$,
- $p(y = 21|H_a) = \binom{30}{21} 0.8^{21}\, 0.2^9 = 0.0676$,

respectively. $BF(21)$ is approximately equal to 0.2 such that (according to Jeffreys) there is 'substantial' evidence to prefer $\theta = 0.8$ over $\theta = 0.5$. With equal prior probabilities, the Bayes factor is equal to the ratio of the two posterior probabilities.

In this scenario, the Bayes factor is exactly equal to the classical likelihood ratio. Unlike in frequentist statistics, though, inference is only based on the observed data.

Scenario 2: $H_0 : \theta \leq 0.5$ **versus** $H_a : \theta > 0.5$
In this scenario, θ is continuous. For the calculation of $p(H_0 \mid y)$, $p(H_a \mid y)$ and the Bayes factor, we need $p(y \mid H_0)$. This likelihood is a weighted average of values $p(y \mid \theta)$ with weights provided by the prior distribution of θ on the interval [0, 0.5]. A similar calculation results in $p(y \mid H_a)$. Suppose that investigators give equal prior probabilities to H_0 and H_a with a uniform $p(\theta \mid H_0)$ and $p(\theta \mid H_a)$. In that case, the averaged likelihoods under H_0 and H_a are

- $p(y = 21 \mid H_0) = \int_0^{0.5} \binom{30}{21} \theta^{21} (1-\theta)^9\, 2\, d\theta = 2\binom{30}{21} B(22, 10)\, 0.01472$,
- $p(y = 21 \mid H_a) = \int_{0.5}^{1} \binom{30}{21} \theta^{21} (1-\theta)^9\, 2\, d\theta = 2\binom{30}{21} B(22, 10)\, (1 - 0.01472)$,

respectively. In the above calculations, $0.01472 = \frac{1}{B(22,10)} \int_0^{0.5} \text{Beta}(\theta \mid 22, 10)\, d\theta$. For this scenario, $BF(21)$ (odds of posterior probabilities) is approximately equal to 0.015. In Jeffreys terminology, there is 'substantial' evidence to favor $\theta > 0.5$ over $\theta \leq 0.5$.

In this scenario, the Bayes factor is not equal to a classical likelihood ratio test. In fact, if different prior distributions $p(\theta \mid H_0)$ and $p(\theta \mid H_a)$ had been chosen, a different Bayes factor would have been obtained. Goodman (1999b) argues that specifying a particular prior for the parameter is part of the specification of the hypothesis and therefore should have an impact on the inference.

The third and last scenario is known as testing a 'sharp' null-hypothesis ($\theta = 0.5$) and represents the most common hypothesis test in practice.

Scenario 3: $H_0 : \theta = 0.5$ **versus** $H_a : \theta \neq 0.5$
In this scenario, we test a *sharp* or a *simple* null-hypothesis. Now it is not immediately clear how to assign prior probabilities to H_0 and H_a, since the former is a simple hypothesis, while the latter is a composite hypothesis. In fact, with a continuous prior distribution the posterior distribution for $\theta = 0.5$ is zero. To bypass this conceptual difficulty it has been suggested, but not without controversy, to assign a 'lump' prior probability to H_0, e.g. 0.5. In that case, the likelihood under H_0 and the averaged likelihood under H_a using a uniform distribution $p(\theta \mid H_a)$ (and thus also $p(\theta)$) are

- $p(y = 21 \mid H_0) = \binom{30}{21} 0.5^{21}\, 0.5^9 = 0.0133$,
- $p(y = 21 \mid H_a) = \int_0^1 \binom{30}{21}\theta^{21}\,(1-\theta)^9\, d\theta = \binom{30}{21} B(22, 10)$,

respectively, such that $BF(21)$ is about 0.41, favoring $\theta \neq 0.5$ over $\theta = 0.5$. According to Jeffreys classification, the preference is, however, 'Not worth more than a bare mention'.

Compare this result with the likelihood ratio test statistic Z equal to $\frac{0.5^{21}\,0.5^9}{(21/30)^{21}\,(9/30)^9} = 0.0847$, favoring again the alternative hypothesis but now with a P-value of 0.026, expressing a much stronger statement against the null hypothesis than obtained with the Bayes factor. □

The Bayes factor occupies a central position in Bayesian statistics and is indispensable in Bayesian model and variable selection. This will be shown in Section 10.2.1 and Chapter 11. However, the use of the Bayes factor in practice is hampered by computational difficulties. In Section 10.2.1, we elaborate on the pros and cons of using a Bayes factor.

We end this introduction to the Bayes factor with a discussion on its relationship with the P-value. In this context, we also discuss the *Jeffreys–Lindley–Bartlett's paradox.*

3.8.3 Bayesian versus frequentist hypothesis testing

3.8.3.1 *P*-value, Bayes factor, and posterior probability

The P-value expresses the evidence that the data provided against H_0 but it does not express the probability that H_0 is true (or false). Thus when the P-value is, say 0.049, the message is not that there is about 0.05 probability that H_0 is true. However, it is a common interpretation of this result and Goodman (1999a, 1999b) called this the *P-value fallacy*. Only the Bayesian approach allows such statements using the posterior probability $p(H_0 \mid \mathbf{y})$ or the Bayes factor. But, in some cases the classical P-value comes close to bringing such a message.

Casella and Berger (1987) examined above scenario 2, i.e. $H_0 : \theta \leq 0$ versus $H_a : \theta > 0$ and compared the P-value with $p(H_0 \mid \mathbf{y})$. Note that in any practical computation $p(H_0 \mid \mathbf{y})$ depends on the choice of the alternative hypothesis, the prior probabilities for the hypotheses and the sample size, so a comparison between the P-value and $p(H_0 \mid \mathbf{y})$ for each specific case would be rather complicated and confusing. Therefore, a different approach is needed. Above, we have seen that the choice of $p(\theta)$ (or $p(\theta \mid H_0)$ and $p(\theta \mid H_a)$) is involved in the hypothesis test. Hence, any sensible comparison between the P-value and $p(H_0 \mid \mathbf{y})$ must specify this prior. Instead of looking at specific choices for $p(\theta)$, Casella and Berger (1987) looked at classes of priors. They demonstrated that if $p(\theta)$ gives equal weight to both hypotheses and belongs to a reasonable class of priors (unimodal and symmetric around zero) then

$$\min p(H_0 \mid \mathbf{y}) = P(\mathbf{y}),$$

where the minimum is taken over the class of above priors and the dependence of the P-value on the data is made explicit. The practical message is that when a small P-value is obtained, it will indeed express a low evidence for H_0 in a Bayesian sense if a reasonable prior $p(\theta)$ is used.

Things are different for the simple hypothesis test (scenario 3). Goodman (1999b) defined the minimum Bayes factor $BF_{\min}(\mathbf{y})$ as the smallest Bayes factor in favor of the null-hypothesis when varying over the alternative hypotheses. In the Gaussian case, Goodman (1999b) showed that $BF_{\min}(\mathbf{y}) = \exp(-0.5z^2)$ with z is the observed test-statistic that yields $P(\mathbf{y})$. This can be easily seen in the following simple case. Assume $y \sim \mathrm{N}(\theta, \sigma^2)$ with σ^2 known and a sample of size n is available. Take $H_0 : \theta = \theta_0$ and $H_a : \theta \neq \theta_0$. Then

$$\frac{p(\bar{y} \mid \theta = \theta_0, \sigma)}{p(\bar{y} \mid \theta = \bar{y}, \sigma)} = \frac{\exp\left[-0.5\left(\frac{\bar{y}-\theta_0}{\sigma/\sqrt{n}}\right)^2\right]}{\exp\left[-0.5\left(\frac{\bar{y}-\bar{y}}{\sigma/\sqrt{n}}\right)^2\right]} = \exp(-0.5z^2).$$

In this case, $P(\mathbf{y}) = 0.05$ corresponds to $BF_{\min}(\mathbf{y}) = 0.15$ and the corresponding minimum posterior probability (under equal priors for H_0 and H_a) is 0.204. This illustrates that there is much less evidence against H_0 than what the observed P-value might suggest. Casella and Berger (1987) and Berger and Sellke (1987) generalized this result and obtained even less extreme values. This leads to the now widely accepted viewpoint (among Bayesians) that, in a simple hypothesis test, P-values exaggerate the evidence against H_0. To make their point more practically appealing, Berger and Sellke (1987) and Sellke *et al.* (2001) illustrated the evidence that is contained in the statement 'P-value is 0.049' in the context of drug research. They demonstrated that for studies with $P \approx 0.05$, at least 23% (and typically close to 50%) of the drugs will have a negligible effect. For this reason, suggestions were made to *calibrate the P-value* which simply means that P-values should be translated into Bayesian measures of evidence. Held (2010) recently proposed a graphical approach that translates the prior probability and P-value to a minimum posterior probability.

Finally, as with the classical P-value, the contour probability also suffers from an 'exaggeration' problem. In the multivariate case, the contour probability is, however, quite useful in quickly picking up important effects (Section 1.1.4). Its similarity to the P-value may also stimulate the medical researchers to accept the Bayesian approach (some will now rightfully think 'for the wrong reasons'). The same is true for the tradition of providing 95% CIs to the estimates, they also appear to be the same as classical CIs.

3.8.3.2 Jeffreys–Lindley–Bartlett's paradox

Lindley (1957) and Bartlett (1957) reported on an apparent paradox where the null hypothesis is rejected in a frequentist analysis with a small P-value while the Bayes factor favors H_0. This is called the *Lindley's paradox*, but also the *Bartlett's paradox*, the *Lindley–Bartlett's paradox* and the *Lindley–Jeffreys's paradox*. The paradox is caused by the different philosophies in hypothesis testing in both paradigms. In the frequentist context, hypothesis testing is done by comparing maximized likelihoods (likelihood ratio statistic), while in the Bayesian approach one compares averaged likelihoods. We borrow the following theoretical example given in Press (2003, pp. 222–225) to explain the paradox.

Example III.16: Illustration of Lindley's paradox
Supose we wish to test $H_0 : \theta = \theta_0$ versus $H_a : \theta \neq \theta_0$ based on an i.i.d. sample $\boldsymbol{y} = \{y_1, \ldots, y_n\}$ with $y_i \sim \mathrm{N}(\theta, \sigma^2)$ for a known σ. The large sample test statistic is given by

$$z = \frac{\overline{y} - \theta_0}{\sigma/\sqrt{n}}.$$

The P-value equals $p = P(|z| > |z_{\text{obs}}|) = 2\,[1 - \Phi(z_{\text{obs}})]$, with z_{obs} the observed z-statistic. For the calculation of the Bayes factor, assign 0.50 prior probability to H_0 and H_a and assume $p(\theta) = \mathrm{N}(\theta \mid \theta_0, \sigma^2)$. Then the marginal distribution of $\overline{y}$ under H_a is $\mathrm{N}\left[\theta_0, (1 + \frac{1}{n})\sigma^2\right]$ and the posterior probability of H_0 given the observed mean $\overline{y}$ (and test statistic z_{obs}) becomes then $p(H_0 \mid \overline{y}) = 1/\left\{1 + \frac{1}{\sqrt{1+n}} \exp\left[z_{\text{obs}}^2/2(1 + 1/n)\right]\right\}$. This allows us to compute the posterior probability $p(H_0 \mid \overline{y})$ for different observed values for the test statistic z and shows that for $z_{\text{obs}} = 1.96$ (two-sided P-value of 0.05) $p(H_0 \mid \overline{y})$ increases from 0.33 to 0.82 when the sample size increases from 5 to 1000. Thus, for a relatively small P-value, H_0 can be accepted in a Bayesian hypothesis with a relatively high probability and this is called Lindley's paradox. It is the result of averaging the likelihood under the alternative hypothesis over a large (infinite) number of unrealistic values of θ which weakens the evidence for H_a. □

Goodman (1999b) argues that the dependence of the Bayes factor on the choice of $p(\theta)$, and hence also Lindley's paradox, is a reflection of our prior imprecision in defining the alternative hypothesis. Thus, a way to avoid Lindley's paradox is to give the distribution $p(\theta \mid H_a)$ not too big a spread. This becomes crucially important in Bayesian variable selection (see Chapter 11).

3.8.3.3 Testing versus estimation

Above computations also make it clear that, unlike in frequentist theory, estimation and testing are not complementary in the Bayesian approach (Kass and Raftery 1995). In testing, Bayesians put positive probabilities on sharp hypotheses, while in estimation one would assign a zero probability to $\theta = \theta_0$. In estimation, the priors often do not have a great impact on the posterior conclusion, but this is not the case in Bayesian testing where the prior can affect the Bayes factor considerably; see Section 10.2.1 for more illustrations on this. Finally, in estimation the model is fitted to the data while in testing only the averaged likelihood is computed.

3.9 Closing remarks

In this chapter, we have reviewed the basic ingredients of the Bayesian 'language'. We have restricted ourselves to the one parameter case, in order to focus on the concepts. The most interesting practical cases involve more than one parameter. This is the topic of Chapter 4, and in fact of all subsequent chapters of the book. We will then also realize that, despite its elegancy, the Bayesian approach also poses great numerical problems.

Exercises

Exercise 3.1 Show that (a) the posterior mean minimizes expression (3.3), (b) the posterior median minimizes expression (3.3) whereby the square loss function is replaced by $a|\theta - \widehat{\theta}|$ with $a > 0$, and (c) the posterior mode minimizes expression (3.3) with a penalty of 1 if we choose the incorrect value and no penalty for the correct value.

Exercise 3.2 Determine the posterior summary measures of Examples III.2 and III.3 using FirstBayes.

Exercise 3.3 Based on the posterior distribution obtained in Example II.3, derive the posterior summary measures for the Signal-Tandmobiel study using FirstBayes.

Exercise 3.4 Show that in the binomial case, the posterior mean is a weighted average of the prior mean and the MLE.

Exercise 3.5 Show that in the binomial case, the variance of the posterior distribution might be in some situations larger than that of the prior distribution, see also Pham-Gia (2004) for a general result in this context.

Exercise 3.6 Explore in the Poisson case the relationship of the variance of the posterior gamma distribution with respect to the variance of the prior gamma distribution.

Exercise 3.7 Show that there is shrinkage of the posterior mode and mean for the gamma-Poisson case.

Exercise 3.8 Write a function in R to determine the HPD interval in Example II.5 for the stroke study and check your result using FirstBayes. Repeat this exercise for the dmft-index in the Signal-Tandmobiel study.

Exercise 3.9 Show that the HPD interval for an odds ratio is not invariant to a switch of the groups by interchanging in Table 1.1 the two columns. More specifically if $[a, b]$ is the HPD interval for the odds ratio in the original setting, then $[1/b, 1/a]$ is not the HPD interval anymore for the odds ratio with the columns switched. However, this property holds for a classical CI. Note also that there is no such difficulty for $\gamma = \log(\text{or})$.

Exercise 3.10 Show that the PPD of a normal likelihood combined with a normal prior yields expression (3.12).

Exercise 3.11 Repeat the analysis of Example III.6 using the data set 'alp.txt' by making use of an R program.

Exercise 3.12 Repeat the analysis of Examples III.7 and III.8 using FirstBayes.

Exercise 3.13 Derive the PPD for the sum of n i.i.d. future counts from a Poisson distribution with a gamma prior for the mean.

Exercise 3.14 Prove the discrete version of expression (3.9). That is, for n possible 'causes' C_i suppose that A_1 and A_2 are two conditionally independent events such that

$$P(A_1 A_2 \mid C_i) = P(A_1 \mid C_i) P(A_2 \mid C_i), i = 1, \ldots, n,$$

and let $P(C_i) = 1/n$. Then show that

$$P(A_1 \mid A_2) = \Sigma P(A_2 \mid C_i) P(C_i \mid A_1).$$

Exercise 3.15 Derive the PPD for the negative binomial likelihood in combination with a beta prior (see Exercise 2.8).

Exercise 3.16 (see Cordani and Wechsler 2006) Consider random sampling without replacement of marbles from an urn having a known composition, 10 red and 5 white marbles. The marbles are selected one by one and if R_i is the event that the ith sampled marble is red and W_i that the ith sampled marble is white, show that $R_1, R_2, \ldots, R_{15}$ (and $W_1, W_2, \ldots, W_{15}$) are exchangeable but not independent random variables. That is, prove that $P(R_1) = P(R_2) = \ldots = P(R_{15}), P(R_1\&R_2) = P(R_1\&R_3) = \ldots,$ etc., but $P(R_1, R_2, \ldots, R_{15}) \neq \prod_{i=1}^{15} P(R_i)$. Show also that if sampling is done with replacement then $R_1, R_2, \ldots, R_{15}$ are exchangeable and independent.

Exercise 3.17 Suppose that the experts in Example III.9 assume that chemotherapy is potentially harmful. Their prior belief on the odds ratio scale is summarized by the median odds ratio equal to 5 and a 95% equal to CI on the odds ratio scale of [1, 25]. Repeat the analysis in Example III.9.

Exercise 3.18 The GUSTO-1 study is a mega-sized RCT comparing two thrombolytics: streptokinase (SK) and rt-PA for the treatment of patients with an acute myocardial infarction. The outcome of the study is 30-day mortality, which is a binary indicator whether the treated patient died after 30 days or not. The study recruited 41 021 acute infarct patients from 15 countries and 1081 hospitals in the period December 1990–February 1993. The basic analysis was reported in The GUSTO Investigators (1993) and found a statistically significant lower 30-day mortality rate for rt-PA compared with SK. Brophy and Joseph (1995) reanalyzed the GUSTO-1 trial results from a Bayesian point of view, leaving out the subset of patients who were treated with both rt-PA and SK. As prior information, the data from two previous studies have been used: GISSI-2 and ISIS-3. In Table 3.1, the data from the GUSTO-1 study and the two historical studies are given. The authors compared the results of streptokinase and rt-PA using the difference of the two observed proportions, equal to absolute risk reduction (ar), of death, nonfatal stroke and the combined endpoint of death or nonfatal stroke. Use the asymptotic normality of ar in the calculations below.

Questions:

1. Determine the normal prior for ar based on the data from (a) the GISSI-2 study, (b) the ISIS-3 study, and (c) the combined data from the GISSI-2 and ISIS-3 studies.

Table 3.1 Data from GUSTO-1, GISSI-2 and ISIS-3 on the comparison between of streptokinase and rt-PA.

Trial	Drug	Number of patients	Number of deaths	Number of nonfatal strokes	Combined deaths or strokes
GUSTO	SK	20 173	1 473	101	1 574
	rt-PA	10 343	652	62	714
GISSI-2	SK	10 396	929	56	985
	rt-PA	10 372	993	74	1 067
ISIS-3	SK	13 780	1 455	75	1 530
	rt-PA	13 746	1 418	95	1 513

2. Determine the posterior for ar for the GUSTO-1 study based on the above priors and a noninformative normal prior.

3. Determine the posterior belief in the better performance of streptokinase or rt-PA based on the above-derived posterior distributions.

4. Compare the Bayesian analyses to the classical frequentist analyses of comparing the proportions in the two treatment arms. What do you conclude?

5. Illustrate your results graphically.

Exercise 3.19 Repeat the analysis in Example III.12 using a sampling approach. Show also the histogram of $\theta/(1-\theta)$.

Exercise 3.20 Repeat the analysis in Example III.12 using a normal prior for θ with prior mean equal to 0.5 and prior standard deviation equal to 0.05.

Exercise 3.21 Repeat the analysis in Example III.14 with $y = 5$. Vary also the prior distribution for θ (stay within the beta-family), e.g. try out some more focused priors and evaluate the change in the Bayes factor.

4

More than one parameter

4.1 Introduction

The majority of statistical models involves more than one parameter, with the most common example being the Gaussian distribution $N(\mu, \sigma^2)$. In this chapter, we review multivariate Bayesian inference involving a statistical model that contains more than one (unknown) parameter, but the data are allowed to be univariate or multivariate. We treat the multivariate Gaussian model (and related models) for continuous data and the multinomial model for categorical data. Finally, we treat the Bayesian linear regression model and the Bayesian generalized linear model (BGLIM). These and more complex models are the topic of subsequent chapters and illustrated therein.

This chapter illustrates the complexity of the computations when more than one parameter is involved. Integration issues will appear almost everywhere in Bayesian calculations. Furthermore, Bayes theorem delivers a multivariate posterior distribution but inference is easier on each parameter separately, and hence, the marginal posterior distributions are required, involving again integration. For the Gaussian model with an appropriate prior, all these computations can be done analytically. This is also true for the multinomial model. However, with a slight glitch in the specification of the prior, the analytical derivations might not be possible anymore, which occurs for instance when a priori information is provided for the mean and variance parameter of the Gaussian model separately.

In addition, a sampling procedure called the *Method of Composition* is treated that allows sampling from a limited class of multivariate distributions. But we need to wait until Chapter 6 for a general method of sampling.

While this chapter is somewhat more technical than the previous ones, for analytical derivations we refer to Box and Tiao (1973), O'Hagan and Forster (2004), or Gelman *et al.* (2004, Chapter 3). The aim of this chapter is merely to concentrate on the ideas behind the derivations, thereby illustrating the complexity of the computations. It will become clear that a different route is needed to tackle practical problems with the Bayesian approach.

Bayesian Biostatistics, First Edition. Emmanuel Lesaffre and Andrew B. Lawson.

4.2 Joint versus marginal posterior inference

Let $\boldsymbol{y}$ represent a sample of n i.i.d. observations (univariate or multivariate) with statistical model characterized by a d-dimensional parameter vector $\boldsymbol{\theta} = (\theta_1, \theta_2, \ldots, \theta_d)^T$. Further, let the corresponding likelihood be $L(\boldsymbol{\theta} \mid \boldsymbol{y})$, then Bayes theorem becomes

$$p(\boldsymbol{\theta} \mid \boldsymbol{y}) = \frac{L(\boldsymbol{\theta} \mid \boldsymbol{y})p(\boldsymbol{\theta})}{\int L(\boldsymbol{\theta} \mid \boldsymbol{y})p(\boldsymbol{\theta})\,\mathrm{d}\boldsymbol{\theta}}, \tag{4.1}$$

with $p(\boldsymbol{\theta})$ now a multivariate prior. Expression (4.1) defines the joint posterior distribution. As in Chapter 3 one can define the posterior mode $\widehat{\boldsymbol{\theta}}_M$ and the posterior mean $\overline{\boldsymbol{\theta}}$. Note that the posterior median is not uniquely defined in higher dimensions; see Niinima and Oja (1999) for some suggestions. The highest posterior density (HPD) interval can easily be generalized to d dimensions. Namely, the region R in the parameter space of $\boldsymbol{\theta}$ is called an *HPD region of content* $(1-\alpha)$ if (a) $P(\boldsymbol{\theta} \in R \mid \boldsymbol{y}) = 1 - \alpha$ and (b) for $\boldsymbol{\theta}_1 \in R$ and $\boldsymbol{\theta}_2 \in / R$: $p(\boldsymbol{\theta}_1 \mid \boldsymbol{y}) \geq p(\boldsymbol{\theta}_2 \mid \boldsymbol{y})$.

In practice, inference is easier in low dimensions. That is, if $\boldsymbol{\theta} = \{\boldsymbol{\theta}_1, \boldsymbol{\theta}_2\}$, then it is simpler to work with the *marginal posterior distribution* of $\boldsymbol{\theta}_1$ defined as

$$p(\boldsymbol{\theta}_1 \mid \boldsymbol{y}) = \int p(\boldsymbol{\theta}_1, \boldsymbol{\theta}_2 \mid \boldsymbol{y})\,\mathrm{d}\boldsymbol{\theta}_2. \tag{4.2}$$

For a one-dimensional θ_1, the graphical display of the marginal posterior is easy and the posterior summary measures based on $p(\theta_1 \mid \boldsymbol{y})$ are convenient. We note in passing that the posterior mean of $\boldsymbol{\theta}$ consists of the marginal posterior means, but this result does not hold for the posterior mode.

Expression (4.2) can be rewritten as

$$p(\boldsymbol{\theta}_1 \mid \boldsymbol{y}) = \int p(\boldsymbol{\theta}_1 \mid \boldsymbol{\theta}_2, \boldsymbol{y})\; p(\boldsymbol{\theta}_2 \mid \boldsymbol{y})\,\mathrm{d}\boldsymbol{\theta}_2,$$

which shows that the marginal posterior of $\boldsymbol{\theta}_1$ is obtained by averaging the *conditional posterior* of $\boldsymbol{\theta}_1$ given $\boldsymbol{\theta}_2$ with a weight function determined by the marginal posterior of $\boldsymbol{\theta}_2$. If $\boldsymbol{\theta}_2$ consists of nuisance parameters, then taking the marginal posterior of $\boldsymbol{\theta}_1$ could be viewed as a way to get rid of the nuisance parameters when drawing posterior inference on $\boldsymbol{\theta}_1$. In other words, inference about $\boldsymbol{\theta}_1$ is obtained by taking into account the uncertainty we have on $\boldsymbol{\theta}_2$. Note the difference with the way nuisance parameters are removed in the likelihood approach using the *profile likelihood* approach (Pawitan 2001). For $\boldsymbol{\theta} = \{\boldsymbol{\theta}_1, \boldsymbol{\theta}_2\}$ with joint likelihood $L(\boldsymbol{\theta})$, the profile likelihood is defined as $pL(\boldsymbol{\theta}_1) = \max_{\boldsymbol{\theta}_2} L(\boldsymbol{\theta}_1, \boldsymbol{\theta}_2)$. As before we see that the Bayesian approach deals with uncertainty via integration, while in the classical approach maximization is the standard approach.

4.3 The normal distribution with μ and σ^2 unknown

We now derive the joint posterior of the normal likelihood with both the mean and variance parameters unknown and based on three different but Gaussian priors. Suppose that $\boldsymbol{y} = \{y_1, \ldots, y_n\}$ is a sample of i.i.d. observations from $\mathrm{N}(\mu, \sigma^2)$. The joint likelihood of (μ, σ^2)

given $\mathbf{y}$ is

$$L(\mu, \sigma^2 \mid \mathbf{y}) = \frac{1}{(2\pi\sigma^2)^{n/2}} \exp\left[-\frac{1}{2\sigma^2}\sum_{i=1}^{n}(y_i - \mu)^2\right]. \tag{4.3}$$

The above expression can be rewritten as a function of $\overline{y}$ and s^2, the sample mean and variance, respectively, since $\sum_{i=1}^{n}(y_i - \mu)^2 = \left[(n-1)s^2 + n(\overline{y} - \mu)^2\right]$. This result simply states that $\overline{y}$ and s^2 are the sufficient statistics for μ and σ^2. The posterior distribution is obtained upon specification of the prior $p(\mu, \sigma^2)$. We consider three cases: (a) there is no prior knowledge on μ and σ^2, (b) a previous study is informative about plausible values for μ and σ^2 and (c) expert knowledge is available on μ and σ^2.

4.3.1 No prior knowledge on μ and σ^2 is available

In the absence of prior knowledge on the mean and variance parameter of the normal model, the popular noninformative joint prior $p(\mu, \sigma^2) \propto \sigma^{-2}$ could be taken. Characteristics of this prior are discussed in Section 5.4.3. This choice of prior leads to the posterior distribution

$$p(\mu, \sigma^2 \mid \mathbf{y}) \propto \frac{1}{\sigma^{n+2}} \exp\left\{-\frac{1}{2\sigma^2}\left[(n-1)s^2 + n(\overline{y} - \mu)^2\right]\right\}, \tag{4.4}$$

shown in Figure 4.1 where n, s and $\overline{y}$ are obtained from Example IV.1. Note that, while a priori the parameters μ and σ^2 of the normal distribution are independent, they are not independent a posteriori anymore.

It is insightful to report the posterior information about the parameters for each parameter separately. This leads to the marginal posterior distributions $p(\mu \mid \mathbf{y})$ and $p(\sigma^2 \mid \mathbf{y})$. They express what is known about each parameter separately in the light of the data and given the available information a priori. Both marginal posterior distributions involve an extra

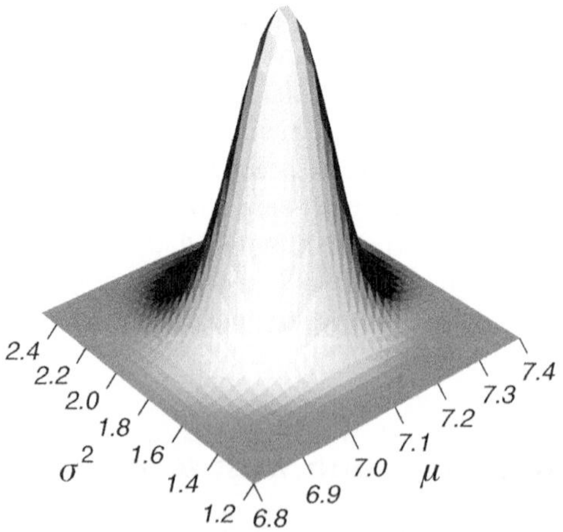

Figure 4.1 Serum alkaline phosphatase study (noninformative prior): joint posterior distribution $p(\mu, \sigma^2 \mid \mathbf{y})$ with $y_i = 100/\sqrt{alp_i}$ $(i = 1, \ldots, 250)$.

integration, e.g.

$$p(\mu \mid \mathbf{y}) = \int p(\mu, \sigma^2 \mid \mathbf{y})\,\mathrm{d}\sigma^2 = \int p(\mu \mid \sigma^2, \mathbf{y}) p(\sigma^2 \mid \mathbf{y})\,\mathrm{d}\sigma^2.$$

The above marginal posterior distribution is a weighted average of conditional posterior distributions $p(\mu \mid \sigma^2, \mathbf{y})$ with weights $p(\sigma^2 \mid \mathbf{y})$. Consequently, the marginal posterior distribution for μ takes into account the uncertainty we have about σ^2. For a large study or a strong prior, σ^2 is known with high precision. In that case $p(\mu \mid \mathbf{y}) \approx p(\mu \mid \sigma^2, \mathbf{y})$ with σ^2 equal to the posterior mode. On the other hand, when there is doubt about the true value of σ^2 the Bayesian way of dealing with this uncertainty is averaging. In a similar manner, the calculation of the marginal posterior distribution for σ^2 takes into account the uncertainty we have about μ.

Applying classical integration rules yields for posterior distribution (4.4), the following results:

- $p(\mu \mid \sigma^2, \mathbf{y})$ is $\mathrm{N}(\overline{y}, \sigma^2/n)$, equal to expression (2.19);
- $p(\mu \mid \mathbf{y})$ is a $t_{n-1}(\overline{y}, s^2/n)$ distribution, which means that μ is distributed as $\overline{y} + t\,(s/\sqrt{n})$ with t following a standard t_{n-1}-distribution. Note that this result implies for μ that, given $\mathbf{y}$,

$$\frac{\mu - \overline{y}}{s/\sqrt{n}} \sim t_{n-1}; \tag{4.5}$$

- $p(\sigma^2 \mid \mathbf{y})$ is a *scaled inverse chi-squared distribution*, denoted $\mathrm{Inv} - \chi^2(n-1, s^2)$. It is illustrative to note that this implies for σ^2 that, given $\mathbf{y}$,

$$\frac{(n-1)s^2}{\sigma^2} \sim \chi^2(n-1); \tag{4.6}$$

  which is equivalent to $\sigma^2 = (n-1)s^2/X^2$, with X^2 following a standard $\chi^2(n-1)$ distribution. The above distribution is a special case of an *inverse gamma distribution* $\mathrm{IG}(\alpha, \beta)$, with $\alpha = (n-1)/2$ and $\beta = 1/2$.

Since $p(\mu, \sigma^2 \mid \mathbf{y}) = p(\mu \mid \sigma^2, \mathbf{y})\; p(\sigma^2 \mid \mathbf{y}) = \mathrm{N}(\mu \mid \overline{y}, \sigma^2/n)\;\mathrm{Inv} - \chi^2(\sigma^2 \mid n-1, s^2)$, the joint posterior distribution is called a *normal-scaled-inverse chi-squared distribution*, denoted by $\mathrm{N\text{-}Inv\text{-}}\chi^2(\overline{y}, n, (n-1), s^2)$. We refer to Section 5.3.2 for more details on this distribution. The above analytical work pays off since it allows us to have explicit mathematical expressions of the posterior summary measures for μ and σ^2:

- For μ, the marginal posterior distribution is symmetrical and all posterior summary measures for location are equal to $\overline{y}$. The posterior variance is equal to $\frac{(n-1)}{n(n-2)}s^2$. The 95% equal tail credible and HPD interval are equal to

$$[\overline{y} - t(0.025; n-1)\, s/\sqrt{n}, \overline{y} + t(0.025; n-1)\, s/\sqrt{n}], \tag{4.7}$$

  with $t(0.025; n-1)$ the 97.5% quantile of the classical t_{n-1}-distribution.

- For σ^2, the posterior mean, mode and median are equal to $\frac{(n-1)}{(n-3)}s^2$, $\frac{(n-1)}{(n+1)}s^2$, $\frac{(n-1)}{\chi^2(0.5,n-1)}s^2$, respectively, with $\chi^2(0.5, n-1)$ the median value of the $\chi^2(n-1)$ distribution. Its posterior variance is equal to $\frac{2(n-1)^2}{(n-3)^2(n-5)}s^4$. Finally, the 95% equal tail CI is

$$\left[\frac{(n-1)s^2}{\chi^2(0.975, n-1)}, \frac{(n-1)s^2}{\chi^2(0.025, n-1)}\right], \tag{4.8}$$

with $\chi^2(0.025, n-1)$, $\chi^2(0.975, n-1)$ the 2.5% and the 97.5% quantile of the $\chi^2(n-1)$ distribution, respectively. The 95% HPD interval is computed numerically using the approach outlined in Section 3.3.2.

The credible intervals (4.7) and (4.8) are the same as the corresponding classical 95% confidence intervals (CIs). This illustrates that with the appropriate priors, a Bayesian analysis can reproduce frequentist results.

Suppose now that it is of interest to know the distribution of a future observation $\widetilde{y}$ (from the same normal distribution as $\mathbf{y}$). In other words, we wish to know the posterior predictive distribution (PPD). The PPD takes into account that we do not know μ and σ^2 and is given by

$$p(\widetilde{y} \mid \mathbf{y}) = \int\int p(\widetilde{y} \mid \mu, \sigma^2)p(\mu, \sigma^2 \mid \mathbf{y})\, d\mu\, d\sigma^2, \tag{4.9}$$

which is equal here to a t_{n-1}- $\left[\bar{y}, s^2\left(1+\frac{1}{n}\right)\right]$ distribution.

The serum alkaline phosphatase data, introduced in Example III.6, are used to illustrate the above-derived results in Example IV.1.

Example IV.1: Serum alkaline phosphatase study: Noninformative prior
The normal range for serum alkaline phosphatase (*alp*) based on a prospective set of 250 'healthy' patients was derived in Example III.6. But since the calculations ignored the uncertainty of σ^2, the reference range is probably too narrow.

The joint posterior distribution for μ and σ^2 given $y_i = 100/\sqrt{alp_i}$ $(i = 1, \ldots, 250)$ is displayed in Figure 4.1. The marginal posterior distributions for μ and σ^2 are shown in Figure 4.2.

On the basis of the above-derived expressions, the posterior location measures for μ are $\overline{\mu} = \widehat{\mu}_M = \overline{\mu}_M = 7.11$ with posterior variance $\overline{\sigma}^2_\mu = 0.0075$. The 95% (equal tail and HPD) CI is [6.94, 7.28]. For σ^2, the posterior summary measures are $\overline{\sigma}^2 = 1.88$ (mean), $\widehat{\sigma}^2_M = 1.85$ (mode), $\overline{\sigma}^2_M = 1.87$ (median) and $\overline{\sigma}^2_{\sigma^2} = 0.029$ (variance). The 95% equal tail CI for σ^2 is equal to [1.58, 2.24], while its 95% HPD interval is equal to [1.56, 2.22].

The distribution of a future observation is a $t_{249}(7.11, 1.37)$ distribution. This leads to a 95% normal range for y equal to [4.41, 9.80] leading to a 95% normal range for *alp* equal to [104.1, 513.2], which is slightly wider than the reference range of Example III.6. □

4.3.2 An historical study is available

The posterior of historical data can be used as a prior to the likelihood of the current data. Suppose that the historical data were combined with a noninformative prior as done in Section 4.3.1, then this yields the N-Inv-$\chi^2(\mu_0, \kappa_0, \nu_0, \sigma_0^2)$ prior for the current data where

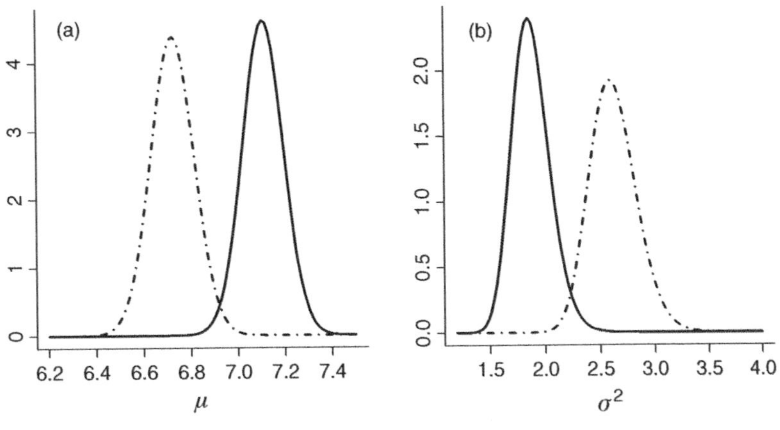

Figure 4.2 Serum alkaline phosphatase study: marginal posterior distributions for (a) μ and (b) σ^2 with a noninformative prior (solid lines) and a data-based informative prior (dashed lines).

the parameters are determined from the past data. That is,

$$\mu \mid \sigma^2 \sim \mathrm{N}(\mu_0, \sigma^2/\kappa_0),$$
$$\sigma^2 \sim \mathrm{Inv} - \chi^2(\nu_0, \sigma_0^2),$$

with $\mu_0 = \overline{y}_0$, $\kappa_0 = n_0$, $\nu_0 = n_0 - 1$ and $\sigma_0^2 = s_0^2$, with $\overline{y}_0$, s_0^2 and n_0 the sample mean, sample variance and size of the historical data, respectively. Note that this prior may also be used when expert knowledge is specified using the above priors. In both cases, μ_0 may be thought of as a prior mean for μ, κ_0 as a prior sample size and ν_0 as a prior mean for σ^2. Thus, when $\kappa_0 = 1$, then the prior sample size is equal to the information in one observation. Combining this prior with likelihood (4.3) results in a N-Inv-$\chi^2(\overline{\mu}, \overline{\kappa}, \overline{\nu}, \overline{\sigma}^2)$ posterior with

$$\overline{\mu} = \frac{\kappa_0\mu_0 + n\overline{y}}{\kappa_0 + n}, \tag{4.10}$$

$$\overline{\kappa} = \kappa_0 + n, \tag{4.11}$$

$$\overline{\nu} = \nu_0 + n, \tag{4.12}$$

$$\overline{\nu\sigma}^2 = \nu_0\sigma_0^2 + (n-1)s^2 + \frac{\kappa_0\, n}{\kappa_0 + n}(\overline{y} - \mu_0)^2. \tag{4.13}$$

Expression (4.10) is similar to expression (2.14) such that the posterior mean is again a weighted average of the prior mean and sample mean. Consequently, there is again shrinkage toward the prior mean. Expression (4.13) shows that the posterior variance is a combination of the prior variance, the sample variance, and the distance between the sample mean and the prior mean.

The next step is to derive marginal posterior distributions:

$$p(\mu \mid \sigma^2, \mathbf{y}) = \mathrm{N}(\mu \mid \overline{\mu}, \sigma^2/\overline{\kappa}), \tag{4.14}$$

$$p(\mu \mid \mathbf{y}) = t_{\overline{\nu}}(\mu \mid \overline{\mu}, \overline{\sigma}^2/\overline{\kappa}), \tag{4.15}$$

$$p(\sigma^2 \mid \mathbf{y}) = \mathrm{Inv} - \chi^2(\sigma^2 \mid \overline{\nu}, \overline{\sigma}^2). \tag{4.16}$$

When $\kappa_0 = \nu_0 = 0$, the aforementioned normal-scaled-inverse χ^2 prior becomes the noninformative prior σ^{-2} and the marginal posteriors reduce to the ones derived in Section 4.3.1.

From expressions (4.13) and (4.15), we observe that the posterior precision of μ is not automatically increased by combining the prior information with the sample data, in contrast to what we have seen in Section 2.7. In fact, if the prior mean is remote from the sample mean, then the posterior precision is likely to decrease. As a consequence, the posterior variance for μ with an informative prior that is in conflict with the sample data might be greater than the one obtained from a noninformative prior. This is illustrated in Example IV.2.

Finally, the PPD is obtained by an extra integration and becomes a $t_{\overline{\nu}}\left[\overline{y}, s^2\left(1+\frac{1}{\kappa_0+n}\right)\right]$-distribution.

Example IV.2: Serum alkaline phosphatase study: Conjugate prior
Prior to the prospective study, a retrospective study was conducted by Topal *et al.* (2003) and delivered data on *alp* from 65 healthy subjects. The mean value and SD for $y = 100/\sqrt{alp}$ obtained from the retrospective study were 5.25 and 1.66, respectively, leading to a N-Inv-χ^2 (5.25, 65, 64, 2.76) conjugate prior. On the basis of this prior and combining with the prospective data, the posterior distribution is N-Inv-χ^2 (6.72, 315, 314, 2.61). The posterior mean (median and mode) 6.72 is a weighted combination of the prior mean 5.25 and the sample mean 7.11. The posterior variance of μ is $\overline{\sigma}^2_\mu = 0.0083$ which is greater than the posterior variance of μ equal to 0.0075 obtained from the noninformative prior specified in Example IV.1. The reason for this peculiar result is that the prior mean, equal to 5.25, is relatively remote from the sample mean. The 95% (equal tail and HPD) CI for μ is [6.54, 6.90]. For σ^2, the posterior mean is equal to $\overline{\sigma}^2 = 2.62$ ($\widehat{\sigma}^2_M = 2.59$, $\overline{\sigma}^2_M = 2.61$) and the posterior variance equals $\overline{\sigma}^2_{\sigma^2} = 0.044$. The 95% equal tail CI is equal to [2.24, 3.07] close to the 95% HPD interval equal to [2.23, 3.04].

The distribution of a future observation is the $t_{314}(6.72, 1.62)$ distribution. This leads to a 95% normal range for y equal to [3.54, 9.91] and corresponds to a 95% normal range for *alp* equal to [101.9, 796.7], which is considerably wider than the reference range computed with the noninformative prior distribution.

The prior information did not have the expected effect of shrinking the posterior uncertainty because of the conflict of the discrepancy between the prospectively collected data and the retrospective data. In Figure 4.2, we contrast the posterior from Example IV.1 and the current posterior. □

4.3.3 Expert knowledge is available

In practice, expert knowledge, if any, is typically available on each parameter separately. For the normal distribution, this means that information is available separately on μ and σ^2. A possible choice for informative priors is

- $\mu \sim \text{N}(\mu_0, \sigma_0^2)$,
- $\sigma^2 \sim \text{Inv} - \chi^2(\nu_0, \tau_0^2)$,

with μ_0, σ_0^2, ν_0 and τ_0^2 obtained from eliciting prior information from experts separately for μ and σ^2. If the prior knowledge on μ and σ^2 is obtained independently, then it is reasonable to take the prior as the product of $p(\mu)$ and $p(\sigma^2)$, i.e.

$$\mathrm{N}(\mu_0, \sigma_0^2)\,\mathrm{Inv} - \chi^2(\nu_0, \tau_0^2). \tag{4.17}$$

This prior is, however, not a normal-scaled-inverse chi-squared distribution. In fact, it is seen in Section 4.3.1. (see also Sections 5.3.2 and 5.3.4) that the N-Inv-$\chi^2(\mu_0, \kappa_0, \nu_0, \sigma_0^2)$ joint prior implies that the prior for μ is dependent on σ^2, a property that is not satisfied by the product prior (4.17). Consequently, with prior (4.17) the posterior cannot be derived analytically. Some partial results are available (Gelman *et al.* 2004, pp. 81–82), namely

$$p(\mu \mid \sigma^2, \mathbf{y}) = \mathrm{N}(\overline{\mu}, \overline{\sigma}^2),$$

with

$$\overline{\mu} = \frac{\frac{1}{\sigma_0^2}\mu_0 + \frac{n}{\sigma^2}\overline{y}}{\frac{1}{\sigma_0^2} + \frac{n}{\sigma^2}} \quad \text{and } \overline{\sigma}^2 = \frac{1}{\frac{1}{\sigma_0^2} + \frac{n}{\sigma^2}}, \tag{4.18}$$

where both $\overline{\mu}$ and $\overline{\sigma}^2$ vary with σ.

For σ^2, the marginal posterior distribution cannot be determined analytically, i.e. the integration constant is not known. It can be shown (Gelman *et al.* 2004) that

$$p(\sigma^2 \mid \mathbf{y}) \propto \overline{\sigma}\,\mathrm{N}(\overline{\mu} \mid \mu_0, \sigma_0^2)\,\mathrm{Inv} - \chi^2(\sigma^2 \mid \nu_0, \tau_0^2) \prod_{i=1}^{n} \mathrm{N}(y_i \mid \overline{\mu}, \sigma^2). \tag{4.19}$$

In spite of the absence of analytical results for the posterior distribution, the posterior distribution can be numerically approximated on a grid. An alternative is to sample from the posterior distribution, which we illustrate in Section 4.6.

4.4 Multivariate distributions

When the response is multivariate, we speak of a multivariate response model. In the continuous case, we distinguish the multivariate normal (MVN) distribution, the multivariate Student's t-distribution, and the Wishart distribution. In the discrete case, we treat the multinomial distribution.

4.4.1 The multivariate normal and related distributions

The most popular multivariate distribution for a p-dimensional continuous response $\mathbf{y}$ is no doubt the *MVN distribution*, denoted by $\mathrm{N}(\boldsymbol{\mu}, \Sigma)$ with mean vector $\boldsymbol{\mu}$ and covariance matrix Σ. We will use the notation $\mathrm{N}_p(\boldsymbol{\mu}, \Sigma)$ when we wish to indicate the dimension of the MVN distribution. The MVN density for a random vector $\mathbf{y}$ is given by

$$p(\mathbf{y} \mid \boldsymbol{\mu}, \Sigma) = \frac{1}{(2\pi)^{p/2}|\Sigma|^{1/2}} \exp\left[-\frac{1}{2}(\mathbf{y} - \boldsymbol{\mu})^T \Sigma^{-1}(\mathbf{y} - \boldsymbol{\mu})\right]. \tag{4.20}$$

It is well known that all marginal and conditional distributions of an MVN distribution are again normal, as well as all linear combinations of $y_1, \ldots, y_p$.

The multivariate Student's t-distribution allows for heavier tails than the MVN distribution. The distribution is obtained as a posterior in a classical Bayesian regression model (see Section 4.7), but it is also used as a data distribution. The multivariate t-distribution $\mathrm{T}_\nu(\boldsymbol{\mu}, \Sigma)$ for a random vector $\boldsymbol{y}$ is given by

$$p(\boldsymbol{y} \mid \nu, \boldsymbol{\mu}, \Sigma) = \frac{\Gamma[(\nu + p)/2]}{\Gamma(\nu/2)(k\pi)^{p/2}} |\Sigma|^{-1/2} \left[1 + \frac{1}{\nu}(\boldsymbol{y} - \boldsymbol{\mu})^T \Sigma^{-1}(\boldsymbol{y} - \boldsymbol{\mu})\right]^{-(\nu+p)/2}, \tag{4.21}$$

which is the multivariate extension of location-scale t-distribution with ν degrees of freedom.

The χ^2-distribution is the distribution of a sum-of-squares of independent normally distributed random variables. In particular, $S^2/\sigma^2 \sim \chi^2(n-1)$ with $S^2 = \sum_{i=1}^n (y_i - \bar{y})^2$. When S^2 is replaced by the matrix $\mathrm{S} = \sum_{i=1}^n (\boldsymbol{y}_i - \bar{\boldsymbol{y}})(\boldsymbol{y}_i - \bar{\boldsymbol{y}})^T$ then the *Wishart-distribution* is obtained with scale matrix Σ and $\nu = n - 1$ degrees of freedom. Hereby, it is seen that the Wishart distribution is the multivariate extension of the χ^2-distribution. The distribution was named after John Wishart (1898–1956) and is denoted as Wishart(Σ, ν). The expression of the distribution is

$$p(\mathrm{S}|\nu, \Sigma) = c|\Sigma|^{-\nu/2}|\mathrm{S}|^{(\nu-p-1)/2} \exp\left[-\frac{1}{2}\mathrm{tr}\,(\Sigma^{-1}\mathrm{S})\right], \tag{4.22}$$

with $c^{-1} = 2^{\nu p/2}\pi^{p(p-1)/4} \prod_{j=1}^p \Gamma\left(\frac{\nu+1-j}{2}\right)$, and tr(A) is the trace of the matrix A. A related distribution is the *inverse Wishart distribution* defined as: $R \sim IW(\Sigma, \nu)$ with Σ a precision matrix if $R^{-1} \sim$ Wishart(Σ, ν).

Illustrations of the use of these distributions are found at many places in the following sections of the book. For an in-depth treatment of multivariate Bayesian models (with proofs of the results), we refer to Rowe (2003).

4.4.2 The multinomial distribution

We consider in this section, the application of the multinomial distribution to explore the association of a row factor with a column factor in a 2×2 contingency table. In the second example, we reanalyze the case-control study of Kaldor *et al.* (1990).

Suppose $\boldsymbol{y} = (y_1, \ldots, y_k)^T$ represents the vector of frequencies falling into k classes, then the *multinomial distribution* Mult(n, θ) is given by

$$p(\boldsymbol{y} \mid \boldsymbol{\theta}) = \frac{n!}{y_1! y_2! \ldots y_k!} \prod_{j=1}^k \theta_j^{y_j}, \tag{4.23}$$

with $n = \sum_{j=1}^k y_j$, $\boldsymbol{\theta} = (\theta_1, \ldots, \theta_k)^T$, $\theta_j > 0$, $(j = 1, \ldots, k)$ and $\sum_{j=1}^k \theta_j = 1$. Clearly, the binomial distribution is a special case of the multinomial distribution with $k = 2$. Further, the marginal distribution of y_j is a binomial distribution Bin(n,θ_j). In addition, the conditional distribution of $y_j (j \in S, S$ subset of $\{1, \ldots, k\})$ given $\boldsymbol{y}_S = \{y_m : m \in S\}$ is Mult$(n_S, \boldsymbol{\theta}_S)$ with $n_S = \sum_{m \in S} y_m$ and $\boldsymbol{\theta}_S = \{\theta_j / \sum_{m \in S} \theta_m : j \in S\}$.

Table 4.1 Young adults study: frequency table of smoking and alcohol consumption.

	Smoking	
Alcohol	No	Yes
No-mild	180	41
Moderate-heavy	216	64
Total	396	105

We now use the multinomial model to explore the association between alcohol drinking and smoking among young adults.

Example IV.3: Young adult study: Association between smoking and alcohol drinking
In Table 4.1, the results are shown of a study examining the life style among young adults. There was interest in knowing the association between smoking and alcohol-consumption. The 2×2 contingency table can be viewed as a multinomial model with parameters $\boldsymbol{\theta} = \{\theta_{11}, \theta_{12}, \theta_{21}, \theta_{22} = 1 - \theta_{11} - \theta_{12} - \theta_{21}\}$, whereby the subscripts indicate the rows and columns, respectively, of the table. More specifically, the multinomial likelihood for observing cell frequencies $\boldsymbol{y} = \{y_{11}, y_{12}, y_{21}, y_{22}\}$ with $\sum_{i=1}^{2}\sum_{j=1}^{2} y_{ij} = n$ is

$$\text{Mult}(n, \boldsymbol{\theta}) = \frac{n!}{y_{11}!\, y_{12}!\, y_{21}!\, y_{22}!}\, \theta_{11}^{y_{11}}\, \theta_{12}^{y_{12}}\, \theta_{21}^{y_{21}}\, \theta_{22}^{y_{22}}.$$

In Section 5.3.3, it is seen that a conjugate prior to this multinomial distribution is given by the *Dirichlet prior*, Dir($\boldsymbol{\alpha}$):

$$\boldsymbol{\theta} \sim \frac{1}{B(\boldsymbol{\alpha})} \prod_{i,j} \theta_{ij}^{\alpha_{ij}-1},$$

with $B(\boldsymbol{\alpha}) = \prod_{i,j} \Gamma(\alpha_{ij}) / \Gamma\left(\sum_{i,j} \alpha_{ij}\right)$ and $\boldsymbol{\alpha}$ stands for all α-parameters. When combined with the multinomial likelihood, the posterior distribution is Dir($\boldsymbol{\alpha} + \boldsymbol{y}$); see Chapter 5 for more details.

The association between smoking and alcohol consumption can be expressed with the cross-ratio

$$\psi = \frac{\theta_{11}\, \theta_{22}}{\theta_{12}\, \theta_{21}}.$$

The posterior distribution of ψ given the observed cell frequencies is difficult to derive analytically, but a sampling procedure can be invoked: Let $W_{ij} (i, j = 1, 2)$ be distributed independently as Gamma(α_{ij}, 1) and $T = \sum_{ij} W_{ij}$, then one can show that $Z_{ij} = W_{ij}/T$ has a Dir($\boldsymbol{\alpha}$) distribution (Exercise 4.1).

For the analysis of the contingency table, we used a noninformative Dirichlet prior with all parameters equal to 1, resulting in a Dir(180+1, 41+1, 216+1, 64+1) posterior. Using the above-suggested sampling procedure, 10 000 ψ-values were generated from its posterior. From the sampled values, we obtained a posterior median for ψ of 1.299 with a 95% equal tail CI of [0.839, 2.014]. Hence, there is no conclusive evidence of a positive association. Note that the above estimates were equal up to 2 decimals to the frequentist estimates. □

One can show that the one-dimensional marginal posteriors of the Dirichlet distribution are all beta distributions $\text{Beta}(\alpha_{ij}, \sum_{kl} \alpha_{kl} - \alpha_{ij})$ (Exercise 5.8). Further, the noninformative Dirichlet prior Dir(1,1,1,1) corresponds to an approximately normal prior for $\log(\psi)$ with mean zero and SD 2.6 (Exercise 4.2). This prior acts as a diffuse prior for $\log(\psi)$.

Example IV.4: Kaldor's *et al.* (1990) case-control study: A reanalysis of Example III.9
We reanalyzed the Hodgkin's survival data using a somewhat different approach to compare the proportion of patients that received chemotherapy among cases (251/411) and controls (138/149). We assumed for controls and cases a binomial likelihood, with probability of receiving chemotherapy denoted as θ_1 for controls and as θ_2 for cases. The likelihood for the total sample is given by a product of binomial likelihoods, i.e.

$$L(\theta_1, \theta_2 \mid \mathbf{y}) \propto \theta_1^{251} (1 - \theta_1)^{160} \, \theta_2^{138} (1 - \theta_2)^{11},$$

where $\mathbf{y}$ stands for $\{251, 160, 138, 11\}$. To test the hypothesis $H_1 : \theta_2 \leq \theta_1$ versus $H_2 : \theta_1 < \theta_2$, we evaluated the posterior distribution of $p(\theta_2 - \theta_1 \mid \mathbf{y})$. As part of a sensitivity analysis, we varied the priors and considered

- Uniform prior for θ_1 and θ_2
- Jeffreys prior (see Chapter 5): $p(\theta_1, \theta_2) \propto \theta_1^{-1/2} (1 - \theta_1)^{-1/2} \, \theta_2^{-1/2} (1 - \theta_2)^{-1/2}$
- Haldane prior: $p(\theta_1, \theta_2) \propto \theta_1^{-1} (1 - \theta_1)^{-1} \, \theta_2^{-1} (1 - \theta_2)^{-1}$

The above priors are products of beta distributions. When combining these priors with the likelihood, the posterior is again a product of beta distributions. Thus, a posteriori θ_1 and θ_2 are independent. To obtain the posterior $p(\theta_2 - \theta_1 \mid \mathbf{y})$, the easiest way is to sample from $p(\theta_2 \mid \mathbf{y})$ and $p(\theta_1 \mid \mathbf{y})$ and to take the difference of each sampled value. On the basis of 1000 sample values, the 95% equal tail CIs for $\theta_2 - \theta_1$ for the three priors were [0.249, 0.373], [0.251, 0.379] and [0.259, 0.381], respectively. □

The above analysis follows the approach of Howard (1998) who treated the problem of comparing the proportions from two independent binomial distributions. Using a variety of priors, he showed that the classical frequentist tests (Fisher's Exact test, chi-squared test, etc.) can be 'reproduced' by Bayesian tests. However, Howard (1998) pleads for a dependent prior $p(\theta_1, \theta_2)$ rather than the independent priors we used here.

4.5 Frequentist properties of Bayesian inference

It is not of prime interest to a Bayesian to know the properties of Bayesian estimators in case the study is repeated (in fact, most often studies in practice are not repeated at all). It might be, however, important to ascertain when Bayesian estimators give on average the correct inference. Indeed, the motivation for looking at the long-run operating characteristics of Bayesian procedures is to assert how frequently a Bayesian procedure will provide a valid answer to the scientific problem taking into account that the chosen prior and model are often not correct. We focus here on objective priors and are interested to know that Bayesian methods perform well in practice if applied repeatedly. We first note that, because of the Bayesian CLT, the posterior measures (mean, mode, median) have asymptotically a normal distribution. For interval estimators, we are interested to know whether they have the correct coverage (Rubin 1984). This can also be interesting from a frequentist point of view. Namely, the Bayesian approach offers alternative interval estimators, not relying on asymptotic properties of the estimators. It might, therefore, be of interest to evaluate the performance of these estimators under the frequentist paradigm and hope for a better coverage in small sample cases than frequentist estimators.

However, there is nothing in the construction of the $100(1-\alpha)\%$ credible interval that guarantees its desired frequentist coverage, at least not for a small sample. For a large sample the Bayesian CLT proves the asymptotic correct coverage for the case of a finite number of parameters. Nevertheless we saw in Section 4.3.1 that the credible intervals obtained from a joint NI prior are exactly the same as the classical 95% CIs. Thus for this case, the coverage of the Bayesian interval estimators is guaranteed. Of course, $100(1-\alpha)\%$ coverage should not be expected anymore when strong subjective priors are taken (but perhaps the coverage is greater than $100(1-\alpha)\%$ for a good choice of the prior).

Other examples of correct coverage of Bayesian procedures will turn up in this and subsequent chapters. For example, when comparing proportions in a 2×2 contingency table, Agresti and Min (2005) explored various noninformative priors on the difference of proportions $\pi_1 - \pi_2$, the ratio π_1/π_2 and the odds ratio $[\pi_1/(1-\pi_1)]\,/\,[\pi_2/(1-\pi_2)]$. Their conclusions were that for the risk difference all considered noninformative priors gave about the correct frequentist coverage, but that for the risk ratio and the odds ratio the uniform prior gave too low a coverage (corresponding to a frequentist analysis). Their recommendation was to use Jeffreys prior for the binomial parameters when a correct coverage in a frequentist sense is aimed for. Rubin (1984) gave other examples where the Bayesian $100(1-\alpha)\%$ CI gives at least $100(1-\alpha)\%$ coverage even when the prior distribution is chosen incorrectly.

Nowadays it becomes more commonplace to explore the frequentist properties of newly proposed Bayesian procedures, see also Chapter 5.

4.6 Sampling from the posterior distribution: The Method of Composition

The *Method of Composition* is a general step-by-step approach to yield a random sample of independent observations from a multivariate distribution. The approach is based on the factorization of the joint distribution into a marginal and one or more conditional distributions. For d parameters, the following factorization of the joint posterior distribution can be established:

$$p(\theta_1, \ldots, \theta_d \mid \mathbf{y}) = p(\theta_d \mid \mathbf{y})\, p(\theta_{d-1} \mid \theta_d, \mathbf{y}) \, \ldots p(\theta_1 \mid \theta_d, \ldots, \theta_2, \mathbf{y}).$$

This factorization yields a natural procedure to sample from the joint posterior distribution. In fact, we first sample $\widetilde{\theta}_d$ from $p(\theta_d \mid \mathbf{y})$, then sample $\widetilde{\theta}_{(d-1)}$ from $p(\theta_{(d-1)} \mid \widetilde{\theta}_d, \mathbf{y})$, etc. until all parameters have been sampled. When repeated K times, an independent sample of size K is obtained from the joint posterior distribution but also from all marginal posterior distributions. The particular ordering of the parameters is, in principle, of no importance, but one ordering may be preferred over another when it results in simpler integrations or when it yields a more elegant sampling procedure. The Method of Composition is particularly useful when a sample of a particular marginal posterior is difficult to obtain, but sampling is easier from another marginal posterior and associated conditional posteriors. Finally, the sampling method also provides a natural and elegant way to sample from a PPD.

As seen in Section 3.7.2, sampling can replace analytical calculations to obtain the posterior distribution and the posterior summary measures. There is, however, a price to pay, namely, the posterior, and the posterior summary measures can only be determined approximately. The quality of the approximation can be evaluated by the classical 95% CI (3.22). The attractive feature of sampling is that if the Monte Carlo (standard) error is judged too large, then the user can simply continue with the sampling until the desired accuracy is achieved.

The Method of Composition will now be illustrated on the normal posterior $p(\mu, \sigma^2 \mid \boldsymbol{y})$. We consider again the three cases with respect to the available knowledge regarding μ and σ^2: (a) no prior knowledge, (b) historical data is available, and (c) expert knowledge is available.

Case 1: No prior knowledge on μ and σ^2 is available
To sample from $p(\mu, \sigma^2 \mid \boldsymbol{y})$, we could first sample from $p(\sigma^2 \mid \boldsymbol{y})$ and then sample from $p(\mu \mid \sigma^2, \boldsymbol{y})$. To sample from $p(\sigma^2 \mid \boldsymbol{y})$, we first sample $\widetilde{\nu}^k$ from a $\chi^2(n-1)$-distribution and then solve $(\widetilde{\sigma}^2)^k$ in $(n-1)s^2/(\widetilde{\sigma}^2)^k = \widetilde{\nu}^k$. In the second step, we sample $\widetilde{\mu}^k$ from a $\text{N}(\overline{y}, (\widetilde{\sigma}^2)^k/n)$-distribution. The sample $\widetilde{\mu}^1, \ldots, \widetilde{\mu}^K$ is automatically a random sample of independent observations from the $t_{n-1}(\overline{y}, s^2/n)$-distribution, which is the marginal posterior distribution for μ. Note that also the reverse ordering could have been taken, i.e. first sample $\widetilde{\mu}$ from $p(\mu \mid \boldsymbol{y})$ and then sample $\widetilde{\sigma}^2$ from $p(\sigma^2 \mid \mu, \boldsymbol{y})$. It turns out, however, that the first ordering is much simpler than the second (see Exercise 4.5).

To sample from the PPD $p(\widetilde{y} \mid \boldsymbol{y})$, we could directly sample from a $t_{n-1}\left[\overline{y}, s^2\left(1+\frac{1}{n}\right)\right]$-distribution or use the Method of Composition. To sample K values from the PPD using the Method of Composition, the following three steps are repeated for $k = 1, \ldots, K$:

1. Sample $(\widetilde{\sigma}^2)^k$ from $\text{Inv-}\chi^2(\sigma^2 \mid n-1, s^2)$
2. Sample $\widetilde{\mu}_k$ from $\text{N}(\mu \mid \overline{y}, (\widetilde{\sigma}^2)^k/n)$
3. Sample $\widetilde{y}_k$ from $\text{N}(y \mid \widetilde{\mu}_k, (\widetilde{\sigma}^2)^k)$

The above sampling procedure is applied to the *alp* data analyzed using the analytical results in Example IV.1.

Example IV.5: Serum alkaline phosphatase study: Sampling the posterior – non-informative prior
Sampling from the joint posterior distribution can be done with the Method of Composition. In Figure 4.3, the sampled posterior distributions are based on $K = 1000$ values. The estimate for the posterior mean (95% CI) based on the sample are for μ: 7.11 ([7.106, 7.117]) and for σ^2: 1.88 ([1.869, 1.890]). The CIs show that these posterior summary measures have been determined with high accuracy. If higher accuracy is needed, one simply increases K.

The 95% equal tail CI for μ is equal to [6.95, 7.27] and for σ^2 equal to [1.58, 2.23]. Again the estimated interval estimators are quite close to the true posterior intervals. For the derivation of the PPD using sampling, see Exercise 4.5. □

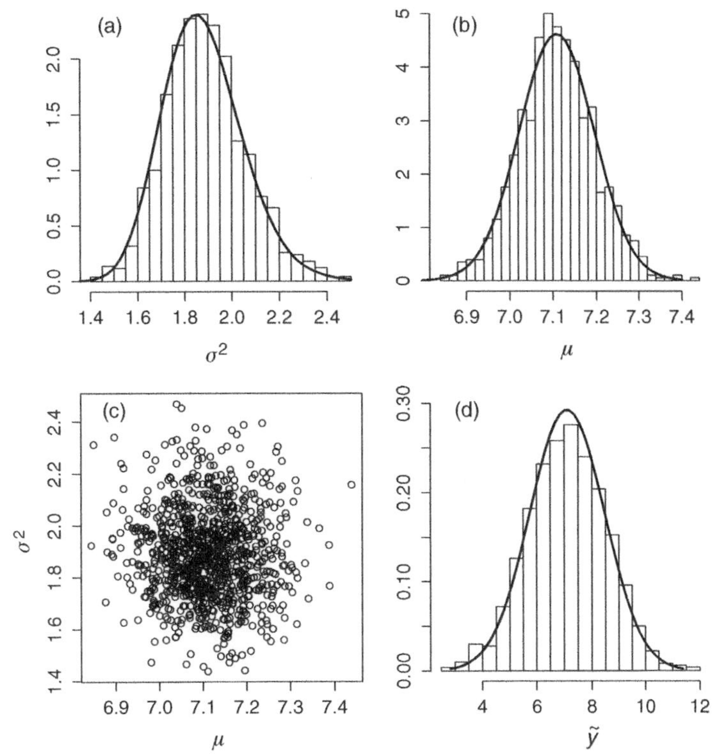

Figure 4.3 Serum alkaline phosphatase study (noninformative prior): sampled posterior distributions for (a) σ^2; (b) μ; (c) μ and σ^2; and (d) future observation $\widetilde{y}$. The solid lines are the true posterior distributions.

Case 2: Historical data are available

The Method of Composition works in exactly the same way as for the noninformative prior with the appropriate change in the parameters of the posterior distribution (see also Example IV.6).

Case 3: Expert knowledge is available

The same sampling procedure could be followed as in the previous two cases. However, $p(\sigma^2 \mid \mathbf{y})$ is not a known distribution because of the nonconjugacy of the prior. Hence, sampling cannot be done using standard routines. We could use expression (4.19) and then the sampling algorithms of Section III.12 will do the job. Then, for a given $\widetilde{\sigma}^2$, sampling $\widetilde{\mu}$ is straightforward using expression (4.18).

Example IV.6: Serum alkaline phosphatase study: Sampling the posterior – product of informative priors

In Section 4.3.3, we have based the prior distributions on the historical *alp* data. That is, the prior distributions for $y = 100/\sqrt{alp}$ are

$$\mu \sim \mathrm{N}(\overline{y}_0, s_0^2/n_0) \;\text{ and }\; \sigma^2 \sim \mathrm{Inv} - \chi^2(n_0 - 1, s_0^2).$$

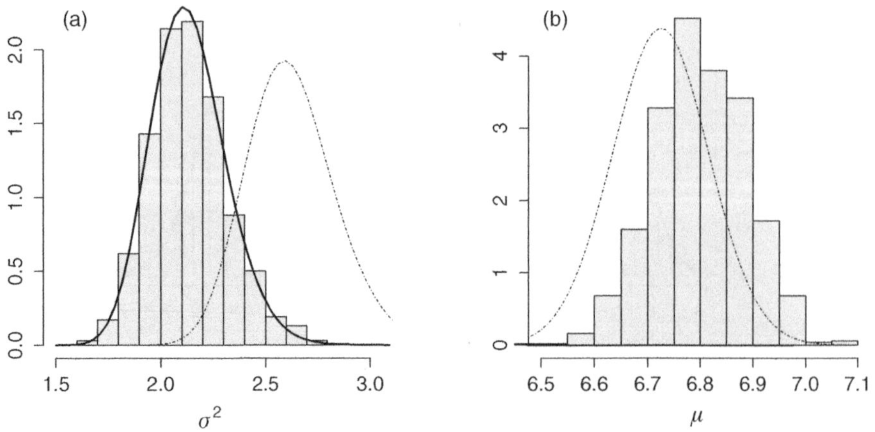

Figure 4.4 Serum alkaline phosphatase study (product of informative marginal conjugate prior distributions): sampled marginal posterior distributions for (a) σ^2 and (b) μ. The solid line corresponds to the standardized version of expression (4.19). The dashed lines correspond to the joint conjugate normal-scaled-inverse-chi-squared prior distribution with corresponding parameters.

With the notation of Section 4.3.3, we have $\mu_0 = \overline{y}_0 = 5.25$, $\nu_0 = n_0 - 1 = 64$, $\sigma_0^2 = s_0^2/n_0 = 0.042$ and $\tau_0^2 = s_0^2 = 2.75$.

To apply the Method of Composition, a sampling procedure is needed to draw from expression (4.19). One possibility is to use the weighted resampling method of Section 3.7.2. This method needs an approximating distribution to expression (4.19). To this end, we evaluated expression (4.19) on a grid and calculated the mean and variance. An excellent approximating distribution $q(\sigma^2)$ is the scaled inverse-chi-squared distribution with the same mean and variance, i.e. the $\text{Inv} - \chi^2(\sigma^2 \mid 294.2, 2.12)$. In Figure 4.4, we show the sampled marginal posterior distributions for σ^2 and μ. For both parameters, the marginal posterior distribution is contrasted with the conjugate marginal posterior distribution.

From the difference in posterior distributions (independent priors versus conjugate prior) shown in Figure 4.4, it is clear that the two priors are quite different although they are based on the same historical data.

The PPD is obtained by sampling $\widetilde{y}$ from $\text{N}(\widetilde{\mu}, \widetilde{\sigma}^2)$. The distribution of $\widetilde{y}$ gives an estimate of the 95% normal range for *y*: [4.05, 9.67] and for *alp*: [106.84, 609.70]. □

4.7 Bayesian linear regression models

4.7.1 The frequentist approach to linear regression

The normal linear regression model assumes a linear relationship between a response *y* and *d* regressors $x_1, x_2, \ldots, x_d$. For a sample of *n* subjects, this model is given by

$$y_i = \boldsymbol{x}_i^T \boldsymbol{\beta} + \varepsilon_i, \ \ (i = 1, \ldots, n), \tag{4.24}$$

with $\boldsymbol{\beta}^T = (\beta_0, \beta_1, \ldots, \beta_d)$, $\boldsymbol{x}_i^T = (1, x_{i1}, \ldots, x_{id})$, and $\varepsilon_i \sim \mathrm{N}(0, \sigma^2)$. In matrix notation, the classical normal linear regression model is written as

$$\boldsymbol{y} = \boldsymbol{X}\boldsymbol{\beta} + \boldsymbol{\varepsilon}, \tag{4.25}$$

with $\boldsymbol{y}$ the $n \times 1$ vector of responses, $\boldsymbol{X}$ the $n \times (d+1)$ design matrix with rows $\boldsymbol{x}_i^T$ and $\boldsymbol{\varepsilon}$ the $n \times 1$ vector of random errors assuming $\mathrm{N}(\boldsymbol{0}, \sigma^2 \mathrm{I})$, with I the $n \times n$ identity matrix. Under these assumptions, the likelihood is

$$L(\boldsymbol{\beta}, \sigma^2 \mid \boldsymbol{y}, \boldsymbol{X}) = \frac{1}{(2\pi\sigma^2)^{n/2}} \exp\left[-\frac{1}{2\sigma^2}(\boldsymbol{y} - \boldsymbol{X}\boldsymbol{\beta})^T(\boldsymbol{y} - \boldsymbol{X}\boldsymbol{\beta})\right]. \tag{4.26}$$

The classical (frequentist) estimate of $\boldsymbol{\beta}$ is the maximum likelihood estimate (MLE) (also equal to least-squares estimate (LSE)) $\widehat{\boldsymbol{\beta}} = (\boldsymbol{X}^T\boldsymbol{X})^{-1}\boldsymbol{X}\boldsymbol{y}$. Further, the residual variability of the observed responses to the fitted responses is expressed by $S = (\boldsymbol{y} - \boldsymbol{X}\boldsymbol{\beta})^T(\boldsymbol{y} - \boldsymbol{X}\boldsymbol{\beta})$, which is called the residual sum of squares. The mean residual sum of squares is $s^2 = S/(n - d - 1)$.

Example IV.7: Osteoporosis study: A frequentist linear regression analysis
A cross-sectional study was set up (Boonen *et al.* 1996) to examine 245 healthy elderly women in a geriatric hospital in order to find determinants for osteoporosis. Osteoporosis is a disease whereby the bone mineral density is reduced so that the bones become fragile. In this study, the average age of the women was 75 years with a range of 70–90 years.

The marker for osteoporosis is total body bone mineral content (TBBMC, in kg), measured for 234 women with dual-energy X-ray absorptiometry. In the original analysis, the regression model contained many regressors, most of which were known determinants. Here, the purpose is to illustrate the use of a Bayesian regression model. Therefore, a simple regression model with only body–mass index (BMI, in kg/m^2) as determinant is considered here. Regressing TBBMC on BMI with a classical frequentist regression analysis gives the following estimates (SE): $\widehat{\beta_0} = 0.813(0.12)$ and $\widehat{\beta_1} = 0.0404(0.0043)$, both highly significant and $s^2 = 0.29$, with $n - d - 1 = 232$; see Figure 4.5 for a graphical depiction of the relationship. The estimated correlation of the $\widehat{\beta_0}$ and $\widehat{\beta_1}$ is -0.99, which is quite high indicating some kind of collinearity problem. □

4.7.2 A noninformative Bayesian linear regression model

A Bayesian regression linear model combines prior information on the regression parameters and residual variance with the above-derived normal regression likelihood. Again prior information may be noninformative as well as informative. Here, we primarily treat the noninformative case.

A common choice for the noninformative prior for $(\boldsymbol{\beta}, \sigma^2)$ is $p(\boldsymbol{\beta}, \sigma^2) \propto \sigma^{-2}$; see Section 5.6 for a motivation. All models are conditional on the design matrix $\boldsymbol{X}$, and therefore, $\boldsymbol{X}$ will be omitted in the notation of the posterior. The joint posterior distribution is $(d+2)$-dimensional: $(d+1)$ dimensions pertain to the regression parameters $\boldsymbol{\beta}$ and one dimension pertains to the residual variance σ^2. With the above choice of the noninformative prior, the posterior distributions become (see Box and Tiao (1973) for mathematical derivations)

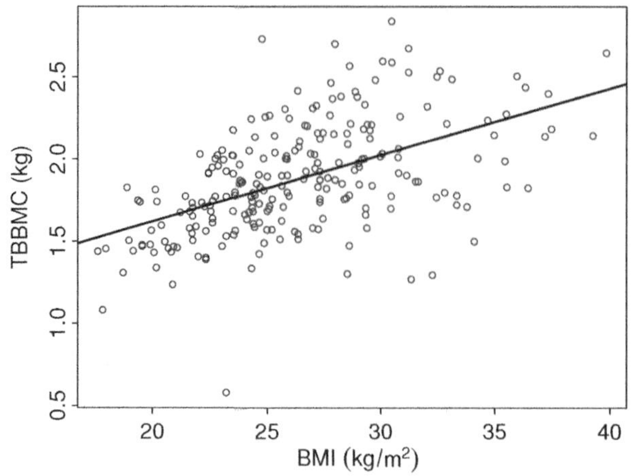

Figure 4.5 Osteoporosis study: scatterplot of TBBMC versus BMI together with the regression line obtained from a frequentist regression analysis.

$$p(\boldsymbol{\beta}, \sigma^2 \mid \boldsymbol{y}) = \mathrm{N}_{d+1}\left[\boldsymbol{\beta} \mid \widehat{\boldsymbol{\beta}}, \sigma^2(\boldsymbol{X}^T\boldsymbol{X})^{-1}\right] \times \mathrm{Inv}-\chi^2(\sigma^2 \mid n-d-1, s^2), \quad (4.27)$$

$$p(\boldsymbol{\beta} \mid \sigma^2, \boldsymbol{y}) = \mathrm{N}_{d+1}\left[\boldsymbol{\beta} \mid \widehat{\boldsymbol{\beta}}, \sigma^2(\boldsymbol{X}^T\boldsymbol{X})^{-1}\right], \quad (4.28)$$

$$p(\sigma^2 \mid \boldsymbol{y}) = \mathrm{Inv}-\chi^2(\sigma^2 \mid n-d-1, s^2), \quad (4.29)$$

$$p(\boldsymbol{\beta} \mid \boldsymbol{y}) = T_{n-d-1}\left[\boldsymbol{\beta} \mid \widehat{\boldsymbol{\beta}}, s^2(\boldsymbol{X}^T\boldsymbol{X})^{-1}\right], \quad (4.30)$$

with $\widehat{\boldsymbol{\beta}}$ the LSE of the regression vector. The marginal posterior distribution of $\boldsymbol{\beta}$ is a $(d+1)$-dimensional t-distribution with $(n-d-1)$ degrees of freedom and mean vector $\widehat{\boldsymbol{\beta}}$ and scale of the matrix $s^2(\boldsymbol{X}^T\boldsymbol{X})^{-1}$. Its jth marginal distribution is a univariate t_{n-d-1}-distribution with location $\widehat{\beta}_j$ and scale $s(\boldsymbol{X}^T\boldsymbol{X})_{jj}^{-1/2}$.

4.7.3 Posterior summary measures for the linear regression model

The posterior summary measures of the $(d+2)$-dimensional posterior distribution (4.27) split up into posterior summary measures for (a) the vector of regression parameters $\boldsymbol{\beta}$ and (b) the parameter of residual variability, σ^2. For σ^2, the posterior summary measures of Chapter 3 can be used and are derived from expression (4.29). When interest lies in each of the regression parameters separately, the marginal posterior summary statistics can be calculated from the marginal t-distributions derived from expression (4.30). On the other hand, when interest lies in the total vector of regression parameters, the multivariate posterior summary measures are based on the $(d+1)$-dimensional marginal posterior (4.30). In that case, multivariate posterior summary measures are needed.

In the case of the NI prior $p(\boldsymbol{\beta}, \sigma^2) \propto \sigma^{-2}$, the following univariate posterior summary measures can be derived from the above marginal posterior distributions (Box and Tiao 1973):

- The marginal posterior mean (mode, median) of β_j $(j = 0, \ldots, d)$ is equal to the classical MLE (LSE) $\widehat{\beta}_j$. The 95% HPD interval for β_j is given by $\widehat{\beta}_j \pm$

$s(X^TX)_{jj}^{-1/2}t(0.025, n-d-1)$ $(j = 0, \ldots, d)$, with $t(0.025, n-d-1)$ the 97.5% quantile of the t_{n-d-1}-distribution.

- The marginal posterior mode of σ^2 is equal to $\frac{n-d-1}{n-d+1}s^2$, and thus not equal to the MLE of σ^2. The posterior mean of σ^2 is equal to $\frac{n-d-1}{n-d-3}s^2$. The 95% HPD-interval for σ^2 is determined from the $\text{Inv}-\chi^2(n-d-1, s^2)$-distribution involving a computational algorithm.

The multivariate posterior summary measures on $\boldsymbol{\beta}$ are based on the marginal posterior distribution (4.30):

- The posterior mean (mode) of $\boldsymbol{\beta}$ is equal to the LSE $\widehat{\boldsymbol{\beta}}$.
- The $100(1-\alpha)\%$-HPD region is a generalization of the $100(1-\alpha)\%$-HPD interval to the multivariate setting and corresponds here to the set:

$$C_\alpha(\boldsymbol{\beta}) = \left\{\boldsymbol{\beta} : (\boldsymbol{\beta} - \widehat{\boldsymbol{\beta}})^T(X^TX)(\boldsymbol{\beta} - \widehat{\boldsymbol{\beta}}) \le d\, s^2 F_\alpha(d+1, n-d-1)\right\}, \quad (4.31)$$

with $F_\alpha(d+1, n-d-1)$ the $100(1-\alpha)\%$ quantile of the $F_{d+1,n-d-1}$-distribution.

- The contour probability introduced in Section 3.8.1 for one parameter can be generalized to a vector of parameters. Letting $H_0 : \boldsymbol{\beta} = \boldsymbol{\beta}_0$, one can determine the HPD-region for $\boldsymbol{\beta}$ with $\boldsymbol{\beta}_0$ on the edge. When the volume of that HPD-region is $1-\alpha_0$, then the contour probability for $\boldsymbol{\beta}_0$ is equal to α_0.

The PPD of a future observation $\widetilde{y}$ with covariate vector $\widetilde{\boldsymbol{x}}$ is a t_{n-d-1}-distribution with location parameter $\widetilde{\boldsymbol{x}}^T\widehat{\boldsymbol{\beta}}$ and scale parameter $s^2\left[1 + \widetilde{\boldsymbol{x}}^T(X^TX)^{-1}\widetilde{\boldsymbol{x}}\right]$. This is equivalent to, given $\boldsymbol{y}$,

$$\frac{\widetilde{y} - \widetilde{\boldsymbol{x}}^T\widehat{\boldsymbol{\beta}}}{s\sqrt{1 + \widetilde{\boldsymbol{x}}^T(X^TX)^{-1}\widetilde{\boldsymbol{x}}}} \sim t_{n-d-1}. \quad (4.32)$$

For a vector of future observations $\widetilde{\boldsymbol{y}}$ with design matrix $\widetilde{X}$ the PPD is a T_{n-d-1}-distribution with mean $\widetilde{X}^T\widehat{\boldsymbol{\beta}}$ and squared scale matrix $s^2\left[\mathrm{I} + \widetilde{X}(X^TX)^{-1}\widetilde{X}^T\right]$.

On the other hand, the conditional distribution of $\widetilde{\boldsymbol{y}}$ given σ^2 is a normal distribution with mean $\widetilde{X}^T\widehat{\boldsymbol{\beta}}$ and variance $\sigma^2\left[\mathrm{I} + \widetilde{X}(X^TX)^{-1}\widetilde{X}^T\right]$. This result can be used to sample future observations using the Method of Composition.

Note that we now have another example where the frequentist results coincide with the Bayesian results, of course, with the obvious difference in interpretation. Consequently, in the noninformative case, credible intervals for the linear regression model have the correct coverage.

4.7.4 Sampling from the posterior distribution

Expressions (4.27), (4.28) and (4.29) enable the use of the Method of Composition for sampling from the joint posterior distribution (4.27). The advantage of the Method of Composition for sampling from the marginal posterior distribution of the regression coefficients is now striking. Indeed, since $p(\boldsymbol{\beta} \mid \boldsymbol{y})$ is a multivariate t-distribution, sampling from this distribution is more complicated (although R functions, such as mvtnorm exist). With the

Method of Composition, the sampling is done in two relatively easy steps. Note that the R function rmvt (in mvtnorm) generates multivariate t-distributed random variables.

We illustrate, below, sampling from a Bayesian linear regression model using the osteoporosis study.

Example IV.8: Osteoporosis study: Sampling from the posterior using the Method of Composition

We consider the regression problem introduced in Example IV.7. The Method of Composition works in two steps. First, sample $\widetilde{\sigma}^2$ from expression (4.29). Given $\widetilde{\sigma}^2$, sample from $\widetilde{\boldsymbol{\beta}}$ from expression (4.28) with σ^2 replaced by $\widetilde{\sigma}^2$. In this way, we sampled 1000 observations from the marginal posterior distribution of β_0 and β_1. The histograms of the sampled values are shown in Figures 4.6(a) and (b). The sampled mean regression vector is equal to (0.816, 0.0403), which is quite close to the true posterior mean. The 95% equal tail CIs are for β_0: [0.594, 1.040] and for β_1: [0.0317, 0.0486]. The contour probabilities for $H_0 : \boldsymbol{\beta} = \mathbf{0}$ are determined using sampling and all result in very small probabilities (<0.001) (see also Exercise 4.9).

In Figure 4.6(c), one can observe that the marginal posterior of (β_0, β_1) has a ridge, i.e. β_0 and β_1 are highly correlated a posteriori which is also reflected in the high correlation of -0.99 between the LSEs of the regression coefficients, as computed in Example IV.5.

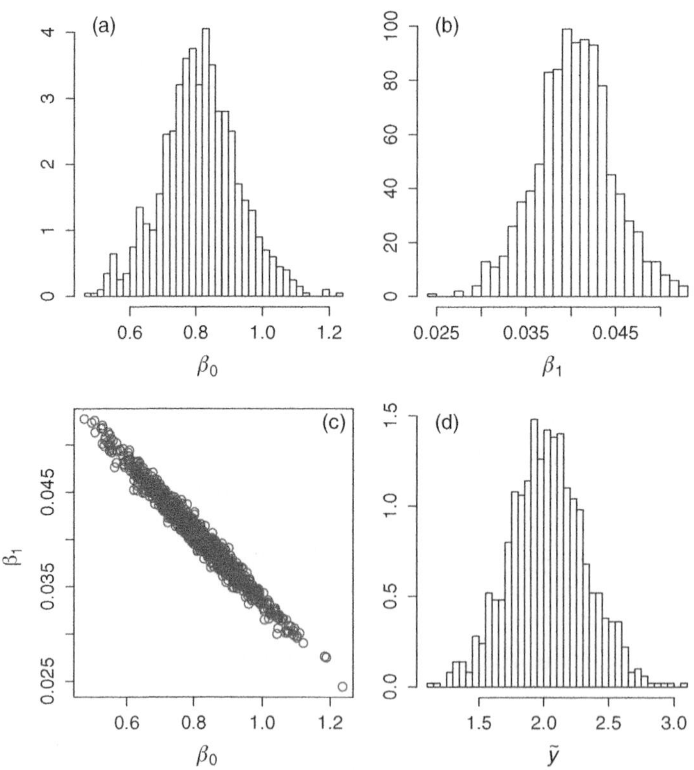

Figure 4.6 Osteoporosis study (noninformative prior): sampled posterior distributions for (a) β_0; (b) β_1; (c) β_0 and β_1; and (d) future observation $\widetilde{y}$ with BMI = 30.

The distribution of a future observation at BMI $= 30$ can be generated by another round of sampling, i.e. based on the sampled $\widetilde{\sigma}^2$, $\widetilde{\beta}_0$ and $\widetilde{\beta}_1$, the future observation $\widetilde{y}$ is obtained from sampling from $\mathrm{N}(\widetilde{\mu}_{30}, \widetilde{\sigma}^2_{30})$, where $\widetilde{\mu}_{30} = \widetilde{\boldsymbol{\beta}}^T(1, 30)$ and $\widetilde{\sigma}^2_{30} = \widetilde{\sigma}^2\left[1 + (1, 30)(\boldsymbol{X}^T\boldsymbol{X})^{-1}(1, 30)^T\right]$. The histogram of sampled values is shown in Figure 4.6(d). The sampled mean and standard deviation are equal to 2.033 and 0.282, respectively. □

Note that simultaneous HPD regions based on Monte Carlo samples can be derived using the approach of Held (2004).

4.7.5 An informative Bayesian linear regression model

Information from historical studies can be reformulated into a prior distribution. This has been shown for the normal distribution in Section 4.3.2. In a similar manner, a normal-inverse-gamma prior (see Section 5.3.2) can be deduced from past data. Another source for prior information is 'expert knowledge'. However, it must be admitted that turning expert knowledge on a regression model into a reasonable prior is not a trivial task. For instance, it is nonsensical to elicit prior information about a single regression coefficient β_j since the value of β_j depends on what other regressors are in the model. In Section 5.5.3, possible ways of shaping expert knowledge into a conjugate prior are described.

4.8 Bayesian generalized linear models

A *generalized linear model* (*GLIM*) provides an extension of the linear regression model to a wide class of regression models. Formally, a GLIM is composed of three parts: (1) a distributional part, (2) a link function, and (3) a variance function. In the classical notation (McCullagh and Nelder 1989), the three parts of a GLIM are as follows:

- *Distributional part*: Let y be a random variable with density

$$p(y \mid \theta; \phi) = \exp\left[\frac{y\theta - b(\theta)}{a(\phi)} + c(y; \phi)\right], \tag{4.33}$$

  with $a(\cdot)$, $b(\cdot)$ and $c(\cdot)$ known functions. Often $a(\phi) = \phi/w$, with w a prior weight. For ϕ known and $w = 1$, one can show that

  $-E(y) = \mu = \frac{d\,b(\theta)}{d\theta}$;

  $-\mathrm{var}(y) = a(\phi)V(\mu)$ with $V(\mu) = \frac{d^2\,b(\theta)}{d^2\theta}$.

- *Link function*: The mean μ is related to covariates via a monotone (differentiable) function g, i.e. $g(\mu) = \eta = \boldsymbol{x}^T\boldsymbol{\beta}$. When $\eta = \theta$, the link function is called *canonical*. One also works with the inverse function $h = g^{-1}$. For a binary response model, e.g. logistic or probit regression, h represents a cumulative distribution function.

- *Variance function*: The parameter ϕ plays the role of an 'extra' dispersion or 'scale' parameter in $\mathrm{var}(y) = a(\phi)V(\mu)$. This expression also shows that the variance can depend on covariates via μ.

Note that the distributional part of a GLIM is an example of the one-parameter exponential family (5.1) expressed in the canonical parameter, but we used a different notation from that in Section 5.3.1.

For a sample of independent observations y_i ($i = 1, \ldots, n$) the GLIM is defined by $p(y_i \mid \theta_i; \phi)$, $E(y_i) = \mu_i$ and $g(\mu_i) = \boldsymbol{x}_i^T \boldsymbol{\beta}$. Examples of a GLIM are (a) the normal linear regression model with a normal distribution $y_i \sim \mathrm{N}(\mu_i, \sigma^2)$, the identity link ($g(\mu_i) = \mu_i$), $\phi = 1$ and $V(\mu_i) = \sigma^2$ assumed known; (b) the Poisson regression model with the Poisson distribution $y_i \sim \mathrm{Poisson}(\mu_i)$, the log link ($g(\mu_i) = \log(\mu_i)$), $\phi = 1$ and $V(\mu_i) = \mu_i$ and (c) the logistic regression model with the Bernoulli (or Binomial) distribution $y_i \sim \mathrm{Bern}(\mu_i)$, the logistic link ($g(\mu_i) = \mathrm{logit}(\mu_i)$), $\phi = 1$ and $V(\mu_i) = \mu_i(1 - \mu_i)$.

Binary response models, especially logistic regression models, constitute the most important subclass of GLIMs in medical applications and hence received the most attention in the literature.

A BGLIM is obtained by providing a prior distribution to all parameters of the GLIM. However, we defer the discussion of GLIM priors to Chapter 5. We also defer numerical examples of Bayesian analyses of GLIMs to later chapters.

4.9 More complex regression models

BGLIMs constitute an important class of regression models, but are by no means sufficient to cover all models needed in practice. Models are required that deal with censoring, truncation, random effects, etc. Almost invariably there will be no analytical solutions for the posterior distribution such that at most some (ad hoc) numericals allow the computation of the posterior summary measures. Gelman *et al.* (2004) explored a variety of such numerical procedures, but to really advance in practice, a more general methodology is needed.

4.10 Closing remarks

This chapter ends before it becomes interesting to the applied statistician, i.e. when tackling nontrivial statistical problems. The reason is that without a powerful numerical framework, it is not really possible to do Bayesian statistical modeling. Currently, almost the only available approach is via complicated sampling techniques, that are provided by Markov chain Monte Carlo methods treated in Chapter 6.

Exercises

Exercise 4.1 Show that when $W_{ij} (i, j = 1, 2)$ are distributed independently as Gamma(α_{ij}, 1) and $T = \sum_{ij} W_{ij}$, then $Z_{ij} = W_{ij}/T$ has a Dir($\boldsymbol{\alpha}$) distribution.

Exercise 4.2 Show by sampling that the noninformative Dirichlet prior Dir(1,1,1,1) corresponds to an approximately normal prior for $\log(\psi)$ with mean zero and SD = 2.6.

Exercise 4.3 Determine in Example IV.4, the contour probability for $H_0 : \theta_1 = \theta_2$ by making use of sampling.

Exercise 4.4 Use the Method of Composition to sample from (a) a mixture of normal distributions and (b) from a t-distribution via sampling from normal distributions. Write an R program to illustrate your procedures.

Exercise 4.5 Serum alkaline phosphatase study: use the Method of Composition to sample from the posterior distributions based on a noninformative prior using an R program based on the data in 'alp.txt'. Sample also from the PPD.

Exercise 4.6 Serum alkaline phosphatase study: reverse the order of sampling in Exercise 4.5. That is, sample first μ and then σ^2.

Exercise 4.7 Serum alkaline phosphatase study: use the Method of Composition to sample from the posterior distributions based on the prior using historical data, as described in Example IV.2. Employ for this an R program and use the data in 'alp.txt'.

Exercise 4.8 Osteoporosis study: based on the data in 'osteop.txt' apply the analytical results of Section 4.7.3 on a regression with response TBBMC and regressors BMI and age.

Exercise 4.9 Osteoporosis study: use the Method of Composition to sample from the regression model specified in Exercise 4.8. Determine via sampling the contour probabilities that the regression parameters are equal to zero.

Exercise 4.10 Osteoporosis study: show that β_0 and β_1 are independent a posteriori in the regression model regressing TBBMC on BMI–$\overline{\text{BMI}}$, with $\overline{\text{BMI}}$, the sample mean of BMI. Use an R program for this.

Exercise 4.11 Serum alkaline phosphatase study: explain why the reference range calculated in Example IV.1 is wider than that obtained in Example III.6.

5

Choosing the prior distribution

5.1 Introduction

Incorporating prior knowledge in a statistical analysis is to its proponents a unique feature that makes the Bayesian approach attractive for empirical research. To its critics, the necessity of specifying a prior makes the Bayesian approach unsuitable for research because of the possible introduction of subjectivity. This split in opinion, which was quite dominant up to a few decades ago, is still a point of discussion nowadays and is likely to remain. This has been addressed in the previous chapters at several occasions. Even among Bayesians, there is a different opinion about the nature of the prior, namely should we strive for an objective or for a subjective prior? Other aspects pertaining to the prior have been introduced in passing, such as conjugacy and the choice of a noninformative prior. In this chapter, our aim is to treat the prior in a more systematic manner. We first treat in generality the three classes of priors: conjugate, noninformative and informative. Since regression models constitute an important class of models requiring a more specific treatment, we will treat these at the end of the chapter.

We start with the sequential nature of Bayes theorem, showing that the Bayesian approach can imitate the process of acquiring knowledge in life.

5.2 The sequential use of Bayes theorem

When a series of independent experiments are performed, at each step the Bayesian approach allows us to use the knowledge gathered in the previous step as a prior for the next step. Namely, the posterior of a parameter obtained in the kth experiment can be used as a prior for that parameter in the $(k+1)$th experiment. The argument for two experiments goes as follows. When $\boldsymbol{y}_k$ represents the data collected in the kth ($k = 1, 2$) experiment, then $p(\theta \mid \boldsymbol{y}_1, \boldsymbol{y}_2) \propto L(\theta \mid \boldsymbol{y}_1, \boldsymbol{y}_2)\, p(\theta) = L(\theta \mid \boldsymbol{y}_1)L(\theta \mid \boldsymbol{y}_2)p(\theta) \propto p(\theta \mid \boldsymbol{y}_1)L(\theta \mid \boldsymbol{y}_2)$, with the first equality obtained as a result of the independence of the two experiments. This shows that the Bayesian approach can mimic our human learning process, i.e. as new information rolls in we combine it with our knowledge obtained from the past. Further, because for m independent experiments

Bayesian Biostatistics, First Edition. Emmanuel Lesaffre and Andrew B. Lawson.

$p(\theta \mid \boldsymbol{y}_1, \ldots, \boldsymbol{y}_m) \propto \prod_{k=1}^{m} L(\theta \mid \boldsymbol{y}_k) p(\theta)$ our initial prior knowledge becomes unimportant when m is large and the prior will be *dominated by the data*. Note that we have assumed above that the experiments were done under identical conditions. The sequential rule still remains true when the experiments have been done under not too grossly different conditions. In that case, the prior for each step can be adapted to allow for the change in condition (see Section 5.5).

Example V.1: Analysis of Ames/Salmonella mutagenic assay data

A mutagen is an agent that is capable of effecting heritable change in genetic material, from one specific DNA base-pair to the chromosome level. Mutagens may exert their effects on germ cells, thereby altering the human gene pool and possibly inducing heritable genetic defects in future generations. To date, there is no evidence of induced heritable genetic damage in humans, but ascertainment of these effects is difficult. It has been demonstrated repeatedly in laboratory animals, however. Mutagens that attack somatic cells may ultimately be implicated in heart disease, aging and developmental birth defects. Finally, there is growing evidence for the role of mutagens in carcinogenesis (see Margolin *et al.* 1989).

The Ames Salmonella/microsome assay was developed to detect mutagenicity. It is used widely in preclinical screening of drug compounds. The Ames test is founded on the existence of auxotrophic and prototrophic strains of *Salmonella typhimurium*. The latter have the property of synthesizing histidine, an amino acid essential for microbial growth. The former cannot grow in an histidine-free environment. The auxotrophic strain can back-mutate and revert to histidine independence. The resulting revertant and its descendants can give rise to cell division until a colony emerges.

In an Ames test, the response from a single plate is the number of visible colonies that result from plating 10^8 microbes. Usually, triplicate plates are examined. For a given condition (dose level), there will be $r \times 3$ plates where r is the replication used. Margolin *et al.* (1989) presents data for an assay of Quinoline where $r = 3$ given in Table 5.1. These data are further analyzed in Chapter 12.

The first replication yields $\boldsymbol{y}_1 = \{15, 21, 29\}$, the second $\boldsymbol{y}_2 = \{19, 21, 24\}$, and the third $\boldsymbol{y}_3 = \{14, 19, 22\}$. The replication of the experiment is made in a sequence (1, 2, 3) and so we have a sequence of experiments that can lead to the sequential Bayesian learning about the assay outcome.

The Poisson distribution might be assumed as the distribution for the counts, but it has been found that it does not provide a good fit to the data. In fact, it appears that the mean of the Poisson distribution does not remain fixed over the counts but has a distribution. A common assumption is then to take a Gamma(α, β) distribution for the mean. Initially the prior distribution would be noninformative and we could assume $\alpha = 0.5$ and $\beta = 0.025$, which gives a prior mean for the gamma distribution of 20 but with a very large variance of

Table 5.1 Quinoline assay counts: revertant counts obtained from the Ames test.

Replication	Revertant count		
1	15	21	29
2	19	21	24
3	14	19	22

800. For the first experiment, the likelihood is

$$L(\mathbf{y}_1 \mid \theta) = \prod_{i=1}^{3} \theta^{y_{i1}} \mathrm{e}^{-\theta} / y_{i1}!,$$

where y_{i1}, $(i = 1, 2, 3)$ denote the data from the first experiment. The posterior distribution is Gamma$(\Sigma y_{i1} + \alpha, 3 + \beta)$ after seeing $\mathbf{y}_1$, so that the posterior mean is $(\Sigma y_{i1} + \alpha)/(3 + \beta) = 21.653$. This is close to the maximum likelihood estimator equal to 21.667.

With the inclusion of the second replication, we can use the posterior distribution from the first replication as our prior distribution for the second. Hence, the posterior distribution for the second replication is Gamma$(\Sigma y_{i2} + 65.5, 3 + 3.025)$ = Gamma(129.5, 6.025) with mean 21.494. For the third replication, $\Sigma y_{i3} = 55$, and so the posterior mean is 20.443, which is very close to the maximum likelihood estimator for the full set of replications, and this demonstrates the gradual dominance of the data over the prior distribution as more data are collected. □

The adjective *prior* in 'prior distribution' gives the impression that it should be defined before data have been collected, but this is not true. The term 'prior' means only that the prior knowledge should be specified independent of the collected data (Cox 1999). The situation is different for comparative clinical trials. In that case, the recommended strategy is to fix the prior distribution in advance in order to avoid possible contamination with gathered data. We address this approach in Section 5.5.4. Finally, note that in the first step of this sequential process the prior could represent minimal information (noninformative prior), but in the second step the prior will always be informative.

5.3 Conjugate prior distributions

An important class of prior distributions is the conjugate family first proposed by Raiffa and Schlaifer (Mc Grayne 2011, p. 125). Conjugate priors can be informative and noninformative and therefore could be treated also in next sections. However, in this section we focus on the technical aspects of specifying a conjugate prior distribution.

5.3.1 Univariate data distributions

In Chapter 2, a binomial likelihood was combined with a beta prior resulting in a beta posterior. Also for the normal likelihood (with σ assumed known or unknown) and the Poisson likelihood, the prior distributions yielded posterior distributions of the same type. This property is called *closed under sampling*. More specifically, suppose that for a random variable y, $p(y \mid \boldsymbol{\theta})$ is a distribution or a density (depending on the nature of y) for a given parameter vector $\boldsymbol{\theta} = (\theta_1, \ldots, \theta_d)^T$, then the family $\Im$ of priors is closed under sampling if for every prior distribution $p(\boldsymbol{\theta}) \in \Im$, the posterior distribution $p(\boldsymbol{\theta} \mid y)$ also belongs to $\Im$.

For an important class of distributions, there exists a recipe of how to choose the class of priors that is closed under sampling. Suppose that $p(y \mid \boldsymbol{\theta})$ belongs to the *exponential family* with distribution

$$p(y \mid \boldsymbol{\theta}) = b(y) \exp\left[c(\boldsymbol{\theta})^T \boldsymbol{t}(y) + \mathrm{d}(\boldsymbol{\theta})\right], \tag{5.1}$$

Table 5.2 Common members of the exponential family and their associated (natural) conjugate prior.

Exponential family member		Parameter	Conjugate prior
	Univariate case		
	Discrete distributions		
Bernoulli	Bern(θ)	θ	Beta(α_0, β_0)
Binomial	Bin(n, θ)	θ	Beta(α_0, β_0)
Negative binomial	NB(k, θ)	θ	Beta(α_0, β_0)
Poisson	Poisson(θ)	θ	Gamma(α_0, β_0)
	Continuous distributions		
Normal-variance fixed	N(μ, σ^2)-σ^2 fixed	μ	N(μ_0, σ_0^2)
Normal-mean fixed	N(μ, σ^2)-μ fixed	μ	IG(α_0, β_0) Inv-$\chi^2(\nu_0, \tau_0^2)$
Normal*	N(μ, σ^2)	μ, σ^2	NIG($\mu_0, \kappa_0, a_0, b_0$) N-Inv-$\chi^2(\mu_0, \kappa_0, \nu_0, \tau_0^2)$
Exponential	Exp(λ)	λ	Gamma(α_0, β_0)
	Multivariate case		
	Discrete distributions		
Multinomial	Mult($n, \boldsymbol{\theta}$)	$\boldsymbol{\theta}$	Dirichlet($\boldsymbol{\alpha}_0$)
	Continuous distributions		
Normal-covariance fixed	N($\boldsymbol{\mu}, \Sigma$)-Σ fixed	$\boldsymbol{\mu}$	N($\boldsymbol{\mu}_0, \Sigma_0$)
Normal-mean fixed	N($\boldsymbol{\mu}, \Sigma$)-$\boldsymbol{\mu}$ fixed	Σ	IW(Λ_0, ν_0)
Normal*	N($\boldsymbol{\mu}, \Sigma$)	$\boldsymbol{\mu}, \Sigma$	NIW($\boldsymbol{\mu}_0, \kappa_0, \nu_0, \Lambda_0$)

IG, inverse-gamma distribution; Inv-χ^2, scaled inverse-chi-squared distribution;
NIG, normal-inverse-gamma distribution; N-Inv-χ^2, normal-scaled-inverse-chi-squared distribution;
IW, inverse Wishart distribution; NIW, normal inverse Wishart distribution.

The distributions indicated with * are an extension of the natural conjugate distribution (O'Hagan and Forster 2004, pp. 140–141).

with $\mathrm{d}(\boldsymbol{\theta})$ is a scalar function of $\boldsymbol{\theta}$, $b(y)$ a scalar function of y, $\boldsymbol{t}(y)$ the d-dimensional sufficient statistic for $\boldsymbol{\theta}$ and $\boldsymbol{c}(\boldsymbol{\theta}) = (c_1(\boldsymbol{\theta}), \ldots, c_d(\boldsymbol{\theta}))^T$. The vector $\boldsymbol{\theta}$ is called the *canonical parameter*. For a random sample, $\boldsymbol{y} = \{y_1, \ldots, y_n\}$ of i.i.d. elements expression (5.1) is replaced by

$$p(\boldsymbol{y} \mid \boldsymbol{\theta}) = b(\boldsymbol{y}) \exp\left[c(\boldsymbol{\theta})^T \boldsymbol{t}(\boldsymbol{y}) + n\mathrm{d}(\boldsymbol{\theta})\right], \tag{5.2}$$

with $b(\boldsymbol{y}) = \prod_1^n b(y_i)$ and $\boldsymbol{t}(\boldsymbol{y}) = \sum_1^n \boldsymbol{t}(y_i)$.

Table 5.2 contains commonly used exponential distributions; see the appendix for the mathematical expression and characteristics of the distributions. That the binomial and Poisson distribution belong to this family is seen as follows:

- Binomial distribution: $p(y \mid \theta) = \binom{n}{y} \theta^y (1-\theta)^{(n-y)}$ becomes expression (5.2) for $b(y) = \binom{n}{y}$, $t(y) = y$, $c(\theta) = \text{logit}(\theta)$ and $\text{d}(\theta) = \log(1-\theta)$.
- Poisson distribution: $p(y \mid \theta) = \frac{1}{y!}\theta^y \exp(-\theta)$ reduces to expression (5.1) for $b(y) = 1/y!$, $c(\theta) = \log(\theta)$, $t(y) = y$ and $\text{d}(\theta) = -\theta$. For a random sample of n Poisson counts, $\boldsymbol{y} = \{y_1, \ldots, y_n\}$ one obtains: $b(\boldsymbol{y}) = \prod_i 1/y_i!$ and $t(\boldsymbol{y}) = \sum_i y_i$.

For a distribution (5.1), the class of prior distributions $\Im$ closed under sampling is given by

$$p(\boldsymbol{\theta} \mid \boldsymbol{\alpha}, \beta) = k(\boldsymbol{\alpha}, \beta) \exp\left[c(\boldsymbol{\theta})^T \boldsymbol{\alpha} + \beta \text{d}(\boldsymbol{\theta})\right], \tag{5.3}$$

where $\boldsymbol{\alpha} = (\alpha_1, \ldots, \alpha_d)^T$ and β are hyperparameters. Expression (5.3) is that of a $(d+1)$-parameter exponential family. The scalar $k(\boldsymbol{\alpha}, \beta)$ is the normalizing constant, i.e. it ensures that expression (5.3) is a distribution:

$$k(\boldsymbol{\alpha}, \beta) = 1 \Big/ \int \exp\left[c(\boldsymbol{\theta})^T \boldsymbol{\alpha} + \beta \text{d}(\boldsymbol{\theta})\right] \text{d}\boldsymbol{\theta}.$$

Expression (5.3) defines a prior closed under sampling for expression (5.1), this follows from the following reasoning. Suppose that the joint density of a random sample $\boldsymbol{y}$ of i.i.d. elements is given by expression (5.1), then

$$\begin{aligned} p(\boldsymbol{\theta} \mid \boldsymbol{y}) &\propto p(\boldsymbol{y} \mid \boldsymbol{\theta}) p(\boldsymbol{\theta}) \\ &= \exp\left[c(\boldsymbol{\theta})^T \boldsymbol{t}(\boldsymbol{y}) + n\,\text{d}(\boldsymbol{\theta})\right] \exp\left[c(\boldsymbol{\theta})^T \boldsymbol{\alpha} + \beta \text{d}(\boldsymbol{\theta})\right] \\ &= \exp\left[c(\boldsymbol{\theta})^T \boldsymbol{\alpha}^* + \beta^* \text{d}(\boldsymbol{\theta})\right], \end{aligned} \tag{5.4}$$

with

$$\boldsymbol{\alpha}^* = \boldsymbol{\alpha} + \boldsymbol{t}(\boldsymbol{y}), \tag{5.5}$$

$$\beta^* = \beta + n. \tag{5.6}$$

The family defined by expression (5.3) is called the *natural conjugate family*. (O'Hagan and Forster 2004, pp. 140–141) extended this family by adding extra parameters leading to the *conjugate family* of distributions which is again closed under sampling (see also Exercise 5.4). Comparing expression (5.2) with expression (5.3) reveals that the conjugate prior has the same functional form as the likelihood. In fact, the conjugate prior of a member of the exponential family is obtained by replacing the data ($\boldsymbol{t}(\boldsymbol{y})$ and n) by parameters ($\boldsymbol{\alpha}$ and β). Note that a conjugate prior is model dependent, in fact likelihood dependent.

In Table 5.2, the conjugate distribution of some common choices of the exponential family is shown, but the list is not exhaustive. A conjugate prior can also be given for, e.g. the gamma distribution (with or without fixed α), the Pareto distribution with $f(y \mid \theta) = \theta y_m^\theta / y^{\theta+1}$ for $y \geq y_m$ and $f(y \mid \theta) = 1$ for $y < 1$, the uniform distribution on $[0, \theta]$, the Inverse Gaussian distribution (Banerjee and Bhattacharyya 1979). Further, conjugate priors can be specified for regression models (see Section 5.6).

In Section 5.3.2, we develop the conjugate for the normal distribution. We now show how the conjugate prior for the binomial and Poisson likelihood can be derived using the above rule:

- Binomial likelihood: For $c(\theta) = \text{logit}(\theta)$ and $\text{d}(\theta) = \log(1-\theta)$, $p(\theta \mid \alpha, \beta) \propto \exp[c(\theta)\alpha + \beta \text{d}(\theta)] = \theta^{\alpha}(1-\theta)^{\beta-\alpha}$. With $\alpha_0 = \alpha + 1$ and $\beta_0 = \beta - \alpha + 1$, the prior is proportional to $\theta^{\alpha_0 - 1}(1-\theta)^{\beta_0 - 1}$ which is the kernel of a beta distribution. The posterior distribution is obtained from $\alpha^* = \alpha + y$ and $\beta^* = \beta + n$, where y is the number of successes and n the size of the study. This results again in a beta distribution with parameters $\overline{\alpha} = \alpha_0 + y$ and $\overline{\beta} = \beta_0 + n - y$.
- Poisson likelihood: For $c(\theta) = \log(\theta)$ and $\text{d}(\theta) = -\theta$, $p(\theta \mid \alpha, \beta) \propto \exp[c(\theta)\alpha + \beta \text{d}(\theta)] = \theta^{\alpha}\exp(-\beta\theta)$, which is the kernel of a Gamma(α_0, β_0) distribution with $\alpha_0 = \alpha + 1$ and $\beta_0 = \beta$. It is left to the reader to check that the posterior is again a gamma distribution (Exercise 5.1).

Taking a (natural) conjugate prior distribution for expression (5.1) is convenient from a mathematical and a numerical viewpoint, but also from an interpretational point of view and is, therefore, also referred to as a *convenience prior*. Namely,

- The likelihood of historical data $\boldsymbol{y}$ can be easily turned into a conjugate prior by taking $\boldsymbol{\alpha} = \boldsymbol{t}(\boldsymbol{y})$ and $\beta = n$. This was illustrated in Chapter 2 for the binomial, the normal (with fixed variance) and the Poisson likelihoods. Conversely, one can also interpret the natural conjugate distribution as equivalent to a fictitious experiment with characteristics $\boldsymbol{\alpha}$ and β, as exemplified in Chapter 2. The correspondence between the likelihood and the conjugate prior is also exploited in Section 5.6 to define conjugate priors in regression models.
- For a natural conjugate prior, the posterior mean is a weighted combination of the prior mean and a sample estimate. This illustrates the impact of the data as well as that of the prior parameters on the posterior mean and helps in interpreting the posterior summary measures; see expressions (2.7), (2.14) and Exercise 2.10 for examples.

Now follows a practical illustration of the convenience of the natural conjugate family with respect to interpretation of the posterior summary measures.

Example V.2: Dietary study: Normal versus *t*-prior
In Example II.2, the IBBENS-2 normal likelihood was combined with the N(328 100) prior distribution. The normal distribution (given σ^2) belongs to the one-parameter exponential family (see also Section 5.3.4) and the normal prior is the conjugate of the normal likelihood. The normal posterior has mean and variance given by expression (2.13). Replacing the normal prior by a t_{30}(128 100)-distribution leaves the posterior distribution practically unchanged, but we loose three elegant features of the conjugate normal prior. Namely, with the t-prior: (1) the posterior cannot be determined analytically, (2) the posterior is not of the same class as the prior and (3) the posterior summary measures are not obvious functions of the prior and the sample summary measures. □

5.3.2 Normal distribution – mean and variance unknown

The Gaussian distribution with unknown μ and σ^2 belongs to the two-parameter exponential family. A standard application of expression (5.3) yields its natural conjugate (Exercise 5.4).

However, in the literature one uses a more flexible conjugate prior, namely the normal-inverse-gamma distribution NIG(μ_0, κ_0, a_0, b_0). This prior is derived as follows. Let $\boldsymbol{y} = \{y_1, \ldots, y_n\}$ be an i.i.d. sample from N(μ, σ^2), where μ and σ^2 are unknown. The joint density of $\boldsymbol{y}$ is factorized as

$$p(\boldsymbol{y} \mid \mu, \sigma^2) \propto \frac{\sqrt{n}}{(\sigma^2)^{1/2}} \exp\left[-\frac{1}{2}\frac{(\overline{y}-\mu)^2}{\sigma^2/n}\right] \frac{1}{(\sigma^2)^{\nu/2}} \exp\left(-\frac{S^2}{2\sigma^2}\right), \tag{5.7}$$

with $S^2 = \sum_{i=1}^n (y_i - \overline{y})^2$ and $\nu = n - 1$. Thus, the joint likelihood factorizes into the product of a N($\mu, \sigma^2/n$)-likelihood and a $\chi^2(\nu, \sigma^2)$-likelihood. Note that the normal likelihood has only two parameters. Consequently, using expression (5.3) yields a natural conjugate with only three parameters so that the NIG(μ_0, κ_0, a_0, b_0) prior cannot be a natural conjugate. To arrive at the NIG prior, we exploit expression (5.7) that suggests factorizing the prior as $p(\mu \mid \sigma^2)\, p(\sigma^2)$, where $p(\sigma^2)$ is an inverse gamma distribution IG($a_0/2$, $b_0/2$) given by

$$\frac{(b_0/2)^{(a_0/2)}}{\Gamma(a_0/2)} (\sigma^2)^{-(a_0+2)/2} \exp\left(-\frac{b_0}{2\sigma^2}\right). \tag{5.8}$$

Further, in Section 2.7, $p(\mu \mid \sigma^2)$ was taken as N(μ_0, σ_0^2) with σ_0^2 fixed because σ^2 was known. Here, the prior variance σ_0^2 must depend on σ^2. It is convenient to take $\sigma_0^2 = \sigma^2/\kappa_0$ with $\kappa_0 > 0$ interpreted as a 'prior sample size' and leading to $p(\mu \mid \sigma^2) = \mathrm{N}(\mu_0, \sigma^2/\kappa_0)$. Multiplying the two prior parts yields the conjugate prior NIG(μ_0, κ_0, a_0, b_0).

The second part of expression (5.7) can alternatively be written as $\frac{1}{(\sigma^2)^{\nu/2}} \exp(-\frac{\nu s^2}{2\sigma^2})$, with $s^2 = S^2/\nu$. In that case, the inverse gamma prior for σ^2 can be reformulated as a *scaled inverse chi-squared distribution*, denoted as Inv-$\chi^2(\nu_0, \tau_0^2)$-distribution and is given by

$$p(\sigma^2) \propto (\sigma^2)^{-(\nu_0/2+1)} \exp\left(-\frac{\nu_0\, \tau_0^2}{2\sigma^2}\right), \tag{5.9}$$

obtained from expression (5.8) by taking $a_0 = \nu_0$ and $b_0 = \nu_0\, \tau_0^2$. In this parameterization, the joint prior is called a *normal-scaled-inverse chi-squared distribution* and is denoted as N-Inv-$\chi^2(\mu_0, \kappa_0, \nu_0, \tau_0^2)$. The posterior distribution is then N-Inv-$\chi^2(\overline{\mu}, \overline{\kappa}, \overline{\nu}, \overline{\tau}^2)$, with parameters defined by expressions (4.10), (4.11), (4.12) and (4.13). Finally, when μ is known but σ^2 unknown, the natural conjugate is given by expression (5.8) or (5.9).

5.3.3 Multivariate data distributions

The results in Section 5.3.2 immediately carry over to multivariate distributions by replacing y by a multivariate vector $\boldsymbol{y}$. Here, we restrict ourselves to two popular multivariate models: (1) the multinomial model and (2) the multivariate normal model. Both models (and the related models) were introduced in Section 4.4.

The multinomial distribution Mult(n, $\boldsymbol{\theta}$) is a member of the exponential family with natural conjugate

$$p(\boldsymbol{\theta} \mid \boldsymbol{\alpha}_0) = \frac{\prod_{j=1}^k \Gamma(\alpha_{0j})}{\sum_{j=1}^k \Gamma(\alpha_{0j})} \prod_{j=1}^k \theta_j^{\alpha_{0j}-1}, \tag{5.10}$$

known as the *Dirichlet distribution* Dirichlet($\boldsymbol{\alpha}_0$) after the German mathematician Peter Lejeune–Dirichlet (1805–1859) who derived the normalizing constant in expression (5.10) (Gupta and Richards 2001). It is readily seen that the posterior distribution is again a Dirichlet distribution with parameters $\boldsymbol{\alpha}_0 + \boldsymbol{y}$ (Exercise 5.7). The beta distribution is a special case of a Dirichlet distribution with $k = 2$. In addition, the marginal distributions of the Dirichlet distribution are beta distributions (Exercise 5.8). Further, note that the prior Dirichlet $(1, 1, \ldots, 1)$ is the extension of the classical uniform prior Beta(1,1) to higher dimensions. In Section 4.4.2, this NI prior was linked to a normal noninformative prior of the log odds-ratio in a 2×2 contingency table.

The likelihood of a sample $\{\boldsymbol{y}_1, \ldots, \boldsymbol{y}_n\}$ drawn from a p-dimensional multivariate normal distribution is given by

$$p(\boldsymbol{y}_1, \ldots, \boldsymbol{y}_n \mid \boldsymbol{\mu}, \Sigma) = \frac{1}{(2\pi)^{np/2}|\Sigma|^{1/2}} \exp\left[-\frac{1}{2}\sum_{i=1}^{n}(\boldsymbol{y}_i - \boldsymbol{\mu})^T \Sigma^{-1}(\boldsymbol{y}_i - \boldsymbol{\mu})\right]. \quad (5.11)$$

When Σ is known but μ unknown, the conjugate for $\boldsymbol{\mu}$ is the normal prior N($\boldsymbol{\mu}_0$, Σ_0). For μ and Σ unknown, we need to generalize the procedure of Section 5.3.2. The term S^2 in expression (5.7) is then replaced by $S = \sum_{i=1}^{n}(\boldsymbol{y}_i - \overline{\boldsymbol{y}})(\boldsymbol{y}_i - \overline{\boldsymbol{y}})^T$, which has a Wishart distribution with $\nu = n - 1$ degrees of freedom denoted as Wishart (Σ, ν) (see Section 4.4.1 for a mathematical expression). The natural conjugate for the covariance matrix in the normal case is then the *inverse Wishart distribution* with $\nu_0 \geq p$ degrees of freedom, IW(Λ_0, ν_0), where Λ_0 is a $p \times p$ positive definite matrix. For $p = 1$ the inverse Wishart distribution is equal to the scaled inverse-chi-squared distribution. The conjugate of N($\boldsymbol{\mu}$, Σ) is then the normal-inverse Wishart distribution NIW($\boldsymbol{\mu}_0$, κ_0, ν_0, Λ_0), but it is not a natural conjugate (for similar reasons as in Section 5.3.2).

To obtain a minimally informative inverse Wishart distribution, $\nu_0 \approx p$ appears an appropriate choice. For $\nu_0 = (p + 1)$, one can show that the prior distribution of the correlation is uniform on $[-1, 1]$. In addition, the scale matrix Λ_0 is often taken diagonal. However, the literature is not clear about the choice of the diagonal elements. On top of this, we note that WinBUGS uses a slightly different formulation of the Wishart distribution with now Λ_0 playing the role of a covariance matrix. This would suggest taking large diagonal elements for Λ_0, but in http://statacumen.com/2009/07/02/wishart-distribution-in-winbugs-nonstandard-parameterization/ it is shown that one should rather take diagonal elements close to zero in order to obtain a NI prior.

When $\boldsymbol{\mu}$ is known but Σ unknown, then we need only a (conjugate) prior for the covariance matrix Σ. It can be readily seen from the above reasoning that in this case the conjugate prior of Σ is again an inverse Wishart distribution.

5.3.4 Conditional conjugate and semiconjugate priors

Suppose the parameter vector $\boldsymbol{\theta}$ splits up into $\boldsymbol{\phi}$ and $\boldsymbol{\nu}$, then the prior distribution $p(\boldsymbol{\phi}) \in \Im$ is a *conditional conjugate* for $\boldsymbol{\phi}$ if the conditional posterior $p(\boldsymbol{\phi} \mid \boldsymbol{\nu}, \boldsymbol{y})$ belongs to the same class $\Im$. Take for example the normal distribution N(μ, σ^2) with μ and σ^2 unknown. Then the natural conjugate for μ, for a given σ^2, is the prior N(μ_0, σ_0^2). In other words, N(μ_0, σ_0^2) is the conditional conjugate of μ. The conditional conjugate for σ^2 given μ is the prior (5.9). The product of the prior distributions N(μ_0, σ_0^2) and Inv-χ^2(ν_0, τ_0^2) is called a *semiconjugate prior* for (μ, σ^2) and was our choice in Section 4.3.3 when independent prior information about μ and σ^2 was available. While a semiconjugate prior will not lead to analytical solutions for the posterior, it proves to be quite useful for the Gibbs sampler, a popular Markov chain Monte Carlo sampling technique.

5.3.5 Hyperpriors

Conjugate prior distributions are restrictive in their ability to represent prior knowledge, but their flexibility can easily be extended by giving the parameters of the conjugate a prior distribution. Namely, suppose that the data have a distribution $p(y \mid \boldsymbol{\theta})$ and the unknown $\boldsymbol{\theta}$ is given a (conjugate) prior $p(\boldsymbol{\theta} \mid \boldsymbol{\phi}_0)$. Instead of fixing the $\boldsymbol{\phi}$-parameters, we could give them also a (prior) distribution $p(\boldsymbol{\phi} \mid \boldsymbol{\omega}_0)$, then $\boldsymbol{\phi}$ is called an *hyperparameter* and $p(\boldsymbol{\phi} \mid \boldsymbol{\omega}_0)$ a *hyperprior* or an *hierarchical prior*. The effect of an hyperprior is that the actual prior for $\boldsymbol{\theta}$ is the mixture prior

$$q(\boldsymbol{\theta} \mid \boldsymbol{\omega}_0) = \int p(\boldsymbol{\theta} \mid \boldsymbol{\phi}) p(\boldsymbol{\phi} \mid \boldsymbol{\omega}_0)\, \mathrm{d}\boldsymbol{\phi}. \tag{5.12}$$

It can then be evaluated whether the prior $q(\boldsymbol{\theta} \mid \boldsymbol{\omega}_0)$ has the desired characteristics. Hyperpriors are extensively used in Chapter 9 where we treat hierarchical models. For a simple illustration, assume that the parameters α and β of the gamma distribution in Example II.3 are given exponential priors $p(\alpha \mid \omega_{\alpha,0})$ and $p(\beta \mid \omega_{\beta,0})$, respectively. These exponential priors are then examples of hyperpriors and α and β are called hyperparameters.

To achieve particular characteristics of the (say shape) of the prior, discrete hyperpriors may be easier to work with. Let the prior distribution of $\boldsymbol{\theta}$ be the finite mixture

$$q(\boldsymbol{\theta} \mid \boldsymbol{\pi}) = \sum_{k=1}^{K} \pi_k p_k(\boldsymbol{\theta}), \tag{5.13}$$

with $\boldsymbol{\pi} = (\pi_1, \ldots, \pi_K)^T$ and $p_k(\boldsymbol{\theta})$ $(k = 1, \ldots, K)$ conjugate for the likelihood. Denote the class of distributions (5.13) as $\Im_M$, then the posterior distribution is $p(\boldsymbol{\theta} \mid \boldsymbol{\pi}^*, \boldsymbol{y}) = \sum_{k=1}^{K} \pi_k^* p_k(\boldsymbol{\theta} \mid \boldsymbol{y})$, with $p(\boldsymbol{\theta} \mid \boldsymbol{\pi}^*, \boldsymbol{y}) \in \Im_M$. The new weights pertaining to the posterior distribution are

$$\pi_k^* = \frac{a_k \pi_k}{\sum_{j=1}^{K} a_j \pi_j},$$

with $a_k = \int L(\boldsymbol{\theta} \mid \boldsymbol{y})\, p_k(\boldsymbol{\theta})\, \mathrm{d}\boldsymbol{\theta}$. In this case, the hyperprior is a discrete distribution and the probabilities $\boldsymbol{\pi}$ represents hyperparameters. Thus for conjugate priors $p_k(\boldsymbol{\theta})$ also $q(\boldsymbol{\theta}|\boldsymbol{\pi})$ is conjugate and $p(\boldsymbol{\theta} \mid \boldsymbol{\pi}^* \boldsymbol{y})$ can be determined analytically. Further, the mean of the mixture prior is simply the weighted sum (with weights π_k^*) of the mixture components. In addition, the variance for $q(\boldsymbol{\theta} \mid \boldsymbol{\omega}_0)$ given by expression (5.12) is

$$\mathrm{var}(\boldsymbol{\theta}) = E_{\boldsymbol{\phi}}[\mathrm{var}(\boldsymbol{\theta} \mid \boldsymbol{\phi})] + \mathrm{var}_{\boldsymbol{\phi}}[E(\boldsymbol{\theta} \mid \boldsymbol{\phi})]. \tag{5.14}$$

Hence, the discrete mixture prior allows for a relatively easy control of the first two moments of the prior $q(\boldsymbol{\theta})$. Moreover, it can be shown that a rich family of distributions can be approximated to any degree by a (possibly infinite) mixture of conjugate priors; see Diaconis and Ylvisaker (1985) and Dalal and Hall (1983). An illustration of this result is provided in Example V.3.

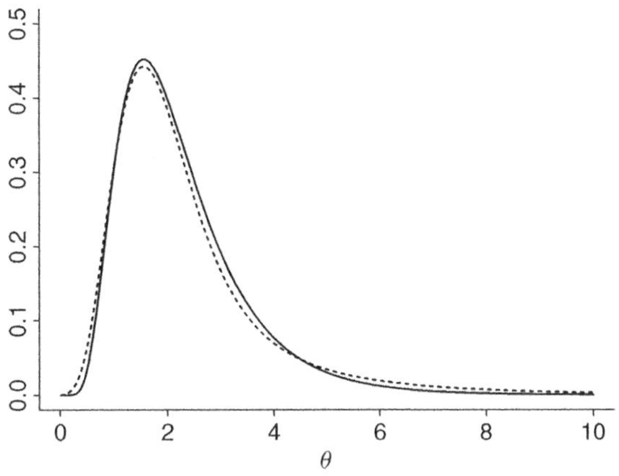

Figure 5.1 Caries study: lognormal prior (solid line) approximated by a mixture of three gamma priors (dashed line).

Note that the FirstBayes program allows for specifying discrete mixtures of some popular conjugate priors.

Example V.3: Caries study: Approximating the lognormal prior
In Example III.11, we have assumed a lognormal prior (see expression (3.20)) for θ representing the mean of the dmft-index. The disadvantage of this prior is that posterior summary measures can only be derived by sampling. The above results of Diaconis and Ylvisaker (1985) and Dalal and Hall (1983) imply that we can approximate to a high degree this prior by a mixture of (possibly a large number of) gamma distributions. We illustrate the performance of a well-chosen mixture of three gamma distributions, i.e. $K = 3$. A grid search minimizing the distance between the mixture and the lognormal prior gave the following components of the mixture: (1) $\pi_1 = 0.15$, $\alpha_1 = 2.5$ and $\beta_1 = 1.75$; (2) $\pi_2 = 0.30$, $\alpha_2 = 3.8$ and $\beta_2 = 0.67$; and (3) $\pi_3 = 0.55$, $\alpha_3 = 6$ and $\beta_3 = 0.3$. In Figure 5.1, it can be seen that the mixture gives an acceptable approximation to the lognormal prior.

The posterior mean and variance obtained from the mixture of gamma distributions is equal to 2.66 and 0.27, respectively, using expression (5.14). An additional important feature of hyperpriors is that they allow for simple full conditional distributions while generalizing the class of prior distributions. This is seen in Example VI.4 in Chapter 6. □

5.4 Noninformative prior distributions

5.4.1 Introduction

The property of allowing prior information into a statistical analysis is a unique feature of Bayesian methods. However, it often happens that researchers cannot or do not wish to make use of prior knowledge. For instance, in the case of pioneering research prior knowledge is largely lacking. Another example is when a drug company seeks for regulatory approval of an experimental medication on the basis of a phase III trial. Registration of the new drug requires the 'data to speak for themselves', i.e. only the obtained results from the phase III trial are allowed to influence the decision.

The prior that expresses lack of information or ignorance was initially called a *noninformative (NI) prior distribution* with the flat prior as an obvious first candidate. However, this choice creates confusion for a continuous parameter since a flat prior for θ implies a nonflat prior for a transformed parameter $\psi = h(\theta)$. This result is particularly disturbing to non-Bayesians and triggered the Bayesian community to find the 'best' noninformative prior. The review article of Kass and Wasserman (1996) illustrates the enormous effort that Bayesian researchers entertained in the search for expressing ignorance. Nowadays, one has contended that a prior always bears some information, even if intended to represent ignorance, and that at best one can hope that the equivalent information is minimal. Consequently, instead of the adjective 'noninformative' terms such as *nonsubjective, objective, default, reference, weak, diffuse, flat, conventional and minimally informative* were used in due time in the literature.

Since each prior implies that some external information creeps into the analysis, one needs to show in practice that the chosen NI prior is indeed minimally informative. This is not always easy, especially when dealing with a complex model involving many parameters. Further, many NI priors are strictly speaking not a distribution and are called *improper* (see Section 5.4.4). When an improper prior causes the posterior to be improper the Bayesian analysis is in trouble, e.g. since the posterior cannot provide summary measures anymore. Impropriety can be hard to detect, as we show in Chapter 7.

In this section, we aim to explain the difficulties in expressing ignorance that lead to the richness in NI priors and the confusion around them. Note that by the adjective 'noninformative' we assume in this book its contemporary meaning of 'weak', 'diffuse', etc.

5.4.2 Expressing ignorance

Bayes and Laplace argued that the *principle of insufficient reason* also called the *principle of indifference* is a logical choice for choosing prior probabilities when one has no prior information. The principle suggests equal prior probabilities for a discrete event and a flat prior in the continuous case (in both cases it may be called a flat prior). The principle is also referred to as the *Bayes–Laplace postulate*.

The flat prior cannot, however, express ignorance. We illustrate this here for the discrete case and the continuous parameter case. For the discrete case, suppose that θ can take values θ_1, θ_2, and θ_3 and that we give equal probabilities $p(\theta_k) = 1/3$ $(k = 1, 2, 3)$ to express our ignorance about the choice of θ. If we are ignorant about θ, then we must be also ignorant about a binary parameter ψ that is equal to ψ_1 when $\theta = \theta_1$ and to ψ_2 when $\theta = \theta_2$ or θ_3. But, if the same principle of indifference is used on ψ, i.e. $p(\psi_k) = 1/2$ $(k = 1, 2)$ then we are in contradiction with the indifference statement on θ. Suppose in the case of a continuous parameter that you are completely ignorant about microorganisms in your body (so you have not experienced any training in biology or medicine) and that you are asked to state your prior probability on (or that you put EUR 100 on either statement) (1) S_1: less than (or equal) 50% of the humans carry prokaryotes in their body or (2) S_2: more than 50% of the humans carry prokaryotes in their body. If you are truly ignorant then your answer must be 'I don't know' equivalent to stating that $p(S_1) = 0.5$ and $p(S_2) = 0.5$ (and betting EUR 50 on each statement). In the next step, we replace in the question 50% by 80%. What is your answer then? If your answer is the same (when you are ignorant) then 0.5 must also be attached to the new statements. But such behavior cannot be turned into a prior distribution. On the other hand with a flat prior, your answer would be $p(S_1) = 0.8$ and $p(S_2) = 0.2$ (and you put

EUR 80 on the first statement). Note that prokaryotes represent a particular class of bacteria present in the gastrointestinal part of your body.

That a flat prior does not express ignorance might still look bizarre given that we showed in Section 2.6 that, with a uniform prior on the binomial parameter θ, the likelihood and the posterior coincided completely. To show that some information must have crept in, suppose that the binomial model was parameterized by $\psi = \log(\theta)$ as in Example II.4 and suppose that a flat prior on ψ was given to express ignorance. Using the transformation rule (2.26), this flat prior is turned into a nonflat prior for θ and since the likelihood is invariant to monotone transformations, the resulting posterior for θ is different. Note that part of our confusion is due to the pointwise interpretation of a density while in fact only statements like $P(a < \theta < b)$ have an interpretation (Edwards 1972).

We conclude that, strictly speaking, there is no prior able to express ignorance and that each prior must bear some knowledge. Consequently, the term noninformative prior is misleading. However, claiming that frequentist methods are not based on any prior at all is incorrect since Bayesian results can reproduce frequentist results under the flat prior, and therefore the frequentist methods assume implicitly a prior.

5.4.3 General principles to choose noninformative priors

5.4.3.1 Jeffreys priors

Bayes proposal of the flat prior lead to the rejection of the Bayesian approach as a whole (Mc Grayne 2011). For instance, to Fisher it was unacceptable that the conclusions of a Bayesian analysis depends on what scale the flat prior was taken on and that there is no clear choice on what scale to take the flat prior on. For example, in the case of a normal likelihood, should we take the flat prior on σ or on σ^2? However, inference based on the likelihood alone does not suffer from this ambiguity.

Thus, in order to preserve the conclusions from a Bayesian analysis when changing from θ to $\psi = h(\theta)$ the transformation rule, i.e. $p(\psi) = p(h^{-1}(\psi))|\frac{dh^{-1}(\psi)}{d\psi}|$, must be applied to the prior. In that case, $p(\theta)\,d\theta = p(\psi)\,d\psi$ and the conclusions from an analysis based on θ are the same as those of ψ. Jeffreys (1946, 1961) proposed a recipe/rule to construct priors that always provide the same conclusion on whatever scale they are specified. His rule is classically referred to as *Jeffreys invariance principle or rule* and is given by: Take the prior proportional to the square root of the Fisher information, i.e.

$$p(\theta) \propto \Im^{1/2}(\theta), \tag{5.15}$$

where $\Im(\theta) = -E\left(\frac{d^2 \log p(y|\theta)}{d\theta^2}\right)$. Thus Jeffreys choice for the (class of) prior(s) depends on the likelihood of the data. That it satisfies the invariance property is seen immediately:

$$p(\psi) \propto \Im^{1/2}(\psi) = \Im^{1/2}(\theta)\left|\frac{d\theta}{d\psi}\right| = p(\theta)\left|\frac{d\theta}{d\psi}\right|. \tag{5.16}$$

Next, for a given likelihood and assuming that the prior $p(\psi)$ is constructed using expression (5.16), the rule indicates how to find the scale where a flat prior can be taken. Indeed, from

$p(\psi)\,\mathrm{d}\psi = p(\theta)\mathrm{d}\theta$ and expression (5.16), we infer that the prior $p(\psi)$ becomes flat for

$$\psi \propto \int \Im^{1/2}(\theta)\,\mathrm{d}\theta. \tag{5.17}$$

Hence, since one can always find a 'flat' element belonging to the class given by expression (5.15) and that the inference from that flat prior is the same as from any other prior of the same class, we could say that Jeffreys rule provides a rule to construct noninformative priors. Formally, Jeffreys rule for choosing a NI prior is, therefore, given by the following: *The prior distribution for a single parameter θ is approximately noninformative if it is taken proportional to the square root of Fisher's information measure.*

Some examples of Jeffreys priors are (except for the binomial model all these priors are improper, see Section 5.4.4) as follows:

- Binomial model: $p(\theta) \propto \theta^{-1/2}(1-\theta)^{-1/2}$ corresponding to a flat prior on $\psi(\theta) \propto \arcsin\sqrt{\theta}$ (Exercise 5.12). This prior is undefined at $\theta = 0$ and 1 and has a higher variance than the uniform prior.
- Poisson model: $p(\theta) \propto \theta^{-1/2}$ corresponding to a flat prior on $\sqrt{\theta}$ (Exercise 5.1).
- Normal model with σ fixed: $p(\mu) \propto c$.
- Normal model with μ fixed: $p(\sigma^2) \propto \sigma^{-2}$ corresponding to a flat prior on $\log(\sigma)$.

Jeffreys extension to multiparameter models was initially to take the prior for $\boldsymbol{\theta}$ equal to

$$p(\boldsymbol{\theta}) \propto |\Im(\boldsymbol{\theta})|^{1/2}. \tag{5.18}$$

Applied to the normal model, this rule gives $p(\mu, \sigma^2) \propto \sigma^{-3}$. However, the popular choice is to take

$$p(\mu, \sigma^2) \propto \sigma^{-2}, \tag{5.19}$$

which is the product of two independent NI prior distributions. Prior (5.19) reflects that prior information on μ and σ^2 arrives independently to us, suggesting a priori independence of the model parameters. In fact, Jeffreys was not too happy himself about his general multiparameter rule (5.18) and he suggested later to treat the location parameters independently from the scale parameters in location-scale problems. This adapted rule gives the location parameters a flat prior and applies the multivariate rule (5.18) to the scale parameters. Jeffreys adapted rule also leads to prior (5.19) for the normal model. Finally, this prior reproduces some classical frequentist results, as seen in Chapter 4. *Jeffreys multiparameter rule* for choosing a NI prior is, therefore, given by

The prior distribution for a parameter vector $(\boldsymbol{\theta}, \boldsymbol{\phi})$ is approximately noninformative if it is taken proportional to the square root of the determinant of Fisher information measure for $(\boldsymbol{\theta}, \boldsymbol{\phi})$. When $\boldsymbol{\theta}$ is a vector of location parameters and $\boldsymbol{\phi}$ represents scale parameters, then the noninformative prior is taken proportional to the product of a flat prior for $\boldsymbol{\theta}$ and the square root of the determinant of Fisher information measure for $\boldsymbol{\phi}$.

Jeffreys rule can be derived using other principles (data-translated likelihood principle, prior that maximizes Kullback–Leibler distance between prior and posterior (reference prior), etc.) and has many attractive properties. However, it has been criticized because of violating the likelihood principle since the prior depends on the expected value of the log-likelihood under the experiment (probability model for the data). As an illustration, in Exercise 5.10 it is shown that Jeffreys prior for the binomial experiment differs from Jeffreys prior for the negative binomial experiment while the two models have the same conjugate prior.

Jeffreys multiparameter rule has been suggested for many (more complex) models (see Section 5.6.2), and thus remains an important tool to construct NI priors. However, when used blindly, it may not have the desired properties. This occurs when Jeffreys rule is applied to parts of the model. As an example: when the prior for the variance of the level-2 observations in a (normal) hierarchical model is given the classical Jeffreys prior for variances, i.e. $p(\sigma^2) \propto \sigma^{-2}$, then the posterior of σ^2 is improper.

5.4.3.2 The data-translated likelihood principle

Jeffreys rule dictates to choose the scale for a flat prior via the invariance principle. Box and Tiao (1973, pp. 25–60) derived Jeffreys prior for location-scale distributions using the *data-translated likelihood (DTL) principle*. Their argument gives a more intuitive explanation for the scale of the flat prior.

Suppose that for $\psi = h(\theta)$, the effect of the data on the likelihood implies only to shift the location of that likelihood, then all information in the data about ψ is contained in the location of that likelihood. Taking an informative prior on this scale would prefer a range of values and hence the posterior would be greatly affected by this prior. On the other hand, taking the prior distribution flat on ψ expresses that we are a priori indifferent about ψ. This is called the *DTL principle*. One can verify that for the normal likelihood with σ known, this happens on the original scale of μ (see Exercise 5.9), while for the normal likelihood in σ with μ known this occurs on the log-scale, as shown in Example V.4.

Example V.4: DTL principle applied to normal likelihood in σ given μ
The normal likelihood for σ with μ given is

$$L(\sigma \mid \mu, \mathbf{y}) \propto \sigma^{-n} \exp\left(-\frac{n S^2}{2\sigma^2}\right), \tag{5.20}$$

with $S^2 = \sum_{i=1}^{n}(y_i - \mu)^2$.

Suppose that we have three data sets each of size $n = 10$, with standard deviations equal to $S = 5$, $S = 10$, and $S = 20$, respectively. Likelihood (5.20) as a function of σ changes in location and in shape with varying S, while as a function of $\log(\sigma)$ the likelihood changes with S only in location (Figure 5.2). According to the DTL principle, one should take the flat prior distribution on the log-scale, as it does not prefer any location over another. Using expression (2.26), a flat prior distribution on $\log(\sigma)$ is equivalent to a prior distribution $p(\sigma) \propto \sigma^{-1}$ and equivalently to $p(\sigma^2) \propto \sigma^{-2}$, which are both Jeffreys priors. □

If the DTL principle cannot be satisfied exactly, perhaps there exists a scale ψ for which the likelihood is approximately data-translated. For moderate to large sample sizes, the log-likelihood of the sample, $\log(L)$, is well approximated by a quadratic function around the

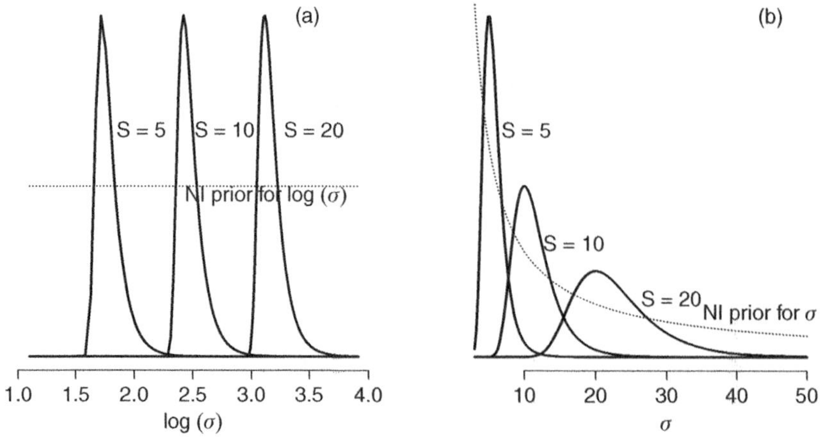

Figure 5.2 Data-translated likelihood principle for N(μ, σ^2)-likelihood given μ. The likelihood is given for three different values of S as a function of (a) $\log(\sigma)$, and (b) σ.

MLE $\widehat{\psi}$ as follows:

$$\log L(\psi \mid \mathbf{y}) \approx \log L(\widehat{\psi} \mid \mathbf{y}) - \frac{n}{2}(\psi - \widehat{\psi})^2 \left(-\frac{1}{n} \frac{\partial^2 \log(L)}{\partial \psi^2} \right)_{\widehat{\psi}}, \tag{5.21}$$

which is a quadratic function in ψ which changes in location and shape (curvature changes with $\widehat{\psi}$). Denote $-\left(\frac{1}{n}\frac{\partial^2 \log(L)}{\partial \psi^2}\right)_{\widehat{\psi}}$ as $J(\widehat{\psi})$, then

$$J(\widehat{\psi}) = -\left(\frac{1}{n} \frac{\partial^2 \log(L)}{\partial \psi^2} \right)_{\widehat{\psi}} = -\left(\frac{1}{n} \frac{\partial^2 \log(L)}{\partial \theta^2} \right)_{\widehat{\theta}} \left(\frac{\mathrm{d}\theta}{\mathrm{d}\psi} \right)^2_{\widehat{\theta}} = J(\widehat{\theta}) \left(\frac{\mathrm{d}\theta}{\mathrm{d}\psi} \right)^2_{\widehat{\theta}}, \tag{5.22}$$

since the first derivative of $\log L(\psi \mid \mathbf{y})$ with respect to ψ, vanishes for $\widehat{\psi}$. Consequently, if ψ satisfies

$$\frac{\mathrm{d}\psi}{\mathrm{d}\theta} \propto J^{1/2}(\theta), \tag{5.23}$$

the coefficient of the quadratic term in ψ will be constant and the likelihood becomes locally data-translated on the ψ scale. In this case, a flat prior could be chosen for ψ and the corresponding NI prior for θ becomes

$$p(\theta) \propto J^{1/2}(\theta). \tag{5.24}$$

The derivation assumes that $J(\widehat{\psi})$ depends only on $\widehat{\psi}$ (and equivalently on $\widehat{\theta}$) and not on the whole sample $\{y_1, \ldots, y_n\}$. If this is not the case, the above arguments are applied to $\Im(\widehat{\theta})$, the Fisher information matrix for a sample.

5.4.3.3 Formal rules to choose noninformative priors

The invariance principle of Jeffreys is one of many formal rules (but an important and influential one) that has been suggested in the literature for constructing NI priors. Another important principle is due to Bernardo (1979) who suggested to take the NI prior that maximizes the Kullback–Leibler distance (for a definition, see expression (10.5)) between the prior and the posterior. He called his proposal a *reference prior* and showed that in important cases, this prior coincides with Jeffreys prior.

The *coverage matching principle* dictates that the prior should be chosen such that it has good frequentist coverage properties. For example, if the $100(1-\alpha)\%$ CI of the parameters has the correct coverage, then the Bayesian analysis mimics the frequentist analysis. In Section 4.3.1, it was seen that the (adapted) Jeffreys prior for the normal distribution with both parameters unknown, results in credible intervals for the mean and variance that are identical to the classical confidence intervals (CIs). In the same section we have reported on the findings of Agresti and Min (2005). They concluded that Jeffreys prior $p(\theta) \propto 1/\sqrt{\theta\,(1-\theta)}$ on the binomial parameter θ has better frequentist coverage for the odds ratio than the uniform prior. Also Berger (2006) reported excellent coverage for the positive predictive value of a diagnostic test with Jeffreys priors (Exercise 5.14). In addition, he reported that the Bayesian approach using Jeffreys priors results in shorter CIs than the classical frequentist approaches.

In Kass and Wasserman (1996), a review is given of a variety of other principles that may lead to a NI prior, but few have found their way into practical applications. Finally, note that many popular NI priors are particular cases of a conjugate distribution. For example in the binomial case the uniform prior, Jeffreys prior and Haldane's prior are special cases of a beta distribution. Similar findings can be derived for the negative binomial likelihood, the Poisson likelihood and the (multivariate) normal likelihood.

5.4.4 Improper prior distributions

Many NI priors are not regular distributions. For instance, Jeffreys prior for the mean parameter μ of a normal distribution, $p(\mu) \propto c$, has an infinite area under the curve (AUC) for each value of $c > 0$. A prior distribution with an infinite AUC is called an *improper prior*. From a technical point of view, improper priors are acceptable as long as the resulting posterior is proper (AUC = 1). For instance, the prior $p(\mu) = c$ (for a normal mean with given σ) gives a proper posterior distribution:

$$p(\mu \mid \mathbf{y}) = \frac{p(\mathbf{y} \mid \mu)\, p(\mu)}{\int p(\mathbf{y} \mid \mu)\, p(\mu)\, \mathrm{d}\mu} = \frac{p(\mathbf{y} \mid \mu)\, c}{\int p(\mathbf{y} \mid \mu)\, c\, \mathrm{d}\mu} = \frac{1}{\sqrt{2\pi}\sigma/\sqrt{n}} \exp\left[-\frac{n}{2}\left(\frac{\mu-\overline{y}}{\sigma}\right)^2\right].$$

The same holds when $p(\sigma^2) \propto \sigma^{-2}$ is taken as prior for the variance parameter of a normal distribution with a given mean (Exercise 5.13).

However, for complex models it is not immediately clear when an improper prior will yield a proper posterior. A well-known example is the variance of the level-2 observations in a Gaussian hierarchical model. In Chapter 9, it is shown that Jeffreys prior $p(\tau^2) \propto \tau^{-2}$ for the variance of the level-2 observations causes the posterior to be improper, but the improper prior $p(\tau) \propto c$ yields a proper posterior (Gelman 2006). When Markov chain Monte Carlo methods are used to derive the posterior, discovering the impropriety of the posterior may be hard (see Chapter 7). To make things even more complex, Ibrahim and Laud (1991) gave an example (their remark 3) of an improper Jeffreys prior yielding a proper posterior distribution but with no finite moments.

Even if the improper prior does not cause problems in estimation, problems may occur elsewhere in a Bayesian analysis. For instance, in Section 10.2.1 it is shown that with improper priors the Bayes factor is undetermined. The reason for this is seen above, namely the marginal likelihoods are not normalizable, i.e. $cp(\theta)$ is equivalent to $p(\theta)$. Also the marginal likelihood $p(\mathbf{y}) = \int p(\mathbf{y} \mid \boldsymbol{\theta})p(\boldsymbol{\theta})\, d\boldsymbol{\theta}$ is improper when $p(\boldsymbol{\theta})$ is improper.

That priors do not need to be a regular distribution may seem a bit weird. However, it is not regarded as a real problem in the Bayesian world. Indeed the improper prior is for Bayesians merely a technical device to express that there is minimal prior information on the parameters and to also ensure that the prior minimally impacts the posterior. Nevertheless, the improper prior has been severely criticized from an interpretational point of view. Take for example a randomized controlled clinical trial (RCT) and suppose that a flat prior is given for the difference Δ of the 2 (true) treatment means on $[-K, K]$. Suppose experts believe that the true difference cannot exceed $[-a, a]$. If $K >> a$ then most of the prior probability lies in the unrealistic part $[-K, -a) \cup (a, K]$. Even worse: when $K \longrightarrow \infty$, an improper flat prior is obtained which puts an infinite mass on unrealistic differences. Greenland (2001) argued that most NI priors used in epidemiological research entail to such absurdities. Similar criticism has been ventilated in the clinical trial area.

5.4.5 Weak/vague priors

For practical purposes, the prior does not need to be uniform over the whole range of parameter values. It is sufficient that the prior is *locally uniform* which means that it is approximately constant on the interval where the likelihood is not (close to) zero. That the effect of a locally uniform prior on the posterior is minimal follows immediately from Bayes theorem, i.e. from $p(\theta \mid \mathbf{y}) \propto p(\mathbf{y} \mid \theta)p(\theta)$ we see that the prior only has impact when $p(\mathbf{y} \mid \theta)$ is not too close to zero. In Chapter 2, locally uniform priors have been used (see Figure 2.9). Note that Box and Tiao (1968) considered Jeffreys prior as locally uniform. They wrote (p. 28) that it would be inappropriate mathematically and meaningless practically to suppose that the prior was uniform over an infinite range. They then continue and speak of Jeffreys prior as a locally uniform prior.

Thus to avoid impropriety of the posterior and for interpretation purposes the improper uniform prior is often replaced in practice by a locally uniform prior that approximates the improper prior. Examples are a $N(0, \sigma_0^2)$ prior for a location parameter with σ_0 large and an $IG(\varepsilon, \varepsilon)$ prior for a variance parameter with ε small. In the latter case, the prior approximates Jeffreys prior $p(\sigma^2) \propto \sigma^{-2}$ when $\varepsilon \rightarrow 0$. Such priors are in the literature loosely referred to as *vague* or *weak*. WinBUGS allows only (proper) vague priors. In the WinBUGS Examples I and II documents, all location parameters are given a $N(0, 10^6)$ prior and for the variance parameter of a Gaussian model the $IG(10^{-3}, 10^{-3})$ prior is taken, except for hierarchical models where the prior of the level-2 standard deviation is taken as uniform (Section 9.5.7).

Cautionary note: unlike Jeffreys priors, vague priors are not invariant to a change in scale of the data. For instance, a $N(0, 10^6)$ prior for the mean of a measurement that varies in an interval [0, 10] is vague, but if the scale of that measurement is changed, say multiplied by 1000 (e.g. changing from kilogram to gram) then this prior is not vague anymore.

5.5 Informative prior distributions

5.5.1 Introduction

The prior distribution describes the available (prior) knowledge about the model parameters. In basically all research, some prior knowledge is available. Box and Tiao (1973) argued that we are almost never in a state of absolute ignorance. The challenge is to incorporate that (possibly little) prior knowledge into a probabilistic framework. The question is whether to include the beliefs of one expert or of a community of experts. This is not important for the application of Bayes theorem, but it is important for the acceptance and the usefulness of the Bayesian analysis.

In this section, we (a) formalize the use of historical data as prior information using the power prior, (b) review the use of *clinical priors*, which are prior distributions based on either historical data or on expert knowledge, and (c) priors that are based on formal rules expressing prior skepticism and optimism. The ensemble of prior distributions that represent prior knowledge are called *subjective* or *informative* priors.

5.5.2 Data-based prior distributions

In Examples II.1 and II.2, the historical data were used to construct the conjugate prior according to expression (5.2). Hereby, we assumed that the historical data were realized under identical conditions as the present data. Combining the prior information from the historical data with the likelihood of the current data is then equivalent to pooling the two sets of data. This assumption is often too strong in practice. In Section 2.7, we downplayed the importance of the Inter-regional Belgian Bank Employee Nutrition Study (IBBENS) prior data for the IBBENS-2 likelihood, hereby we kept the location of the IBBENS prior but inflated its variance. This is called *discounting* the prior information. Ibrahim and Chen formalized this process in the *power prior distribution* (Ibrahim and Chen 2000; Ibrahim *et al.* 2003). Their approach is quite general and can be applied to Bayesian generalized linear (mixed) models, survival models, and nonlinear models. Here, we introduce their approach for simple statistical models.

Let the historical data be $\boldsymbol{y}_0 = \{y_{01}, \ldots, y_{0n_0}\}$, $\boldsymbol{\theta}$ represent the model parameters and $L(\boldsymbol{\theta} \mid \boldsymbol{y}_0)$ represent the likelihood of the historical data. Ibrahim and Chen (2000) proposed the following prior based on the historical data

$$p(\boldsymbol{\theta} \mid \boldsymbol{y}_0, a_0) \propto L(\boldsymbol{\theta} \mid \boldsymbol{y}_0)^{a_0}\, p_0(\boldsymbol{\theta} \mid \boldsymbol{c}_0), \tag{5.25}$$

with $p_0(\boldsymbol{\theta} \mid \boldsymbol{c}_0)$ an initial prior for the historical data with chosen parameters $\boldsymbol{c}_0$. The parameter a_0 is taken between zero and one and is in the first instance assumed known. Further, suppose that the likelihood of the current data $\boldsymbol{y} = \{y_1, \ldots, y_n\}$ is given by $L(\boldsymbol{\theta} \mid \boldsymbol{y})$, then the posterior obtained from the above power prior is

$$p(\boldsymbol{\theta} \mid \boldsymbol{y}, \boldsymbol{y}_0, a_0) \propto L(\boldsymbol{\theta} \mid \boldsymbol{y}) L(\boldsymbol{\theta} \mid \boldsymbol{y}_0)^{a_0}\, p_0(\boldsymbol{\theta} \mid \boldsymbol{c}_0). \tag{5.26}$$

When $a_0 = 0$, the historical data are ignored, and while for $a_0 = 1$, the historical data are given the same weight as the current data. When $a_0 \to 0$ the tails of the prior become heavier and more uncertainty is introduced in the prior.

Some special cases of the power prior are (a) binomial case: the power prior is proportional to $\theta^{a_0 y_0}(1-\theta)^{a_0 n_0 - a_0 y_0}$, which is the likelihood of a sample of size $a_0 n_0$ with

$a_0 y_0$ successes, and combined with a uniform initial prior for θ, the power prior becomes $p(\theta \mid y_0, a_0) = \text{Beta}(\theta \mid a_0 y_0 + 1, a_0(n_0 - y_0) + 1)$; (b) Gaussian case given σ^2: with an initial flat prior the power prior becomes $p(\mu \mid y_0, a_0) = \text{N}\left(\mu \mid \overline{y}_0, a_0^{-1}\sigma^2/n_0\right)$; (c) Poisson case: with $p_0(\theta) \propto \theta^{-1}$ (limiting gamma prior with α and $\beta \to 0$) the power prior becomes $\text{Gamma}(\theta \mid n\overline{y} + a_0 n_0, n + a_0 n_0)$.

It is not immediately clear on what basis a_0 should be chosen. The choice could be subjective, or a_0 could be given a (beta) prior with the parameters determined from the data. Applications of the power prior may be found in the use of historical controls in toxicological studies (Ibrahim *et al.* 1998) and Bayesian variable selection (Chen *et al.* 1999) (see also Chapter 11). The power prior does not, however, cover the situation where the historical data have a different model than the current data, e.g. when secular changes in the society have happened.

5.5.3 Elicitation of prior knowledge

5.5.3.1 Elicitation techniques

Expert knowledge can replace or augment the information that comes from historical data. The process of extracting information from experts is called *elicitation of prior information*. The main activity of the elicitation process is to turn the often qualitative knowledge of the experts into a probabilistic language. This will be illustrated in Example V.5. An in-depth treatment of elicitation is found in O'Hagan *et al.* (2006).

Example V.5: Stroke study: Prior distribution for the first interim analysis from expert knowledge

Prior to the first interim analysis one wishes to establish the available prior knowledge on the incidence of SICH (θ) for rt-PA treated patients, but no historical data were available.

The elicitation of expert knowledge typically collects two pieces of information: (1) the most likely value for θ (interpreted as a prior mode, mean or median) according to the expert and (2) the uncertainty of the expert on θ expressed as, e.g. a prior equal-tail 95% CI. Let the expert's prior mode for θ be 0.10 with 95% prior equal-tail CI equal to [0.05, 0.20]. A conjugate beta prior distribution could be computed with approximately the same summary measures. A quick exploration shows that a Beta(7.2, 56.2) density has roughly the desired characteristics. This prior is displayed in Figure 5.3 as the dashed curve. Alternatively, the experts could be asked about their prior belief p_k on each of the K intervals $I_k \equiv [\theta_{k-1}, \theta_k)$ covering [0,1]. Suppose that for our example, the experts produced prior probabilities equal to 0.025, 0.40, 0.45, 0.10 and 0.025, respectively, for the intervals [0,0.05), [0.05,0.10), [0.10,0.15), [0.15,0.20) and [0.20,0.25) and zero for the remaining intervals. This prior is shown in Figure 5.3 as the step function. Again an approximate conjugate prior distribution was fitted and this exercise produced (on purpose here) the same continuous prior in Figure 5.3. Note that in the above example the experts are not directly asked for their opinion about the hyperparameters α and β of the beta distribution since this is a much harder exercise. □

Eliciting expert knowledge in practice is challenging. The following problems have been reported:

- *Turning expert knowledge into probabilistic language*: Most experts do not have enough statistical background which makes the translation of their beliefs into a probabilistic

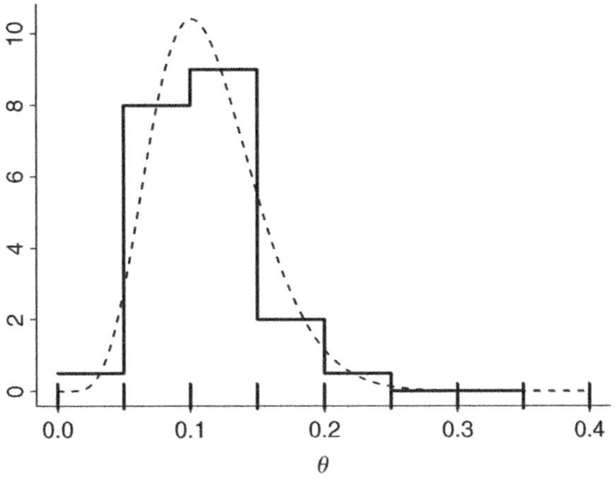

Figure 5.3 Stroke study: elicitation of prior knowledge on the incidence of SICH in rt-PA treated patients. The discrete prior is obtained from elicitation of prior probabilities on intervals. The continuous prior is obtained from elicitation of prior mode and prior 95% CI.

form a challenging task (Andrews *et al.* 1993; Chaloner 1996; Kadane and Wolfson 1997).

- *The construction of the prior distribution*: Details such as whether a best guess of θ represents prior mode, mean or median, may have an effect on determining the prior distribution. Also, choosing to express prior uncertainty via extremes (2.5%-ile and 97.5%-ile) or via a more general description of the prior (quartiles, mean, SD) may impact the easiness with which the expert knowledge is transformed into a prior. Chaloner *et al.* (1993) reported that better results were obtained with extreme quantiles, while O'Hagan (1998) reported the opposite. Finally, Chaloner (1996) mentioned that some probability statements are easier to elicit than others. This is illustrated in Example V.6.

A subjective Bayesian analysis is probably better digested if the prior is obtained from a community of experts rather than from a single expert. A community of priors allows us to evaluate the robustness of the conclusions based on the posterior distribution. But, the different prior opinions also allow the construction of a *community prior* that represents the (prior) viewpoint of a community of experts. The community prior can be established by averaging the priors of the experts, leading to a mixture prior distribution as in Example V.7. Another possibility is that the community prior is established via a consensus process and then it is called a *consensus* prior.

In the multiparameter case, the expert's opinion is needed for each parameter which requires the elicitation of a multivariate prior. When historical data are available, a multivariate prior distribution can be constructed as in Example IV.2. But, expressing expert knowledge jointly for several parameters is quite hard, if not impossible. In Example IV.4, prior knowledge on the normal mean and variance was treated separately. In practice, priors for a multiparameter model are often the product of priors of the individual parameters. But, in regression problems the prior knowledge must be specified jointly as the meaning of a regression coefficient depends on which other covariates are in the model. This is treated in Section 5.6. In some high-dimensional models, elicitation of prior information is basically impossible, for instance in the case of nonparametric regression models involving splines. In this case, it is absolutely unclear in which way prior information can be incorporated, hence a default prior appears to be the only option.

Including prior information in an analysis is one of the selling arguments of the Bayesian approach. Yet, when browsing through the statistical and medical/epidemiological literature revealed that Bayesian applications which include available knowledge are rather sparse. One reason to refrain from including prior information in the analysis, is the difficulty to turn knowledge into a probabilistic framework. For this reason, Johnson *et al.* (2010) reviewed methods published in the medical literature to elicit prior information from clinicians. The studies were evaluated on, e.g. their validity, reliability and responsiveness of the elicitation methods. From their review, the authors provided the guidelines to produce better accepted (by the general community) priors. They suggested: 'sampling from groups of experts, use clear instructions and a standardized script, provide examples and/or training exercises, avoid use of scenarios or anchoring data, ask participants to state the baseline rate in untreated patients, provide feedback and opportunity for revision of the response, and use simple graphical methods'.

5.5.3.2 Identifiability issues

A well-chosen informative prior allows for more accurate statements a posteriori about the parameters of interest than a noninformative prior. In some situations, strong subjective prior information is indispensable to arrive at posterior estimates. This is illustrated in Example V.6 on diagnostic testing. The model is overspecified, i.e. the data are not sufficient to estimate all parameters of the model and the model is then called *nonidentifiable*. By an *identifiable* model we mean that it is likelihood-identifiable, i.e. the likelihood is sufficient to provide a unique estimate of the model parameters. Strong prior information allows us to obtain reasonably precise posterior information on all parameters, but some of the parameters will not be updated by collecting data and estimation of these parameters will highly depend on the choice of the priors.

Example V.6: Cysticercosis study: Estimating prevalence in the absence of a gold standard

Pigs harbor a range of parasites and diseases that can be easily transmitted to humans. These include cysticercosis. Cysticercosis is the most common parasitic disease in the world affecting the central nervous system. Relatively accurate estimates of the prevalence of cysticercae in fattening pigs are essential to appraise the risk for human infection. Several diagnostic tests are used in practice, but none of them is a gold standard and exact information about test sensitivity and specificity is unavailable.

A total of 868 pigs were tested in Zambia with an antigen Enzyme-linked Immunosorbent Assay (Ag-ELISA) diagnostic test (see Dorny *et al.* 2004). The results of the study are summarized in Table 5.3. Of the 868 pigs, 496 pigs showed a positive test. The goal of the study was to estimate the prevalence π of cysticercosis in Zambia among pigs. If an estimate of the sensitivity α and of the specificity β are available, then the prevalence can be estimated as

$$\widehat{\pi} = \frac{p^+ + \widehat{\beta} - 1}{\widehat{\alpha} + \widehat{\beta} - 1}, \tag{5.27}$$

Table 5.3 Cysticercosis study: theoretical characteristics and observed results of the Ag-ELISA diagnostic test on pigs collected in Zambia.

		Disease (true)		Observed
		+	−	
Test	+	$\pi\alpha$	$(1-\pi)(1-\beta)$	$n^+ = 496$
	−	$\pi(1-\alpha)$	$(1-\pi)\beta$	$n^- = 372$
Total		π	$(1-\pi)$	$n = 868$

Notes: π is the true prevalence of cysticercosis. α and β are the sensitivity and specificity of the Ag-ELISA diagnostic test, respectively. n^+ (n^-) is the observed number of subjects with a positive (negative) Ag-ELISA test.

where $p^+ = n^+/n$ is the proportion of subjects with a positive test, and $\widehat{\alpha}$ and $\widehat{\beta}$ are the estimated sensitivity and specificity, respectively.

The results in Table 5.3 alone do not allow the estimation of π, α or β. The estimation needs the 2×2 contingency table of test versus true results. In fact, Table 5.3 contains only the diagnostic test results collapsed over the true disease status. It is customary that prior to the field experiment, the diagnostic test has been evaluated in the lab yielding estimates for α and β and hence allowing the use of expression (5.27). There is abundant evidence, though, that sensitivity and specificity are not intrinsic qualities of a diagnostic test but vary geographically (see Berkvens *et al.* 2006). Therefore, only expert knowledge can make the estimation of π possible. For this, we need to specify a prior distribution on π, α, and β. The posterior distribution is then

$$p(\pi, \alpha, \beta \mid n^+, n^-) \propto \binom{n}{n^+} [\pi\alpha + (1-\pi)(1-\beta)]^{n^+}$$
$$\times [\pi(1-\alpha) + (1-\pi)\beta]^{n^-} p(\pi)p(\alpha)p(\beta), \qquad (5.28)$$

with $p(\pi)$, $p(\alpha)$, and $p(\beta)$, the prior distribution for π, α, and β, respectively. Even for beta priors the marginal posterior distributions cannot be derived analytically. We used WinBUGS to produce the posterior summary measures and a graphical display of the marginal posterior distribution of the prevalence.

With uniform prior distributions for π, α and β, we produced Figure 5.4(a) and obtained [0.03, 0.97] as a 95% equal tail CI for π. Clearly, the uncertainty on the prevalence is huge. In fact, it must be said that with the above noninformative priors, the parameters of the model cannot be estimated because of identifiability problems. Extra information about the parameters is necessary to make the estimation of parameters work. Berkvens *et al.* (2006) reported that an additional 65 pigs were slaughtered and yielded estimates for sensitivity (20/31) and specificity (31/34). This data can be turned into a beta prior distribution for α (β) equal to Beta(21,12) (Beta(32,4)). The result of combining this prior knowledge with the likelihood is shown in Figure 5.4(b). Now the 95% equal tail CI for π is reduced to [0.66,0.99].

Finally, in order to solve the identifiability problem, we initially plugged-in some elicited values for sensitivity and specificity from experts. However, we discovered that they resulted in prior distributions that are in conflict with the observed data. This problem was largely

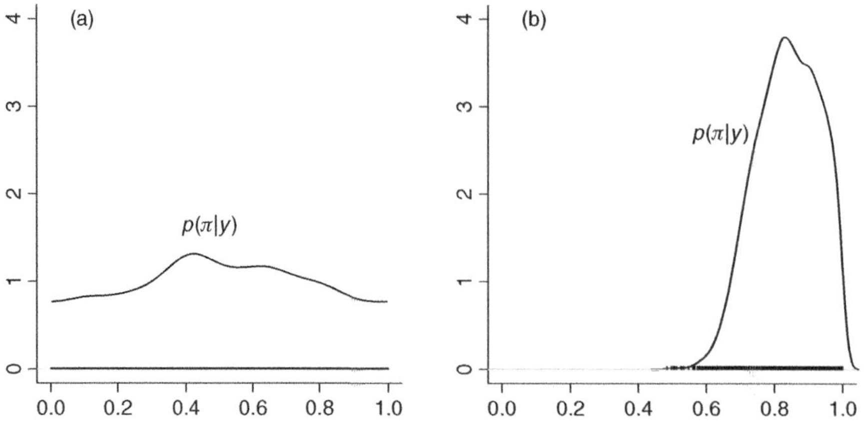

Figure 5.4 Cysticercosis study: posterior density of π for noninformative priors (a) of the parameters and informative priors (b).

removed when the experts were elicited in a different manner. That is, instead of directly asking their opinion on the sensitivity and specificity of the diagnostic test, we elicited their conditional probability of a positive test result given a positive or negative result on another test (Berkvens *et al.* 2006). □

Example V.6 showed both the strength and the weakness of the Bayesian approach. Prior knowledge provides a practical answer to the nonidentifiability problem but there is a price to pay since the posterior estimates of some of the parameters are dominated by the prior information. If this prior information is not adequate, then the posterior information is worthless. There is a vast literature (Gustafson 2009) on the estimation of parameters (sensitivity, specificity, and prevalence) in studies involving diagnostic tests that lack a gold standard.

5.5.4 Archetypal prior distributions

Among the different application areas, clinical trials are probably the toughest for the Bayesian philosophy to penetrate. While the Bayesian methodology has made its entrance via medical device clinical trials (see the FDA guidance document at http://www.fda/gov/cdrh/osb/guidance/1601.pdf), it is much harder to find Bayesian applications in phase III clinical trials. Indeed, such a trial is the pivotal step in convincing the regulatory authorities about the value of the drug for registration. The process of registering new drugs is (rightly) conservative and driven by regulatory requirements laid down by the Food and Drug Administration (FDA) in United States and by the EMEA (European Agency for the Evaluation of Medicinal Products) in Europe. Hence, despite the fact that at the phase III developmental stage of the drug there is a lot of information from previous stages (phases I and II) and that there is often abundant information from other similar drugs, in general, there is skepticism about the usefulness of that prior knowledge. In a special issue of Clinical Trials (Vols. 2, 4, 2005) reporting on the FDA Conference on the usefulness of Bayesian approaches in studying new treatments, Dr. Temple (FDA) states on page 302: 'We have seen many things that were "true" turn out not to be true. So it seems difficult to judge how much credit to give for prior evidence.' A Bayesian reply to such a statement may be that one should try out a community of priors and assess the sensitivity of the conclusion to the choice of the prior. However, this might not be satisfying to everyone, especially when the conclusions vary wildly. There is a need, as argued in Berger (2006), to keep up the appearance of objectivity. This pleas for an objective Bayesian analysis in this context. But formal rules can also be given to establish subjective priors in the context of clinical trials. Spiegelhalter *et al.* (1994) suggested two archetypal priors in addition to the vague prior: the *skeptical* and the *enthusiastic* prior.

5.5.4.1 The skeptical prior

Suppose that a drug company developed a cure for a disease but that prior to the present study five trials in a row failed to show any benefit. Even when the present trial turns out to be positive, the scientific community is likely to remain skeptical especially when there is no immediate evidence for this positive result. In that case, the scientists will likely combine their personal negative opinion with the result of the trial and might not accept the claimed benefit of the drug. This is illustrated below.

Example V.7: The use of a skeptical prior in a phase III randomized trial
Tan *et al.* (2003) reported on a phase III trial for treating cancer patients with either of two treatments. The standard treatment for hepatocellular carcinoma is surgical resection. A randomized trial was set up to compare surgery (standard therapy) with surgery + adjuvant radioactive iodine treatment (adjuvant therapy) on the rate of recurrence. The trial planned to recruit 120 patients. Frequentist interim analyses for efficacy were planned and at the first interim analysis, a significantly better result for the experimental treatment was obtained ($P = 0.01$), smaller than specified by a predefined frequentist stopping rule ($P < 0.029$). Despite the significant better performance of the experimental treatment, the scientific community was skeptical about the claimed effect of the adjuvant therapy. Consequently, a new, larger multicentric trial (300 patients) was set up to clarify the results of the earlier single-center trial.

Prior to the start of the subsequent trial, the pretrial opinions of the 14 clinical investigators were elicited. The prior distributions of each investigator were constructed by eliciting the prior belief on the treatment effect (adjuvant versus standard) on a grid of intervals. The average of the prior distributions yielded a community prior, while the average distribution of the five most skeptical investigators was called a skeptical prior. To exemplify the use of the skeptical prior, Tan *et al.* (2003) combined this prior with the interim analysis results of the previous trial and showed that the one-sided contour probability for superiority of the experimental treatment was only 0.49. Clearly, if one had combined this skeptical prior with the interim results, the trial would not have been stopped for efficacy. □

The choice of the skeptical prior in the above example depends on the selected investigators in the trial. In his special *Clinical Trials*', Dr. Temple states on page 323: 'It is a pain in the neck to have to discuss and agree on your priors every time you do a trial.' This statement pleas for a more formal choice of the skeptical prior distribution. The proposal of Spiegelhalter *et al.* (1994) for a skeptical prior in the normal case addresses this problem. More specifically, assume that θ expresses the true effect of treatment (A versus B) and that $\theta = 0$ means that the two treatments do not differ in performance. A skeptical normal prior could be concentrated around the (null-hypothesis) value of zero. The choice for the variance of the prior, σ_0^2, is motivated as follows. Suppose that the sample size calculation was done under the alternative hypothesis $\theta = \theta_a$. Since, the choice of θ_a is often optimistic, it is assumed that there is a small prior probability γ that the treatment effect exceeds θ_a. Then $P(\theta > \theta_a) = 1 - \Phi(\frac{\theta_a}{\sigma_0}) = \gamma$ implying that $\sigma_0 = -\theta_a/z_\gamma$, with $\gamma = \Phi(z_\gamma)$.

Example V.8: A lipid-lowering RCT: Use of skeptical prior
The Lescol Intervention Prevention Study (LIPS) study (Serruys *et al.* 2002) was a placebo-controlled randomized clinical trial set up to demonstrate that fluvastatin induces a reduction of major adverse cardiac events (MACE) in patients with coronary artery disease, without major hypercholesterolemia following successful completion of their first percutaneous coronary intervention (PCI). The sample size calculation was based on the assumption that after 3 years following PCI the incidence rate of MACE is 25% in the placebo group and that fluvastatin reduces this incidence rate by 25% to arrive at 18.75%. While the original study used a survival technique, we assume here for simplicity that the relative risk (placebo/fluvastatin) at the third year was taken as the primary endpoint. Let the true log(relative risk) be denoted as θ and suppose that the log-scale is used to specify prior information on the relative risk. Further, let the value of θ under the alternative hypothesis (θ_a) be equal to $\log(25/18.75) = 0.288$.

Using Spiegelhalter's *et al.* (1994) suggestion with $\gamma = 0.05$, the skeptical prior can be calculated and is shown in Figure 5.5. This prior assumes that it is unlikely ($P = 0.05$) that θ is greater than 0.288. The LIPS study used a frequentist stopping rule while a Bayesian approach may consist in combining this skeptical prior with the likelihood at each interim analysis to avoid early stopping in case of an overly optimistic interim result. □

In Exercise 5.15, another example of the use of a skeptical prior is given, but now the variance of the prior is determined by $P(\theta > \widehat{\theta}) = 1 - \Phi(\frac{\widehat{\theta}}{\sigma_0}) = \gamma$. Thus σ_0 is computed using the observed result in the study, rather than a prespecified result.

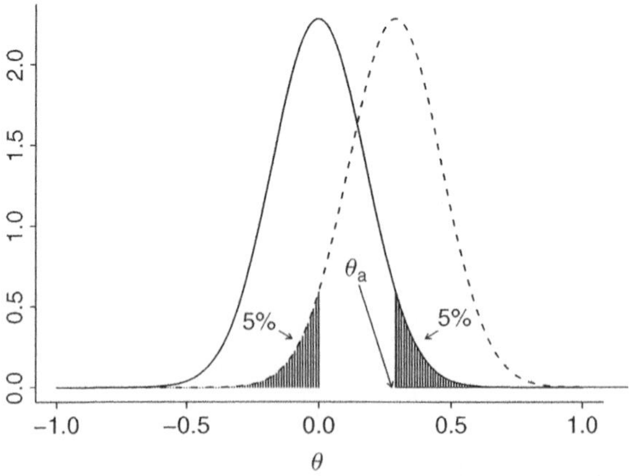

Figure 5.5 Lipid-lowering RCT: skeptical (solid line) and enthusiastic prior (dashed line) corresponding to $\theta_a = \log(25/18.75)$.

5.5.4.2 The enthusiastic prior

Spiegelhalter *et al.* (1994) also suggested an enthusiastic prior which is the counterbalance of the skeptical prior defined above. In this case, the normal prior has mean θ_a and σ_0^2 is determined such that $P(\theta < 0) = \gamma$. Thus, the enthusiastic prior specifies that a priori there is little evidence that the true effect is less or equal to zero.

Example V.9: A lipid-lowering RCT: Use of enthusiastic prior
The first patient was enrolled in the LIPS study in April 1995. At the planning stage of the LIPS study, the results of the 4S study were made public (The Scandinavian Simvastatin Survival Study Group (1994)). This study was a major step forward in demonstrating that a statin not only reduces the serum cholesterol level, but also saves lives in secondary prevention. The purpose of the LIPS study was similar to that of the 4S study, but now for PCI patients. With the results of the 4S study in mind, some of the investigators questioned whether the LIPS study was still needed and ethically feasible given that some patients were put at risk when allocated to the placebo treatment. After lengthy discussions, it was concluded that there was an ethical and a scientific basis to conduct the LIPS study. Given the intensive discussions at the start of the LIPS study, the use of an enthusiastic prior (Figure 5.5) might have been useful. Indeed, given the historical information from the 4S study and the positive results with fluvastatin in earlier stages of the development, the enthusiastic prior can protect the investigators from inadvertently stopping the trial if an early LIPS interim analysis had shown less promising results for fluvastatin (which was not the case, however). □

5.6 Prior distributions for regression models

5.6.1 Normal linear regression

In Section 4.7, the normal linear regression model

$$y = X\beta + \epsilon$$

was introduced. We refer to that section for further details.

5.6.1.1 Noninformative priors

A popular NI prior for the linear regression is obtained from Jeffreys multiparameter rule. It is the product of a flat prior for the regression parameters and the classical Jeffreys prior for the scale parameter, i.e. $p(\boldsymbol{\beta}, \sigma^2) \propto \sigma^{-2}$. In practice, often a normal prior with a large variance is chosen for the regression coefficients and for σ^2 an IG(ε, ε) prior with ε small.

5.6.1.2 Conjugate priors

The conjugate prior for a normal linear regression model is an extension of the conjugate prior for the basic normal model with both parameters unknown, seen in Section 5.3.2. Similar to expression (5.7), the joint density (likelihood) can be factorized into the product of $\chi^2(s^2 \mid \nu, \sigma^2)$ and $\text{N}[\widehat{\boldsymbol{\beta}} \mid \boldsymbol{\beta}, \sigma^2(\boldsymbol{X}^T\boldsymbol{X})^{-1}]$, with $\boldsymbol{X}$ as the design matrix. The conjugate prior is therefore the product of a normal prior $\text{N}(\boldsymbol{\beta}_0, \sigma^2\Sigma_0)$ for the regression coefficients and an inverse-gamma $\text{IG}(a_0, b_0)$ for the residual variance (or equivalently an Inv-$\chi^2(\nu_0, \tau_0^2)$-

distribution). The product yields again a normal-inverse-gamma prior NIG($\boldsymbol{\beta}_0$, Σ_0, a_0, b_0) (or equivalently N-Invχ^2($\boldsymbol{\beta}_0$, Σ_0, ν_0, τ_0^2)) given by the following complex expression:

$$\frac{(b_0/2)^{(a_0/2)}}{(2\pi)^{(d+1)/2} \mid \Sigma_0 \mid ^{1/2}\Gamma(a_0/2)(\sigma^2)^{(a_0+d+3)/2}} \exp\left[-\frac{(\boldsymbol{\beta}-\boldsymbol{\beta}_0)^T\Sigma_0^{-1}(\boldsymbol{\beta}-\boldsymbol{\beta}_0)+b_0}{2\sigma^2}\right]. \tag{5.29}$$

The posterior based on the above NIG prior and data $\boldsymbol{y}$ is a NIG($\overline{\boldsymbol{\beta}}$, $\overline{\Sigma}$, $\overline{a}$, $\overline{b}$) with

$$\overline{\Sigma} = \left(\Sigma_0^{-1} + \boldsymbol{X}^T\boldsymbol{X}\right)^{-1}, \tag{5.30}$$

$$\overline{\boldsymbol{\beta}} = \left(\Sigma_0^{-1} + \boldsymbol{X}^T\boldsymbol{X}\right)^{-1}\left(\Sigma_0^{-1}\boldsymbol{\beta}_0 + \boldsymbol{X}^T\boldsymbol{y}\right), \tag{5.31}$$

$$\overline{a} = a_0 + n, \tag{5.32}$$

$$\overline{b} = b_0 + \boldsymbol{\beta}_0^T\Sigma_0^{-1}\boldsymbol{\beta}_0 + \boldsymbol{y}^T\boldsymbol{y} - \overline{\boldsymbol{\beta}}^T\overline{\Sigma}^{-1}\overline{\boldsymbol{\beta}}. \tag{5.33}$$

Marginal posteriors are of the same type as described in Section 4.3, e.g. the marginal posterior distribution of $\boldsymbol{\beta}$ is a multivariate t-distribution with mean $\overline{\boldsymbol{\beta}}$. Further, as mentioned in Section 4.3.3, the NIG-prior is problematic as a tool to express our (subjective) prior information since prior knowledge on the regression parameters is related to prior knowledge on the residual variance.

Despite the difficulties of the NIG prior, a particular NIG-prior has become quite popular for instance in Bayesian variable selection. Zellner (1986) suggested as priors $\boldsymbol{\beta} \mid \sigma^2, \boldsymbol{X} \sim \mathrm{N}\left[\boldsymbol{\beta}_0, g\sigma^2(\boldsymbol{X}^T\boldsymbol{X})^{-1}\right]$ and $\sigma^2 \sim \mathrm{IG}(a_0, b_0)$ which implies that $\Sigma_0 = g(\boldsymbol{X}^T\boldsymbol{X})^{-1}$ in the normal prior for $\boldsymbol{\beta}$. This is known as *Zellner's g prior* (he actually suggested to put g in the denominator). Zellner's g prior can be seen as carrying information equivalent to pseudo-data $\boldsymbol{y}_0$ with the same design matrix as for $\boldsymbol{y}$ (and hence correlation structure) but with variance $\sigma_0^2 = g\sigma^2$. More precisely, if the pseudo $n \times 1$ data vector $\boldsymbol{y}_0 = \boldsymbol{X}\boldsymbol{\beta} + \varepsilon_0$ with $\varepsilon_0 \sim \mathrm{N}(\boldsymbol{0}, \sigma_0^2)$ is given a flat prior for $\boldsymbol{\beta}$ and an independent inverse gamma prior for σ^2, then the conditional posterior $p(\boldsymbol{\beta} \mid \sigma^2, \boldsymbol{y}_0)$ is $\mathrm{N}\left[(\boldsymbol{X}^T\boldsymbol{X})^{-1}\boldsymbol{X}^T\boldsymbol{y}_0,\ g\sigma^2(\boldsymbol{X}^T\boldsymbol{X})^{-1}\right]$. For $\boldsymbol{y}_0 = \boldsymbol{X}\boldsymbol{\beta}_0$ Zellner's g prior is obtained. This prior can also be interpreted as a particular case of the power prior (Chen *et al.* 2000; Ibrahim and Chen 2000) introduced in Section 5.5 when the pseudo-data $\boldsymbol{y}_0$ are assumed to have variance σ^2 and the likelihood is raised to a power $1/g$. Note that from expression (5.31) we conclude that the posterior mean of $\boldsymbol{\beta}$ with Zellner's g prior and $\boldsymbol{\beta}_0 = \boldsymbol{0}$ is equal to the LSE times a shrinkage factor $g/(g+1)$. Different values have been suggested for g, a popular choice being $g = n$. Other choices of g that offer a vague prior useful for Bayesian variable selection are reviewed in Chapter 11.

5.6.1.3 Priors based on historical data and expert knowledge

Prior knowledge on a single regression coefficient is rarely meaningful, since its meaning depends on what other regressors are in the model. Consequently, when prior knowledge is provided it must be done for the whole vector of regression parameters, but this is quite difficult in practice. Kadane *et al.* (1980) and Kadane and Wolfson (1996) proposed a predictive elicitation process, i.e. they offered the experts a set of design points and asked them to provide the 50th, 75th and 90th percentiles of the response distribution at these covariate values. With enough design points, the parameters of the conjugate prior can be computed.

Zellner's g prior can also be used to construct a prior based on historical data or expert knowledge, and is by far the most popular informative prior in regression models.

5.6.2 Generalized linear models

The Bayesian generalized linear model (BGLIM) for a sample $\boldsymbol{y} = \{y_1, \ldots, y_n\}$ was introduced in Section 4.8 and is given by

$$p(y_i \mid \theta_i; \phi) = \exp\left[\frac{y_i\theta_i - b(\theta_i)}{a_i(\phi)} + c(y_i; \phi)\right], \tag{5.34}$$

with $a_i(\phi) = \phi/w_i$ where w_i is a prior weight and $b(\cdot)$ and $c(\cdot)$ known functions. Further, $E(y_i) = \mu_i = \frac{d\,b(\theta_i)}{d\theta_i}$, $\text{var}(y_i) = a_i(\phi)V(\mu_i)$ with $V(\mu_i) = \frac{d^2\,b(\theta_i)}{d^2\theta_i}$, $g(\mu_i) = \eta_i = \boldsymbol{x}_i^T\boldsymbol{\beta}$ and for the canonical link $\eta_i = \theta_i$. In addition, all model parameters are given prior distributions.

5.6.2.1 Noninformative priors

A popular diffuse prior for the regression coefficients in any regression model and hence also for a BGLIM is to take a product of independent normal proper priors with a large variance. This is probably still the most frequently used NI prior for a BGLIM. For instance such a prior is used for location parameters in basically all examples in the WinBUGS Examples volumes I and II. However, for logistic (or other binary outcome) regression models, some concern has been raised against too dispersed normal priors in Markov chain Monte Carlo sampling. Indeed, when the prior variance is too large, sampling may occur too often in areas of low prior probability. Gelman *et al.* (2008) suggested as default prior a Cauchy density with center 0 and scale parameter equal to 2.5 for standardized continuous covariates (mean zero and SD $= 0.5$). This prior is weakly enough in practice and has good properties in case of separation problems (see Section 5.7).

Another possibility is to make use of Jeffreys multiparameter rule. For ϕ known, Ibrahim and Laud (1991) derived Jeffreys prior for the regression coefficients of a BGLIM. They suggested to use the following prior:

$$p(\boldsymbol{\beta}) \propto \left|\boldsymbol{X}^T \mathrm{W}\mathrm{V}(\boldsymbol{\beta})\Delta^2(\boldsymbol{\beta})\boldsymbol{X}\right|^{1/2}, \tag{5.35}$$

with W a $n \times n$ diagonal matrix of the weights w_i, $\mathrm{V}(\boldsymbol{\beta})$ a $n \times n$ diagonal matrix of $v_i = \mathrm{d}^2 b(\theta_i)/\mathrm{d}\theta_i^2$ and $\Delta(\boldsymbol{\beta})$ a $n \times n$ diagonal matrix of $\delta_i = \mathrm{d}\,b(\theta_i)/\mathrm{d}\eta_i$ (identity matrix for the canonical link). This prior follows easily from the Fisher information matrix of $\boldsymbol{\beta}$ which is expression (5.35) times ϕ^{-1} and can be readily computed for each GLIM. For normal linear regression with known residual variance, $p(\boldsymbol{\beta}) \propto \left|\boldsymbol{X}^T\boldsymbol{X}\right|^{1/2}$ which is an improper flat prior but yielding a Gaussian posterior for $\boldsymbol{\beta}$. It is the only GLIM for which the prior does not depend on $\boldsymbol{\beta}$. For logistic regression $p(\boldsymbol{\beta}) \propto \left|\boldsymbol{X}^T\mathrm{V}(\boldsymbol{\beta})\boldsymbol{X}\right|^{1/2}$ with $\mathrm{V}(\boldsymbol{\beta}) = \text{diag}(v_1, \ldots, v_n)$ and $v_i = \mu_i(1 - \mu_i)$. For Poisson regression with the canonical link, the same expression for $p(\boldsymbol{\beta})$ is obtained with $v_i = \mu_i$. Ibrahim and Laud (1991) proved the propriety of the posterior for several BGLIMs. Prior (5.35) has been implemented in two Bayesian SAS procedures (see Section 5.6.3).

5.6.2.2 Conjugate priors

Without the regression structure, distribution (4.33) belongs to the one-parameter exponential family for $a(\phi)$ known. Hence, the conjugate prior distribution can be derived from expression (5.3). However, the covariate structure complicates matters. Chen and Ibrahim (2003) suggested a conjugate prior for a BGLIM. Applied to the case without a regression structure and assuming that $a_i(\phi) = 1/\phi$ is known, they specified as joint prior for expression (5.34):

$$p(\boldsymbol{\theta} \mid \boldsymbol{y}_0, a_0, \phi) \propto \prod_{i=1}^{n} \exp\{a_0\phi[y_{0i}\theta_i - b(\theta_i)]\} = \exp\left\{a_0\phi[\boldsymbol{y}_0^T\boldsymbol{\theta} - \boldsymbol{j}^T\boldsymbol{b}(\boldsymbol{\theta})]\right\}, \qquad (5.36)$$

with $a_0 > 0$ a scalar prior parameter, $\boldsymbol{y}_0 = (y_{01}, \ldots, y_{0n})^T$ a vector of prior parameters, $\boldsymbol{j}$ a $n \times 1$ vector of ones, and $\boldsymbol{b}(\boldsymbol{\theta}) = (b(\theta_1), \ldots, b(\theta_n))^T$. That this prior is conjugate to (5.34) can be readily derived from expression (5.3) with an appropriate change in notation. The regression structure is introduced by allowing $\theta_i = \theta(\eta_i)$ and $\eta_i = \boldsymbol{x}_i^T\boldsymbol{\beta}$, $(i = 1, \ldots, n)$. Then the authors defined the prior $D(\boldsymbol{y}_0, a_0)$ for $\boldsymbol{\beta}$ (given ϕ) as

$$p(\boldsymbol{\beta} \mid \boldsymbol{y}_0, a_0, \phi) \propto \exp\left\{a_0\phi[\boldsymbol{y}_0^T\boldsymbol{\theta}(\boldsymbol{\eta}) - \boldsymbol{j}^T\boldsymbol{b}(\boldsymbol{\theta}(\boldsymbol{\eta}))]\right\} \equiv \exp\left\{a_0\phi[\boldsymbol{y}_0^T\boldsymbol{\theta}(\boldsymbol{X\beta}) - \boldsymbol{j}^T\boldsymbol{b}(\boldsymbol{\theta}(\boldsymbol{X\beta}))]\right\}. \qquad (5.37)$$

Chen and Ibrahim (2003) proved the conjugacy of $D(\boldsymbol{y}_0, a_0)$, i.e. the posterior is equal to $D\left(\frac{a_0\boldsymbol{y}_0+\boldsymbol{y}}{a_0+1}, a_0 + 1\right)$ after combining the prior with the likelihood (5.34) for a sample $\boldsymbol{y}$. With ϕ random, conjugacy can be proved again, but conjugacy is lost when a_0 is also random. The use of $D(\boldsymbol{y}_0, a_0)$ requires to supply the vector $\boldsymbol{y}_0$ and the parameter a_0. The vector $\boldsymbol{y}_0$ could be elicited as a prior for $E(\boldsymbol{y})$ with a_0 representing the prior sample size. However, $\boldsymbol{y}_0$ must be of same length as $\boldsymbol{y}$ with the same design matrix. The prior $D(\boldsymbol{y}_0, a_0)$ can also be seen as the posterior density of $(\boldsymbol{\beta} \mid a_0, \boldsymbol{y}_0, \phi)$ with $\boldsymbol{y}_0$ seen as (pseudo-)data and an initial flat prior for $\boldsymbol{\beta} \mid \phi$. This makes this conjugate prior in principle suitable for use with historical data, with the limitation that $n_0 = n$.

5.6.2.3 Priors based on historical data and expert knowledge

The power prior introduced in Section 5.5.2 was originally proposed for a regression structure. It has the advantage that, unlike the above conjugate prior, the historical data do not have to have the same size as the data at hand.

The next two informative BGLIM priors require that expert prior knowledge is elicited about the predicted response at k representative covariate vectors $\boldsymbol{x}_{01}, \ldots, \boldsymbol{x}_{0k}$ in the sense of Kadane *et al.* (1980) and Kadane and Wolfson (1996). The two approaches differ in the number and the choice of the covariate vectors and in the way the predictive distribution at the covariate locations is included in the Bayesian model. To fix ideas we will focus on the logistic regression case. We distinguish between data augmentation prior and conditional means prior:

- *Data augmentation prior* (*DAP*): the number of design points k is equal to the size of the observed data set. Let $\boldsymbol{x}_{0i}$ $(i = 1, \ldots, n)$ denote the design points with pseudo-observations y_{0i} (in this case, say, prior proportions), which could be elicited from experts or derived from historical data and given a weight n_{0i} proportional to their importance (say prior sample size). The pseudo-sample $\boldsymbol{y}_0 = \{y_{01}, \ldots, y_{0n}\}$ yields a likelihood

$L_P(\boldsymbol{\beta} \mid \boldsymbol{y}_0)$ proportional to $\prod_{i=1}^n F(\boldsymbol{x}_{0i}^T\boldsymbol{\beta})^{n_{0i}y_{0i}}[1 - F(\boldsymbol{x}_{0i}^T\boldsymbol{\beta})]^{n_{0i}(1-y_{0i})}$. The DAP is then defined as proportional to $L_P(\boldsymbol{\beta} \mid \boldsymbol{y}_0)$. Further, suppose that the likelihood of the observed data $\{(y_i, \boldsymbol{x}_i, n_i),\ (i = 1, \ldots, n)\}$ is $L(\boldsymbol{\beta} \mid \boldsymbol{y}) \propto \prod_{i=1}^n F(\boldsymbol{x}_i^T\boldsymbol{\beta})^{n_i y_i}[1 - F(\boldsymbol{x}_i^T\boldsymbol{\beta})]^{n_i(1-y_i)}$. When $\boldsymbol{x}_i = \boldsymbol{x}_{0i}$, $(i = 1, \ldots, n)$, the posterior $p(\boldsymbol{\beta} \mid \boldsymbol{y})$ is proportional to

$$\prod_{i=1}^{n} F(\boldsymbol{x}_i^T\boldsymbol{\beta})^{n_{0i}y_{0i}+n_i y_i}[1 - F(\boldsymbol{x}_i^T\boldsymbol{\beta})]^{n_{0i}(1-y_{0i})+n_i(1-y_i)}$$

and hence the DAP is conjugate to the logistic likelihood. The posterior mode can be obtained from a maximum likelihood program, but for other posterior measures sampling algorithms (e.g. Markov chain Monte Carlo) might be needed. The attractiveness of the prior is that it can be directly interpreted as containing the information from a pseudo-sample in a similar way as with Zellner's g prior. Clogg *et al.* (1991) introduced the DAP as an alternative to MLE for logistic regression models with sparse data.

Greenland (2001, 2003, 2007) used a DAP for a Bayesian regression analysis of epidemiological data. For instance, for logistic regression, the normal prior on the log-odds ratio, β, is turned into a 2×2 prior contingency table of pseudo-data with odds ratio approximately equal to the specified prior mean of β and the sampling variance of the odds ratio of the pseudo-data equal to the specified prior variance of β. This approach allows us to use standard frequentist software for the approximate determination of the posterior for β.

- *Conditional means prior* (CMP): another approach is suggested by Bedrick *et al.* (1996). For logistic regression, they suggested to elicit prior information on $\pi_{0i} = E(y_{i0} \mid x_{0i})$ $(i = 1, \ldots, k)$ the success probabilities at the design points x_{0i}, e.g. one might specify beta priors $\pi_{i0} \sim \text{Beta}(\alpha_i, \beta_i)$. This yields the joint prior for the k success probabilities, i.e.

$$p(\boldsymbol{\pi}_0) \propto \prod_{i=1}^{k} \pi_{0i}^{\alpha_i - 1}(1 - \pi_{0i})^{\beta_i - 1}.$$

In their proposal k is equal to $d + 1$, the number of regression coefficients and the $\boldsymbol{x}_{0i} (i = 1, \ldots, d + 1)$ are linearly independent. The above prior yields the conditional means prior (CMP) for $\boldsymbol{\beta}$ by the transformation rule. Bedrick *et al.* (1996) showed that the CMP prior is in some cases also a DAP. For example, the above-induced prior on $\boldsymbol{\beta}$ is a DAP, which means that it has the functional form of the likelihood. Other connections between a CMP and a DAP can be found in Bedrick *et al.* (1996). As for the DAP sampling techniques are needed to derive posterior inference.

As seen above, eliciting prior knowledge directly on regression parameters does not work in practice. For a GLIM there is an extra challenge in that the meaning of regression coefficients changes with the link function. For example, when prior knowledge is available for logistic regression parameters, then it is not immediately clear how this translates into prior knowledge on the regression parameters for the complementary log–log link. Despite the attractiveness of the above data-based priors, their application in practice is still sparse.

5.6.3 Specification of priors in Bayesian software

As seen in Section 5.4.5, WinBUGS only allows proper priors. Regression coefficients are given in WinBUGS most often independent normal priors, with a large variance if their impact must be minimal. For noninformative priors on the variance parameters, the uniform prior and the inverse gamma IG(ε, ε) prior with $\varepsilon = 10^{-3}$ are the most popular.

The SAS® program offers from version 9.2 on a variety of Bayesian regression models and the user is allowed to provide a great range of priors including improper priors. The procedures GENMOD and MCMC allow for the fitting of a BGLIM. Both procedures accept Jeffreys priors for the regression coefficients and therefore one needs the propriety results derived by Ibrahim and Laud (1991) to ensure that the posterior is proper. Indeed, SAS leaves this check up to the responsibility of the user. Other aspects on Bayesian software are dealt with in Chapter 8.

5.7 Modeling priors

Every informative prior impacts the estimation of the model parameters, but a prior can also direct the model to address computational difficulties or to achieve computational properties. We call these *modeling priors* because their intention is to adapt the characteristics of the statistical model. We consider here priors that address multicollinearity, convergence issues, parameter constraints and variable selection.

In the case where there is multicollinearity in the regressors, i.e. $\boldsymbol{X}^T\boldsymbol{X}$ is nearly rank-deficient and regression coefficients and standard errors are inflated. Ridge regression provides a way to stabilize the estimates, which involves replacing $\boldsymbol{X}^T\boldsymbol{X}$ with $\boldsymbol{X}^T\boldsymbol{X} + \lambda\mathrm{I}$ with $\lambda > 0$ the ridge parameter and yields $\widehat{\boldsymbol{\beta}}^R(\lambda) = (\boldsymbol{X}^T\boldsymbol{X} + \lambda\mathrm{I})^{-1}\boldsymbol{X}^T\boldsymbol{y}$ as estimator. The estimator is obtained by minimizing

$$(\boldsymbol{y}^* - \boldsymbol{X\beta})^T(\boldsymbol{y}^* - \boldsymbol{X\beta}) + \lambda\boldsymbol{\beta}^T\boldsymbol{\beta} \tag{5.38}$$

for a given λ, with $\boldsymbol{y}^* = \boldsymbol{y} - \overline{y}\mathbf{1}_n$. This implies shrinkage of the regression coefficients toward zero. Note that the centered response is taken such that the intercept is not taking part in the shrinkage process. The ridge solution can also be obtained from the posterior mode of a Bayesian normal linear regression analysis with a normal prior $\mathrm{N}(\mathbf{0}, \tau^2\mathrm{I})$ for $\boldsymbol{\beta}$ and $\tau^2 = \sigma^2/\lambda$, keeping σ and τ fixed. Thus, in the Bayesian formulation, the *normal ridge prior* restricts the parameter vector (with high probability) to a sphere of radius determined by λ. Note that the R function rmvt (in mvtnorm) generates multivariate t-distributed random variables. Note also that the ridge estimator is the posterior mean in expression (5.30) for $\boldsymbol{\beta} \sim \mathrm{N}(\mathbf{0}, \frac{\sigma^2}{\lambda}\mathrm{I})$. Ridge regression is easily extended to GLIMs; see Van Houwelingen and Le Cessie (1992) for an example in logistic regression. We elaborate further on the ridge estimator and other shrinkage procedures in Chapter 11.

With GLIMs other numerical problems may occur. For instance in binary response models, the regression coefficient estimates fail to converge (to a finite value) when the diagnostic classes show a high degree of separation in the covariate space. This problem has been addressed in Albert and Anderson (1984); Lesaffre and Albert (1989); and Lesaffre and Kaufmann (1992) and occurs frequently especially with categorical covariates and small sample sizes. To avoid such numerical difficulties, Gelman *et al.* (2008) suggested independent

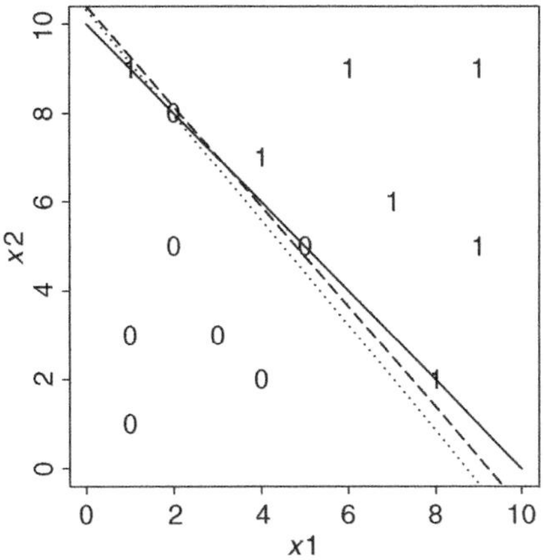

Figure 5.6 Quasi-complete separation in logistic regression: line of quasi-complete separation (solid line), estimated discrimination rule obtained from the normal prior with variance 10^2 (dotted line) and estimated discrimination rule using Gelman *et al.* (2008) (dashed line).

weakly informative Cauchy priors for the regression parameters and recommended these priors as a default. In the next example, we illustrate the numerical problems when separation occurs in a logistic regression model.

Example V.10: Computational difficulties in binary response models
In Figure 5.6, we show a case of quasi-complete separation between two diagnostic classes involving two regressors x_1 and x_2. Complete separation means that the two classes can be separated by a hyperplane in the covariate space, while quasi-complete separation means that there is complete separation for all observations except for observations lying on the hyperplane. In both cases, it can be shown that (some of) the regression parameter estimates diverge. The problem looks similar to that caused by multicollinearity, but there are differences (Lesaffre and Marx 1993).

A WinBUGS logistic regression analysis with diffuse priors equal to $\text{N}(0, \tau^2)$ with $\tau = 10^3$ for all three regression parameters, aborted immediately. For $\tau = 10$ a stable and reasonable discrimination rule was obtained and is shown in Figure 5.6. In fact, this is a ridge-regression solution since we penalize large regression coefficients, a consequence of the separation problem. In addition, we applied the proposal of Gelman *et al.* (2008) but had to use a $t(2)$-distribution since WinBUGS does not provide a Cauchy distribution. The estimated discrimination rule is again reasonable and close to the previous one. □

When a statistical model has a built-in constraint on the parameters, the estimation of the parameters needs to be done under this restriction. As a practical example let θ_k be the probability of showing caries experience (caries in the past or at present) among Flemish children in the Signal-Tandmobiel® study at the kth ($k = 1, \ldots, 6$) school year. These probabilities must satisfy $\theta_1 \leq \theta_2 \leq \ldots \leq \theta_6$ since caries experience is defined in a cumulative manner. An estimation procedure which takes this constraint into account is isotonic regression. Many other algorithms have been written to determine the ML estimates under the constraints

(Barlow *et al.* 1972; de Leeuw *et al.* 2009). In a Bayesian approach, inequality constraints on parameters are easily dealt with by choosing a prior distribution that puts zero weight on the parameter vectors that are not allowed. For instance, the prior on $\boldsymbol{\theta} = (\theta_1, \ldots, \theta_6)^T$ in the dental example that maps all $\boldsymbol{\theta}$s that violate the constraint to zero, is a good choice. This ensures that $p(\boldsymbol{\theta} \mid \mathbf{y}) \propto p(\boldsymbol{\theta})p(\mathbf{y} \mid \boldsymbol{\theta})$ will satisfy this constraint. In addition, the Bayesian constrained theory remains the same as the unconstrained unlike in the frequentist world. Chen and Deely (1996) used this approach in an agricultural example and concluded that the Bayesian results look more reasonable than the frequentist solutions. Note that there is another possible way to deal with the constraint and that is to neglect the values that are not allowed in the posterior. This can be particularly handy when the posterior summary measures are obtained by sampling.

Other priors may be specified which direct the model to exhibit a specific characteristic. For instance when we replace the normal ridge priors $p(\beta_j) \sim \mathrm{N}(0, \tau^2)$ for the regression parameters by double exponential (Laplace) distributions $p(\beta_j) \sim \frac{\lambda}{2}\exp(-\lambda|\beta_j|)$ one obtains the Bayesian *LASSO estimator* introduced by Tibshirani (1996) in the frequentist context. With this prior the regression coefficients of unimportant regressors are more shrunk than the regression coefficients of unimportant regressors; see Sections 11.2.2 and 11.8 for an extensive treatment of this topic.

5.8 Other regression models

The literature on priors is extensive and we had to limit here to a few important classes of models, thereby realizing that we left out other quite important models used in epidemiologic research such as the conditional logistic regression model, the Cox proportional hazards model, the generalized linear mixed effects model, etc. Some of the above approaches for constructing priors have been extended to these models. For instance, Chaloner *et al.* (1993) applied the approaches of Kadane *et al.* (1980) and Kadane and Wolfson (1996) to proportional hazards models. Further, DAPs and CMPs have been proposed for survival models by Bedrick *et al.* (1996); Greenland and Christensen (2001) and Greenland (2003).

5.9 Closing remarks

While the choice of the prior lies at the heart of the Bayesian approach, specifying appropriate subjective and objective priors may be difficult in complex models. In this chapter, we have reviewed the Bayesian literature on the choice of the prior. Increasingly, the prior is interacting with the statistical model, as exemplified in Section 5.7. It illustrates that in a Bayesian model, both the likelihood and the prior shape the final model.

It has been repeatedly stated that the use of a prior distribution is a major objection to use Bayesian methods because of the fear that it will pollute inference with subjective information. But subjectivity is lurking in every statistical analysis, frequentist or Bayesian. A striking example is the use of smoothing approaches for sparse data. Clearly, when restricting the behavior of the estimates by penalty constraints (Eilers and Marx 1996) expert knowledge is incorporated into analysis and the 'data don't speak for themselves' anymore as one regularly claims in a frequentist approach.

Exercises

Exercise 5.1 Show that Jeffreys prior for the mean parameter θ of a Poisson likelihood is given by $\sqrt{\theta}$.

Exercise 5.2 Let y be uniformly distributed given θ on $[0, \theta]$, find the conjugate distribution for $f(y \mid \theta) = \theta^{-1}$.

Exercise 5.3 Show graphically when the normal prior distribution with mean = 328 and variance = 100 and a $t(\nu)$-prior distribution for varying ν (but with same mean and variance) give a noticeably different posterior distribution when combined with the IBBENS likelihood. Note that to obtain the posterior distribution for a $t(\nu)$-prior distribution one requires numerical integration.

Exercise 5.4 Show that the normal model with unknown mean and variance belongs to the two-parameter exponential family. Use expression (5.3) to derive the natural conjugate prior of the normal distribution. Finally, show that the extended conjugate family is needed

$$p(\boldsymbol{\theta} \mid \boldsymbol{\alpha}, \beta, \boldsymbol{\gamma}) = k(\boldsymbol{\alpha}, \beta, \boldsymbol{\gamma}) \exp\left[c(\boldsymbol{\theta})^T \boldsymbol{\alpha} + \beta d(\boldsymbol{\theta}) + \boldsymbol{\gamma} e(\boldsymbol{\theta})\right], \tag{5.39}$$

where $\boldsymbol{\alpha}$, β are hyperparameters as in expression (5.3) and $\boldsymbol{\gamma}$ an extra set of parameters, to yield the normal-inverse-gamma prior (O'Hagan and Forster 2004, pp. 140–141).

Exercise 5.5 Derive the posterior mean and variance of the mixture distribution in Example V.3.

Exercise 5.6 Sample from the mixture distribution in Example V.3 and report the summary statistics.

Exercise 5.7 Show that the natural conjugate for the multinomial distribution is the Dirichlet distribution and derive Jeffreys prior and the resulting posterior distribution.

Exercise 5.8 Prove that all one-dimensional marginal distributions of a Dirichlet distribution are beta distributions.

Exercise 5.9 Show graphically that the data-translated likelihood principle is satisfied on the original scale of μ for a normal likelihood with σ given.

Exercise 5.10 Show that Jeffreys rule for the negative binomial model gives $\theta^{-1}(1-\theta)^{-1/2}$ and thereby violates the likelihood principle which states that inference should be based only on the observed data.

Exercise 5.11 Show that for the multinomial model, Jeffreys rule suggests to take for a noninformative prior $p(\boldsymbol{\theta}) \propto (\theta_1 \times \ldots \times \theta_p)^{-1/2}$.

Exercise 5.12 Show that in the binomial case the arcsin($\sqrt{\cdot}$)-transformation yields an approximate data-translated likelihood. Show also that this prior is locally uniform in the original scale for proportions that are not too close to 0 and 1.

Exercise 5.13 Show that Jeffreys prior distribution for σ^2 of a normal distribution with given mean, results in a proper posterior distribution when there are at least two observations.

Exercise 5.14 Berger (2006) reported on a Bayesian analysis to estimate the positive predictive value θ of a diagnostic test for a disease from (a) the prevalence of the disease (p_0),

(b) the sensitivity of the diagnostic test (p_1) and (c) 1-specificity of the diagnostic test (p_2). Bayes theorem states that

$$\theta = \frac{p_0\, p_1}{p_0\, p_1 + (1 - p_0)\, p_2}.$$

Suppose that data x_i ($i = 0, 1, 2$) are available with binomial distributions Bin(n_i, p_i). Show that an equal tail interval CI for θ based on Jeffreys priors $\pi(p_i) \propto p_i^{-1/2}(1 - p_i)^{-1/2}$ enjoys good coverage properties. Employ sampling for this and compare the 95% equal-tail CI with a classical 95% CI.

Exercise 5.15 Holzer *et al.* (2006) analyzed a retrospective cohort study for the efficacy and safety of endovascular cooling in unselected survivors of cardiac arrest compared to controls. The authors found that the patients in the endovascular cooling had a 2-fold increased odds of survival (67/97 patients versus 466/941 patients; odds ratio 2.28, 95% CI, 1.45 to 3.57) compared to the control group. After adjustment for baseline imbalances, the odds ratio was 1.96 (95% CI = [1.19, 3.23]). In the final step, the authors took account of the fact that their study was nonrandomized and wished to discount their results for the study design. More specifically, they discounted their cohort study data by assuming that the observed effect on the logarithmic scale (log odds ratio) was actually 0 and the probability of exceeding the observed effect was 5% (skeptical prior). Determine the normal skeptical prior and compute the posterior distribution assuming that the log odds ratio has a normal likelihood.

Exercise 5.16 Derive the conjugate prior for the distribution (4.33) using the rule explained in Section 5.3.1.

6

Markov chain Monte Carlo sampling

6.1 Introduction

In Chapter 4, we illustrated that the analytical calculation of the posterior distribution (and its summary measures) is often not feasible due to the difficulty in determining the integration constant. Calculating the integral using numerical integration methods is a practical alternative if only a few parameters are involved, but it becomes prohibitive for real-life applications where the dimensionality is often high.

In Chapters 3 and 4, we illustrated that sampling from the posterior can be an elegant alternative procedure to analytical calculations. To sample from standard univariate distributions (normal, t, χ^2, etc.) routines are available in statistical software such as R, S+ and SAS®. For nonstandard distributions, general procedures, e.g. the accept–reject algorithm, are required. To sample from a d-dimensional distribution, the Method of Composition may be used if the distribution can be factorized into a product of a univariate marginal and conditional distributions of dimensions $d-1$, $d-2$, etc. But these distributions (except for one) can only be determined after integration, and therefore, this sampling approach cannot work in most practical problems.Thus for basically each practical problem, an alternative approach is required. In this chapter, we explore an attractive class of sampling algorithms, called *Markov chain Monte Carlo (MCMC) methods*. Integration is not needed anymore, which makes MCMC algorithms applicable to virtually all (highly multivariate) problems. The two most important MCMC procedures are (a) the *Gibbs sampler* and (b) the *Metropolis(–Hastings) algorithm*. No doubt, it is the introduction of these two sampling algorithms that revolutionized Bayesian statistics and created an immense revival of the Bayesian idea by offering solutions to practical problems. Without exaggeration, MCMC techniques allow for tackling statistical modeling problems which are hard (or even impossible) to solve with maximum likelihood procedures, thereby offering the applied statistician a rich toolbox of statistical modeling techniques. In addition, the introduction of the MCMC approaches initiated an impressive line of new

Bayesian Biostatistics, First Edition. Emmanuel Lesaffre and Andrew B. Lawson.

statistical research. Historical notes on the development of MCMC can be found in Hitchcock (2003).

While the Gibbs sampler is mathematically a special case of the Metropolis–Hastings (MH) algorithm, the two MCMC procedures are treated separately in the literature because their sampling mechanisms are quite different. The choice between the two methods often depends on the particular problem at hand as will be illustrated in this chapter.

The aim of this chapter is to introduce the reader to MCMC sampling techniques. Hereby, we focus on the intuition behind the techniques. A variety of numerical examples serve as first illustrations, where other more practical illustrations will be given in subsequent chapters. The justification of the MCMC approaches, i.e. why they give a sample from the posterior distribution, is treated in Section 6.4. The reader is introduced to Markov Chain terminology and the most important theorems which justify the MCMC approach as a method to extract information from the posterior distribution are stated.

6.2 The Gibbs sampler

The *Gibbs sampler* was introduced by Geman and Geman (1984) in the context of image processing. They assumed that the intensity of the pixels in an image have a *Gibbs distribution*, which is a classical distribution in statistical mechanics. Since this distribution is analytically intractable involving easily a million unknowns, Geman and Geman developed a sampling algorithm to explore the distribution. The sampler was called after the distribution. However, the Gibbs sampler became only popular in the statistical world when Gelfand and Smith (1990) showed its ability to tackle complex estimation problems in a Bayesian manner.

We first treat the two-dimensional Gibbs sampler and illustrate the method on three elementary examples.

6.2.1 The bivariate Gibbs sampler

The Method of Composition (Section 4.6) provides a tool to sample from a bivariate posterior distribution $p(\theta_1, \theta_2 \mid \boldsymbol{y})$. The approach is based on the property that the joint posterior $p(\theta_1, \theta_2 \mid \boldsymbol{y})$ is completely determined by the marginal $p(\theta_2 \mid \boldsymbol{y})$ and the conditional posterior $p(\theta_1 \mid \theta_2, \boldsymbol{y})$ distribution. A sample from $p(\theta_1, \theta_2 \mid \boldsymbol{y})$ is then obtained by sampling first from the marginal posterior distribution $p(\theta_2 \mid \boldsymbol{y})$ yielding a sampled value $\widetilde{\theta}_2$ and then from the conditional $p(\theta_1 \mid \widetilde{\theta}_2, \boldsymbol{y})$ yielding $\widetilde{\theta}_1$ and hence $(\widetilde{\theta}_1, \widetilde{\theta}_2)$ is also obtained.

The Gibbs sampler, on the other hand, uses the property that (under fairly general regularity conditions) a multivariate distribution is uniquely determined by its conditional distributions (Section 6.2.3). In a Bayesian context, this implies for two dimensions that $p(\theta_1, \theta_2 \mid \boldsymbol{y})$ is uniquely determined by $p(\theta_1 \mid \theta_2, \boldsymbol{y})$ and $p(\theta_2 \mid \theta_1, \boldsymbol{y})$. The sampling approach is initiated using a starting value for the parameters, say θ_1^0 and θ_2^0 (in fact only one is needed) and then 'explores' the posterior distribution by generating θ_1^k and θ_2^k $(k = 1, 2, 3, \ldots)$ in a sequential manner. Formally, given θ_1^k and θ_2^k at iteration k, the $(k+1)$th value for each of the parameters is generated according to the following iterative scheme:

- Sample $\theta_1^{(k+1)}$ from $p(\theta_1 \mid \theta_2^k, \boldsymbol{y})$
- Sample $\theta_2^{(k+1)}$ from $p(\theta_2 \mid \theta_1^{(k+1)}, \boldsymbol{y})$

Hereby, the Gibbs sampler generates a sequence of values $\theta_1^1, \theta_2^1, \theta_1^2, \theta_2^2, \ldots$ such that the vectors $\boldsymbol{\theta}^k = (\theta_1^k, \theta_2^k)^T, k = 1, 2, \ldots$ are dependent and create a chain. The chain has the Markov property which means that given $\boldsymbol{\theta}^k$, $\boldsymbol{\theta}^{(k+1)}$ is independent of $\boldsymbol{\theta}^{(k-1)}$, $\boldsymbol{\theta}^{(k-2)}$, etc. In a probabilistic notation, $p(\boldsymbol{\theta}^{(k+1)} \mid \boldsymbol{\theta}^k, \boldsymbol{\theta}^{(k-1)}, \ldots, \mathbf{y}) = p(\boldsymbol{\theta}^{(k+1)} \mid \boldsymbol{\theta}^k, \mathbf{y})$.

The aim of the Gibbs sampler is to generate samples from the posterior distribution. But this sampling procedure differs from the sampling techniques seen in the previous chapters. First, the chain of sampled values depends on a starting value. Second, the generated values are dependent. Therefore, it is not immediately clear that the Gibbs sampler gives a sample from the posterior distribution and that the summary measures from the chain estimate consistently the true summary posterior measures. Because of the Markov property and the fact that Monte Carlo techniques are used to generate new values, the Gibbs sampler is called a *Markov chain Monte Carlo* method. In Section 6.4, it is demonstrated that the Gibbs sampler delivers, under mild regularity conditions, ultimately samples from the posterior distribution, called the *target distribution*. However, an initial portion of the chain, called the *burn-in part*, is discarded.

Summarized, the Gibbs sampler generates a Markov chain $\boldsymbol{\theta}^1, \boldsymbol{\theta}^2, \ldots$ which constitutes a dependent sample from the posterior distribution starting from a well chosen iteration k_0 and the summary measures calculated from the chain consistently estimate the true posterior measures. In the next three examples, we illustrate the mechanics of the Gibbs sampler. First, we determine the posterior distribution of Example IV.5 via Gibbs sampling.

Example VI.1: Serum alkaline phosphatase study: Gibbs sampling the posterior – non-informative prior

In Example IV.5, we sampled from the posterior distribution of the normal likelihood based on 250 *serum alkaline phosphatase* (*alp*) measurements of 'healthy' patients. We assumed for both parameters a noninformative prior. To apply the Gibbs sampler, we need to establish the two conditional distributions $p(\mu \mid \sigma^2, \mathbf{y})$ and $p(\sigma^2 \mid \mu, \mathbf{y})$ from expression (4.4). The first conditional distribution is equal to $\mathrm{N}(\mu \mid \overline{y}, \sigma^2/n)$, while $p(\sigma^2 \mid \mu, \mathbf{y})$ is obtained by fixing μ in expression (4.4) and verifying that we are dealing with an $\mathrm{Inv}-\chi^2(\sigma^2 \mid n, s_\mu^2)$-distribution, with $s_\mu^2 = \frac{1}{n}\sum_{i=1}^n (y_i - \mu)^2$.

Upon initialization, the Gibbs sampler explores the posterior distribution (4.4) using the following iterative scheme at iteration $(k+1)$:

1. Sample $\mu^{(k+1)}$ from $\mathrm{N}(\overline{y}, (\sigma^2)^k/n)$
2. Sample $(\sigma^2)^{(k+1)}$ from $\mathrm{Inv}-\chi^2(n, s^2_{\mu^{(k+1)}})$

One Gibbs step thus consists of two substeps and the sampling procedure creates a zigzag pattern in the (μ, σ^2)-plane. In the first substep, a move is made from $(\mu^k, (\sigma^2)^k)$ to $(\mu^{(k+1)}, (\sigma^2)^k)$. In the second substep, a move is made to $(\mu^{(k+1)}, (\sigma^2)^{(k+1)})$. Note that only every second generated vector belongs to the chain.

To exemplify the sampling procedure in detail, we describe the first steps of one realized chain. The starting value for the parameter vector (μ, σ^2) was taken as (6.5, 2). The value $\mu^1 = 7.19$ was then generated using $\mathrm{N}(7.11, 2/250)$ ($\overline{y} = 7.11, \sigma^2 = 2$) yielding an intermediate vector (7.19, 2). This constitutes the first substep of the Gibbs chain. In the next substep, the value $(\sigma^2)^1 = 1.78$ was generated from $\mathrm{Inv}-\chi^2(250, s^2_{7.19})$. Therefore, the first genuine element of the Gibbs chain is (7.19, 1.78). Similarly, the vectors (7.20, 1.74), (7.22, 1.95), (7.03, 1.62) were generated in three further Gibbs steps (six substeps). The path of the sampled vectors $(\mu^k, (\sigma^2)^k)$, $(k = 1, \ldots, 6)$ is displayed in Figure 6.1(a). The zigzag behavior of the

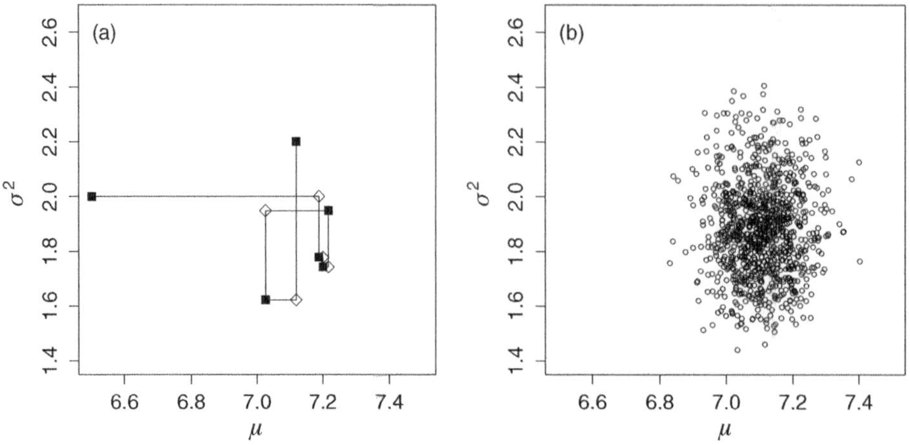

Figure 6.1 Serum alkaline phosphatase study (noninformative prior): (a) first six steps when Gibbs sampling the joint posterior distribution for μ and σ^2 with a noninformative prior. The squares represent elements of the Gibbs chain, while the diamonds represent intermediate stages, and (b) last 1000 Gibbs sampled parameter vectors (μ, σ^2) from a chain of total size equal to 1500.

path illustrates that the chain explores the posterior distribution along the coordinate axes. In the graph, a square symbol pertains to a genuine element of the chain, while a diamond indicates an intermediate vector.

We stopped sampling at $k = 1500$. Except for an initial portion, the elements of the chain constitute a sample from $p(\mu, \sigma^2 \mid \mathbf{y})$. We ignored the first 500 sampled parameter vectors, and hence, the size of the burn-in part is here 500. The remaining 1000 sampled vectors are displayed in Figure 6.1(b). To demonstrate that the Gibbs sampler delivers a sample from the correct posterior distribution, we show in Figure 6.2 the histogram of μ^k and of $(\sigma^2)^k$ for $k \geq 501$ together with the correct marginal posterior distributions determined in an analytical way. □

Note that the choice of the chain length of 1500 and the length of the burn-in part of 500 were not motivated. General guidelines for choosing the chain length and the burn-in part will be extensively dealt with in Chapter 7. These guidelines indicate that the above-chosen lengths are appropriate. The following example from Casella and George (1992) illustrates that the Gibbs sampler is not restricted to the Bayesian context.

Example VI.2: Sampling from a discrete × continuous distribution
Assume that the joint distribution of x and y is given by

$$f(x, y) \propto \binom{n}{x} y^{x+\alpha-1}(1-y)^{(n-x+\beta-1)},$$

with x a discrete random variable taking values in $\{0, 1, \ldots, n\}$, y a random variable on the unit interval and $\alpha, \beta > 0$ parameters. To sample from the marginal distribution $f(x)$, one

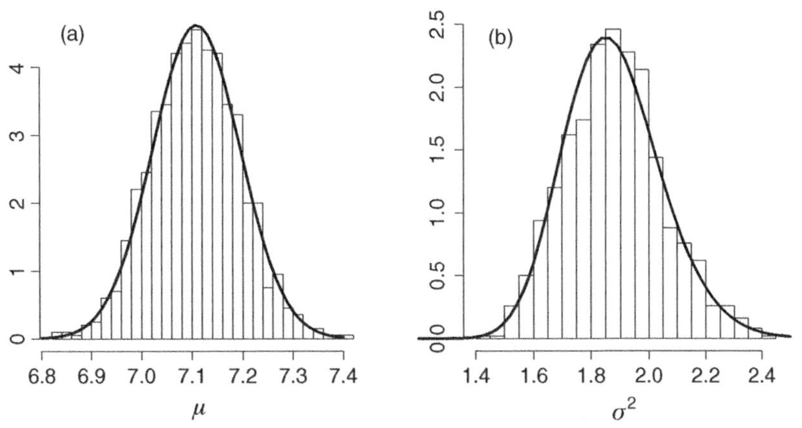

Figure 6.2 Serum alkaline phosphatase study (noninformative prior): marginal posterior distribution of (a) μ and (b) σ^2 corresponding to the generated sample in Figure 6.1(b). The solid lines pertain to the true posterior distributions.

can use the Gibbs sampler by generating samples from $f(x, y)$ and retaining only the sampled values for x. To this end, the conditional distributions $f(x \mid y)$ and $f(y \mid x)$ are needed. To establish the conditional distribution $f(x \mid y)$, it is handy to write $f(x, y)$ as

$$f(x, y) \propto \binom{n}{x} y^x (1-y)^{(n-x)} y^{\alpha-1}(1-y)^{(\beta-1)}.$$

For $f(x \mid y)$, we remove the part that does not depend on x, which is $y^{\alpha-1}(1-y)^{(\beta-1)}$. This shows that $f(x \mid y)$ is a Bin(n, y) distribution. Similarly, $f(y \mid x)$ is Beta$(x+\alpha, n-x+\beta)$. The Gibbs iterative sampling scheme is therefore at iteration $(k+1)$:

1. Sample $x^{(k+1)}$ from Bin(n, y^k)
2. Sample $y^{(k+1)}$ from Beta$(x^{(k+1)} + \alpha, n - x^{(k+1)} + \beta)$

The true marginal distribution $f(x)$ is equal to the beta-binomial distribution BB(n,α,β) defined in expression (3.14), allowing us to compare the generated histogram with the true probability histogram.

We illustrate the Gibbs sampler for $n = 30$, $\alpha = 2$ and $\beta = 4$. Figure 6.3 is based on $x = 0, y = 0.5$ as starting values generating first x and then y. It can be seen from the figure that the sampled histogram is relatively close to the true distribution even with these extreme starting values. Further, it can easily be verified that it does not matter which starting values are chosen or whether (x, y) are generated in the reversed order. □

For the third example, we return to the serum alkaline phosphatase study, but now we assume that there is prior information available, as in Section 4.3.3.

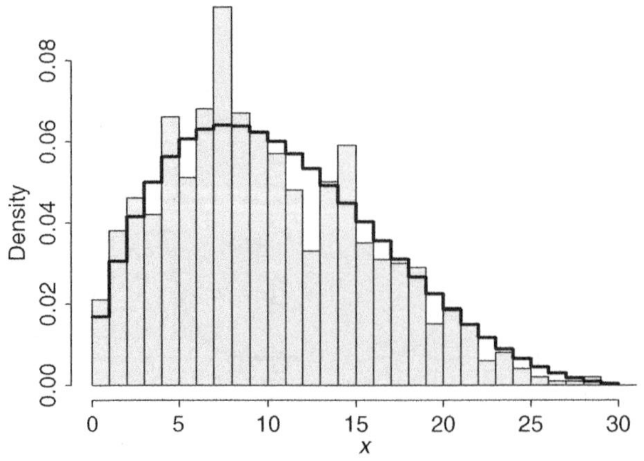

Figure 6.3 Beta-binomial BB(30, 2, 4)-distribution: histogram of Gibbs sampled x based on starting values $x = 0, y = 0.5$, 1500 iterations and burn-in part of 500 iterations; the solid line shows true distribution.

Example VI.3: Serum alkaline phosphatase study: Gibbs sampling the posterior – semi-conjugate prior

We repeat here the analysis of Example VI.1 with independent informative priors for the parameters:

- $\mu \sim \text{N}(\mu_0, \sigma_0^2)$
- $\sigma^2 \sim \text{Inv} - \chi^2(\nu_0, \tau_0^2)$

The posterior distribution for μ and σ^2 is (up to a proportionality constant) the product of the likelihood with the two independent priors:

$$\begin{aligned} p(\mu, \sigma^2 \mid \mathbf{y}) &\propto \frac{1}{\sigma_0} e^{-\frac{1}{2\sigma_0^2}(\mu-\mu_0)^2} \\ &\times (\sigma^2)^{-(\nu_0/2+1)} e^{-\nu_0 \tau_0^2/2\sigma^2} \\ &\times \frac{1}{\sigma^n} \prod_{i=1}^{n} e^{-\frac{1}{2\sigma^2}(y_i-\mu)^2} \\ &\propto \prod_{i=1}^{n} e^{-\frac{1}{2\sigma^2}(y_i-\mu)^2} e^{-\frac{1}{2\sigma_0^2}(\mu-\mu_0)^2} (\sigma^2)^{-\left(\frac{n+\nu_0}{2}+1\right)} e^{-\nu_0 \tau_0^2/2\sigma^2}. \end{aligned}$$

To obtain the conditional distribution $p(\mu \mid \sigma^2, \mathbf{y})$, we remove in the above expression all terms that do not involve μ. Thus, only the term $\prod_{i=1}^{n} e^{-\frac{1}{2\sigma^2}(y_i-\mu)^2} e^{-\frac{1}{2\sigma_0^2}(\mu-\mu_0)^2}$ remains. Then we recognize that this is the kernel of a density given by expression (2.13). For $p(\sigma^2 \mid \mu, \mathbf{y})$, we find that it is the kernel of $\text{Inv} - \chi^2\left(\nu_0 + n, \frac{\sum_{i=1}^{n}(y_i-\mu)^2+\nu_0\tau_0^2}{\nu_0+n}\right)$. The Gibbs sampling procedure at iteration $(k+1)$, therefore, consists of the following steps:

1. Sample $\mu^{(k+1)}$ from $\text{N}(\overline{\mu}^k, (\overline{\sigma}^2)^k)$, with

$$\overline{\mu}^k = \frac{\frac{1}{\sigma_0^2}\mu_0 + \frac{n}{(\sigma^2)^k}\overline{y}}{\frac{1}{\sigma_0^2} + \frac{n}{(\sigma^2)^k}} \quad \text{and} \quad (\overline{\sigma}^2)^k = \frac{1}{\frac{1}{\sigma_0^2} + \frac{n}{(\sigma^2)^k}}.$$

   Note that $\overline{\mu}^k$ does not depend on the generated μ-values despite what the notation might suggest.

2. Sample $(\sigma^2)^{(k+1)}$ from

$$\text{Inv} - \chi^2\left(\nu_0 + n, \frac{\sum_{i=1}^{n}(y_i - \mu^{(k+1)})^2 + \nu_0\tau_0^2}{\nu_0 + n}\right).$$

The priors are conditional conjugate distributions, and hence, the product is a semi-conjugate prior (see Section 5.3.4).

As in Example IV.6, the historical data were used to establish independent priors. One chain of size 1500 was generated using the above iterative scheme, with starting values (5.5, 3) and a burn-in part of size 500. The posterior distributions for μ and σ^2 as well as their posterior means and medians were close to those obtained by the Method of Composition in Example IV.6. The 95% CIs differed somewhat more, illustrating that extreme quantiles show greater variability. With the Gibbs sampler, we obtained for the posterior mean (95% equal tail CI) of μ and σ^2 the values 6.79 ([6.73, 6.85]) and 2.14 ([2.01, 2.25]), respectively, which are basically the same as obtained from the Method of Composition. □

The three examples enjoy the luxury that the output of the Gibbs sampler can be checked against either an analytical result or a result obtained from another independent sampling approach. In general, this will not be possible and we need some reassurance that we are exploring the posterior distribution appropriately. This will be given by the theory in Section 6.4. However, these theoretical results do not tell us how long the chain should be. A chain of length 1500 may be too short and may have produced an empirical histogram quite different from the true posterior distribution. To get an idea of how fast the chain explores the posterior distribution, one uses a simple graphical tool called the *trace plot*. The trace plot is a time series plot with the iteration number on the x-axis and the sampled value on the y-axis. In Figure 6.4, we have shown the trace plots for both parameters of the previous example. The figure shows (a) that we have chosen extreme starting values and (b) that the chain moves for both parameters quickly through the distribution. The erratic behavior of these trace plots is also characteristic for classical (independent) sampling procedures. Strictly speaking, trace plots cannot prove that the posterior is sampled appropriately, convergence diagnostics are needed for this (see Section 7.2).

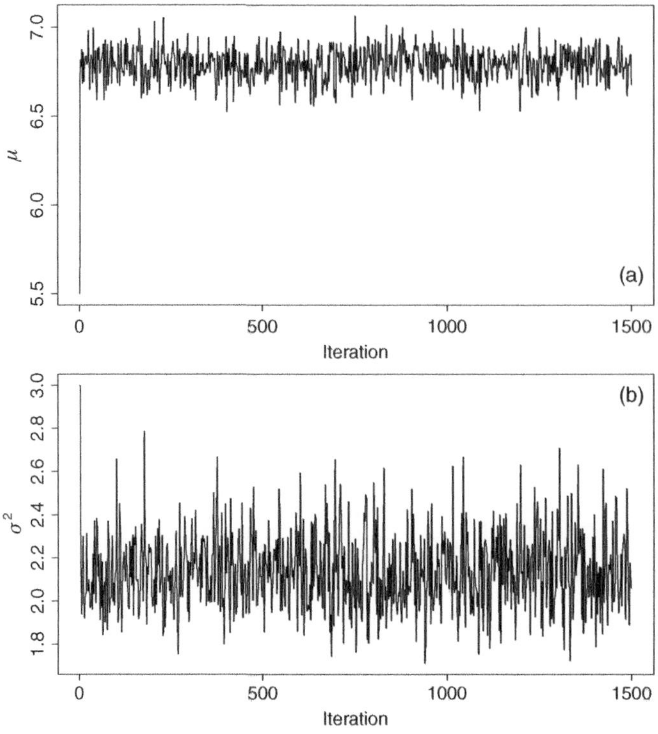

Figure 6.4 Serum alkaline phosphatase study (informative prior): trace plots for (a) μ and (b) σ^2 when using a semi-conjugate prior.

6.2.2 The general Gibbs sampler

Given a starting position $\boldsymbol{\theta}^0 = (\theta_1^0, \ldots, \theta_d^0)^T$, the multivariate version of the Gibbs sampler has the following iterative scheme. At iteration $(k + 1)$, the sampling procedure performs the following d steps:

1. Sample $\theta_1^{(k+1)}$ from $p(\theta_1 \mid \theta_2^k, \ldots, \theta_{(d-1)}^k, \theta_d^k, \mathbf{y})$
2. Sample $\theta_2^{(k+1)}$ from $p(\theta_2 \mid \theta_1^{(k+1)}, \theta_3^k, \ldots, \theta_d^k, \mathbf{y})$

$\vdots$

d. Sample $\theta_d^{(k+1)}$ from $p(\theta_d \mid \theta_1^{(k+1)}, \ldots, \theta_{(d-1)}^{(k+1)}, \mathbf{y})$

The conditional distributions $p(\theta_j \mid \theta_1^k, \theta_2^k, \ldots, \theta_{(j-1)}^k, \theta_{(j+1)}^k, \ldots, \theta_{(d-1)}^k, \theta_d^k, \mathbf{y})$ are called *full conditional distributions* or shorter *full conditionals*, because θ_j is conditioned on all other parameters. It is shown in Section 6.4 that, under mild regularity conditions, the generated values $\boldsymbol{\theta}^k, \boldsymbol{\theta}^{(k+1)}, \ldots$ ultimately can be regarded as observations from the posterior distribution. Two examples illustrate the mechanism of the multivariate Gibbs sampler. We start with a well-known, but not biostatistical, example. It is an example of a change-point model.

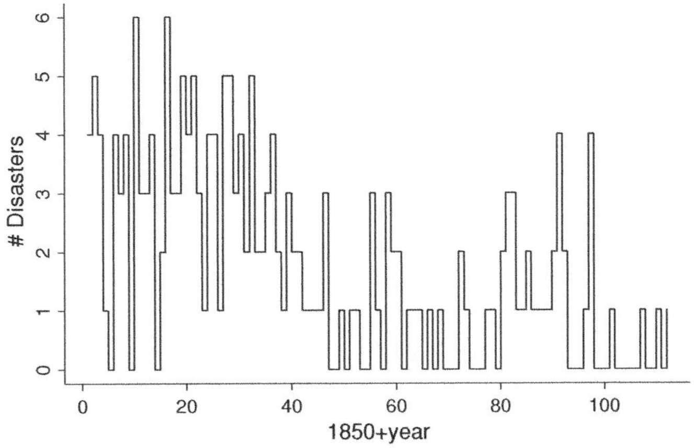

Figure 6.5 British coal mining data: frequency of disasters per year.

Change-point models are important in longitudinal studies when the aim is to detect the onset of a disease.

Example VI.4: British coal mining disasters data: Finding the change point using the Gibbs sampler

The well-known British coal-mining disasters data set contains the number of severe accidents in British coal mines from 1851 to 1962. This data set has been analyzed by many; see Tanner (1993) and references therein. The frequency of disasters per year is plotted in Figure 6.5. This figure indicates a possible decrease in frequency of disasters from year 40 (+ 1850) onward. We now wish to see whether there is statistical evidence for this claim.

The count in the ith year, y_i, is assumed to have a Poisson distribution with mean θ until year k, the change point. Afterward, y_i has a Poisson distribution with mean λ. Thus, a Poisson process with a change point at k is assumed, given by

$$y_i \sim \text{Poisson}(\theta) \text{ for } i = 1, \ldots, k \text{ and } y_i \sim \text{Poisson}(\lambda) \text{ for } i = k+1, \ldots, n,$$

with $n = 112$. Conditional conjugate priors are chosen for θ and λ, i.e.

$$\theta \sim \text{Gamma}(a_1, b_1) \text{ and } \lambda \sim \text{Gamma}(a_2, b_2),$$

with a_1, a_2, b_1, b_2 parameters. The prior for k is taken as uniform on $\{1, \ldots, n\}$, i.e. $p(k) = 1/n$. The a- and b-parameters can be given a hyperprior, but Tanner (1993) assumed only b_1 and b_2 to be stochastic with distribution

$$b_1 \sim \text{Gamma}(c_1, d_1) \text{ and } b_2 \sim \text{Gamma}(c_2, d_2),$$

and c_1, c_2, d_1, d_2 fixed.

The full conditionals are determined as before, i.e. we multiply the likelihood with all priors and for each parameter we remove the part that does not depend on it. The goal is again to recognize a standard distribution (at least a distribution from which we can sample). This

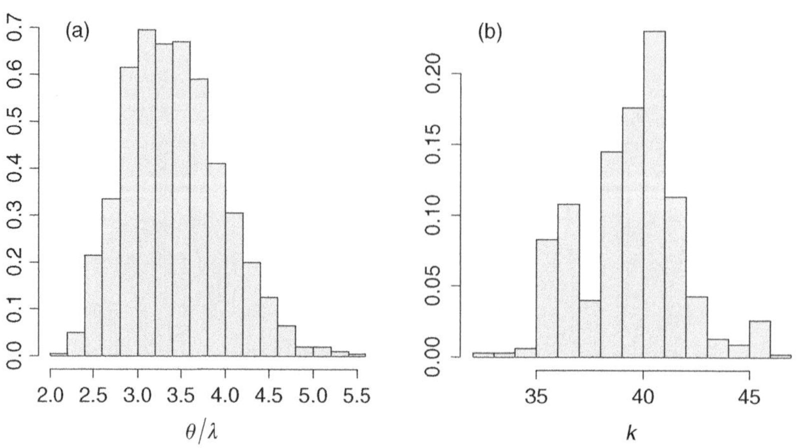

Figure 6.6 British coal mining data: posterior distribution for (a) θ/λ and (b) k.

gives

$$p(\theta \mid \mathbf{y}, \lambda, b_1, b_2, k) = \text{Gamma}(a_1 + \sum_{i=1}^{k} y_i, k + b_1),$$

$$p(\lambda \mid \mathbf{y}, \theta, b_1, b_2, k) = \text{Gamma}(a_2 + \sum_{i=k+1}^{n-k} y_i, n - k + b_2),$$

$$p(b_1 \mid \mathbf{y}, \theta, \lambda, b_2, k) = \text{Gamma}(a_1 + c_1, \theta + d_1),$$

$$p(b_2 \mid \mathbf{y}, \theta, \lambda, b_1, k) = \text{Gamma}(a_2 + c_2, \lambda + d_2),$$

$$p(k \mid \mathbf{y}, \theta, \lambda, b_1, b_2) = \frac{\pi(\mathbf{y} \mid k, \theta, \lambda)}{\sum_{j=1}^{n} \pi(\mathbf{y} \mid j, \theta, \lambda)},$$

$$\text{with } \pi(\mathbf{y} \mid k, \theta, \lambda) = \exp[k(\lambda - \theta)] \left(\frac{\theta}{\lambda}\right)^{\sum_{i=1}^{k} y_i}.$$

The full conditional distributions determine the iterative Gibbs sampling scheme together with a choice for the a, c and d-parameters. Here, we take the values assumed by Tanner, i.e. $a_1 = a_2 = 0.5$, $c_1 = c_2 = 0$ and $d_1 = d_2 = 1$. One Markov chain was run with length 1500. The posterior summary measures were based on the last 1000 values. On the basis of this chain, we can derive the posterior summary measures of original and derived parameters. For instance, in Figure 6.6(a) the posterior distribution of θ/λ is shown. The posterior distribution of k shows that most likely in 1891 the frequency of coal mining disasters was drastically reduced with approximately a factor of 3.5, obtained from the posterior mean for θ/λ equal to 3.42 with 95% CI = [2.48, 4.59]. □

In the next example, we reanalyze the osteoporosis study analyzed in Example V.7 with the Method of Composition.

Example VI.5: Osteoporosis study: Exploring the posterior with the Gibbs sampler
Take the regression model specified in Section 4.7.1 with noninformative priors for the parameters as in Section 4.7.2. Further, suppose that there is only one regressor x (BMI)

Table 6.1 Osteoporosis study: posterior summary measures obtained from the Method of Composition and the Gibbs sampler, both based on 1000 sampled values.

Parameter	Method of Composition						
	2.5%	25%	50%	75%	97.5%	Mean	SD
β_0	0.57	0.74	0.81	0.89	1.05	0.81	0.12
β_1	0.032	0.038	0.040	0.043	0.049	0.040	0.004
σ^2	0.069	0.078	0.083	0.088	0.100	0.083	0.008
	Gibbs Sampler						
	2.5%	25%	50%	75%	97.5%	Mean	SD
β_0	0.67	0.77	0.84	0.91	1.10	0.77	0.11
β_1	0.030	0.036	0.040	0.042	0.046	0.039	0.0041
σ^2	0.069	0.077	0.083	0.088	0.099	0.083	0.0077

to predict the response y (TBBMC). Both have been measured on n individuals to yield $\boldsymbol{x} = (x_1, \ldots, x_n)^T$ and $\boldsymbol{y} = (y_1, \ldots, y_n)^T$. For the three parameters, intercept β_0, slope β_1 and residual variance σ^2, the full conditionals are derived in the usual manner and are

$$p(\sigma^2 \mid \beta_0, \beta_1, \boldsymbol{y}) = \text{Inv} - \chi^2(n, s_{\beta}^2),$$

$$p(\beta_0 \mid \sigma^2, \beta_1, \boldsymbol{y}) = \text{N}(r_{\beta_1}, \sigma^2/n),$$

$$p(\beta_1 \mid \sigma^2, \beta_0, \boldsymbol{y}) = \text{N}(r_{\beta_0}, \sigma^2/\boldsymbol{x}^T\boldsymbol{x}),$$

with $s_{\beta}^2 = \frac{1}{n}\sum(y_i - \beta_0 - \beta_1 x_i)^2$, $r_{\beta_1} = \frac{1}{n}\sum(y_i - \beta_1 x_i)$, and $r_{\beta_0} = \sum(y_i - \beta_0)x_i/\boldsymbol{x}^T\boldsymbol{x}$.

One Markov chain of size 1500 was generated using the Gibbs iterative scheme making. The above full conditionals dictate the sampling procedure. An initial 500 iterations were discarded.

In Table 6.1, the posterior summary measures obtained from the converged Markov chain are compared with the corresponding measures obtained from the Method of Composition (based on 1000 independent sampled values). The summary measures for the two sampling approaches match relatively well, with an even better correspondence for σ^2. An explanation for this different behavior is found in the trace plots of the parameters.

Figure 6.7 shows the index plots of the sampled values of β_1 and σ^2 based on the Method of Composition. Note that the index has no sequential interpretation here since the values are sampled independently. This index plot illustrates what graph one may expect in case of independent sampling. Comparing the index plots in Figure 6.7 with the corresponding ones obtained with Gibbs sampling (Figure 6.8) highlights that σ^2 is sampled with the MCMC approach in an almost independent manner, in contrast to β_1 (similar for β_0) where sampling with the MCMC approach is quite dependent. Indeed, the trace plot for β_1 points to a relatively high correlation between β_1^k and $\beta_1^{(k-1)}, \beta_1^{(k-2)}, \ldots$. In that case one speaks of a chain with high *autocorrelation(s)*. In general, more initial iterations must be removed when there is high autocorrelation. In addition, the remaining part of the Markov chain needs to be longer to obtain a stable estimate of the marginal posterior distribution. However, upon convergence, the chain should have forgotten its starting position which evidently takes longer for highly

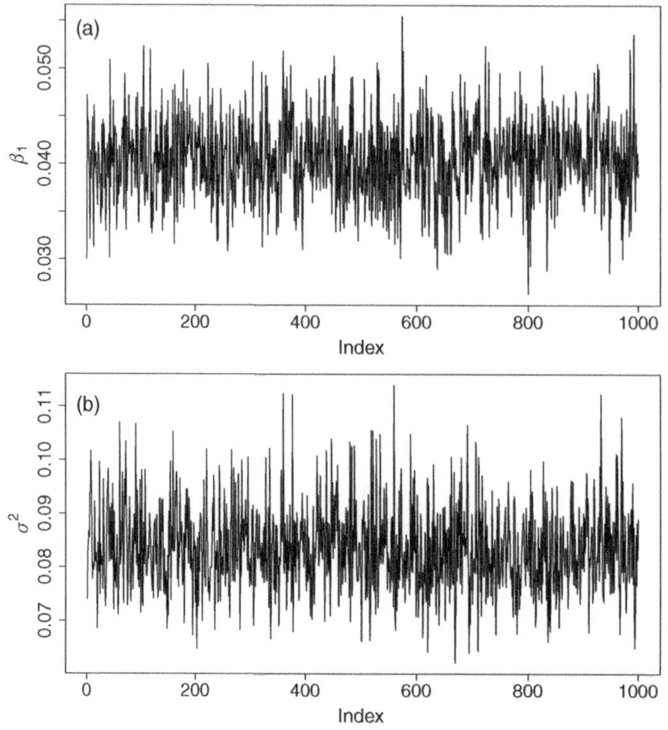

Figure 6.7 Osteoporosis study: index plots of 1000 sampled values of (a) β_1 and (b) σ^2 obtained using the Method of Composition.

correlated chain values. Hence, the chain for the regression coefficients needs to be longer than for σ^2. To illustrate this, Figure 6.9 shows two histograms for β_1 obtained from different parts of the same Markov chain. Clearly, the summary measures for β_1 obtained from these two parts are quite different. In contrast, the summary measures for σ^2 do not differ substantially for the corresponding parts of the chain (results not shown). Further illustrations of the sampling behavior of the regression parameters, more specifically of the difficulty to converge, are given in Section 7.2. □

6.2.3 Remarks*

Central to the Gibbs sampler is the property that the full conditionals determine the joint distribution. This result was shown in Besag (1974) but appears to date back to an unpublished result of Hammersley and Clifford in 1971. Proofs of this theorem are given by Robert and Casella (2004) for the bivariate case (Theorem 9.3) and for the general case (Theorem 10.5). The proof of the bivariate case is reproduced here. To simplify notation, we omit the dependence on $\boldsymbol{y}$ in the formulas. Since $p(\theta_1, \theta_2) = p(\theta_2 \mid \theta_1)p_1(\theta_1) = p(\theta_1 \mid \theta_2)p_2(\theta_2)$, $\int \frac{p(\theta_2|\theta_1)}{p(\theta_1|\theta_2)}\, d\theta_2 = \int \frac{p_2(\theta_2)}{p_1(\theta_1)}\, d\theta_2 = \frac{1}{p_1(\theta_1)}$, $p(\theta_1, \theta_2) = p(\theta_2 \mid \theta_1)/\int [p(\theta_2 \mid \theta_1)/p(\theta_1 \mid \theta_2)]\, d\theta_2$ which demonstrates that the joint distribution is determined by its two conditional distributions. The implicit assumption in the above proof is that the

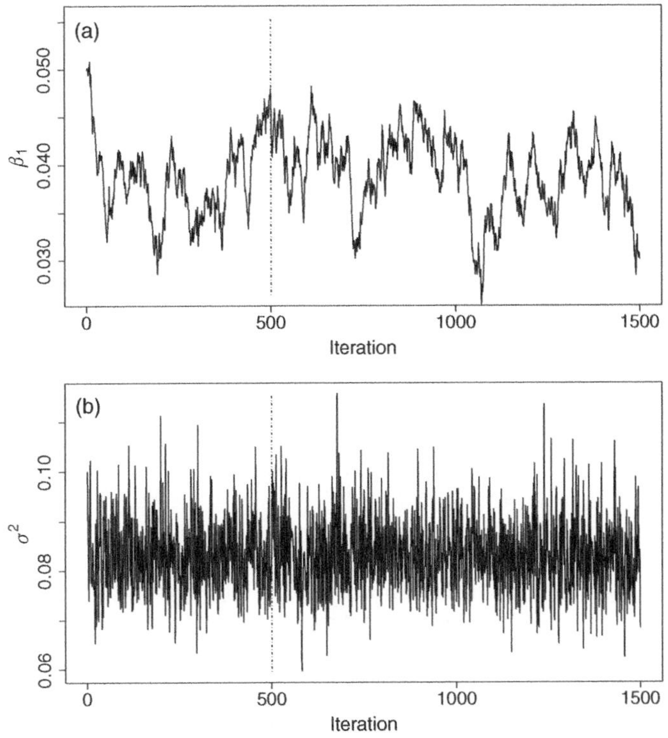

Figure 6.8 Osteoporosis study: trace plot of (a) β_1 and (b) σ^2 based on 1500 sampled values using the Gibbs sampler (vertical lines indicate the end of the burn-in part).

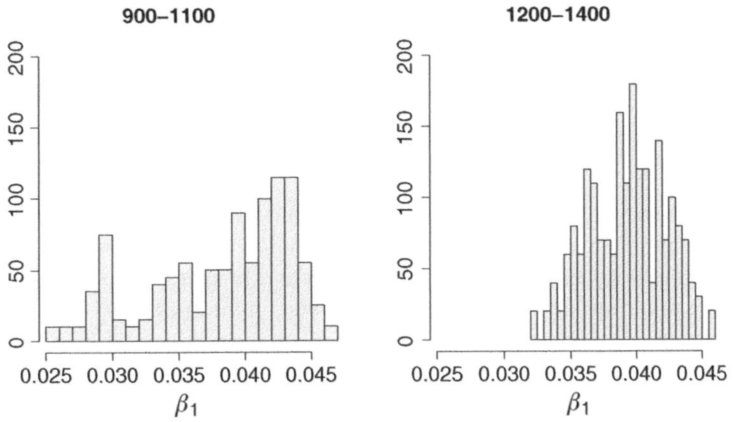

Figure 6.9 Osteoporosis study: posterior distribution for β_1 obtained from the Gibbs sampler, from iterations 900 to 1100 and 1200 to 1400.

joint distribution exists. It becomes more complicated when is not known whether the joint distribution exists (Arnold *et al.* 2001).

Proving the existence of the joint distribution is not enough to determine the distribution. Casella and George (1992) show for $d = 2$ that, if the conditional distributions $p(\theta_1 \mid \theta_2)$ and $p(\theta_2 \mid \theta_1)$ are known, the marginal distribution $p_1(\theta_1)$ and hence the joint distribution $p(\theta_1, \theta_2)$ can be determined. Indeed, by definition, $p_1(\theta_1) = \int p(\theta_1, \theta_2)\,\mathrm{d}\theta_2$, since $p(\theta_1, \theta_2) = p(\theta_1 \mid \theta_2)p_2(\theta_2)$, $p_1(\theta_1) = \int p(\theta_1 \mid \theta_2)p_2(\theta_2)\,\mathrm{d}\theta_2$. A similar expression holds for θ_2 and can be imputed in the previous expression leading to

$$\begin{aligned} p_1(\theta_1) &= \int p(\theta_1 \mid \theta_2)\left[\int p(\theta_2 \mid \phi_1)p_1(\phi_1)\,\mathrm{d}\phi_1\right]\mathrm{d}\theta_2 \\ &= \int\left[\int p(\theta_1 \mid \theta_2)p(\theta_2 \mid \phi_1)\,\mathrm{d}\theta_2\right]p_1(\phi_1)\,\mathrm{d}\phi_1 \\ &= \int K_1(\phi_1, \theta_1)\,p_1(\phi_1)\,\mathrm{d}\phi_1, \end{aligned} \tag{6.1}$$

where $K_1(\phi_1, \theta_1) = \int p(\theta_1 \mid \theta_2)p(\theta_2 \mid \phi_1)\,\mathrm{d}\theta_2$. This result shows that, if the conditional distributions are known, the marginal distribution $p_1(\theta_1)$ can be solved by finding the (fixed point) solution of an integral equation. The Gibbs sampler is a stochastic version of this iterative algorithm.

The 'engine' that generates a move from $\boldsymbol{\theta} \equiv \boldsymbol{\theta}^k$ to $\boldsymbol{\phi} \equiv \boldsymbol{\theta}^{(k+1)}$ is called the *transition kernel* or the *transition function*. The transition kernel expresses the probability (density) of the move and is given for the Gibbs sampler by

$$K(\boldsymbol{\theta}, \boldsymbol{\phi}) = p(\phi_1 \mid \theta_2, \ldots, \theta_d) \times p(\phi_2 \mid \phi_1, \theta_3, \ldots, \theta_d) \times p(\phi_d \mid \phi_1, \ldots, \phi_{(d-1)}).$$

Note that $K_1(\phi_1, \theta_1)$ in expression (6.1) is also a transition kernel expressing the probability of a move from ϕ_1 to θ_1. The integration in the expression of K_1 creeps in because a move from ϕ_1 to θ_1 can be made via all possible values for θ_2. The transition kernel is simply a prescription to generate a Markov chain converging to $p(\boldsymbol{\theta} \mid \boldsymbol{y})$. For a Gibbs sampler, the transition kernel is completely determined by the posterior in contrast to the Metropolis(–Hastings) algorithm.

6.2.4 Review of Gibbs sampling approaches

For a given problem, the Gibbs sampler can be combined with different algorithms to sample from the full conditionals. In the above examples, the full conditionals were classical distributions, so that sampling was done with standard software. In general, the full conditionals are known only up to a constant requiring general purpose algorithms, such as those of Section III.12. The choice of the sampling algorithm depends on the (shape of the) full conditional but also on the personal preference of the software developer. For instance, the Bayesian SAS procedures GENMOD, LIFEREG and PHREG all use the ARMS algorithm, while WinBUGS makes use of a variety of samplers depending on the actual full conditional.

There are several versions of the basic Gibbs sampler depending on how the sampler travels in the d dimensions. We distinguish these samplers as follows:

- *Deterministic- or systematic scan Gibbs sampler*: The d dimensions are visited in a fixed order. This is the standard (above described) Gibbs sampler.

- *Random-scan Gibbs sampler*: The d dimensions are visited in a random order.
- *Reversible Gibbs sampler*: The d dimensions are visited in a particular order and then the order is reversed. One step consists of $(2d - 1)$ substeps.
- *Block Gibbs sampler*: The d dimensions are split up into m blocks of parameters with respective sizes $d_1, d_2, \ldots, d_m$ and corresponding parameter vectors $\boldsymbol{\theta}_1, \boldsymbol{\theta}_2, \ldots, \boldsymbol{\theta}_m$. Then the distributions $p(\boldsymbol{\theta}_k \mid \boldsymbol{\theta}_1, \ldots, \boldsymbol{\theta}_{k-1}, \boldsymbol{\theta}_{k+1}, \ldots, \boldsymbol{\theta}_m)$, $(k = 1, \ldots, m)$ are sampled in a (most often) fixed order.

Most popular is the deterministic Gibbs sampler. The block Gibbs sampler is especially useful when the parameters are highly correlated a posteriori. For instance, the Gibbs sampler in Example VI.5 may be replaced by the block Gibbs sampler, which processes the whole vector (β_0, β_1) instead of its components, using the conditional distributions:

1. $p(\sigma^2 \mid \beta_0, \beta_1, \mathbf{y})$
2. $p(\beta_0, \beta_1 \mid \sigma^2, \mathbf{y})$

We show in Chapter 7 that sampling blocks of parameters instead of each of the parameters separately may speed up the convergence to the target distribution considerably. However, the time needed to complete each iteration is in general greater. The block Gibbs sampler is implemented in WinBUGS and treats location and scale parameters as separate blocks. The SAS® procedure MCMC makes intensive use of blocking and allows the user to specify the blocks.

6.2.5 The Slice sampler*

Suppose that we wish to sample from a density $f(x)$. From $f(x) = \int_0^{f(x)} \mathrm{d}y$, it is seen that f is the marginal density (in x) of the (bivariate) joint uniform density $g(x, y)$ on the region

$$(x, y) : 0 < y < f(x). \tag{6.2}$$

By adding the variable y, the univariate sampling problem is translated into a bivariate sampling problem. Classically, y is referred to as an *auxiliary variable*.

Samples from $f(x)$ can be obtained by simulating (x, y) from a uniform density on the set (6.2). If $f(x)$ is defined on a finite interval $[a, b]$ and is bounded above by a finite value m, then simulating from $f(x)$ could be done by a uniform simulation from the rectangle $[a, b] \times [0, m]$ and retaining only the pairs (x, y) that satisfy the constraint (6.2). In the general case, a bivariate Gibbs sampling algorithm may be applied. In the first case, we assume that $f(x)$ is unimodal. In this case, the *Slice sampler* consists of repeatedly sampling from two uniform conditional distributions which satisfy constraint (6.2):

- $y \mid x \sim \mathrm{U}(0, f(x))$
- $x \mid y \sim \mathrm{U}(\min_y, \max_y)$, with $\min_y, \max_y$ are the minimal and maximal x-values, respectively, of the solution $y = f(x)$

The stochastic intervals $S(y) = [\min_y, \max_y]$ are called *slices* hereby naming the sampler. The slice sampler is an example of the Gibbs sampling procedure and hence requires only the density up to a proportionality factor. In addition, the properties of the Gibbs sampler are inherited which implies that the sampler will yield (ultimately) samples from $f(x)$. The Slice sampler is implemented in WinBUGS to sample from (nonstandard) densities with a finite support. When the density is multimodal, then sampling requires more care. Indeed, for such

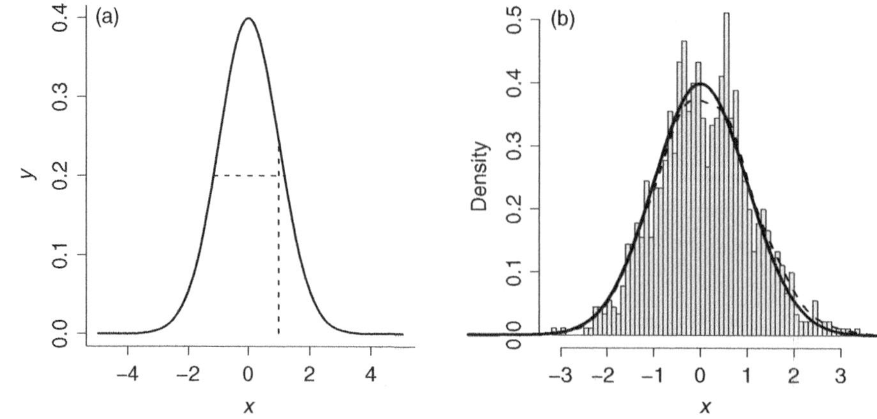

Figure 6.10 Normal density: (a) sampling mechanism of slice sampler and (b) histogram of 5000 sampled values (dashed line = smoothed histogram, solid line = true density).

a density one needs to establish the total set of solutions to the equation $y = f(x)$. In addition, uniform sampling needs to be done on multiple intervals.

Example VI.6: Slice sampling applied to the normal density
We wish to sample from a standard normal density. The slices are, therefore, $S(y) = [-\sqrt{-2\log(y)}, \sqrt{-2\log(y)}]$ and sampling involves the following two conditional sampling steps:

- $y \mid x \sim \text{U}\left(0, \text{e}^{-x^2/2}\right)$
- $x \mid y \sim \text{U}\big(-\sqrt{-2\log(y)}, \sqrt{-2\log(y)}\big)$

In Figure 6.10(a), we show two typical intervals in the x- and y-directions which define the two uniform distributions in the above Gibbs sampling procedure. The histogram based on 5000 sampled values with the Slice sampler is shown in Figure 6.10(b). As one can readily see, the smoothed histogram and the true density are quite close. In addition, no burn-in values were removed which illustrates the fast convergence of the algorithm. □

6.3 The Metropolis(–Hastings) algorithm

The Metropolis–Hastings *(MH) algorithm* is a general Markov chain Monte Carlo technique to sample from the posterior distribution which, in contrast to the Gibbs sampler, does not require the full conditionals. The *Metropolis algorithm* is a special case of the MH algorithm. We refer to both algorithms as the MH algorithm.

The Metropolis algorithm was proposed more than 50 years ago by Metropolis *et al.* (1953). Two decades later Hastings (1970) extended the approach to what is now called the Metropolis–Hastings approach and introduced the method into the statistical world. But, only after the publication of Gelfand and Smith (1990)'s paper (again two decades later) this MCMC approach became popular among statisticians. The MH algorithm shows some similarity with the AR algorithm of Section III.12. Below, it is shown that the Gibbs sampler is in a mathematical sense a special case of the MH algorithm, but for a variety of reasons, the two algorithms are treated separately in the literature. We elaborate in this section on the philosophy behind the Metropolis and the Metropolis–Hastings approach and on their properties.

6.3.1 The Metropolis algorithm

Suppose that a Markov chain is at position $\boldsymbol{\theta}^k$ at the kth iteration when exploring the posterior distribution $p(\boldsymbol{\theta} \mid \boldsymbol{y})$. The general idea behind the Metropolis algorithm goes as follows. The next position in the chain, $\widetilde{\boldsymbol{\theta}}$, is sampled from a density q having typically its central location at $\boldsymbol{\theta}^k$. However, $\widetilde{\boldsymbol{\theta}}$ is only a proposal for the new position (if it were automatically the next value we would be exploring q and not the posterior). The new position will always be accepted when it is located in an area of higher posterior mass, otherwise it will be accepted with a certain probability. Clearly, positions with a lower posterior mass must also be visited otherwise the algorithm would be searching for the (posterior) mode and not exploring the posterior distribution. The probability of accepting the proposed position should be taken such that, at the end of the day, the Markov chain explores $p(\boldsymbol{\theta} \mid \boldsymbol{y})$. The density q is called the *proposal density* and the proposal density evaluated in $\widetilde{\boldsymbol{\theta}}$ at iteration k is denoted as $q(\widetilde{\boldsymbol{\theta}} \mid \boldsymbol{\theta}^k)$. When the proposal density is symmetric, i.e. $q(\widetilde{\boldsymbol{\theta}} \mid \boldsymbol{\theta}^k) = q(\boldsymbol{\theta}^k \mid \widetilde{\boldsymbol{\theta}})$, we speak of the Metropolis algorithm.

A popular choice for q is the multivariate normal distribution (or the multivariate t-distribution) with mean equal to the current position $\boldsymbol{\theta}^k$ and a user-chosen covariance matrix Σ. In that case, we sample $\widetilde{\boldsymbol{\theta}}$ from $\mathrm{N}(\boldsymbol{\theta}^k, \Sigma)$ at the kth iteration to obtain the proposed subsequent value.Obviously, the location parameter $\boldsymbol{\theta}^k$ of the proposal density changes with k. Further, just as for the AR algorithm, an appropriate decision rule is needed to accept or reject the 'proposed' $\widetilde{\boldsymbol{\theta}}$. Upon acceptance, $\widetilde{\boldsymbol{\theta}}$ becomes the next value in the Markov chain, i.e. $\boldsymbol{\theta}^{(k+1)} = \widetilde{\boldsymbol{\theta}}$ and we move to $\widetilde{\boldsymbol{\theta}}$. If rejected we stay at $\boldsymbol{\theta}^k$, hence $\boldsymbol{\theta}^{(k+1)} = \boldsymbol{\theta}^k$. The probability of accepting the proposed value depends on the posterior distribution. When the candidate lies in an area where the posterior distribution has a higher value, i.e. when $p(\widetilde{\boldsymbol{\theta}} \mid \boldsymbol{y})/p(\boldsymbol{\theta}^k \mid \boldsymbol{y}) > 1$, then the move will always be made and hence $\boldsymbol{\theta}^{(k+1)} = \widetilde{\boldsymbol{\theta}}$. In contrast, when the candidate value lies in an area where the posterior distribution has a lower value, i.e. when $p(\widetilde{\boldsymbol{\theta}} \mid \boldsymbol{y})/p(\boldsymbol{\theta}^k \mid \boldsymbol{y}) < 1$, then the move will be made with probability $r = p(\widetilde{\boldsymbol{\theta}} \mid \boldsymbol{y})/p(\boldsymbol{\theta}^k \mid \boldsymbol{y})$ and then $\boldsymbol{\theta}^{(k+1)} = \widetilde{\boldsymbol{\theta}}$ with probability r. This procedure ensures that the posterior distribution will be 'visited' more often at locations where the posterior likelihood is relatively higher. The proof that this is the correct procedure is shown in Section 6.4. The above-described procedure is called the *Metropolis algorithm* and satisfies again the Markov property.

Formally, when the chain is at $\boldsymbol{\theta}^k$, the Metropolis algorithm samples the chain values as follows:

1. Sample a candidate $\widetilde{\boldsymbol{\theta}}$ from the symmetric proposal density $q(\widetilde{\boldsymbol{\theta}} \mid \boldsymbol{\theta})$, with $\boldsymbol{\theta} = \boldsymbol{\theta}^k$.
2. The next value $\boldsymbol{\theta}^{(k+1)}$ will be equal to
   - $\widetilde{\boldsymbol{\theta}}$ with probability $\alpha(\boldsymbol{\theta}^k, \widetilde{\boldsymbol{\theta}})$ (accept proposal),
   - $\boldsymbol{\theta}^k$ otherwise (reject proposal),

   with

$$\alpha(\boldsymbol{\theta}^k, \widetilde{\boldsymbol{\theta}}) = \min\left(r = \frac{p(\widetilde{\boldsymbol{\theta}} \mid \boldsymbol{y})}{p(\boldsymbol{\theta}^k \mid \boldsymbol{y})}, 1\right). \tag{6.3}$$

The function $\alpha(\boldsymbol{\theta}^k, \widetilde{\boldsymbol{\theta}})$ is called the *probability of a move*.

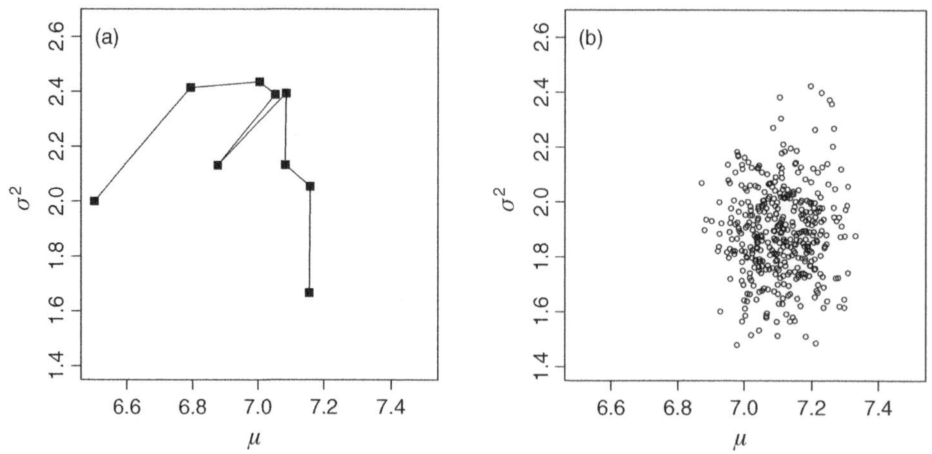

Figure 6.11 Serum alkaline phosphatase study (noninformative prior): (a) first 15 steps when using Metropolis algorithm ($\tau_1^2 = \tau_2^2 = 0.03$) to explore the joint posterior distribution for μ and σ^2 with a noninformative prior, and (b) last 1000 parameter vectors (μ, σ^2) from a chain of total size equal to 1500.

We now illustrate the Metropolis algorithm using the serum alkaline phosphatase study. In particular, we replace the Gibbs sampler in Example VI.1 with the Metropolis algorithm.

Example VI.7: Serum alkaline phosphatase study: Exploring the posterior with the Metropolis algorithm – noninformative prior

Take the same settings as in Example VI.1. To use the Metropolis algorithm, a proposal density is needed, which should be two-dimensional here since proposals are expected for μ and σ^2. We have taken the bivariate normal density as the proposal density. In principle, this choice can present difficulties since negative values for σ^2 might be generated, but this choice of q did not pose problems here. At iteration k the proposal density is $\text{N}(\boldsymbol{\theta}^k, \Sigma)$ where $\boldsymbol{\theta}^k = (\mu^k, (\sigma^2)^k)^T$ and $\Sigma = \text{diag}(\tau_1^2, \tau_2^2)$. First we have taken $\tau_1^2 = \tau_2^2 = 0.03$ for the variances of the proposal density.

With the same starting position as in Example VI.1 and using the proposal density at $\boldsymbol{\theta}^0$, the vector $\widetilde{\boldsymbol{\theta}} = (6.76, 1.94)^T$ was generated yielding a ratio of $r = 5.84 \times 10^{-6}$. Given such a small ratio the decision was to stay at the starting position (6.5, 2.0), i.e. $\boldsymbol{\theta}^1 = \boldsymbol{\theta}^0$. In the second iteration, the vector $\widetilde{\boldsymbol{\theta}} = (6.79, 2.41)^T$ was generated, now yielding a ratio of $r = 1,483,224$ and the move was made. Hence, $\boldsymbol{\theta}^2 = (6.79, 2.41)^T$. In the third step the suggested move was again not accepted with $r = 0.00049$. The positions taken in the plane up to $k = 15$ are shown in Figure 6.11(a). In contrast to the Gibbs sampler, now the moves go in any direction. In Figure 6.11(b), we show the last 1000 values of the Markov chain (from $k \geq 501$).

In Figure 6.12, the marginal posterior distributions based on the retained part of the Markov chain are shown, together with the true posterior distributions. The fit to the true distributions appears less satisfactory than with the Gibbs procedure. Nevertheless, the posterior summary measures were about the same.

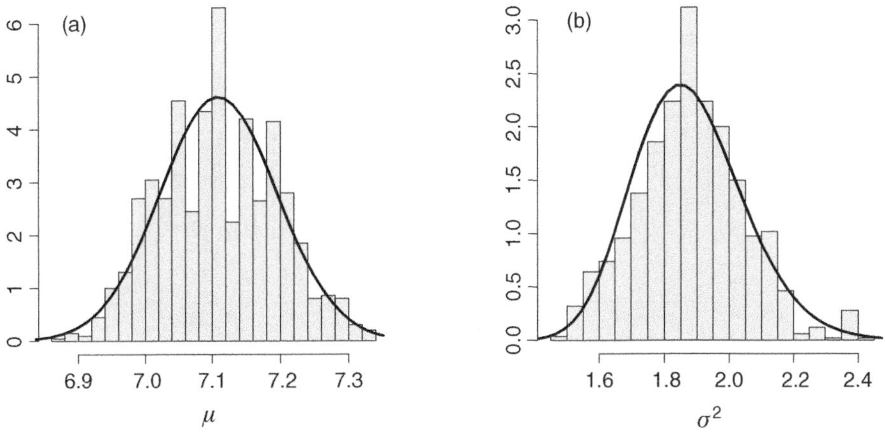

Figure 6.12 Serum alkaline phosphatase study (noninformative prior): marginal posterior distribution of μ and σ^2 corresponding to the retained part of the Markov chain shown in Figure 6.11(b). The solid lines represent the true posterior marginals.

The trace plots in Figure 6.13 show horizontal lines indicating when the proposed move was not accepted. The percentage of accepted moves, i.e. the *acceptance rate* (or *acceptance probability*), was 40%. Thus the posterior measures were based on roughly 400 different values.

Next, we have taken the variance parameters of the proposal density equal to $\tau_1^2 = \tau_2^2 = 0.001$. Consequently, the proposal density can only suggest small steps. On its turn, this implies a high acceptance rate (steps are small and thus r is often close to 1). We obtained now an acceptance rate of 84%. The implication is that the Markov chain explores the posterior distribution slowly, as seen in Figure 6.14(a). The negative effect of this slow exploration is illustrated in Figure 6.14(b) which shows that the Markov chain provides a poor approximation to the true marginal distribution. □

The above examples illustrate the flexibility of the Metropolis algorithm. But the examples also stress that one needs to be careful in choosing the proposal density, especially its dispersion. We will return to this issue in Section 6.3.4.

6.3.2 The Metropolis–Hastings algorithm

For the Metropolis algorithm, the proposal density $q(\widetilde{\boldsymbol{\theta}} \mid \boldsymbol{\theta})$ is symmetric. In some cases, it might be more advantageous to choose an asymmetric proposal density. In that case, moving from $\boldsymbol{\theta}$ to $\widetilde{\boldsymbol{\theta}}$ is not as easy as moving in the opposite direction. To ensure that the posterior distribution is equally accessible in all corners, the asymmetric nature of the proposal density needs to be compensated for. Hastings (1970) extended Metropolis' proposal to an asymmetric proposal density and the approach is referred to as the *MH algorithm*.

The first step in the MH algorithm is to suggest a candidate for a move. At the kth step $\widetilde{\boldsymbol{\theta}}$ will be sampled from q. As in the Metropolis algorithm, one needs to decide whether to 'move' or to 'stay'. However, in order to ensure that the posterior distribution will be explored equally well in all directions, one should compensate for the fact that moving from $\boldsymbol{\theta}^k$ to $\widetilde{\boldsymbol{\theta}}$ is

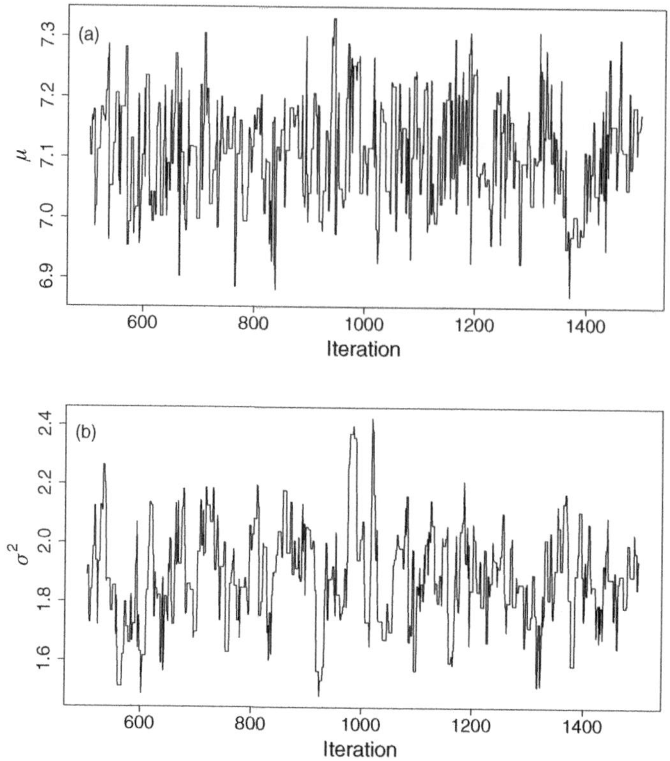

Figure 6.13 Serum alkaline phosphatase study (noninformative prior): trace plots for (a) μ and (b) σ^2 based on the Metropolis algorithm.

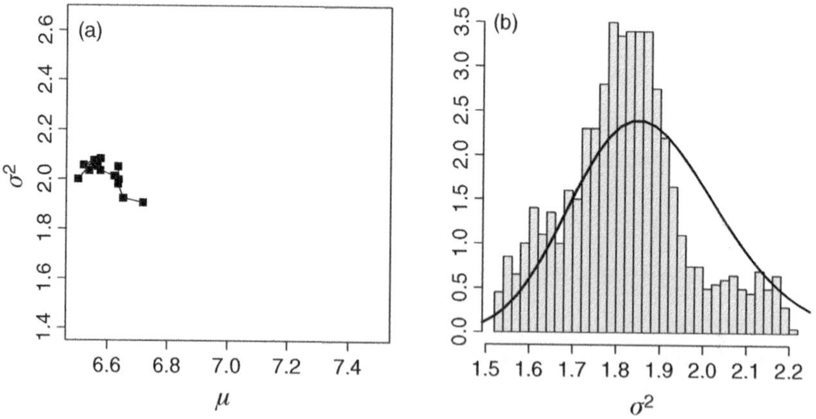

Figure 6.14 Serum alkaline phosphatase study (noninformative prior): (a) first 15 steps when using Metropolis algorithm ($\tau_1^2 = \tau_2^2 = 0.001$) to explore the joint posterior distribution for μ and σ^2 with a noninformative prior, and (b) marginal posterior distribution of σ^2 corresponding to the generated sample as in (a). The solid line pertains to the true posterior distribution.

easier or more difficult than in the opposite direction. This is done by changing the probability of making a move at the kth iteration, as follows:

1. Sample a candidate $\widetilde{\boldsymbol{\theta}}$ from the proposal density $q(\widetilde{\boldsymbol{\theta}} \mid \boldsymbol{\theta})$, with $\boldsymbol{\theta} = \boldsymbol{\theta}^k$.
2. The next value $\boldsymbol{\theta}^{(k+1)}$ will be equal to
   - $\widetilde{\boldsymbol{\theta}}$ with probability $\alpha(\boldsymbol{\theta}^k, \widetilde{\boldsymbol{\theta}})$ (accept proposal),
   - $\boldsymbol{\theta}^k$ otherwise (reject proposal),

   with

$$\alpha(\boldsymbol{\theta}^k, \widetilde{\boldsymbol{\theta}}) = \min\left(r = \frac{p(\widetilde{\boldsymbol{\theta}} \mid \mathbf{y})\, q(\boldsymbol{\theta}^k \mid \widetilde{\boldsymbol{\theta}})}{p(\boldsymbol{\theta}^k \mid \mathbf{y})\, q(\widetilde{\boldsymbol{\theta}} \mid \boldsymbol{\theta}^k)}, 1\right). \tag{6.4}$$

The change in acceptance probability was needed in order to ensure that the probability of moving from $\boldsymbol{\theta}$ to $\widetilde{\boldsymbol{\theta}}$ is equal to the probability of the opposite move. This is called the *reversibility condition*, and the resulting chain is called a *reversible Markov chain*; see Section 6.3.3 for a more formal definition and Section 6.4 for a justification. Note that also the Markov chain created by the Metropolis algorithm is reversible.

An example of an asymmetric proposal density is one that does not depend on the current position, i.e. $q(\widetilde{\boldsymbol{\theta}} \mid \boldsymbol{\theta}^k) \equiv q(\widetilde{\boldsymbol{\theta}})$, is asymmetric since $q(\boldsymbol{\theta}^k) \neq q(\widetilde{\boldsymbol{\theta}})$ for $\boldsymbol{\theta}^k \neq \widetilde{\boldsymbol{\theta}}$. With this proposal density the generated value $\widetilde{\boldsymbol{\theta}}$ does not dependent on the position in the chain and the sampling algorithm is called the *Independent MH algorithm*. Note that the proposed values of the chain are generated independently from one distribution, yet the elements of the chain are dependent. The reason is that acceptance of $\widetilde{\boldsymbol{\theta}}$ depends on $\alpha(\boldsymbol{\theta}^k, \widetilde{\boldsymbol{\theta}})$, which is now equal to $\min\left(\frac{p(\widetilde{\boldsymbol{\theta}}|\mathbf{y})\, q(\boldsymbol{\theta}^k)}{p(\boldsymbol{\theta}^k|\mathbf{y})\, q(\widetilde{\boldsymbol{\theta}})}, 1\right)$.

The next example makes use of the MH algorithm to sample from a univariate distribution. The Gibbs sampler applied to a univariate problem is just a standard one-dimensional sampler.

Example VI.8: Sampling a t-distribution using the Independent MH algorithm
Suppose the target distribution is the $t_3(3, 2^2)$-distribution. Sampling from this distribution was done using the Independent MH algorithm with proposal density $\mathrm{N}(3, 4^2)$. 1500 values were generated and we retained the last 1000 elements. The sampling procedure accepted 48% of the proposed moves. This histogram of sampled values approximated well the true distribution (Figure 6.15(a)). But when the variance of the proposal density was reduced to 2^2, the approximation became quite poor (Figure 6.15(b)). This exercise reinforces the statement that the MH algorithm needs to be used with care and that its success depends on (the variability of) the proposal density. □

6.3.3 Remarks*

As with the Gibbs sampler, the MH algorithm only needs the posterior distribution up to a constant, which can be verified from expression (6.4). In Gelman *et al.* (2004, p. 293) and in Chib and Greenberg (1995), it is shown that the Gibbs sampler is a special case of the MH algorithm. Robert and Casella (2004, p. 381) give a more precise statement, namely that the Gibbs sampler is equivalent to the composition of d MH algorithms with acceptance probabilities all equal to 1. The proof in Gelman *et al.* (2004) is repeated here.

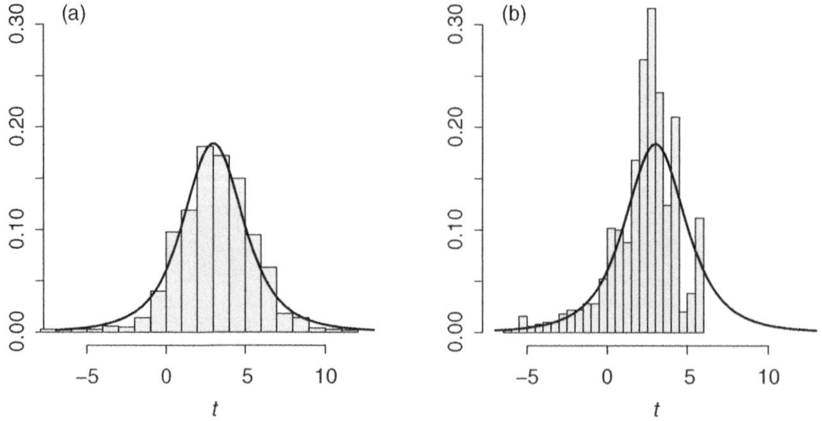

Figure 6.15 Sampling $t_3(3, 2^2)$-distribution based on: (a) Independent MH algorithm using proposal density $\mathrm{N}(3, 4^2)$ and (b) Independent MH algorithm using proposal density $\mathrm{N}(3, 2^2)$. The solid line pertains to the true $t_3(3, 2^2)$-distribution.

Define d transition functions

$$q_j^G(\widetilde{\boldsymbol{\theta}} \mid \boldsymbol{\theta}^k) = p(\widetilde{\theta}_j \mid \boldsymbol{\theta}^k_{-j}, \mathbf{y}) \text{ if } \widetilde{\boldsymbol{\theta}}_{-j} = \boldsymbol{\theta}^k_{-j} \tag{6.5}$$

$$= 0 \text{ otherwise,} \tag{6.6}$$

with $\boldsymbol{\theta}_{-j}$ equal to $\boldsymbol{\theta}$ without the jth component. Hence, the only possible jumps are to parameter vectors $\widetilde{\boldsymbol{\theta}}$ that match $\boldsymbol{\theta}^k$ on all components other than the jth. Under this transition function, the ratio r is given in the jth substep by

$$r = \frac{p(\widetilde{\boldsymbol{\theta}} \mid \mathbf{y}) q_j^G(\boldsymbol{\theta}^k \mid \widetilde{\boldsymbol{\theta}})}{p(\boldsymbol{\theta}^k \mid \mathbf{y}) q_j^G(\widetilde{\boldsymbol{\theta}} \mid \boldsymbol{\theta}^k)} = \frac{p(\widetilde{\boldsymbol{\theta}} \mid \mathbf{y}) p(\boldsymbol{\theta}^k_j \mid \widetilde{\theta}_{-j}, \mathbf{y})}{p(\boldsymbol{\theta}^k \mid \mathbf{y}) p(\widetilde{\theta}_j \mid \boldsymbol{\theta}^k_{-j}, \mathbf{y})} \tag{6.7}$$

$$= \frac{p(\widetilde{\boldsymbol{\theta}} \mid \mathbf{y}) / p(\widetilde{\theta}_j \mid \boldsymbol{\theta}^k_{-j}, \mathbf{y})}{p(\boldsymbol{\theta}^k \mid \mathbf{y}) / p(\boldsymbol{\theta}^k_j \mid \widetilde{\theta}_{-j}, \mathbf{y})} = 1, \tag{6.8}$$

which implies that each jump is accepted.

Despite the above result, the distinction between the two samplers is still made in the literature because of their different sampling strategies. In addition, the Gibbs sampler is a very important specific type of MH algorithm that requires separate mathematical arguments to establish its performance.

The transition kernel of the MH algorithm expresses the probability to move from $\boldsymbol{\theta} \equiv \boldsymbol{\theta}^k$ to $\boldsymbol{\phi} \equiv \boldsymbol{\theta}^{(k+1)}$ with $\boldsymbol{\theta}, \boldsymbol{\phi} \in \Theta$. The jump is done in two steps and the transition kernel therefore consists of two components. The first component $K(\boldsymbol{\theta}, \boldsymbol{\phi}) = \alpha(\boldsymbol{\theta}, \boldsymbol{\phi}) q(\boldsymbol{\phi} \mid \boldsymbol{\theta})$ describes the move to $\boldsymbol{\phi} = \widetilde{\boldsymbol{\theta}}$, whereby $\boldsymbol{\phi}$ is suggested by the proposal density $q(\boldsymbol{\phi} \mid \boldsymbol{\theta})$ and accepted with probability $\alpha(\boldsymbol{\theta}, \boldsymbol{\phi})$. The suggested move is, however, rejected with probability equal to

$$r(\boldsymbol{\theta}) = 1 - \int_{I\!R^d} \alpha(\boldsymbol{\theta}, \boldsymbol{\phi}) q(\boldsymbol{\phi} \mid \boldsymbol{\theta}) \, \mathrm{d}\boldsymbol{\phi},$$

and then no move is made, i.e. $\boldsymbol{\phi} = \boldsymbol{\theta}$. Thus the probability that $\boldsymbol{\phi} \in B$, with B a set in Θ, equals

$$p(\boldsymbol{\theta}, B) = \int_B K(\boldsymbol{\theta}, \boldsymbol{\phi})\, \mathrm{d}\boldsymbol{\phi} + r(\boldsymbol{\theta}) I(\boldsymbol{\theta} \in B),$$

with $I(\cdot)$ the indicator function. This probability is composed of two parts. The first term $\int_B K(\boldsymbol{\theta}, \boldsymbol{\phi})\, \mathrm{d}\boldsymbol{\phi}$ expresses the probability of moving into B when originally outside B and the second term expresses the probability of staying in B.

A reversible Markov chain is a sufficient condition (Section 6.4) for the chain to converge to the posterior distribution. The reversibility condition requires that the probability of moving from set A to set B is equal to the probability of moving from set B to set A, for any two sets A and B in Θ. This is translated into

$$\int_A p(\boldsymbol{\theta}, B)\, \mathrm{d}\boldsymbol{\theta} = \int_B p(\boldsymbol{\phi}, A)\, \mathrm{d}\boldsymbol{\phi}.$$

The above condition is satisfied when the *detailed balance condition* is satisfied

$$\int_A \int_B K(\boldsymbol{\theta}, \boldsymbol{\phi})\, \mathrm{d}\boldsymbol{\phi}\, \mathrm{d}\boldsymbol{\theta} = \int_B \int_A K(\boldsymbol{\phi}, \boldsymbol{\theta})\, \mathrm{d}\boldsymbol{\theta}\, \mathrm{d}\boldsymbol{\phi}, \tag{6.9}$$

for any two sets A and B in Θ. It can be shown that this condition is achieved optimally by taking the acceptance probability as in expression (6.4) (Hastings 1970).

Finally, the MH algorithm shows some resemblance with the AR algorithm. Indeed, both algorithms make use of an instrumental distribution which produces sampled values that are evaluated and subsequently accepted or rejected. The most important difference is that the AR algorithm generates independent samples while the MH algorithm generates a Markov chain and thus dependent samples. Exploring the posterior with an MCMC approach leaves out a trace of visited positions in the joint posterior space. Hence, when the MH algorithm rejects a proposal, the chain will stay at the current position and that is recorded. On the other hand, when the AR algorithm rejects a proposed value no record of that proposal is kept. Thus, the two methods also differ in the way rejection impacts the generated values.

6.3.4 Review of Metropolis(–Hastings) approaches

A variety of Metropolis(–Hastings) algorithms are in use differing according to the choice of the proposal density. We review the three most common algorithms which are as follows:

The Random-Walk Metropolis(–Hastings) algorithm: the proposal density satisfies $q(\widetilde{\boldsymbol{\theta}} \mid \boldsymbol{\theta}) = q(\widetilde{\boldsymbol{\theta}} - \boldsymbol{\theta})$. For $q(\widetilde{\boldsymbol{\theta}} - \boldsymbol{\theta}) \equiv q(|\widetilde{\boldsymbol{\theta}} - \boldsymbol{\theta}|)$ the proposal density is symmetric and gives the Metropolis algorithm. Popular choices for the proposal density are the multivariate normal density $\mathrm{N}_d(\widetilde{\boldsymbol{\theta}} \mid \boldsymbol{\theta}, c^2\Sigma)$ (implemented in WinBUGS and different SAS procedures) and the multivariate t-distribution (SAS PROC MCMC). The t-proposal density is better for sampling long tailed posterior distributions. Analytical results and simulations in Roberts *et al.* (1997) suggested that for a normal proposal density the acceptance rate should be around 45%

for $d = 1$ and 23.4% for $d > 1$. For the normal proposal density the acceptance rate depends highly on the covariance matrix $c^2\Sigma$ (Σ is often taken as the identity matrix) as was illustrated in Example VI.7. Robert and Casella (2004) suggested adapting the variance of the proposal density in the iterative process to improve the sampling performance. This procedure is called *tuning the proposal density* and is implemented in WinBUGS when the one-dimensional MH algorithm is used. In that case, the standard deviation of the proposal density is tuned by default in the first 4000 iterations to produce an acceptance rate between 20% and 40%; see Figure 8.3 for a graphical illustration. On the other hand, the SAS procedure MCMC tunes the proposal density in several loops.

The Independent MH algorithm: the proposal density does not depend on the position in the chain, e.g. $q(\widetilde{\boldsymbol{\theta}} \mid \boldsymbol{\theta}) = \mathrm{N}_d(\widetilde{\boldsymbol{\theta}} \mid \boldsymbol{\mu}, \Sigma)$, with $\boldsymbol{\mu}$ and Σ fixed or tuned throughout the MCMC run. The Independent MH algorithm is similar to the AR algorithm but accepts $\widetilde{\boldsymbol{\theta}}$ when $p(\widetilde{\boldsymbol{\theta}} \mid \mathbf{y})/q(\widetilde{\boldsymbol{\theta}}) > p(\boldsymbol{\theta}^k \mid \mathbf{y})/q(\boldsymbol{\theta}^k)$. As for the AR algorithm, a high acceptance rate is desirable and is obtained when the proposal density $q(\theta)$ is close to the posterior density. This could be achieved by taking for the proposal density a normal or a t-distribution with the posterior mode as mean and as covariance matrix the inverse of minus the observed Fisher information matrix evaluated at the posterior mode. Robert and Casella (2004) showed that if the proposal density satisfies $p(\theta \mid \mathbf{y}) \leq A\, q(\theta)$ for all θ, then the Markov chain generated by the Independent MH algorithm enjoys excellent convergence properties (Theorem 7.8) and that the expected acceptance probability exceeds that of the AR algorithm (Lemma 7.9). Note that this condition was not satisfied in Example VI.8. The Independent MH algorithm is one of the possible samplers of the SAS procedure MCMC.

The Block MH algorithm: In Section 6.2.4, we have introduced the block Gibbs sampler and mentioned that it can speed up the sampling process considerably. Within the m blocks, occasionally independent sampling might be applied (as in the osteoporosis regression analysis) but usually it will be a Metropolis(–Hastings) algorithm. This combination of the Gibbs and MH algorithm is called *Metropolis-within-Gibbs*. Chib and Greenberg (1995) showed that this procedure is valid. In the SAS procedure MCMC, blocks are specified by the user. WinBUGS puts automatically the regression coefficients into one block (if the blocking option is not switched off) and the variance parameters in another block.

A sampler of a different nature is the *Reversible Jump MCMC (RJMCMC) algorithm* (see Section 6.6). This algorithm is a special case of the MH algorithm whereby the proposal density suggests moves as with an ordinary MH algorithm, but also jumps between spaces of different dimensions. RJMCMC is useful, e.g. in Bayesian variable selection.

6.4 Justification of the MCMC approaches*

The results of this chapter are based on the property that the MCMC techniques generate a Markov chain that ultimately provides a sample from the posterior distribution and that the summary measures calculated from this chain consistently estimate the corresponding true posterior summary measures. The proof of these results is based on Markov chain theory. Robert and Casella (2004) reviewed in their Chapter 4 the most important results. A rigorous treatment of the topic is found in Meyn and Tweedie (1993). A detailed treatment of Markov chain theory is certainly beyond the aim of this book but we believe that it is useful to review the most important Markov chain concepts and results for a better understanding of (the terminology used in) the literature on MCMC methods.

A Markov chain is a sequence of discrete or continuous random variables θ with the property that, given the present outcome, the past and future outcomes are independent:

$$p(\theta^{(k+1)} = y \mid \theta^k = x, \theta^{(k-1)} = x_{k-1}, \ldots, \theta^0 = x_0) = p(\theta^{(k+1)} = y \mid \theta^k = x).$$

When the above probabilities do not depend on k, the Markov chain is called *homogeneous*. For a homogenous Markov chain, a constant transition kernel $K(x, A)$ describes the probability of generating a value in A when starting in x, i.e. $K(x, A) = p(\theta^{(k+1)} \in A \mid \theta^k = x) = p(\theta^1 \in A \mid \theta^0 = x)$. In other words, the transition kernel describes how the moves are made.

What happens with the Markov chain when k goes to infinity? One can show that if the generated chain has a limiting distribution π, then the distribution is also *stationary* which means that further elements of the chain also have π as distribution. Further, we speak of a *reversible* Markov chain if the rate at which the Markov chain moves from x to y is the same as the rate at which it moves from y to x, which is the detailed balance condition (6.9). Furthermore, we say that a Markov chain satisfies the *ergodicity criteria* if it satisfies the following three criteria: (1) *irreducibility*: the chain can reach each possible outcome whatever the starting position; (2) *aperiodicity*: there is no cyclic behavior in the chain and (c) *positive recurrence*: the chain visits every possible outcome an infinite number of times and the expected time to return to a particular outcome, irrespective of where we start in the chain, is finite. In practical terms, ergodicity means that the chain will explore the posterior distribution exhaustively.

The Law of Large Numbers (LLN) and the Central Limit Theorem (CLT) are fundamental to statistical theory and known by all statisticians. But these results are based on i.i.d. random variables. The central question is how these results carry-over to the case where the random variables are dependent as in Markov chains. Many results have been proven in the probabilistic and statistical literature that generalize the LLN and the CLT to the dependent case; see Meyn and Tweedie (1993), Tierney (1994) or Robert and Casella (2004). Below, the three most important results are given.

Theorem 6.4.1 *When $(\theta^k)_k$ is an ergodic Markov chain with stationary distribution π, then the limiting distribution is also π.*

Further, suppose that $t(\theta)$ is function of θ, e.g. $t(\theta) = \theta, t(\theta) = \theta^2, t(\theta) = I(\theta = x)$ with $I(a) = 1$ if a is true and 0 otherwise, etc. Then the sample average of $t(\theta)$ based on the Markov chain up to k is called the *ergodic average* and is defined as

$$\bar{t}_k = \frac{1}{k}\sum_{j=1}^{k} t(\theta^j).$$

One can show the equivalent of the classical Law of Large Numbers but now for dependent observations.

Theorem 6.4.2 *(Markov Chain Law of Large Numbers) For an ergodic Markov chain with a nite expected value for $t(\theta)$, $\bar{t}_k$ converges to the true mean.*

Theorem 6.4.2 states that for a properly behaving Markov chain the sample average of the chain can be used to estimate the true mean values. Thus, the sample mean, the sample median, the standard deviation, etc. estimate their true values and the estimation improves as $k \to \infty$. Clearly, this is a most important result because it implies that we can use the converged Markov chain to draw inference about the unknown (stationary) distribution.

Although the elements of a Markov chain are conditionally independent given the immediate past, they are dependent unconditionally. The *autocovariance of lag m* ($m \geq 0$) of the Markov chain $(t^k)_k \equiv (t(\theta)^k)_k$ is defined as $\gamma_m = \text{cov}(t^k, t^{k+m})$. The variance of $(t^k)_k$, defined as the autocovariance for $m = 0$ and denoted as γ_0. Finally, the *autocorrelation of lag m* is defined as $\rho_m = \gamma_m/\gamma_0$.

If the Markov chain is reversible and enjoys an additional property, i.e. when the convergence to the limiting distribution goes quickly enough for all starting positions (geometrical or uniform ergodicity), then the following CLT for Markov chains holds.

Theorem 6.4.3 *(Markov Chain CLT) For a uniformly (or geometrically) ergodic Markov chain with $t^2(\theta)$ (or $t^{2+\epsilon}(\theta)$, for some $\epsilon > 0$ in the geometric case) integrable with respect to π then*

$$\sqrt{k}\frac{\bar{t}_k - E_\pi\left[t(\theta)\right]}{\tau} \text{ converges in distribution to } N(0,1) \text{ as } k \to \infty,$$

with

$$\tau^2 = \gamma_0\left(1 + 2\sum_{m=1}^{\infty}\rho_m\right). \tag{6.10}$$

Theorem 6.4.3 allows for the construction of a classical confidence interval for the true mean of $t(\theta)$ based on $\bar{t}_k$.

The above results hold for discrete Markov chains. Tierney (1994) proved Theorems 6.4.2 and 6.4.3 for Markov chains with a general outcome under appropriate regularity conditions. Further, to know whether these theorems apply in practice, one needs to verify whether the regularity conditions are satisfied. Luckily, this is most often the case.

6.4.1 Properties of the MH algorithm

The MH algorithm creates a reversible Markov chain, i.e. a Markov chain that satisfies the detailed balance condition. This will be shown here for the discrete case as an illustration. The proof of the general case can be found, e.g. in see Chib and Greenberg (1995) or Robert and Casella (2004, Theorem 7.2). The proof goes as follows: Suppose that π is a discrete distribution with $\pi_j = p(\theta = x_j)$ with possible values $S = \{x_1, x_2, \ldots, x_r\}$. Further, suppose that $Q = (q_{ij})_{ij}$ is a matrix that describes the moves, i.e. if the chain is in state x_i, then state x_j is drawn with probability q_{ij}. Now, one can either move from x_i to a different x_j or stay at x_i. The discrete version of the MH algorithm states that the move should happen with probability

$$\alpha_{ij} = \min\left(1, \frac{\pi_j q_{ji}}{\pi_i q_{ij}}\right). \tag{6.11}$$

The probability to move from x_i to x_j is therefore $p_{ij} = \alpha_{ij} q_{ij}$. The detailed balance condition, which implies here that $\pi_i p_{ij} = \pi_j p_{ji}$ is satisfied because

$$\begin{aligned}\pi_i p_{ij} &= \pi_i \alpha_{ij} q_{ij} = \pi_i \min\left(1, \frac{\pi_j q_{ji}}{\pi_i q_{ij}}\right) q_{ij} \\ &= \min\left(\pi_i q_{ij}, \pi_j q_{ji}\right) = \min\left(1, \frac{\pi_i q_{ij}}{\pi_j q_{ji}}\right) \pi_j q_{ji} \\ &= \pi_j p_{ji}.\end{aligned}$$

Further, it can be shown that reversibility of the Markov chain implies that π is the stationary distribution for that chain. Consequently, the MH algorithm creates a Markov chain where the target distribution is also the stationary distribution.

Hastings (1970) notes that the above α_{ij} are not the only ones that make the Markov chain reversible. However, Peskun (1973) proves that the optimal choice (in terms of the sampling variance of summary measures) is given by expression (6.11).

To apply Theorems 6.4.1 and 6.4.2 for an appropriate function $t(\theta)$, the Markov chain must be ergodic. A sufficient (and mild) condition for this is that $q(\boldsymbol{\phi} \mid \boldsymbol{\theta})$ is strictly positive if $\boldsymbol{\phi}$ and $\boldsymbol{\theta}$ are close (see Lemma 7.6 and Corollary 7.7 in Robert and Casella (2004) for more formal conditions). It can easily be seen that this condition is satisfied in Examples VI.7 and VI.8. The above results, however, do not imply that convergence to the target distribution goes fast. This is illustrated by the second proposal density in Example VI.7.

Theorem 6.4.3 applies to suitable functions $t(\theta)$ when geometric or uniform ergodicity holds. For the Independent MH algorithm Robert and Casella (2004)(Theorem 7.8) show that uniform ergodicity holds whenever $p(\theta \mid \mathbf{y}) \leq A\, q(\theta)$ for all θ and A finite. But apart from this result, general practical conditions for geometric or uniform ergodicity do not seem to be available.

6.4.2 Properties of the Gibbs sampler

To show that the Gibbs sampler generates a Markov chain for which Theorems 6.4.1 and 6.4.2 hold (for an appropriate function $t(\theta)$), the target distribution must be equal to the stationary distribution. This is shown in general in Theorem 10.10 of Robert and Casella (2004) for ergodic Markov chains generated by the Gibbs sampler. Robert and Casella (2004) also demonstrate that ergodicity of the chain holds when the full conditionals are strictly positive (for a formal and less restrictive condition, see Lemma 10.11 in Robert and Casella (2004)). It can be checked that the necessary conditions for convergence hold in Examples VI.1 to VI.5.

6.5 Choice of the sampler

With the availability of the Gibbs sampler and the MH algorithm we must choose between the two algorithms. Some may automatically opt for the Gibbs sampler especially when the full conditionals are relatively easy to sample from. Others may always prefer a Metropolis(–Hastings) algorithm because of its generality. For each of the two methods some further choices need to be made. For example, for the MH algorithm one needs to select a proposal density while for the Gibbs sampler one needs to pick the sampling algorithms for the full conditionals. In practice, the choice will be often dictated by the available software. But, most likely our ultimate choice of the sampler will depend on its convergence properties, i.e. how fast the algorithm will provide the posterior summary measures. In fact, even if one has chosen the Gibbs sampler because the full conditionals are easy to sample, the Gibbs sampler will not be our choice if is globally inefficient (see osteoporosis example).

In the next example, we illustrate the use of three sampling approaches for a Bayesian logistic regression problem. The first algorithm is based on a self-written R program, the second is a WinBUGS program and the third is based on a SAS procedure.

Example VI.9: Caries study: MCMC approaches for a logistic regression problem
We illustrate the Bayesian sampling procedures on a subset of $n = 500$ children of the Signal-Tandmobiel® study at their first annual dental examination. Suppose we wish to know whether girls have a different risk for developing caries experience than boys in the first year of primary school. For this analysis, we binarized the variable caries experience (CE) which is defined as $dmft > 0$ (CE = 1) or $dmft = 0$ (CE = 0). Of the 500 children, 51% were girls and 53.6% had CE at their first examination. Some analyses (Mwalili *et al.* 2005) showed that there is a east-west gradient in CE (higher in the east of Flanders). We wished to confirm also this result with our analysis. For this reason we added the x-coordinate (of the centroid of the municipality of the school of the child) to the logistic regression model.

Suppose that the first n_1 children have CE=1 and let the binary response (CE) for the ith child be denoted as y_i. For our logistic regression model, there are three covariates: x_{1i} (constant = 1), x_{2i} (gender) and x_{3i} (x-coordinate). The logistic regression likelihood is, therefore,

$$L(\boldsymbol{\beta} \mid \boldsymbol{y}) \propto \prod_{i=1}^{n_1} \exp(\boldsymbol{x}_i^T \boldsymbol{\beta}) \prod_{i=1}^{n} \left[\frac{1}{1 + \exp(\boldsymbol{x}_i^T \boldsymbol{\beta})} \right], \tag{6.12}$$

with $\boldsymbol{\beta} = (\beta_1, \beta_2, \beta_3)^T$. Independent normal priors for the regression coefficients were chosen, i.e. $\beta_j \sim \mathrm{N}(\beta_{j0}, \sigma_{j0}^2)$, $(j = 1, 2, 3)$ (with $\beta_{j0} = 0$ and $\sigma_{j0} = 10$). The jth full conditional is obtained by considering $\beta_k (k \neq j)$ as fixed in the posterior and is equal to

$$p(\beta_1 \mid \widetilde{\beta}_2, \widetilde{\beta}_3, \boldsymbol{y}) \propto \prod_{i=1}^{n_1} \exp(\beta_1 x_{1i}) \prod_{i=1}^{n} \left[\frac{1}{1 + \exp(\beta_1 x_{1i}) \widetilde{a}_{1i}} \right] \times \exp\left[-\frac{(\beta_1 - \beta_{10})^2}{2\sigma_{10}^2} \right], \tag{6.13}$$

with $\widetilde{a}_{1i} = \exp(\widetilde{\beta}_2 x_{2i}) \exp(\widetilde{\beta}_3 x_{3i})$ and $\widetilde{\beta}_2$, $\widetilde{\beta}_3$ the parameter values of the two other regression coefficients obtained at a previous iteration in the MCMC algorithm. The full conditionals do not correspond to any classical distribution function, hence a general purpose sampler is needed.

We used three MCMC programs to arrive at the Bayesian solution:

- *R program*: a self-written R program based on the Gibbs sampler that evaluates the full conditionals (like in expression (6.13)) on a grid. Function (6.13) is standardized on the grid to have AUC = 1 and the cdf, say F, is established numerically. To sample from F we used the ICDF method (see Section III.12). This is a simple but relatively time consuming approach, since at each iteration the full conditional needs to be computed at all grid points. For all regression coefficients a 50-point grid was taken on the interval

$[\widehat{\beta}_j - 4\,\widehat{SE}(\widehat{\beta}_j), \widehat{\beta}_j + 4\,\widehat{SE}(\widehat{\beta}_j)]$, with $\widehat{\beta}_j$ the MLE of the jth regression coefficient and $\widehat{SE}(\widehat{\beta}_j)$ its asymptotic frequentist standard error.

- *WinBUGS*: For a (logistic) regression problem, the default option in WinBUGS is a multivariate MH algorithm (taken here) which samples all regression coefficients jointly (*blocking mode* on). An alternative sampling approach can be invoked by switching off the blocking mode, then the derivative-free ARS algorithm is used.
- *SAS PROC MCMC*: The procedure uses the MH algorithm and allows for different proposal densities. Here the default sampler is the Random-Walk MH algorithm with a trivariate normal proposal density with mean equal to the current value of the parameters and a multiple of the identity matrix as covariance matrix, tuned during the MCMC run.

The covariates are standardized (mean = 0, SD = 1) to improve convergence of the MCMC algorithm, but the results are reported on the original scale. There was rapid convergence. For all MCMC analyses 500 burn-in iterations were discarded and the summary measures were based on 1000 extra iterations. The results of the MCMC analyses are shown in Table 6.2. Taking into account the posterior SD, the posterior means/medians of the three samplers are close (to the MLE). However, the precision with which the posterior mean was determined (high precision = low MCSE, see Section 7.2.5) differs considerably with the SAS algorithm having the lowest precision and WinBUGS the highest.

Table 6.2 Caries study (random sample of 500 children): comparison of the summary measures obtained by three Bayesian logistic regression programs predicting caries experience (CE) from gender and the geographical location of the school to which the child belongs (x-coord). A comparison is also made with the MLE solution.

Program	Parameter	Mode	Mean	SD	Median	MCSE
	Intercept	−0.5900		0.2800		
MLE	gender	−0.0379		0.1810		
	x-coord	0.0052		0.0017		
	Intercept		−0.5880	0.2840	−0.5860	0.0104
R	gender		−0.0516	0.1850	−0.0578	0.0071
	x-coord		0.0052	0.0017	0.0052	6.621E-5
	Intercept		−0.5800	0.2810	−0.5730	0.0094
WinBUGS	gender		−0.0379	0.1770	−0.0324	0.0060
	x-coord		0.0052	0.0018	0.0053	5.901E-5
	Intercept		−0.6530	0.2600	−0.6450	0.0317
SAS	gender		−0.0319	0.1950	−0.0443	0.0208
	x-coord		0.0055	0.0016	0.0055	0.00016

MCSE, Monte Carlo standard error.

The clinical conclusion from our analyses was though the same, i.e. that girls do not show a different risk for CE than boys and children from the east of Flanders appear to have a higher risk for CE. □

The previous exercise shows that samplers may have quite a different efficiency. It may be, however, hard to imagine in advance which MCMC sampler to use for a problem at hand; see Example VII.9 for an example where the choice between the Gibbs sampler and MH algorithm comes natural.

6.6 The Reversible Jump MCMC algorithm*

The *Reversible Jump MCMC (RJMCMC) algorithm* is an extension of the standard MH algorithm suggested by Green (1995) to allow sampling from target distributions on spaces of varying dimension. This is called the *trans-dimensional case*. Examples of problems where the RJMCMC algorithm is useful are: (a) mixtures with an unknown number of components and hidden Markov models; (b) change-point problems with an unknown number of change-points and/or with unknown locations; (c) in model and variable selection problems and (d) analysis of quantitative trait locus (QTL) data.

In Hastie and Green (2012), the standard MH algorithm is explained to connect better with the RJMCMC algorithm. This is the approach we adopted here. Another good source is Waagepetersen and Sorensen (2001).

Standard MH algorithm: The purpose is to sample from $p(\boldsymbol{\theta} \mid \boldsymbol{y})$ with $\boldsymbol{\theta} \in \Theta$ of d dimensions. When in state $\boldsymbol{\theta}$, the proposal density $q(\cdot \mid \boldsymbol{\theta})$ generates $\tilde{\boldsymbol{\theta}}$ which is accepted with probability $\alpha(\boldsymbol{\theta}, \tilde{\boldsymbol{\theta}})$. This sampling process can be described alternatively as follows. Given $\boldsymbol{\theta}$, a vector $\boldsymbol{u}$ of r (possibly $< d$) random numbers is generated according to a density g and the new state $\tilde{\boldsymbol{\theta}}$ is obtained by $h(\boldsymbol{\theta}, \boldsymbol{u}) = \tilde{\boldsymbol{\theta}}$. The function h should have good properties in order to ensure reversibility. However, defined as earlier, h goes from an $(d+r)$-dimensional space to a d-dimensional space. Since reversibility implies that it must be as easy to go from $\boldsymbol{\theta}$ to $\tilde{\boldsymbol{\theta}}$ as from $\tilde{\boldsymbol{\theta}}$ to $\boldsymbol{\theta}$, the function h is taken bijective with $h(\boldsymbol{\theta}, \boldsymbol{u}) = (\tilde{\boldsymbol{\theta}}, \tilde{\boldsymbol{u}})$ and an inverse function $\tilde{h}$ combined with $\tilde{\boldsymbol{u}}$, a r-dimensional vector of random numbers generated by $\tilde{g}$. For instance, the Random Walk MH algorithm satisfies $\tilde{\boldsymbol{\theta}} = \boldsymbol{\theta} + \boldsymbol{u}$, $\boldsymbol{\theta} = \tilde{\boldsymbol{\theta}} + \tilde{\boldsymbol{u}}$ with $\tilde{\boldsymbol{u}} = -\boldsymbol{u}$ and g, $\tilde{g}$ are normal densities with mean zero and a chosen covariance matrix.

To achieve reversibility condition, expression (6.9) needs to be fulfilled, which translates here into $(d+r)$-dimensional integrals that satisfy

$$\int_{(\boldsymbol{\theta}, \tilde{\boldsymbol{\theta}}) \in A \times B} p(\boldsymbol{\theta} \mid \boldsymbol{y}) g(\boldsymbol{u}) \alpha(\boldsymbol{\theta}, \tilde{\boldsymbol{\theta}})\, \mathrm{d}\boldsymbol{\theta} \mathrm{d}\boldsymbol{u} = \int_{(\boldsymbol{\theta}, \tilde{\boldsymbol{\theta}}) \in A \times B} p(\tilde{\boldsymbol{\theta}} \mid \boldsymbol{y}) \tilde{g}(\tilde{\boldsymbol{u}}) \alpha(\tilde{\boldsymbol{\theta}}, \boldsymbol{\theta})\, \mathrm{d}\boldsymbol{\theta} \mathrm{d}\tilde{\boldsymbol{u}}. \tag{6.14}$$

If both h and $\tilde{h}$ are differentiable, then from the change-of-variable trick we know that condition (6.14) is satisfied when

$$p(\boldsymbol{\theta} \mid \boldsymbol{y}) g(\boldsymbol{u}) \alpha(\boldsymbol{\theta}, \tilde{\boldsymbol{\theta}}) = p(\tilde{\boldsymbol{\theta}} \mid \boldsymbol{y}) \tilde{g}(\tilde{\boldsymbol{u}}) \alpha(\tilde{\boldsymbol{\theta}}, \boldsymbol{\theta}) \left| \frac{\partial(\tilde{\boldsymbol{\theta}}, \tilde{\boldsymbol{u}})}{\partial(\boldsymbol{\theta}, \boldsymbol{u})} \right|,$$

with the last term being the Jacobian of the transformation from$(\boldsymbol{\theta}, \boldsymbol{u})$ to $(\tilde{\boldsymbol{\theta}}, \tilde{\boldsymbol{u}})$. From Section 6.3.3 we know that this happens when

$$\alpha(\boldsymbol{\theta}, \tilde{\boldsymbol{\theta}}) = \min\left(1, \frac{p(\tilde{\boldsymbol{\theta}} \mid \boldsymbol{y})\tilde{g}(\tilde{\boldsymbol{u}})}{p(\boldsymbol{\theta} \mid \boldsymbol{y})g(\boldsymbol{u})}\left|\frac{\partial(\tilde{\boldsymbol{\theta}}, \tilde{\boldsymbol{u}})}{\partial(\boldsymbol{\theta}, \boldsymbol{u})}\right|\right). \tag{6.15}$$

The somewhat different explanation of the standard MH algorithm provides a better basis for understanding RJMCMC.

Reversible Jump MH algorithm: Suppose that the parameter space is more complex now. For instance, suppose that there are two (or more) statistical models to choose from. Below, we examine whether the dmft-index in Signal-Tandmobiel® study has a Poisson distribution or a negative binomial distribution. The first distribution has one parameter, while the second has two parameters. Thus the two parameter spaces have unequal dimensions. A sampling algorithm that needs to sample from both distributions must be able to move between models of different dimensions.

We now suppose that the parameter space is given by $\Theta = \bigcup_m (m, \Theta_m)$ and that the posterior distribution of interest is $p(m, \boldsymbol{\theta}_m \mid \boldsymbol{y})$. Thus we wish to draw joint inference on both the model choice and the parameters of the models. In analogy with the standard MH algorithm, assume that $h_{m,\tilde{m}} : R^d \times R^r \rightarrow R^{\tilde{d}} \times R^{\tilde{r}}$transforms the $(d+r)$-dimensional vector $\boldsymbol{\psi}_m = (m, \boldsymbol{\theta}_m)$ into the $(\tilde{d}+\tilde{r}) = (d+r)$-dimensional vector $\tilde{\boldsymbol{\psi}}_{\tilde{m}} = (\tilde{m}, \tilde{\boldsymbol{\theta}}_{\tilde{m}})$. It is further assumed that $h_{m,\tilde{m}}$ is a bijective function with inverse $\tilde{h}_{\tilde{m},m}$ and differentiable. The equality $(\tilde{d}+\tilde{r}) = (d+r)$ is called the *dimension matching condition*. Let the proposal distribution to move from $\boldsymbol{\psi}_m$ to $\tilde{\boldsymbol{\psi}}_{\tilde{m}}$ be denoted as $j_{(m,\tilde{m})}(\boldsymbol{\psi}_m \mid \tilde{\boldsymbol{\psi}}_{\tilde{m}})$, then the probability to move from A to B (both sets in Θ) involves a sum of terms given by the LHS of expression (6.16) over the moves (from the different submodels m in A to the different submodels $\tilde{m}$ in B). The reversibility condition for each of these moves follows from expression (6.14):

$$\begin{aligned}
&\int_{(\boldsymbol{\psi}_m, \tilde{\boldsymbol{\psi}}_{\tilde{m}}) \in A \times B} p(\boldsymbol{\psi}_m \mid \boldsymbol{y}) j_{(m,\tilde{m})}(\boldsymbol{\psi}_m \mid \tilde{\boldsymbol{\psi}}_{\tilde{m}}) g(\boldsymbol{u}) \alpha(\boldsymbol{\psi}_m, \tilde{\boldsymbol{\psi}}_{\tilde{m}})\, d\boldsymbol{\psi}_m d\boldsymbol{u} \\
&= \int_{(\boldsymbol{\psi}_m, \tilde{\boldsymbol{\psi}}_{\tilde{m}}) \in A \times B} p(\tilde{\boldsymbol{\psi}}_{\tilde{m}} \mid \boldsymbol{y}) j_{(\tilde{m},m)}(\tilde{\boldsymbol{\psi}}_{\tilde{m}} \mid \boldsymbol{\psi}_m) \tilde{g}(\tilde{\boldsymbol{u}}) \alpha(\tilde{\boldsymbol{\psi}}_{\tilde{m}}, \boldsymbol{\psi}_m)\, d\tilde{\boldsymbol{\psi}}_{\tilde{m}} d\tilde{\boldsymbol{u}}.
\end{aligned} \tag{6.16}$$

The detailed balance condition is then satisfied if the acceptance probability is given by

$$\alpha(\boldsymbol{\psi}_m, \tilde{\boldsymbol{\psi}}_{\tilde{m}}) = \min\left(1, A_{m,\tilde{m}}(\boldsymbol{\psi}_m, \tilde{\boldsymbol{\psi}}_{\tilde{m}})\right), \tag{6.17}$$

with

$$A_{m,\tilde{m}}(\boldsymbol{\psi}_m, \tilde{\boldsymbol{\psi}}_{\tilde{m}}) = \frac{p(\tilde{\boldsymbol{\psi}}_{\tilde{m}} \mid \boldsymbol{y}) j_{(\tilde{m},m)}(\tilde{\boldsymbol{\psi}}_{\tilde{m}} \mid \boldsymbol{\psi}_m) \tilde{g}(\tilde{\boldsymbol{u}})}{p(\boldsymbol{\psi}_m \mid \boldsymbol{y}) j_{(m,\tilde{m})}(\boldsymbol{\psi}_m \mid \tilde{\boldsymbol{\psi}}_{\tilde{m}}) g(\boldsymbol{u})}\left|\frac{\partial(\tilde{\boldsymbol{\theta}}_m, \tilde{\boldsymbol{u}})}{\partial(\boldsymbol{\theta}_m, \boldsymbol{u})}\right|. \tag{6.18}$$

The Jacobian expresses the transition from $\boldsymbol{\psi}_m$ to $\tilde{\boldsymbol{\psi}}_{\tilde{m}}$ and depends on the move type.

The above description determines the RJMCMC algorithm, though only partially, since the function $h_{m,\tilde{m}}$ needs to be chosen. The actual choice of $h_{m,\tilde{m}}$ will greatly impact the performance of the RJMCMC algorithm.

To fix ideas we now illustrate the RJMCMC algorithm with the example in Hastie and Green (2012) but applied to the dmft-index in the Signal-Tandmobiel® study of Example II.3.

Example VI.10: Caries study: Choosing between a Poisson and a negative binomial distribution using RJMCMC
In Example II.3, we analyzed the dmft-index with a Poisson distribution. There is evidence for overdispersion since the mean dmft is equal to 2.24, while the variance is equal to 7.93. A candidate for fitting overdispersed counts is the negative binomial distribution. Therefore, we applied the RJMCMC to choose between the Poisson and negative binomial distribution based on the dmft-indices.

The Poisson likelihood for the sample of n dmft-indexes is

$$L(\lambda \mid \mathbf{y}) = \prod_{i=1}^{n} \frac{\lambda^{y_i}}{y_i!} \exp(-n\lambda),$$

derived from expression (2.20). For the negative binomial model, there exist several parameterizations, we deviate slightly from expression (3.15) here and express the negative binomial likelihood as

$$L(\lambda, \kappa \mid \mathbf{y}) = \prod_{i=1}^{n} \frac{\Gamma(1/\kappa + y_i)}{\Gamma(1/\kappa)\, y_i!} \left(\frac{1}{1+\kappa\lambda}\right)^{1/\kappa} \left(\frac{\lambda}{1/\kappa+\lambda}\right)^{y_i}, \tag{6.19}$$

where the above expression is derived from expression (3.15) using the relations $\kappa = 1/\alpha$ and $\lambda = \alpha/\beta$. The parameter λ is the mean for both distributions while the variance of the negative binomial distribution equals $\lambda(1+\kappa\lambda)$. Hence κ measures the overdispersion, and for $\kappa = 0$ the Poisson model is obtained.

We have two models, for $m = 1$: Poisson(λ) with $\theta_1 \equiv \lambda$ and for $m = 2$: NB(λ,κ) with $\boldsymbol{\theta}_2 = (\theta_{21}, \theta_{22}) \equiv (\lambda, \kappa)$. The trans-dimensional moves are thus between $\psi_1 = (1, \theta_1)$ and $\psi_2 = (2, \boldsymbol{\theta}_2)$. To complete the model specification we need to give priors to the parameters. First, gamma distributions were assumed for the model parameters: θ_1 and $\theta_{21} \sim \text{Gamma}(\alpha_\lambda, \beta_\lambda)$, and $\theta_{22} \sim \text{Gamma}(\alpha_\kappa, \beta_\kappa)$. Second, the prior probabilities for the models were taken as equal: $p(m = 1) = p(m = 2) = 0.5$. The posterior distribution then splits up into two posteriors:

- $(m = 1)$: $p(1, \theta_1 \mid \mathbf{y}) = 0.5\,\text{Gamma}(\alpha_\lambda, \beta_\lambda) L(\lambda \mid \mathbf{y})$
- $(m = 2)$: $p(2, \boldsymbol{\theta}_2 \mid \mathbf{y}) = 0.5\,\text{Gamma}(\alpha_\lambda, \beta_\lambda)\,\text{Gamma}(\alpha_\kappa, \beta_\kappa) L(\lambda, \kappa \mid \mathbf{y})$

The choices for the hyperparameters are $\alpha_\lambda = \overline{y} \times a = 22.43$, $\beta_\lambda = a$ and $\alpha_\kappa = (2/\overline{y}) \times a = 11.69$, $\beta_\kappa = a$. In this way λ has a prior mean equal to the observed mean dmft-index. The choice of a for β_λ and β_κ determines the prior knowledge on the mean parameter λ, we have taken $a = 1$ here but varied a from 0.5 to 10 with similar results. Finally, the choice of α_κ takes into account that the observed variance is about three times the observed mean. Further information and the R program can be found in 'chapter 6 dmft index Poisson vs negative bin.R'.

There are four types of moves: (1) Poisson to Poisson, (2) Poisson to negative binomial, (3) negative binomial to Poisson, and (4) negative binomial to negative binomial. Only moves 2 and 3 are trans-dimensional. Moves 1 and 4 are done using standard sampling approaches.

For move 2, we need to increase the dimension of the parameter vector to jump from one dimension to two dimensions. Suppose the Markov chain is in state $(1, \theta_1)$, then jumping to the negative binomial distribution can be done by generating u from a density g, e.g. $\mathrm{N}(0, \sigma^2)$ with σ fixed but well chosen combining it with θ_1 to propose $(2, \tilde{\boldsymbol{\theta}}_2)$. Hastie and Green (2012) suggested $\tilde{\boldsymbol{\theta}}_2 = (\tilde{\theta}_1, \tilde{\theta}_2) = h_{1,2}(\theta_1, u) = (\theta_1, \mu \exp(u))$ with μ fixed. This choice keeps the parameter λ fixed when switching between models. The overdispersion parameter κ is a lognormal random variable varying around μ. For the reverse move 3 we go back to the Poisson space but we need to make sure that the $h_{2,1}$ is the inverse of $h_{1,2}$. This is achieved by taking $h_{2,1}(\tilde{\boldsymbol{\theta}}_2) = (\tilde{\theta}_1, \log(\tilde{\theta}_2/\mu)) = (\theta_1, u)$. The Jacobian is equal to $\mu \exp(u)$. Two acceptance probabilities are used. For a move 2, it is $\min(1, A_{1,2})$ whereby

$$A_{1,2} = \frac{p(2, \tilde{\boldsymbol{\theta}}_2 \mid \boldsymbol{y})}{p(1, \theta_1 \mid \boldsymbol{y})} \left[\frac{1}{\sqrt{2\pi\sigma^2}} \exp\left(-\frac{u^2}{2\sigma^2}\right)\right]^{-1} \mu \exp(u), \tag{6.20}$$

and for the reciprocal move 3, it is $\min(1, A_{2,1})$ whereby

$$A_{2,1} = \frac{p(1, \theta_1 \mid \boldsymbol{y})}{p(2, \tilde{\boldsymbol{\theta}}_2 \mid \boldsymbol{y})} \frac{1}{\sqrt{2\pi\sigma^2}} \exp\left[-\frac{(\log(\tilde{\theta}_2/\mu))^2}{2\sigma^2}\right] \frac{1}{\tilde{\theta}_2}. \tag{6.21}$$

For the RJMCMC machinery to be complete we need to choose σ and μ. For move 3, κ was sampled from a right-skewed distribution varying around μ. The choice of σ and μ must reflect roughly what is observed in the data, otherwise too many unrealistic κ values are chosen (both parameters too large) or the sampled negative binomial distribution will not be much different from the Poisson distribution (both parameters too small). We experimented with three values of σ: 0.5, 1 and 2. Four combinations were taken with μ, such that the average value for κ was either equal to that obtained from the data or twice as much. For each of the four scenarios 10 000 iterations were generated and we removed 2000 initial iterations.

For each of the four scenarios, the negative binomial distribution was preferred. Preference was measured by the percentage of times the Markov chain was in model 1 (Poisson) or model 2 (negative binomial). The preference for model 2 varied between 56% and 74%. Surprisingly for some of the scenarios this preference is not overwhelming. However, with all scenarios a suggested move from model 1 to model 2 was always accepted. The median value for λ in the two models is around two, which is close to the observed mean value of the dmft-index. The median value of κ varied between 0.78 and 1.75 hence exhibiting quite some dependence on the settings. The percentage of trans-dimensional moves varied between 32% and 55%. The trace plots and posterior densities of the parameters for the within-space moves for the first scenario are shown in Figure 6.16. The parameter λ enters twice in the figures, once for the Poisson model and once for the negative binomial model.

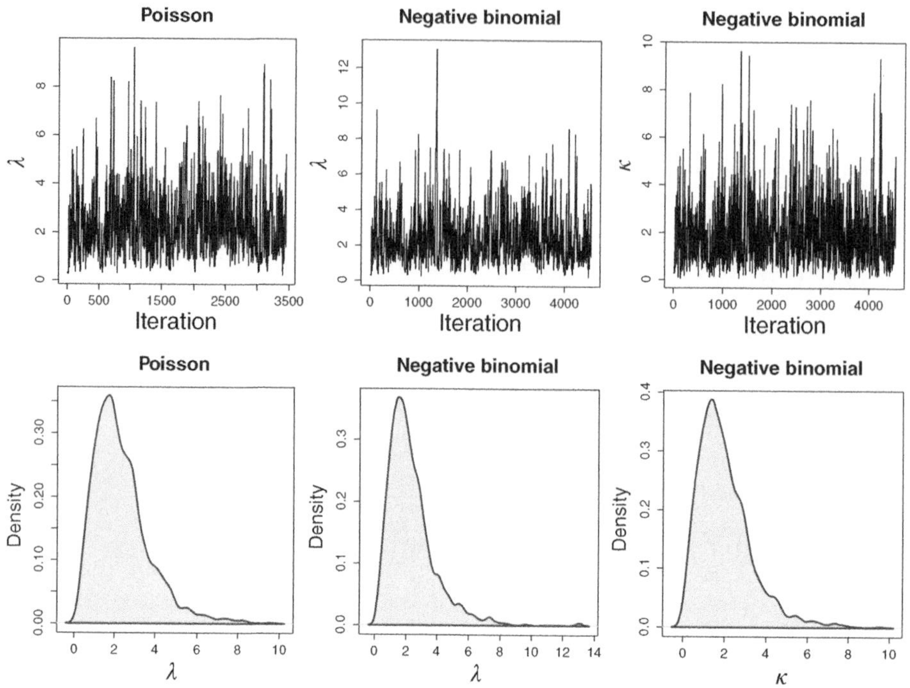

Figure 6.16 Caries study: choosing between Poisson distribution and negative binomial distribution using a RJMCMC approach. The trace plots and densities are based on the converged part of the chains and are model-specific.

We conclude that the negative binomial distribution appears best for the dmft-index, but surprisingly the evidence is not overwhelming. In addition, the RJMCMC appeared to be quite sensitive to the choices of σ and μ. □

To summarize, the idea behind the RJMCMC algorithm is to replace the jumps between spaces of different dimensions by jumps of spaces of greater but equal dimension. The RJMCMC algorithm needs for this reason bijective functions that ensure the reversibility of each move that is made. In general, a RJMCMC algorithm involves moves within the current space corresponding to a classical MH algorithm, moves between different spaces of the same dimension and moves between spaces of different dimensions. In the latter two cases, the RJMCMC algorithm requires an extension of the classical MH algorithm. The RJMCMC allows a lot of flexibility in constructing the jumps, e.g. the bijective function $h_{m,\tilde{m}}$ is not specified, nor the dimension r or the function g. This creates a lot of freedom and at the same time possibilities for refinements and extensions, but it often requires a lot of tuning to find the optimal choices. We return to the RJMCMC algorithm for variable selection in Chapter 11.

6.7 Closing remarks

Markov chain Monte Carlo techniques have greatly enlarged the class of problems we can now tackle with (Bayesian) statistical methods. However, there is a price to pay. Namely, often (much) longer execution times are needed and checking the convergence of the algorithm is more difficult than with likelihood approaches. Nevertheless, many (but not all) are prepared to pay this price to gain flexibility in fitting models to data.

Exercises

Exercise 6.1 Derive the posterior distribution (with the same NI priors as in the chapter) of $(\beta_0, \beta_1, \sigma^2)$ in the osteoporosis study (data are in 'osteop.txt') by: (a) Gibbs sampler and (b) the Random Walk Metropolis Sampler with proposal density $\mathrm{N}(\boldsymbol{\theta}^k, c^2 I)$ on $(\beta_0, \beta_1, \log(\sigma))$ and vary the value of c. Compare the performance of the two samplers.

Exercise 6.2 Derive the full conditionals of Example VI.4 and derive the posterior summary measures of all parameters and of derived parameters such as $\theta - \lambda$. Raftery and Akman (1986) used as priors for θ and λ

$$\theta \sim \text{Gamma}(a_1, b_1) \text{ and } \lambda \sim \text{Gamma}(a_2, b_2),$$

with $a_1 = a_2 = 0.5, b_1 = b_2 = 0$. Show that this Bayesian model gives virtually the same posterior summary measures as the analysis done by Tanner (1993).

Exercise 6.3 Sample from the auto-exponential model of Besag (1974) which is defined for positive (y_1, y_2, y_3) with density

$$f(y_1, y_2, y_3) \propto \exp\left[-(y_1 + y_2 + y_3 + \psi_{12}y_1y_2 + \psi_{13}y_1y_3 + \psi_{23}y_2y_3)\right],$$

with known $\psi_{ij} > 0$.

Exercise 6.4 Write an R program for the reversible Gibbs sampler introduced in Section 6.2.4. Apply the procedure on the osteoporosis data (see also Exercise 6.1) and compare the performance of the basic Gibbs sampler to the reversible version.

Exercise 6.5 Program the random-scan Gibbs sampler introduced in Section 6.2.4. Apply the procedure on the osteoporosis data (see also Exercise 6.1) and compare the performance of the basic Gibbs sampler to the random scan version.

Exercise 6.6 Apply the block Gibbs sampler introduced in Section 6.2.4 to the osteoporosis data (see also Exercise 6.1), with blocks (β_0, β_1) and σ^2. Compare its performance to the basic Gibbs sampler.

Exercise 6.7 Apply the Slice sampler to a beta distribution. Compare its performance to the classical R built-in sampler `rbeta`. Apply the Slice sampler also to a mixture of two beta distributions whereby the mixture exhibits a bi-modal shape.

Exercise 6.8 Perform a Bayesian logistic regression on the caries data of Example VI.9 (data in 'caries.txt') and with the same priors. Make use of the R function `ars` to apply the basic Gibbs sampler. Do the same for probit regression.

Exercise 6.9 Repeat Exercise 6.8 but now employ a Random Walk Metropolis algorithm.

Exercise 6.10 Perform a Bayesian regression of TBBMC on age, length, weight, and BMI (data in 'osteoporosismultiple.txt') with the classical NI priors using the following:

- Basic Gibbs sampler and block Gibbs sampler with the regression parameters in one block and the residual variance parameter in another block.
- Block Random Walk Metropolis sampler for the regression parameters. Use a normal proposal density and look for an appropriate scale parameter. Further, replace the normal proposal density by a multivariate t_3-density.
- Block Independent MH sampler for the regression parameters. Use as proposal density a normal distribution with mean the MLE and covariance matrix proportional to minus the inverse of the Hessian matrix at the MLE. Look for an appropriate proportionality factor.

Exercise 6.11 Vary in the RJMCMC program of Example VI.10 the settings of the prior distributions and evaluate the sensitivity of the results. Evaluate also the dependence of the results to the choice of σ and μ.

Exercise 6.12 Consult Waagepetersen and Sorensen (2001) which gives a more elaborate explanation of the Reversible Jump MCMC approach. In that paper, Example 4.2 describes the use of RJMCMC to choose between a gamma and a lognormal distribution for a positive-valued random variable. Adapt the R program of Exercise 6.11 to the above case and apply it the IBBENS data 'diet.txt' of Example 11.2.

7

Assessing and improving convergence of the Markov chain

7.1 Introduction

The generality of the MCMC sampling procedures comes with a cost: the sampled values are not immediately taken from the posterior distribution and assessing convergence of the Markov chain is more difficult than for the likelihood case. In addition, one needs to monitor the chain to ensure that the posterior summary measures are computed with enough accuracy. While the convergence theorems in Chapter 6 ensure that the Markov chain generated by a MCMC algorithm will (under weak regularity conditions) converge to the posterior distribution, it might not be immediately clear that the conditions are satisfied for the particular problem at hand especially when a complex model is involved. Moreover, the convergence theorems do not tell us when convergence will occur. In the examples of Chapter 6, we did not motivate the choice of the burn-in size and the total size of the chain. In this chapter, we look at a variety of graphical and formal diagnostics to assess convergence of the chain.

When convergence is slow, one can either let the MCMC procedure run longer or one could try to accelerate the algorithm. We explore in this chapter, the general purpose techniques to speed up the MCMC sampling procedure. In Chapter 9, specific acceleration techniques for hierarchical models are discussed.

The well-known likelihood-based EM-algorithm introduced by Dempster *et al.* (1977) is a particular case of *data augmentation*. Data augmentation reformulates an original, non-standard, likelihood into a standard one. By reformulating the problem, data augmentation can also accelerate the sampling procedure but at the very least it will simplify the sampling procedure. In this chapter, we look at the Bayesian implementation of data augmentation.

For most of the illustrations, we used WinBUGS in combination with CODA. In some examples, we used the recently released Bayesian routines in SAS®.

Bayesian Biostatistics, First Edition. Emmanuel Lesaffre and Andrew B. Lawson.

7.2 Assessing convergence of a Markov chain

7.2.1 Definition of convergence for a Markov chain

It goes without saying that convergence is not an issue when the posterior is determined analytically. When numerical procedures as in Section 3.7.1 are involved, then convergence only deals with the accuracy with which the integrals are computed. It is also important to see the difference between convergence for likelihood-based procedures and convergence for a Markov chain. In the first case, convergence has to do with how close we are to the MLE, while convergence for an MCMC algorithm checks how close we are to the true posterior distribution.

More formally, convergence in a MCMC context is an asymptotic property which implies for a Markov chain that $p_k(\boldsymbol{\theta})$, the distribution of $\boldsymbol{\theta}^k$, grows to the target distribution $p(\boldsymbol{\theta} \mid \mathbf{y})$ for $k \to \infty$. In other words it means that, for k large and small $\varepsilon, d_k \equiv d[p_k(\boldsymbol{\theta}), p(\boldsymbol{\theta} \mid \mathbf{y})] < \varepsilon$, with $d(f, g)$ the distance between two distributions f and g. Theoretical research has focused on establishing conditions under which convergence can be guaranteed. In some simple cases one can provide an expression for k_0 such that $d_k < \varepsilon$ for $k > k_0$. For example, Jones and Hobert (2001) showed that for the Gaussian case with μ and σ^2 unknown, a k_0 can be specified for the *total variation* discrepancy measure between two distributions, i.e. $d(f_k, f) = \frac{1}{2}\int |f_k(\boldsymbol{\theta}) - f(\boldsymbol{\theta})| d\boldsymbol{\theta}$. But such theoretical results are hard to establish in most practical cases (Jones and Hobert 2001). Note that most often evaluating the convergence of the chain involves checking convergence of the marginal posterior distributions. This means that we will be looking at one parameter at the time. For notation simplicity we denote this parameter as θ. The posterior $p(\theta \mid \mathbf{y})$ then refers to the marginal posterior for that parameter and $p_k(\theta)$ refers to the marginal sampling distribution of that component.

A variety of practical procedures have been suggested to check convergence via *convergence diagnostics*. The diagnostics involve two aspects: checking *stationarity* of the chain and verifying the *accuracy* of the posterior summary measures. In the stationarity step one determines the iteration k_0 such that for $k \geq k_0$, θ^k is sampled from the correct posterior distribution. This is equivalent to assessing the burn-in part of the Markov chain ($k = 1, \ldots, k_0$). Most convergence diagnostics (graphical and formal) appeal to the stationarity property of a converged chain. In the accuracy step it is verified that the posterior summary measures of interest based on θ^k ($k = k_0 + 1, \ldots, n$) are computed with the desired accuracy. Note that it is customary to base the summary measures on only the converged part of the chain (i.e. on θ^k with $k > k_0$). This is strictly speaking not necessary according to the ergodic theorems, but in practice it is recommended to do so since it results in more stable estimates especially for variance parameters.

7.2.2 Checking convergence of the Markov chain

The theoretical developments have had a limited impact on practice. Rather procedures based on the output of the Markov chain(s) (ignoring how this output has been generated) are in use. These methods verify the stationarity of the chain, in some cases in combination with checking the accuracy, and were called *output analysis* techniques by Ripley (1987). Comparative reviews of the methods can be found in Ripley (1987), Cowles and Carlin (1996), Brooks and Roberts (1998) and Mengersen *et al.* (1999). Their conclusions were that (a) a battery of diagnostics is necessary to assess convergence since none of the methods are fool-proof; (b) many diagnostics are too complicated for practical use and show too little evidence of success and (c) only diagnostics that are implemented in readily available software are likely to be applied in practice. More than 10 years later only a handful of diagnostics are in use, namely those that are implemented in WinBUGS (or related software). Both single chain and multiple chain diagnostics are in use.

We largely restrict ourselves to convergence diagnostics that are implemented in WinBUGS, CODA, BOA, and the Bayesian SAS procedures. Two sets of divergence diagnostics can be distinguished: graphical and formal. Both procedures will be illustrated using the osteoporosis study introduced in Example VI.5.

We have used $\overline{\theta}$ for the true posterior mean, but when sampling only an estimate of the posterior mean is available. Therefore the correct notation for the posterior mean obtained from a MCMC chain should be $\widehat{\overline{\theta}}$. However, to simplify the notation we will continue to denote the sampled posterior mean as $\overline{\theta}$ and hence here $\overline{\theta} = (1/n)\sum_{k=1}^{n}\theta^k$.

7.2.3 Graphical approaches to assess convergence

Trace plot: A simple exploration of the trace plot (Section 6.2) gives a first and insightful impression of the characteristics of the Markov chain. Trace plots are produced for each parameter separately and evaluate the chain univariately, but it is also useful to monitor the Markov chains jointly, i.e. the total parameter vector $\boldsymbol{\theta}$. This can be done by monitoring the (log) of the likelihood or of the posterior density. In WinBUGS, the deviance, which is equal to $-2\times$ log(likelihood), is automatically created, while in SAS a variable LogPost equal to the log of the posterior is by default added when an output file with sampled values is requested. In case of stationarity, the trace plot appears as a horizontal strip and the individual moves are hardly discernable. This is the basis of the informal *thick pen test* (Gelfand and Smith 1990). The test involves checking that the trace plot can be covered by a thick pen. The trace plot in Figure 6.8 passed this test. Gross deviations from stationarity are easily picked up in a trace plot, such as a dependence of the chain on its initial state by revealing an initial (up- or downward) trend. Further, the trace plot also shows how fast the chain explores the posterior distribution, i.e. it shows the *mixing rate* of the chain. The thick pen test is still a popular way to claim stationarity, and for some perhaps the only test that they apply in practice.

Autocorrelation plot: When future positions in the chain are highly predictable from the current position, then the posterior is slowly explored and one says that the chain has a *low mixing rate*. The mixing rate is measured by *autocorrelations* of different lags. The autocorrelation of lag m, denoted as ρ_m, is defined as the correlation between θ^k and $\theta^{(k+m)}$ (for $k = 1, \ldots$) and can be simply estimated by the Pearson correlation or a time series approach (see Section 6.4). The *autocorrelation function* (abbreviated as *ACF*) is the function that relates m to $\widehat{\rho}_m$ ($m = 0, 1, \ldots$) and is graphically depicted in the *autocorrelation plot*. When the autocorrelation decreases only slowly with increasing lag, the mixing rate is low. Note that the autocorrelation plot can also indicate the minimum number of iterations for the chain to 'forget' its starting position.

The autocorrelation plot is a useful tool but cannot be used as a convergence diagnostic. Indeed, even if ρ_m is relatively high for large m, this does not imply absence of convergence, but only slow mixing. In addition, once converged, the ACF does not change anymore, irrespective of the magnitude of the autocorrelations. When all autocorrelations are close to zero then MCMC sampling is done in an almost independent manner and stationarity will be attained quickly.

Running mean plot: Upon stationarity at k_0, the mean (and all other characteristics) of $p_k(\theta)$ shows stability for $k > k_0$. The *running mean* or *ergodic mean* plot can display this stability. It is a time-series plot of the running mean $\overline{\theta}^k$, i.e. the mean of all sampled values up to and including iteration k. The initial variability of the running-mean plot is always relatively high (even when sampling from the correct posterior), but stabilizes with increasing k in case of stationarity.

Q–Q plot: In the case of stationarity one expects that the distribution of the chain is stable irrespective at which part one is looking. Gelfand and Smith (1990) suggested a Q–Q plot with the first half of the chain on the x-axis and the second half of the chain on the y-axis. A Q–Q plot deviating from the bisecting line is an indication of nonstationarity of the chain.

Brooks plot: Brooks (1998) suggested two plots based on *cusums*, i.e. cumulative sums, to assess stationarity. His first suggestion is a time-series plot of the cumulative sum

$$T_m = \sum_{k=1}^{m}(\theta^k - \overline{\theta}), \ (m = 1, 2, \ldots, n), \tag{7.1}$$

with $T_0 \equiv 0$. A smooth plot with large excursions of T_m (before returning to zero) implies a slowly changing chain and thus low mixing, while hairy plots indicate good mixing (Brooks 1998). Labeling a plot 'smooth' is subjective and to give more guidance Brooks suggested a time-series plot based on $D_t = \frac{1}{t-k_0-1}\sum_{m=k_0+1}^{t-1} d_m$ $(k_0 + 2 \leq t \leq n)$ with $d_m = 1$ when the point (m, T_m) corresponds to a local minimum or maximum and 0 otherwise. D_t is the average number of times θ^k has crossed $\overline{\theta}$ up to iteration t. Assuming that the elements of the Markov chain are i.i.d. and symmetrically distributed around $\overline{\theta}$, Brooks derived (approximate) bounds for the plot against which the realized plot of (t, D_t) can be judged. In this way, the D_t-statistic is approximately a formal diagnostic to assess stationarity.

Cross-correlation plot: The correlation between θ_1^k with θ_2^k $(k = 1, \ldots, n)$ is called the *cross-correlation* of θ_1 with θ_2. The scatterplot of θ_1^k versus θ_2^k produces a *cross-correlation plot*. This plot is useful in case of convergence problems to indicate if model parameters are strongly related and thus is a diagnostic for an overspecified model.

Example VII.1: Osteoporosis study: Assessing convergence graphically
Recall that in WinBUGS, the third monitored variable, is practically equivalent to the automatically computed deviance, while in SAS the variable LogPost provides this information. In Example IV.7, TBBMC was regressed on BMI. This analysis involves three parameters: two regression coefficients β_0 (intercept) and β_1 (regression coefficient of BMI) and the residual variance σ^2. We monitored here β_1, σ^2 and $\log\left[p(\boldsymbol{\beta}, \sigma^2 \mid \boldsymbol{y})\right] \propto -0.5\left[(n+2)\log(\sigma^2) + (\boldsymbol{y} - \boldsymbol{\beta}^T\boldsymbol{x})^T(\boldsymbol{y} - \boldsymbol{\beta}^T\boldsymbol{x})/\sigma^2\right]$, the log(posterior). As before, we neglect the intercept for most plots since it shows similar behavior to the slope.

The trace plots in Figure 6.8 show quite a different sampling behavior for the regression parameters than for the variance parameter. In fact, the trace plots for the regression parameters exhibit low mixing, but there is rapid mixing for the variance parameter. The posterior distribution is therefore rapidly explored in the direction of σ^2 but slowly explored in the (β_0, β_1)-subspace. The trace plot of log(posterior) in Figure 7.1 behaves somewhat better. Namely, after a steep rise from its starting values, it evolves to a relatively stable pattern (although there are some excursions toward areas of low posterior evidence). The cross-correlation plot is similar to Figure 4.6(c) and highlights collinearity of BMI with the intercept.

The autocorrelation plots in Figure 7.2 confirm the low mixing for β_1 and the good mixing for σ^2. The autocorrelation for β_1 is around zero only from $m = 200$ onward. For σ^2 the autocorrelation drops immediately to zero demonstrating again the almost independent

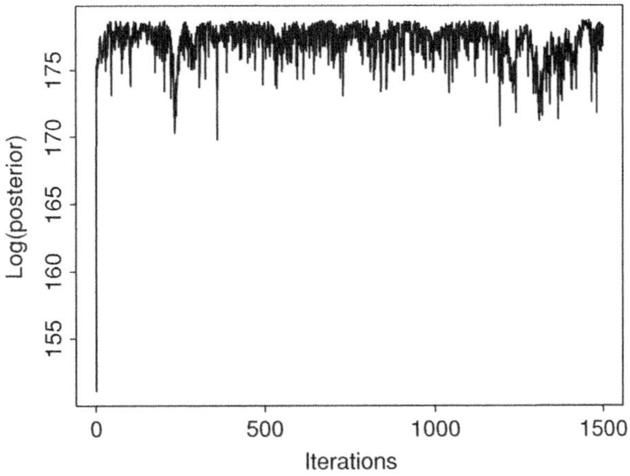

Figure 7.1 Osteoporosis study: trace plot for log(posterior) obtained from WinBUGS and plotted with the CODA function `trace plot`.

sampling of σ^2. Its initial state is almost immediately forgotten. Thus the burn-in part of 500 initial values looks excessive for σ^2, but not for the regression parameters. However, we would like to see this confirmed with formal diagnostics. Finally, that the ACFs look the same after 150 000 iterations illustrates that the autocorrelation plot is itself not an indicator for convergence.

The running-mean plots show a nonstable behavior for β_1 in contrast to the running mean plot for log(posterior) and σ^2. From the Q–Q plots (not shown), we infer that the sampled

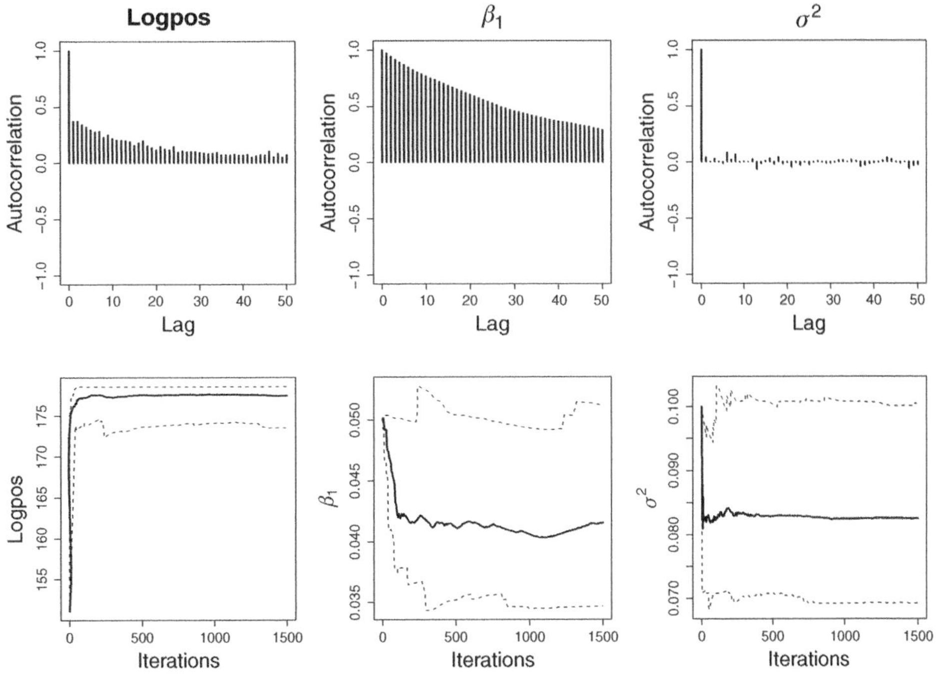

Figure 7.2 Osteoporosis study: autocorrelation plot and running-mean plot of log(posterior), β_1 and σ^2 obtained from WinBUGS + CODA.

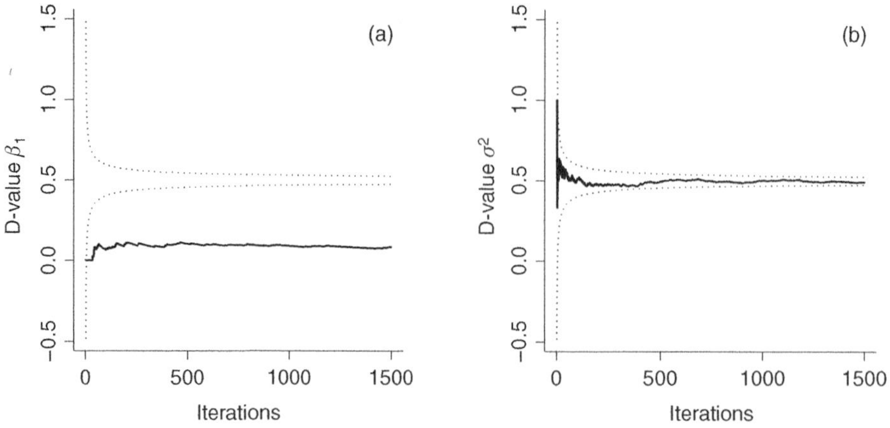

Figure 7.3 Osteoporosis study: Brooks' plot for (a) β_1 and (b) σ^2.

distribution of both regression parameters is quite different in the first half compared to the second half illustrating again nonstationarity.

Brooks' plot shows nonstationarity for β_1 but good behavior for σ^2 from the start on (see Figure 7.3).

We conclude that for the regression parameters stationarity is not quickly achieved, while it is almost instantly obtained for σ^2. We will postpone our final conclusion until we have applied more formal diagnostics. □

In addition to graphical procedures more formal guidelines are useful to conclude about the stationarity of the chain and the precision with which the posterior means are determined.

7.2.4 Formal diagnostic tests

Let $(\boldsymbol{\theta}^k)_k$ be a Markov chain obtained from a MCMC procedure. Four diagnostic tests for assessing stationarity and/or accuracy are introduced here. The first three tests assess convergence on a single chain and are based on the time-series or stochastic process properties of a Markov chain. The fourth diagnostic evaluates the discrepancy between multiple Markov chains to detect nonstationarity. Two diagnostics evaluate stationarity (size of burn-in part k_0) and accuracy (number of extra iterations k_1). All tests can be applied on the total chain or on the chain whereby an initial portion is removed automatically. Again we apply the diagnostic tests on the individual parameters denoted as θ.

Geweke diagnostic: This diagnostic test looks only for k_0. Geweke (1992) suggests to formally test the stationarity of a Markov chain by comparing the means of an early and a late part of the chain using a (frequentist) significance test. If the n values θ^k were i.i.d. and split up into two different parts: A (early part) with n_A elements and B (late part) with n_B elements, then their respective (posterior) means $\overline{\theta}_A$ and $\overline{\theta}_B$ could be compared with an unpaired Z-test given by

$$Z = \frac{\overline{\theta}_A - \overline{\theta}_B}{\sqrt{s_A^2/n_A + s_B^2/n_B}}, \tag{7.2}$$

with s_A^2, s_B^2 the classical estimates of the respective variances. For n_A and n_B large, Z would then be evaluated against a standard normal distribution. However, the elements of the Markov chain are dependent, which implies that (a) the means $\overline{\theta}_A$ and $\overline{\theta}_B$ are dependent and (b) s_A^2/n_A (s_B^2/n_B) underestimates the variance of $\overline{\theta}_A$ ($\overline{\theta}_B$) (Ripley 1987). In fact, $\text{var}(\overline{\theta})$, the limiting variance of $\overline{\theta}$, is equal to τ^2/n with τ^2 given by expression (6.10).

Hence another estimator of $\text{var}(\overline{\theta})$ is needed in expression (7.2). The method of batch means is one approach (see Section 7.2.5). Here, we look at an estimator that is based on a time-series approach. A central concept in time series is the *spectral density*, which characterizes the time series $f(\cdot)$ in the frequency domain and is given by

$$f(\omega) = \frac{\gamma_0}{2\pi} \sum_{m=-\infty}^{\infty} \rho_m \cos(m\,\omega).$$

One can show that $2\pi f(0) = \tau^2$ (Diggle 1990), so that the spectral density at 0 produces the variance of $\overline{\theta}$. The spectral density can be estimated from the chain by the periodogram (Diggle 1990). A time series estimate of τ^2 is then obtained by evaluating the periodogram in a window around 0, called the *spectral window*. This is the approach taken by Geweke.

To use test statistic of expression (7.2), the two means $\overline{\theta}_A$ and $\overline{\theta}_B$ must be independent (assertion (a) above). Geweke (1992) suggests to take for A the initial 10% of the iterations ($n_A = n/10$) and for B the last 50% ($n_B = n/2$) to create a distance between the two parts.

Summarized, with a time series estimate of the denominator in expression (7.2) and $n \to \infty$ with $(n_A + n_B)/n < 1$, the Z-score has a standard normal distribution and can be used to test stationarity of the Markov chain.

When the overall Z-test is significant at say, $\alpha = 0.05$, either the burn-in part (i.e. k_0) was taken too small and/or the total chain is too short. A dynamic version of Geweke diagnostic might also help to find a better value for k_0. For the dynamic version of the test, the Z-test is applied on $100(K - m)/K\%$ ($m = 0, \ldots, K$) last iterations of the chain. This produces Z_m ($m = 0, \ldots, K$) test statistics that are plotted in a time-series plot.

Heidelberger–Welch (HW) diagnostic: Heidelberger and Welch (1983) proposed a fully automated method that tests the stationarity of the chain (k_0) and evaluates whether the length of the chain is sufficient to guarantee a desired accuracy for the posterior mean of the parameter(s) (k_1). For a multivariate and multiple-chain extension of this test, we refer to Brooks and Roberts (1998).

Step 1 – Checking stationarity: Let the cumulative sums be $S_m = \sum_{k=1}^{m} \theta^k$ for $m = 1, 2, \ldots, n$ and $S_0 \equiv 0$. In the case of stationarity, S_m should fluctuate in a random way around $m\overline{\theta}$. This is equivalent to T_m in expression (7.1) fluctuating around zero. This fluctuation varies with m and must, by construction, be zero for $m = 0$ and $m = n$. For $0 \le t \le 1$, let m be equal to $[nt]$ which is the integer part of nt. HW used a standardized version of $T_{[nt]}$, i.e.

$$B_n(t) = \frac{S_{[nt]} - [nt]\overline{\theta}}{\sqrt{n}\tau}, \quad 0 \le t \le 1, \tag{7.3}$$

and is therefore related to Brooks' plot. Under stationarity $B_n = \{B_n(t), 0 \le t \le 1\}$ converges in distribution to a Brownian bridge $B = \{B(t), 0 \le t \le 1\}$ for $n \to \infty$. Briefly, a Brownian bridge B (Ross 2000, Chapter 10) satisfies that (a) $B(t)$ has Gaussian distribution for each t, (b) $B(0) = B(1) = 0$ and (c) $\text{cov}(B(s), B(t)) = s(1 - t)$ for $s < t < 1$.

To flag nonstationarity, HW suggested to use the Cramer–von Mises statistic given by

$$\int_0^1 B_n(t)^2 dt = \frac{1}{n}\sum_{m=1}^{n-1}\frac{(S_m - m\overline{\theta})^2}{n\tau^2}, \tag{7.4}$$

since its asymptotic distribution is known under stationarity. Stationarity will be rejected at, say significance level $\alpha_0 = 0.05$, which will happen with long excursions away from zero. In practice, $B_n(t)$ is replaced by

$$\widehat{B}_n(t) = \frac{S_{[nt]} - [nt]\overline{\theta}}{\sqrt{n}\widehat{\tau}}, \quad 0 \leq t \leq 1, \tag{7.5}$$

with $\widehat{\tau}$ obtained from the periodogram.

Step 2 – Determining accuracy: When stationarity is established, the size of (remaining part of the) chain should be large enough to ensure a desired accuracy of the estimated posterior means. Thus, we now look for the extra number of iterations k_1 beyond k_0, but for notational simplicity we denote the size of the stationary part of the chain by n.

Let $\widehat{d}(\alpha_1, \theta) = z_{(1-\alpha_1/2)}\widehat{\tau}/\sqrt{n}$ be the estimated width of the $100(1-\alpha_1/2)\%$ (classical) confidence interval for the true posterior mean of θ with $z_{(1-\alpha_1/2)}$ equal to 1.96 for $\alpha_1 = 0.05$. HW suggested to use the relative half-width of this interval,

$$\text{ERHW}(\alpha_1, \theta) = \frac{1/2\ \widehat{d}(\alpha_1, \theta)}{\overline{\theta}},$$

to ascertain the accuracy. If the desired accuracy (ERHW$< \varepsilon$) is not met, extra iterations are needed.

In practice, testing for (initial) nonstationarity is done in steps of, say, 10% of the chain. First, stationarity is tested on the initial 10% of the chain. If there is evidence of nonstationarity, the test is repeated on the remaining 90% portion of the chain. This process continues (with steps of 10%) until the remaining chain passes the test or more than 50% of the iterations have been discarded. In the first case, the procedure enters the second step. In the second case, the procedure stops and the Markov chain did not pass the test.

Raftery–Lewis (RL) diagnostic: The above convergence diagnostics were all based on the posterior mean. But, when the posterior distribution is skewed, the preferred summary measure is the posterior median. Further, the 95% credible interval requires the computation of the 0.025 and 0.975 quantile. This motivates to look for a diagnostic that ensures a desired accuracy of the estimated posterior quantiles.

Raftery and Lewis (1992) suggested a procedure to estimate the posterior quantile u_q, defined by $P(\theta < u_q \mid \mathbf{y}) = q$, for a prespecified q with a desired accuracy. Let $\widehat{u}_q$ be the estimate of u_q, then the implemented procedure gives the necessary number of iterations such that $P(\theta < \widehat{u}_q \mid \mathbf{y}) = \widehat{q}$ lies in the interval $[q - \delta, q + \delta]$ (with δ equal to say 0.005) with (a frequentist) probability $(1 - \alpha)$ (e.g. 0.95). Note that the desired accuracy is specified on $\widehat{q}$ and not on $\widehat{u}_q$.

The RL diagnostic is based on two steps. In the first step, the stationarity of the chain is checked on a binarized chain Z^k derived from the original Markov chain using $Z^k = I_{(\theta^k < \widehat{u}_q)}$. Since the binary chain $(Z^k)_k$ does not satisfy the Markov property, the authors suggested taking a subchain to again achieve (approximately) the Markov property (see also *thinning* in Section 7.3). That is, the smallest value of s is chosen such that for the subchain $(Z^m)_m$ with $m = 1, 1+s, 1+2s, \ldots$ a first-order Markov model is preferred over a second-order Markov model with the BIC (see Chapter 10). For this binary subchain one can easily determine n_0, the number of burn-in iterations to be discarded, yielding $k_0 = s \times n_0$ for the original chain. In the second step the number of extra iterations (k_1) is computed to arrive at a desired accuracy of the estimated posterior quantile. Based on the asymptotic normality of $\widehat{q}$, the extra k_1 iterations are taken such that $P(q - \delta \leq \widehat{q} \leq q + \delta) = (1 - \alpha)$ is satisfied.

Finally, RL calculated the necessary size of the chain for independent Z^k to achieve the desired accuracy. In that case, no iterations need to be discarded ($k_0 = 0$) and no thinning ($s = 1$) is required yielding the minimum size of the chain, denoted by $n_{\min}$. The ratio $(k_0 + k_1)/n_{\min}$ is called the *dependence factor* and quantifies 'the damage' of the dependence in the binary sequence. A dependence factor greater than 5 is, according to the authors, a sign of problems with the implementation of the chain (bad starting values, high autocorrelations, etc.).

Brooks–Gelman–Rubin (BGR) diagnostic: When the posterior is multi-modal, a single Markov chain might get stuck for a very long time in an area around a local mode. Convergence to a local mode is a well-known problem in classical optimization routines. To circumvent this problem it is advised to start up the optimization routine from various initial positions. In the same spirit, Gelman and Rubin (1992) suggested a convergence diagnostic based on multiple chains with 'overdispersed' (relative to the posterior distribution) starting positions. Their diagnostic is based on an ANOVA idea where the chains play the role of groups. We classified the diagnostic as 'formal' but we could also have classified it as 'graphical'.

The Gelman and Rubin (GR) ANOVA diagnostic: Take M widely dispersed starting points θ_m^0 ($m = 1, \ldots, M$) and suppose that M parallel chains are run for $2n$ iterations. The first n iterations are discarded and regarded as burn-in. The M chains $(\theta_m^k)_k$ ($m = 1, \ldots, M$) of length n produce means $\overline{\theta}_m = (1/n)\sum_{k=1}^{n} \theta_m^k$ ($m = 1, \ldots, M$). The overall mean (across the chains) is $\overline{\theta} = (1/M)\sum_m \overline{\theta}_m$. As in classical ANOVA one calculates the within- and between-chain variability. Let

$$W = \frac{1}{M}\sum_{m=1}^{M} s_m^2, \quad \text{with } s_m^2 = \frac{1}{n}\sum_{k=1}^{n}(\theta_m^k - \overline{\theta}_m)^2,$$

$$B = \frac{n}{M-1}\sum_{m=1}^{M}(\overline{\theta}_m - \overline{\theta})^2.$$

Two estimates of the posterior variance of θ^k in the target distribution can be constructed from W and B. First,

$$\widehat{V} \equiv \widehat{\text{var}}(\theta^k \mid \mathbf{y}) = \frac{n-1}{n}W + \frac{1}{n}B$$

is an unbiased estimate of the variance when there is stationarity (in which case all $\overline{\theta}_m$ are unbiased estimates of the true posterior mean). However, when the M chains are not mixing well $\widehat{V}$ overestimates $\text{var}(\theta^k \mid \mathbf{y})$ and W often underestimates this variance as long as the chains have not yet explored the whole target distribution. When $n \to \infty$ both $\widehat{V}$ and W

approach $\text{var}(\theta^k \mid \boldsymbol{y})$ but from opposite directions. GR suggested therefore the ratio

$$\widehat{R} = \frac{\widehat{V}}{W}$$

as a convergence diagnostic. $\widehat{R}$ is called *the estimated potential scale reduction factor (PSRF)* since if $\widehat{R}$ is substantially greater than 1, further iterations are needed either to reduce $\widehat{V}$ or to increase W. To take the sampling variability of the variance estimates into account, a corrected version $\widehat{R}_c = (\widehat{d}+3)/(\widehat{d}+1)\widehat{R}$ with $\widehat{d} = 2\widehat{V}/\widehat{\text{var}}(\widehat{V})$ is suggested. In addition, a 97.5% upper confidence bound of $\widehat{R}_c$ can be computed. GR advised to continue sampling until $\widehat{R}_c$ is smaller than 1.1 or 1.2. In that case, the M chains are mixing well and will have (hopefully) converged to the posterior distribution. In addition, GR advised that $\widehat{V}$ and W be monitored, both of which must stabilize. In the case of convergence, the posterior summary measures are taken from the second half of the total chain.

A dynamic/graphical version of the diagnostic is proposed in Brooks and Gelman (1998). The M chains are divided into batches of length b and $\widehat{V}^{1/2}(s)$, $W^{1/2}(s)$ and $\widehat{R}_c(s)$ are calculated based upon the second half of the (cumulative) chains of length $2sb$, for $s = 1, \ldots, [n/b]$. In addition, a 97.5% upper pointwise confidence bound is computed. Note that the GR diagnostic is implemented in the R packages CODA and BOA. Other versions of the diagnostic including a multivariate version of $\widehat{R}$ have been proposed by Brooks and Gelman (1998). One of these extensions is implemented in WinBUGS and is discussed in the next paragraph.

The Brooks–Gelman–Rubin (BGR) interval diagnostic: The ANOVA diagnostic assumes a Gaussian behavior of the sampled parameter values. For σ^2, the variance of a normal distribution, a log-transformation is required prior to the application of the GR-diagnostic. Alternatively one might use a nonparametric version of the GR-diagnostic as follows. We take from each chain the empirical $100(1-\alpha)\%$ interval, i.e. the $100\alpha/2\%$ and the $100(1-\alpha/2)\%$ points of the last n iterations of M chains of length $2n$. This yields M within-chain intervals. The average of these M intervals is then contrasted with the empirical total equal-tail $100(1-\alpha)\%$ interval obtained in a similar way across all chains to yield the interval-based $\widehat{R}_I$:

$$\widehat{R}_I = \frac{\text{length of total-chain interval}}{\text{average length of the within-chain intervals}} \equiv \frac{\widehat{V}_I}{W_I}.$$

In WinBUGS, a dynamic version of $\widehat{R}_I$ is implemented. Based on $\alpha = 0.20$, the chain is divided into cumulative subchains based on iterations 1–100, 1–200, 1–300, etc. For each part WinBUGS computes on the second half of the subchain: (a) $\widehat{R}_I$, (b) $\widehat{V}_I/\max(\widehat{V}_I)$, and (c) $W_I/\max(W_I)$. Thereby, three curves are produced. As for the GR-diagnostic the three curves are monitored and in the case of convergence the posterior summary measures are taken on the second half of the total chain.

In the remainder of the book, we will refer both multiple-chain diagnostics as the BGR-diagnostics. In the next example, we apply the formal diagnostic tests to the osteoporosis data.

Example VII.2: Osteoporosis study: Assessing convergence using formal diagnostic tests
First, we assessed convergence of the chain of length 1500, analyzed in Example VII.1. For this we used the R package CODA. Under the standard settings of 10% (first part) and 50% (second part), the R program `geweke.diag` did not converge. With 20% for the

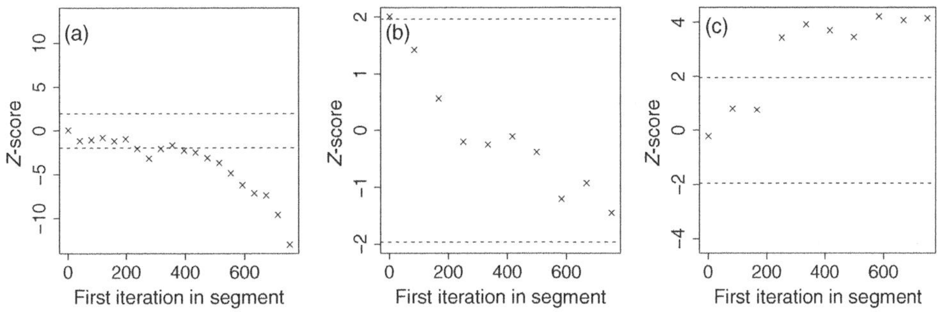

Figure 7.4 Osteoporosis study: Geweke diagnostic dynamic plot for (a) β_1, (b) σ^2 and (c) log(posterior) obtained from WinBUGS+CODA.

first part, the results of Geweke diagnostic were for β_1: $Z = 0.057$ and for σ^2: $Z = 2.00$. Surprisingly, the diagnostic did reject stationarity for σ^2 but not for β_1. The dynamic version of the Geweke diagnostic (with $K = 20$) is shown in Figure 7.4. Most of the Z-values for β_1 are outside the $[-1.96, 1.96]$ interval indicating nonstationarity. The same is true for log(posterior), which implies that the behavior seen in the trace plot was not yet stable enough to conclude stationarity. For σ^2 all values except for the first were within the $[-1.96, 1.96]$ interval.

The HW diagnostic was applied with the R program `heidel.diag` with default settings of $\alpha_0 = 0.05$ and $\alpha_1 = 0.05$ (yielding a 95% confidence interval). The stationary test was passed only for σ^2 ($P = 0.29$). In addition, the posterior mean for σ^2 was estimated with the desired relative accuracy since the half-width test was also passed with the halfwidth equal to 0.000504. Note that the half-width test applied to log(posterior) has no practical value.

The RL diagnostics were calculated for $q = 0.025$ and $q = 0.975$ with the standard settings being $\delta = 0.005$, $\alpha = 0.05$, and $\varepsilon = 0.001$ (precision with which the burn-in part is estimated) using the R program `raftery.diag`. A warning was given that at least $3746 = n_{min}$ iterations are needed to achieve the desired accuracy.

For the BGR diagnostics, we used the output of a classical linear regression program to suggest overdispersed starting values for the parameters, i.e. the eight corners of the 99.9% confidence intervals of the three parameters were taken as starting positions. For each of the eight chains 1500 iterations were run. The CODA program `gelman.diag` produced $\widehat{R}_c = 1.06$ (with 97.5% upper bound equal to 1.12) for β_1. Thus, for $\beta_1, \widehat{R}_c$ is below the threshold, but the 97.5% upper bound is above 1.1. For σ^2, $\widehat{R}_c = 1.00$ with 97.5% upper bound equal to 1. All of this shows that mixing is worse for the regression parameters. In Figure 7.5, the dynamic version of the GR ANOVA diagnostic is shown. The plots are based on 20 batches. The plot of $\widehat{R}_c$ stabilizes fast for σ^2, but the plot for β_1 has not yet stabilized after 1500 iterations and the 0.975 quantile of $\widehat{R}$ is fluctuating around 1.2. Further iterations appear necessary.

In Figure 7.6, the dynamic version of GR interval diagnostic as obtained from WinBUGS is displayed. Three curves are given: a top curve representing $\widehat{R}_I$, a middle curve representing the total-chain 80% confidence interval and a bottom curve representing the averaged within-chain 80% confidence interval. The reported values for the numerator and denominator of $\widehat{R}_I$ are standardized in WinBUGS. The values of $\widehat{R}_I$ (obtained by ctrl-left mouse clicking on the BGR graph) dropped quickly below 1.1 for β_1 with increasing iterations and varied around 1.03 from iteration 600 onward. Further, from iteration 500 onward the three curves stabilized. Thus, now no extra iterations appear necessary and posterior summary measures

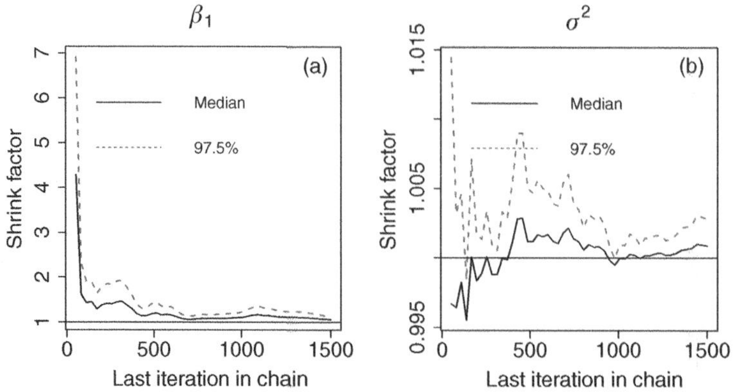

Figure 7.5 Osteoporosis study: dynamic version of Gelman and Rubin ANOVA diagnostic plot applied to (a) β_1 and (b) σ^2 obtained from WinBUGS+CODA.

can be taken from 500 onward. For σ^2, $\widehat{R}_I$ was quickly around 1.003 and the curves stabilized almost immediately.

We conclude that a single chain of length 1500 seemed inadequate for achieving convergence of the regression parameters. Therefore, we increased the number of iterations to 15 000. Convergence was then obtained, but for accurately estimating certain quantiles, the Markov chain was still not large enough. The convergence problems seem odd given that the considered model is the simplest one can imagine. The reason for the difficulties is a multicollinearity problem in regression which also causes numerical and statistical difficulties in a classical regression analysis (see also Example IV.7). □

7.2.5 Computing the Monte Carlo standard error

MCMC algorithms produce dependent random variables. Thus, we cannot use the classical standard error of the mean $s/\sqrt{n}$, with s the posterior standard deviation and n the length of the chain, to estimate the Monte Carlo standard error (MCSE) of the posterior mean. A correct limiting expression of the Monte Carlo variance of $\overline{\theta}$ is equal to τ^2/n with τ given by expression (6.10) and estimated with a time series approach.

The *method of batch means* is another approach to estimate the Monte Carlo variance of $\overline{\theta}$. Under the assumption that the Markov chain $(\theta^k)_k$ has converged, we split the chain up into

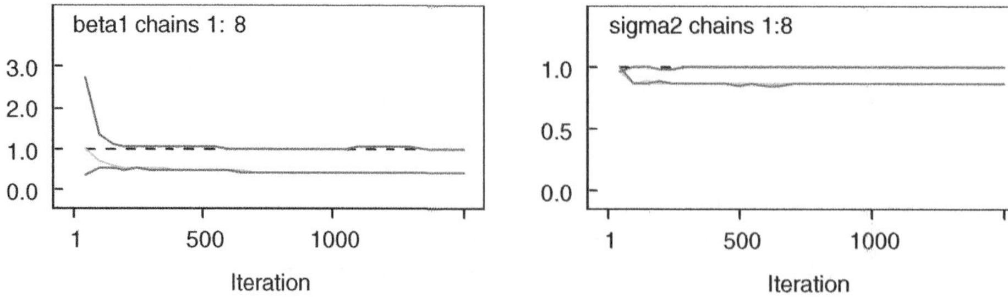

Figure 7.6 Osteoporosis study: Brooks–Gelman–Rubin diagnostic plot for β_1 and σ^2 from WinBUGS.

b batches each of size m, i.e. $\{\theta^1, \theta^2, \ldots, \theta^m\}$, $\{\theta^{(m+1)}, \ldots, \theta^{2m}\}, \ldots, \{\theta^{(b-1)m+1}, \ldots, \theta^{bm}\}$, with $bm = n$. Taking for each batch the average value of the θ-values in that batch, yields batch means $\{\overline{\theta}^1, \ldots, \overline{\theta}^b\}$. Note that the posterior mean $\overline{\theta}$ is also the mean of the b batch means. The autocorrelation among the batch means is in general lower than that of the original chain elements and must decrease with the size of the batch. Suppose that m is taken such that the correlation between $\overline{\theta}^k$ and $\overline{\theta}^{(k+1)}$ is small, say < 0.1. Since these batch means are practically uncorrelated (and assuming that this implies independence), the standard error of the posterior mean can be approximated by

$$s_{\overline{\theta}}^B = \sqrt{\frac{\sum_{k=1}^{b}(\overline{\theta}^k - \overline{\theta})^2}{(b-1)b}}. \tag{7.6}$$

The calculation of expression (7.6) involves the choice of m and b. The higher the autocorrelation in the original chain, the greater m must be to satisfy that the correlation < 0.1, the lower b must be and the less precise the true posterior mean will be estimated. From the classical 95% confidence interval

$$[\overline{\theta} - 1.96\, s_{\overline{\theta}}^B, \overline{\theta} + 1.96\, s_{\overline{\theta}}^B]$$

we can compute the length of the chain in order to get the required precision. Note that the method of batch means is considered less precise than the time-series approach.

To measure the inflation of the Monte Carlo standard error due to dependency in the chain, the RL diagnostic reports the dependence factor. A high value indicates highly dependent sampling. A measure of the same kind is the *effective sample size (ESS)*. In the case of independence $\widehat{\text{var}}(\overline{\theta}) = s^2/n$. According to expression (6.10), the dependence in the chain increases this variance to at least $\widehat{\text{var}}(\overline{\theta}) = (s^2/n) \times (1 + 2\sum_{m=1}^{\infty} \rho_m)$. The effective sample size is therefore estimated as $n/(1 + 2\sum_{m=1}^{M} \widehat{\rho}_m)$, with M chosen such that $|\widehat{\rho}_M|$ is small enough.

The Monte Carlo estimate based on the time series approach is implemented in the SAS procedure MCMC, while the method of batch means is implemented in WinBUGS. CODA and BOA report both estimates.

Example VII.3: Osteoporosis study: Calculating the Monte Carlo standard error of the posterior mean

Since the Markov chain converges only slowly, 40 000 iterations were taken in total and we discarded the first 20 000 iterations. Further, we computed the Monte Carlo standard error for β_1 using three programs: WinBUGS, CODA and SAS. We obtained from (1) WinBUGS: MCSE = 2.163E−4 (method of batch means), (2) from SAS: MCSE = 6.270E−4 (time series), and (3) CODA: no estimate for batch means was obtained due to computational difficulties, but for the time series estimate MCSE = 1.788E−4. The effective sample size obtained by CODA was 312, while for SAS it was 22.9. Thus in both cases there is an enormous loss of information by the dependent sampling algorithms compared to independent sampling.

The MCSE and ESS differed considerably between WinBUGS, CODA and SAS. The explanation for this difference is the different sampling procedures in WinBUGS (Gibbs) and SAS (Metropolis) in combination with the extremely slow convergence for the regression parameters. In fact, the HW and the Geweke diagnostic indicated no stationarity for the SAS run. Only after 500 000 burn-in iterations and an additional 500 000 iterations, stationarity could be claimed by the two diagnostics (stationarity could have been achieved earlier, but we were bored running SAS over-and-over again). □

7.2.6 Practical experience with the formal diagnostic procedures

We now summarize our experience with each of the diagnostics, based on many Bayesian analyses (not only of the osteoporosis data).

Geweke diagnostics: This procedure is popular and easy to understand. However, it suffers from a high dependence on the choice of the early and late part especially in the presence of high autocorrelations. For this reason, it is recommended to explore in addition its dynamic version. The test can also highly depend on the method to compute spectral window when determining τ^2, and hence different software implementations might yield different test outcomes.

HW diagnostics: This procedure determines both k_0 and k_1 and is relatively easy to use in practice. Heidelberger and Welch (1983) tested their procedure extensively and concluded that, when the initial transient part is longer than the run length of the chain, good performance can be expected.

RL diagnostics: Brooks and Roberts (1999) argued against the RL procedure when the interest does not lie in a quantile because the method tends to underestimate k_0, especially when the popular 0.025 quantile is used. The criticism on the RL approach is unfortunate, since we should test extreme quantiles if the 95% CI is the basis for Bayesian hypothesis testing.

GR diagnostics: There is an animated discussion in the literature whether or not to use multiple chains to assess convergence. Gelman and coauthors advocate multiple chains with overdispersed starting values to avoid that a single chain might get stuck in a local mode. Based on our experience, we believe that the BGR diagnostic should be part of each test for convergence especially in complex models; see Chapter 9 for additional examples. The only problem with the approach is that it is not always clear how to pick overdispersed but also realistic starting values.

It is impossible in practice to prove convergence. Geyer (1992) reported on a MCMC analysis of a hierarchical model. At the time of publication of his paper he realized, though, that his NI prior must yield an improper posterior. Only . . . a million iterations were not enough to discover it. It is not without reason that the WinBUGS manual has the following warning: *MCMC sampling can be dangerous!* (although WinBUGS does not allow improper priors). In the analyses of next chapters, we also occasionally observed that the chains behaved well until a few thousands iterations and then started to deteriorate. An example of this behavior is seen in Figure 7.7 that represents the trace plot of one of the regression coefficients in one of the joint models (but not final) developed in Section 15.4. One can observe an initially well-behaved Markov chain, followed by an excursion to other parts of the posterior distribution (this happened with all parameters) and then coming back to the original stable behavior. This trace plot remained then stable until 500 000 iterations (thinning=10), but it is not guaranteed that the chain will not start another excursion afterward. This is a frightening idea but reality (see also Exercise 9.17).

In Section 7.4, we expand on some practical guidelines on testing convergence. We now explore techniques to accelerate convergence in case convergence is prohibitively low as in the case of our regression example.

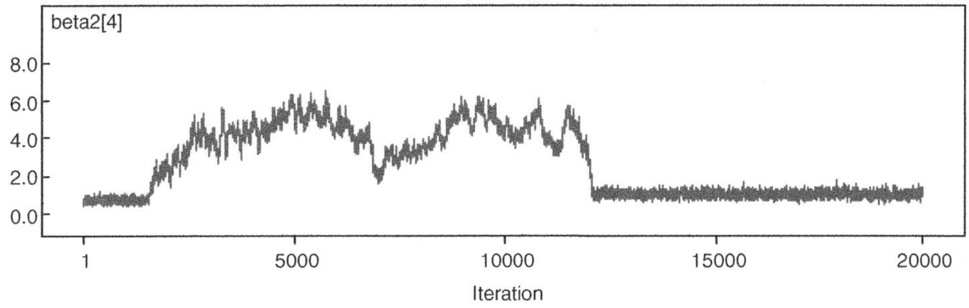

Figure 7.7 AZT clinical trial: trace plot obtained from WinBUGS of one of the regression coefficients based on 200 000 iterations (thinning=10).

7.3 Accelerating convergence

7.3.1 Introduction

In this section, we review some simple tricks to speed up convergence. They are not guaranteed to work in all circumstances, but if applicable they may accelerate convergence considerably. Approaches to speed up convergence may be classified into (a) choosing better starting values, (b) transforming the variables, (c) blocking, (d) algorithms that suppress the purely random behavior of the MCMC sample, and (e) reparameterization of the parameters. We focus here on techniques that can be used in combination with standard software such as WinBUGS and SAS. Novel MCMC algorithms as in Green and Han (1990), Gustafson (1998b), and Barone *et al.* (2002) illustrate that other, more sophisticated, MCMC algorithms can be developed that could accelerate convergence greatly. However, these techniques are beyond the scope of this book.

7.3.2 Acceleration techniques

A trivial, but important remark, is that the convergence rate heavily depends on the chosen model. Indeed, exchanging one model for another can completely alter the mixing rate. This is illustrated in Exercise 7.3 where the Weibull survival distribution in the Mice example of *WinBUGS Manual* Vol I is replaced by a lognormal survival distribution. With the second distribution the autocorrelations dropped quickly to zero with increasing lag.

The following tricks can accelerate convergence of the Markov chain:

Choosing better starting values: When the starting values are taken in an area where the posterior probability is low, it may take a long time to escape from the starting positions and mixing could be low initially. This can be spotted by an initial decreasing or increasing trend in the trace plot. A simple and obvious remedy is to try out other starting values.

Transforming the data: When the regressors differ greatly in magnitude, computational difficulties may be expected in a classical (frequentist) regression analysis. For this reason, it is recommended to render the regressors unit-free, which can be done by dividing the regressor values by their sample standard deviation. This trick is also recommended for MCMC computations. Another problem that affects the speed of convergence is multicollinearity (in the regressors). Let $\boldsymbol{X}$ be the design matrix of the regression model, then $|\boldsymbol{X}^T\boldsymbol{X}| \approx 0$ in case of multicollinearity. It can be seen that multicollinearity affects the conditional distribution (4.28) and the marginal posterior distribution (4.30) of the regression model. But $|X^T X| \approx 0$ also implies that the posterior surface has a ridge since one of the eigenvalues of $X^T X$ is around zero. In that case the Gibbs sampler, but also the MH algorithm, will only make small steps when exploring the posterior distribution. Classical solutions to avoid high correlations are centering or more generally Gram–Schmidt orthogonalization. These tricks may help to accelerate convergence of a Markov chain especially in linear regression problems (see Example VII.4). They might also work in nonlinear regression models (Exercises 7.4 and 8.1) but care is needed since they might even reduce the speed of convergence (Exercise 8.4). Another solution to the problem is blocking; see below.

Thinning: The aim of acceleration methods is to lower the autocorrelations. A simple trick to lower the autocorrelations consists in retaining only every Mth value in the chain, which is called *thinning* the chain. In fact, the thinned Markov chain can even be turned into a chain with all autocorrelations equal to zero for lags greater than one. This is done by taking the thinning factor equal to the lag for which the original Markov chain has autocorrelation equal to (roughly) zero. However, the thinned Markov chain has a higher Monte Carlo error than the original one. In fact, in almost all cases, the gain is only with respect to computer storage (see Example VII.4).

Blocking: In Section 6.2.3, the block Gibbs sampler was introduced as a Gibbs sampler applied on blocks of parameters. In a regression model, the regression coefficients are often put into one block and the variance parameters in another block. The advantage of this choice is seen in normal linear regression where the conditional posterior of the regression coefficients (given the residual variance) is a multivariate normal given by expression (4.30). Sampling the whole vector of regression coefficients from this conditional distribution is simple and sampling is not affected by the ridge in the posterior surface. In fact, with the use of a multivariate normal sampler, the vector of regression coefficients is sampled independently. From this example, it is clear that block sampling may accelerate the convergence of the Gibbs sampler considerably. However, a necessary condition for an accelerated convergence is that the blocks are well chosen; see Section 8.2.2 for an example where a bad choice of blocks decreased the convergence rate dramatically. In WinBUGS, the blocks are chosen by the program when the blocking option is switched on, while with the SAS procedure MCMC the blocks are specified by the user.

Overrelaxation: When the autocorrelations are high (and positive) the subsequent values in the Markov chain are highly predictable from the current position and the exploration of the posterior distribution is slow. *Overrelaxation* can break up this high positive dependence. This acceleration technique was introduced by Adler (1981) for Gaussian distributions. Let the full-conditional of θ be $N(\mu, \sigma^2)$ with current value θ^k, then Adler (1981) suggested to take the subsequent value as: $\theta^{k+1} = \mu + \alpha(\theta^k - \mu) + \sigma(1 - \alpha^2)^{1/2}\nu$, with $\nu \sim N(0, 1)$ and α a parameter between -1 and 1. For α negative, θ^{k+1} lies at the other side of μ. For $\alpha = 0$, the method is equivalent to Gibbs sampling. The ordered overrelaxation approach of Neal (1995) is based on a similar philosophy but can be applied to all conditional distributions and is implemented in WinBUGS. At step $(k + 1)$, M (around 20) values $\theta^{k+1,1}, \theta^{k+1,2}, \ldots, \theta^{k+1,M}$ are sampled and the current value θ^k is added to this set. The $(M + 1)$ values are then sorted and are given ranks $0, 1, 2, \ldots, M$. The next value in the chain, θ^{k+1}, is chosen from this set and is the value with rank $(M - m)$ when m is the rank of θ^k. Hence, the ordered overrelaxation approach takes in the above set the mirror image of θ^k, thereby reducing the correlation with the current value. Overrelaxation methods leave the conditional distribution invariant, which is an essential property otherwise one would be sampling from the wrong distribution. The effect of overrelaxation is seen in the autocorrelation plot which may exhibit a series of alternating negative and positive autocorrelations. However, note that overrelaxation methods imply M times more sampled values, retaining only one of them and therefore acts as a thinning approach but with the advantage that the positive autocorrelation is broken. Several extensions of the basic overrelaxation techniques have been proposed in the literature (Barone *et al.* 2002). Another approach that induces negative correlations is based on *antithetic sampling*, whereby two related values θ^{k+1} and $\theta^{*,k+1}$ (e.g. opposite to μ) are sampled together; see Ripley (1987) for a general treatment of this topic and Green and Han (1990) and Gustafson (1998b) for some recent developments.

Reparameterization: Centering the regressors in the linear regression model $y = \beta_0 + \beta_1\, x + \varepsilon$ implies a change of parameters from $\boldsymbol{\theta} = (\beta_0, \beta_1, \sigma)^T$ to $\boldsymbol{\theta}^* = (\beta_0^*, \beta_1, \sigma)^T$, with $\beta_0^* = \beta_0 + \beta_1\, \overline{x}$. We say that the model has been *reparameterized*. Reparameterizations may be helpful in removing constraints on parameters. For instance, the logarithmic transformation maps variance parameters onto the real axis. A logit-transformation does a similar job for parameters constrained on a finite interval. In the context of Gibbs sampling, such reparameterizations will have primarily an effect on the ease with which the full conditional is sampled since up to a transformation the full conditionals remain the same. For the MH procedure such a reparameterization may simplify sampling (e.g. allowing a Gaussian or t-like proposal distribution) and may avoid generating impossible parameter values. But to have an impact on the convergence rate, parameters must be transformed jointly. Example VII.5 shows that a simple joint reparameterization can have an important effect on the convergence of the MCMC procedure. Finally, proposals have been made for reparameterizations in normal-like or log-concave posterior distributions (Hills and Smith 1992), but they are difficult to apply in practice.

Miscellaneous acceleration approaches: Roberts and Sahu (1997) showed that for Gaussian target distributions, the rates of convergence may be different for the various types of a Gibbs sampler (systematic, reversible, and random scan). Thus, in order to accelerate convergence one could opt for a different sampling algorithm instead of trying to improve upon an existing approach. Unfortunately, Roberts and Sahu (1997) concluded for Gaussian models that the winning strategy depends on the true correlation structure of the Gaussian distribution. Wilks and Roberts (1996) described other variations of the Gibbs sampler such as the *hit-and-run algorithm* and generalizations, and methods which modify the stationary distribution such as generalizations of importance sampling and data augmentation. Most of these refinements imply quite some extra programming and are therefore beyond the aims of this book.

Finally, we have seen that the acceptance rate for MH algorithms is indicative for the speed of convergence. In WinBUGS, the Metropolis algorithm is imbedded in the Gibbs sampler and by default 4000 iterations are used to adjust the proposal density such that the acceptance rate varies between 20% and 40% (see also Section 8.1.2). The SAS procedure MCMC dynamically adjusts the proposal density to achieve an optimal acceptance rate.

Example VII.4: Osteoporosis study: Accelerating convergence

Consider again regressing TBBMC on BMI with a simple linear regression model. First, to illustrate the effect of bad starting values, we have taken the value of 100 as starting value for both regression coefficients. This has the effect that for about 200 iterations the trace plots of all parameters showed a monotonic behavior.

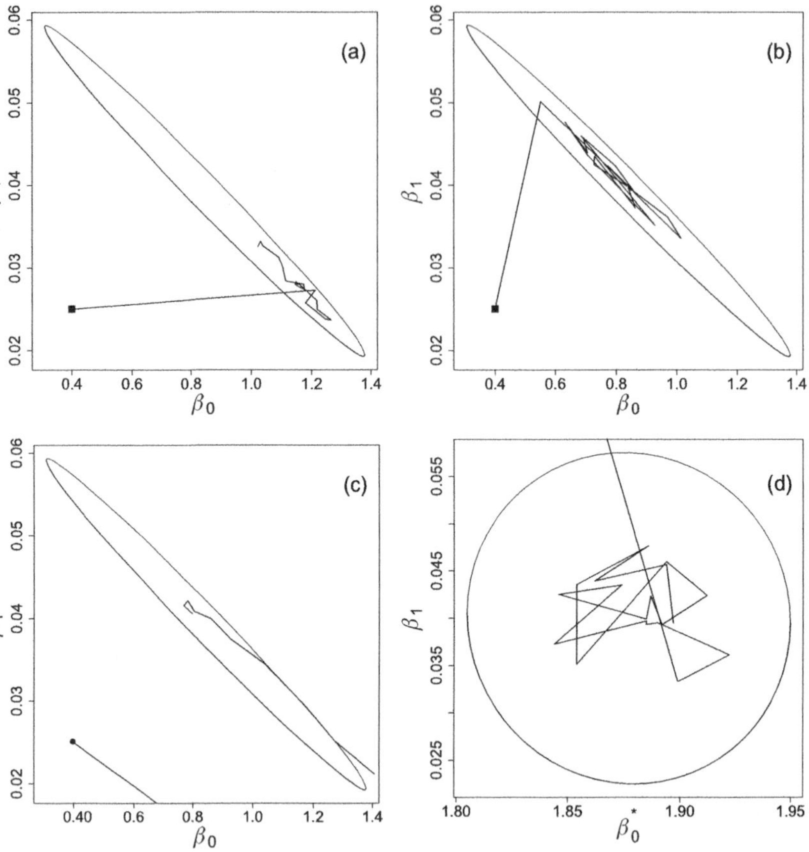

Figure 7.8 Osteoporosis study: 20 initial chain values (starting value indicated by square) obtained from WinBUGS for Bayesian linear regression based on (a) original Gibbs sampling, (b) block Gibbs sampling, (c) Gibbs sampling with overrelaxation, and (d) Gibbs sampling with centered BMI.

In Figure 7.8, we illustrate graphically the exploration of the posterior distributions for three acceleration techniques. Figure 7.8(a) shows the first 20 iterations obtained from WinBUGS without an acceleration technique. The posterior density has a ridge caused by a phenomenon called 'multicollinearity with the intercept'. The problem is that the regressor BMI is concentrated between 20 and 30 and thus relatively 'far away' from the origin. The ridge forces the Gibbs sampler to make small steps which creates high correlations between the subsequent steps. Switching on the blocking mode in WinBUGS produced independent sampling of the two regression parameters conditional on the sampled value for σ^2. That sampling is better with the blocking option is seen from the first 20 positions in Figure 7.8(b), which are more dispersed than in the original graph. The effect of overrelaxation is shown in Figure 7.8(c). The overrelaxation technique in WinBUGS is based on the approach of Neal (1995) with $M = 16$ for this sampler (see also Section 8.1.2). This speeds up the exploration of the posterior surface. However, the first ten iterations are outside the graph indicating that the chain might have some uncontrolled explorations. Finally, when the regressor is centered, the contour plot of the posterior surface turns into a circle and the regression coefficients were sampled independently (see Figure 7.8(d)). In Figure 7.9, the effect of the

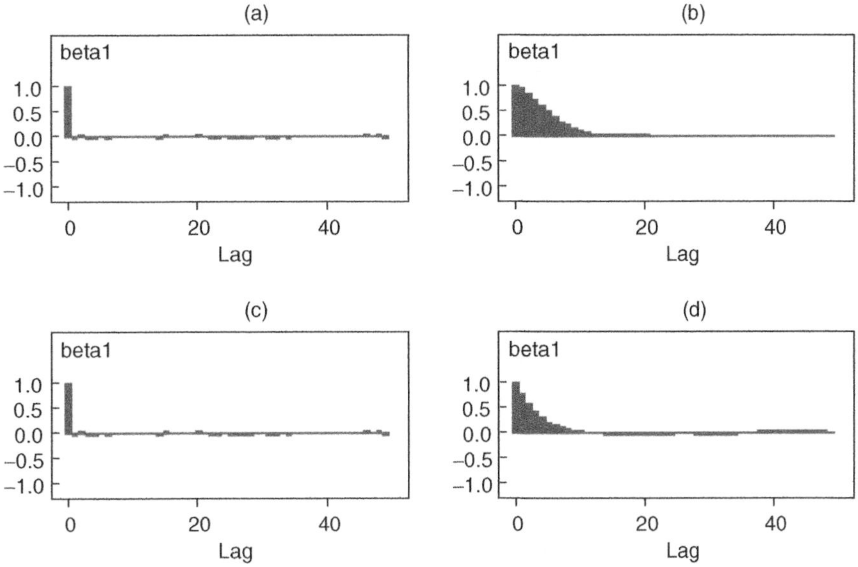

Figure 7.9 Osteoporosis study: autocorrelation plot based on (a) block Gibbs sampling, (b) Gibbs sampling with overrelaxation, (c) Gibbs sampling with centered BMI, and (d) using thinning with factor 10, obtained from WinBUGS.

different acceleration techniques on the autocorrelation function is shown. Clearly, block Gibbs sampling and centering BMI reduced the autocorrelation the most.

Further, we compared the effect of the acceleration techniques on MCSE. The conclusions from this exercise are the following. First, centering and blocking had the same effect on the MCSE of β_0 and β_1. Second, overrelaxation also reduced the MCSE but to a lesser extent without needing more time to converge than the original analysis. Finally when thinning was applied, the MCSE of the regression coefficients increased.

We conclude that simple tricks can speed up the convergence of the chain dramatically but not all tricks will have the same effect. □

The following example illustrates that a simple reparameterization of the model can imply a drastic change in the rate of convergence.

Example VII.5: Effect of reparameterization on convergence

Consider two exponential distributions: (a) $f_1(x) = \lambda e^{-\lambda x}$ and (b) $f_2(x) = \phi e^{-\phi x}$ and suppose that interest lies in the parameter $\psi = \lambda/\phi$.

We sampled twenty observations from each of these distributions with $\lambda = 3$ and $\phi = 1$, respectively. Two models were fitted to the data. The first is based on the parameters λ and ϕ. For the second model $f_2(x)$ is replaced by $f_2^*(x) = (\lambda/\psi)\, e^{-(\lambda/\psi)x}$ and the parameters of interest are now λ and ψ. Thus, the two models differ only in their parameterization. We used WinBUGS for estimating the parameters. For each model 11 000 iterations were run with 1000 burn-in iterations. Sampling the first model yielded MCSE = 0.01484 for ψ. For the second model, the posterior summary measures were based only on the 7000 final iterations. The reason is that WinBUGS uses a Metropolis step within Gibbs and the default number of iterations to calibrate, the acceptance rate is 4000. Now, we obtained MCSE = 0.07901 for

ψ which is about five times more than for the first model. When the first model was run for 7000 iterations, we obtained MCSE = 0.01649. This exercise illustrates the importance of a good parameterization and its impact on the convergence rate of the Markov chain. □

7.4 Practical guidelines for assessing and accelerating convergence

In practice, assessing convergence could be quite laborious. This makes it impractical to check convergence each time a new model is fitted since for a statistical modeler switching from one model to another model should go rather smoothly. So we question in this section which practical procedure can guarantee a reasonable probability that divergence of the Markov chain does not go undetected. It is illustrative to see in this sense how experienced Bayesians look upon assessing convergence in practice. Kass *et al.* (1998) reported on a panel discussion held in 1996 on checking convergence. At first it is surprising to read that some of the discussants admitted to monitor the Markov chain by merely inspecting the trace plots and autocorrelations or made use of only a very limited number of convergence diagnostics. For instance, Geyer (1992) mentioned that 'routinely throwing away the initial 1% or 2% of runs will usually suffice'. Others reported to use only the thick pen test.

When numerous statistical models are tried out, inevitably corners must be cut. Therefore, we propose below some guidelines which aim to assess and improve convergence of the Markov chain in a reasonable amount of time. Some of the guidelines have WinBUGS/OpenBUGS in mind, since with the Bayesian SAS procedures the convergence checks come basically for free. We propose the following:

- It is best to start with a pilot run to detect quickly some trivial problems, such as starting values that were taken too remote. For relatively simple problems a single-chain analysis may be sufficient, but experience shows that taking multiple (3–5) chains often highlights the problems faster. When in the second step a longer chain is initiated, the trace and other graphical plots (such as the BGR plot) should be used as guidance.
- One may check convergence of each parameter separately or jointly. A joint evaluation of all parameters may be done by monitoring the log(likelihood) (in WinBUGS by the deviance) or the log(posterior) (in SAS by LogPost).
- Start with a more formal assessment of convergence only when the trace plots show good mixing, say when they passed the thick pen test. For a single chain use Geweke and HW diagnostics while for multiple chains it is recommended to use in addition the BGR diagnostics.
- When convergence is slow, check whether one of the above acceleration tricks may help. Standardization is one of the tricks one should always have in mind.
- When convergence cannot be achieved despite all tricks, you may need to let the sampler run longer and apply thinning to reduce the amount of information stored. Or … you may need to change the software or … write your own sampler.
- Extensive convergence checking is often impractical in a model building exercise. In that case, it is often enough to use the thick pen test before the final model is chosen.

- Establish the MCerror that you wish to attain for the parameters of interest and let the chain run as long as needed to achieve the accuracy. As a rule of thumb, the Markov chain is run until the MCerror is at most 5% of the posterior standard deviation.
- When many parameters are involved such as in hierarchical models, it is challenging to monitor all of them for convergence. In the *WinBUGS Manual*, it is advised to choose a random selection of relevant parameters to monitor. For example, rather than checking convergence for every element of a vector of random effects, one could take a random subset.

Depending on the chosen model it might be sufficient to focus on the convergence of only the parameters of interest. For instance, if in the regression analysis of the osteoporosis data the parameter of interest is the residual variance, then a single chain of maximally 1000 iterations would have been sufficient. The reason is that fast convergence for the variance parameter irrespective of the poor convergence of the regression coefficients. Whether this will happen in other models depends on how orthogonal the parameters of interest are to the nuisance parameters. Further, in Section 9.7, we explore the technique of parameter expansion to improve the convergence of the Markov chains of interest. To this end extra parameters are created which are, however, nonestimatble. The chains of the fabricated parameters will never converge but this not a problem, on the contrary, since the parameters of interest will converge more rapidly.

7.5 Data augmentation

Data augmentation (DA) is a term that is reserved for estimation techniques (frequentist or Bayesian) which augment the observed data with fictive data. The fictive data are often referred to as missing data, although they do not need to be missing in a strict sense. A DA technique is an iterative procedure that consists of two parts which are repeated until convergence. In the first part, one assumes that the missing data z are available, and thus that one can rely on all data (complete data) $\boldsymbol{w} = \{\boldsymbol{y}, z\}$ with $\boldsymbol{y}$ representing the actually observed data. In the second part, one takes into account that part of the (complete) vector $\boldsymbol{w}$ is not available. The motivation for using a DA technique is that it may simplify the estimation procedure considerably.

The Expectation–Maximization (EM)-algorithm Dempster *et al.* (1977) is the default likelihood-based DA procedure. In the case of truly missing data, the iterative procedure determines plausible values for the data that are missing (E-step), imputes these plausible values into the likelihood and maximizes the *completed likelihood*, i.e. the likelihood of all data (observed and fictive) as if they were observed (M-step). The plausible values of the missing data are obtained by taking the expectation of the missing data given the observed data and the current values of the parameters.

In a seminal paper, Tanner and Wong (1987) suggested a DA approach in the Bayesian context to compute the posterior distribution in an iterative manner. In fact, the term 'data augmentation' was introduced by them. The argument for using a Bayesian DA approach is similar to using an EM algorithm in the likelihood case, namely sampling from $p(\boldsymbol{\theta} \mid \boldsymbol{y}, z)$ may often be easier than from $p(\boldsymbol{\theta} \mid \boldsymbol{y})$. The E-step is replaced here by sampling the missing data z from the conditional distribution $p(z \mid \boldsymbol{\theta}, \boldsymbol{y})$, and the M-step by sampling $\boldsymbol{\theta}$ from the completed posterior $p(\boldsymbol{\theta} \mid \boldsymbol{y}, z)$. Thus the DA approach of Tanner and Wong (1987) consists of repeatedly sampling from $p(\boldsymbol{\theta} \mid \boldsymbol{y}, z)$ and from $p(z \mid \boldsymbol{\theta}, \boldsymbol{y})$. This is in fact the block Gibbs sampler, whereby the missing data are viewed as extra parameters also called *auxiliary variables*. In the original approach of Tanner and Wong (1987) more than one value for z were generated, which combined with one value for $\boldsymbol{\theta}$ generates a smooth estimate of the posterior at convergence.

In a variety of applications the data augmentation approach may be useful. Besides the obvious case of genuine missing data, the DA approach is recommended, e.g. when the observations are censored or misclassified, and in mixture models. In the hierarchical models of Chapter 9, the DA approach enters in a quite natural way via the latent (unobserved) random effects. While in a frequentist context, the random effects are integrated out to maximize the marginal likelihood, in a Bayesian context the random effects are sampled from their full conditionals which take the form of $p(\mathbf{z} \mid \boldsymbol{\theta}, \mathbf{y})$. Below, we treat three examples where the DA approach implies a simplified Gibbs sampling procedure. The first example is the famous genetic linkage example introduced by Rao (1973) and used by many afterward (see Tanner 1993, p. 368). There are no missing data in this example, but assuming that more data were available simplifies the Gibbs sampler.

Example VII.6: Genetic linkage model: Estimating the recombination fraction using the DA approach

If two factors are linked with a recombination fraction π, the intercrosses $Ab/aB \times Ab/aB$ (repulsion) result in the following probabilities: (a) for AB: $0.5 + \theta/4$, (b) for Ab: $(1 - \theta)/4$, (c) for aB: $(1 - \theta)/4$, and (d) for ab: $\theta/4$ with $\theta = \pi^2$. Suppose that in a study one has collected n subjects, which can be classified according to the above four classes and that one has observed the frequencies $\mathbf{y} = \{y_1, y_2, y_3, y_4\}$, with $\sum_k y_k = n$. The frequencies follows a multinomial distribution Mult(n, $(0.5 + \theta/4, (1 - \theta)/4, (1 - \theta)/4, \theta/4)$). Based on 197 animals with $\mathbf{y} = (125, 18, 20, 34)^T$, Tanner (1993) estimated θ. With a flat prior for θ, $p(\theta \mid \mathbf{y})$ is proportional to $(2 + \theta)^{y_1}(1 - \theta)^{y_2+y_3}\theta^{y_4}$. Although $p(\theta \mid \mathbf{y})$ is a unimodal function of θ, it has a nonstandard expression and needs a dedicated sampler to obtain the posterior distribution.

Imagine that more information was available, namely that the first cell was split up into two cells with probabilities $1/2$ and $\theta/4$ and that we observed the corresponding frequencies $(y_1 - z)$ and z. The (completed) vector of frequencies then becomes $\mathbf{w} = (y_1 - z, z, y_2, y_3, y_4) = (125 - z, z, 18, 20, 34)^T$. Assuming that z is known, the posterior $p(\theta \mid \mathbf{w})$ is proportional to $\theta^{z+y_4}(1 - \theta)^{y_2+y_3}$ which is simply a binomial distribution. On the other hand, given θ and the observed data the posterior of z is $p(z \mid \theta, \mathbf{y}) = \text{Bin}(y_1, \theta/(2 + \theta))$. These two posteriors are the full conditionals of the posterior obtained from combining the multinomial likelihood Mult(n, $(0.5, \theta/4, (1 - \theta)/4, (1 - \theta)/4, \theta/4)$) based on frequencies $(125 - z, z, 18, 20$ and $34)$ with a flat prior for θ and a discrete uniform prior for z on the set $\{0, 1, \ldots, 125\}$.

The Gibbs sampler follows from the above-derived full conditionals. Using starting values $\theta_0 = 0.5$ and $z_0 = 50$ convergence was quickly obtained. After 100 iterations and leaving out the first 10 initial iterations the posterior mean for θ and z were 0.6250 (posterior mode obtained by Tanner (1993) is 0.6268) and 28.63, respectively. In Figure 7.10, the trace plots of θ and z are shown, together with their marginal posterior densities. □

Example VII.7: Cysticercosis study: Estimating the prevalence in the absence of a gold standard

In Example V.6, we showed that prior information is necessary to estimate the prevalence of cysticercosis and the sensitivity and specificity of the Ag-ELISA diagnostic test. The analysis

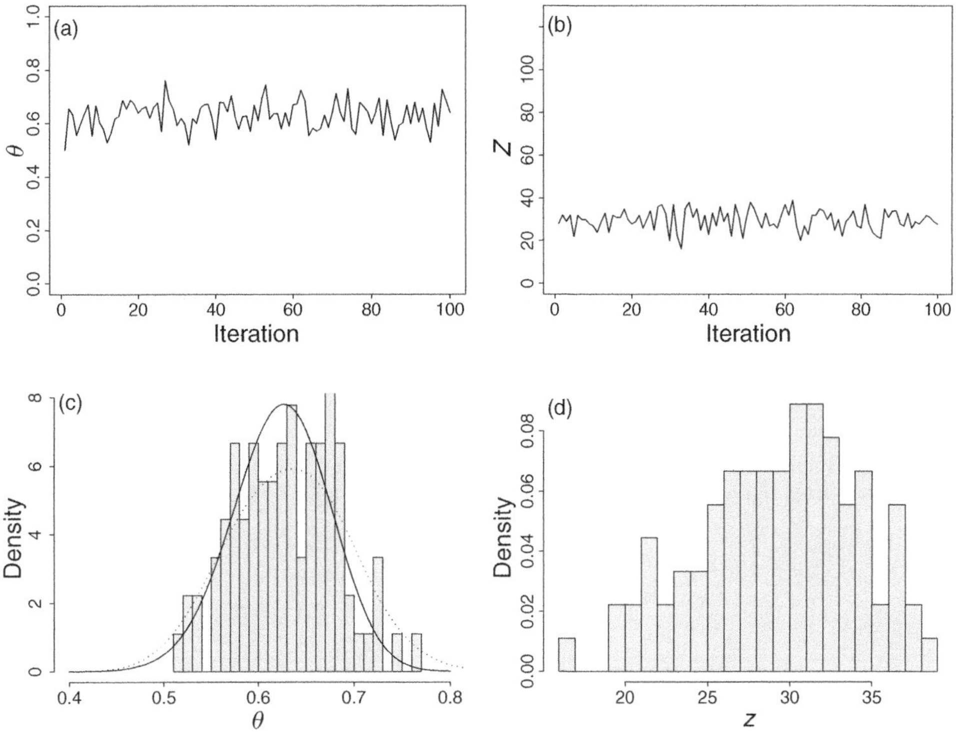

Figure 7.10 Genetic linkage model: (a) trace plot of θ, (b) trace plot of z, (c) histogram of θ (overlayed with numerically computed posterior (solid line) and smoothed version of histogram (dotted line)), and (d) histogram of z.

was done with WinBUGS 1.4.3. Here, we show how data augmentation can simplify the MCMC procedure.

Recall that in total 868 pigs were tested in Zambia with the Ag-ELISA diagnostic test and that 496 pigs showed a positive test. Let the prevalence of cysticercosis in Zambia among pigs be π and the sensitivity and specificity of the Ag-ELISA diagnostic test be α and β, respectively. In Table 7.1, we reproduced Table 5.3, but (a) added two columns indicating the missing information, and (b) changed the notation somewhat.

The following beta priors were taken on the parameters: Beta(ν_π, η_π) for π, Beta$(\nu_\alpha, \eta_\alpha)$ for α and Beta(ν_β, η_β) for β. The posterior is the product of the multinomial likelihood with probabilities given in Table 7.1 with the beta priors. On the other hand, the posterior based on the completed data is proportional to

$$\pi^{z_1+z_2+\nu_\pi-1}(1-\pi)^{n-z_1-z_2+\eta_\pi-1}\,\alpha^{z_1+\nu_\alpha-1}(1-\alpha)^{z_2+\eta_\alpha-1}\,\beta^{(n-y)-z_2+\nu_\beta-1}(1-\beta)^{y-z_1+\eta_\beta-1},$$

which results in a marginal posterior for the prevalence equal to Beta$(z_1 + z_2 + \nu_\pi, n - z_1 - z_2 + \eta_\pi)$.

Table 7.1 Cysticercosis study: theoretical characteristics and observed results of the Ag-ELISA diagnostic test on pigs collected in Zambia.

		Disease (true)		Observed		
		+	−	+	−	Total
Test	+	$\pi\alpha$	$(1-\pi)(1-\beta)$	z_1	$y-z_1$	$y = 496$
	−	$\pi(1-\alpha)$	$(1-\pi)\beta$	z_2	$(n-y)-z_2$	$n-y=372$
Total		π	$(1-\pi)$			$n = 868$

Note: π is the true prevalence of cysticercosis. α and β are the sensitivity and specificity of the Ag-ELISA diagnostic test, respectively. y $(n-y)$ is the observed number of subjects with a positive (negative) Ag-ELISA test. z_1 and z_2 are the missing frequencies.

The full conditionals based only on the observed data are complex, while the full conditionals based on the completed data are of a standard type, i.e.

$$
\begin{aligned}
z_1 \mid y, \pi, \alpha, \beta &\sim \text{Bin}\left(y, \frac{\pi\,\alpha}{\pi\,\alpha + (1-\pi)(1-\beta)}\right),\\
z_2 \mid y, \pi, \alpha, \beta &\sim \text{Bin}\left(n-y, \frac{\pi\,(1-\alpha)}{\pi\,(1-\alpha) + (1-\pi)\beta}\right),\\
\alpha \mid y, z_1, z_2, \pi, \nu_\alpha, \eta_\alpha &\sim \text{Beta}(z_1 + \nu_\alpha, z_2 + \eta_\alpha),\\
\beta \mid y, z_1, z_2, \pi, \nu_\beta, \eta_\beta &\sim \text{Beta}((n-y) - z_2 + \nu_\beta, y - z_1 + \eta_\beta),\\
\pi \mid y, z_1, z_2, \pi, \nu_\pi, \eta_\pi &\sim \text{Beta}(z_1 + z_2 + \nu_\pi, n - z_1 - z_2 + \eta_\pi).
\end{aligned}
$$

We have taken a Beta(1, 1) prior for π, a Beta(21, 12) prior for α and a Beta(32, 4) prior for β. 100 000 iterations (burn-in = 10 000) were necessary to achieve convergence with a self-written R-program. The posterior mean for the prevalence was 0.84 with 95% equal tail CI of [0.65, 0.99]. For the sensitivity we obtained 0.66 ([0.57, 0.80]) and for the specificity 0.88 ([0.76, 0.97]). These are basically the same results as obtained from WinBUGS. However, the WinBUGS program in Chapter 5 does not make use of the DA technique. As a result, the samplers were not conjugate. How to detect this, will be seen in Section 8.1.2. One may force WinBUGS to make use of DA. The file 'chapter 7 prevalence Ag Elisa test Cysticercosis.odc' contains two programs: one program using the DA mechanism and one without (used in Chapter 5). When the DA approach is used all samplers become conjugate.

Note that in this problem another identifiability problem pops up. Namely when π, α, and β are replaced by $1-\pi$, $1-\alpha$, and $1-\beta$ it results in the same model but with modified definitions of 'diseased' and 'positive test'. To avoid this problem one needs to restrict π, α, and β to one half of the unit interval. □

Example VII.8: Caries study: Analysis of interval-censored data

The children of the Signal-Tandmobiel® study were annually examined for their oral health status. There was interest to document the distribution of the emergences of permanent teeth of children from Flanders. Here we look at tooth 22 (incisor) located in the upper left part of the mouth and we have selected a random sample of 500 children to limit computation time. However, the true distribution of the emergence times could not be read off from the observed data since emergence was never recorded exactly. For some children the teeth had already emerged before their first annual examination (left-censored), for others the teeth had not emerged at their last examination (right-censored) but most often emergence was recorded in-between two examinations (interval-censored). Consequently, for the ith child it was only observed that tooth 22 emerges between L_i (annual examination) and R_i (next annual examination). Hence the true emergence time of tooth 22, y_i, must lie in the interval (L_i, R_i) whereby L_i is equal to $-\infty$ for left censoring an R_i equal to ∞ for right censoring.

The data augmentation approach is now based on the completed data y_i, $(i = 1, \ldots, n)$. Explorative procedures indicated that a normal distribution for the latent true emergence time is a reasonable choice. Therefore we assumed that for the ith child $y_i \sim N(\mu, \sigma^2)$. The Gibbs sampler is based on two types of full conditionals. The first type consists of the conditional distributions of the model parameters assuming that the true emergence times y_i are known. The second type consists of the conditional distributions of y_i given (L_i, R_i) and the model parameters, which are in fact truncated normal distributions.

An R program based on the DA principle was written. Note that WinBUGS can also easily handle this type of data. The censored character (left-, right- or interval) of the emergence time is specified in WinBUGS by the indicator function I with boundary values given in the data part of the program.

Initial explorations indicated that mixing was fast. So we decided on a single-chain analysis with 10 000 iterations and a burn-in part of 2000 iterations. Convergence was checked with the classical convergence diagnostics. Based on the converged part of the chain the posterior mean (SD) of μ and σ are 8.03 (0.044) and 0.90 (0.037), respectively. Since the latent data y_i are generated as a by-product of the DA algorithm we obtained predicted emergence times (and 95% prediction intervals) from the converged part of the chain. In Figure 7.11, we show these predictions for the first 50 children in the study together with the intervals (L_i, R_i). □

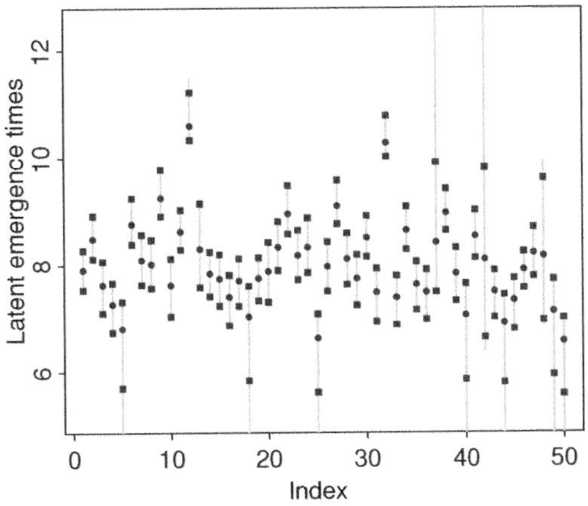

Figure 7.11 Caries study: interval-censored emergence times of tooth 22 of first 50 children. The grey bars represent the intervals (L_i, R_i). The symbol • represents the average predicted emergence time based on the converged part of the chain, the symbols ■ represent the 2.5% and 97.5% predicted quantiles of the true emergence time, respectively.

In the final example, we return to the question of when to choose the Gibbs sampler or the MH-algorithm. Although this question is largely academic when Bayesian software like WinBUGS or SAS is used since they employ their own built-in sampler, it becomes important when the user wishes to write his own sampler. The next example shows that sometimes the choice comes natural. The example is again an illustration of the DA approach.

Example VII.9: MCMC approaches for a probit regression problem
In Example VI.9, several MCMC approaches were applied to estimate the parameters of a logistic regression model. Now we focus on a probit regression model and show that the Gibbs sampler is the natural choice here. For a probit regression model, the probability of success for the ith subject is $P(y_i = 1 \mid \boldsymbol{x}_i) = \Phi(\boldsymbol{x}_i^T \boldsymbol{\beta})$, with y_i the binary response, $\boldsymbol{x}_i$ a vector of covariates and Φ the standard normal cdf.

Albert and Chib (1993) proposed the DA approach to sample from a probit regression model using the relationship between a normally distributed latent random variable and the binary response. Suppose n independent continuous random variables $z_i = \boldsymbol{x}_i^T \boldsymbol{\beta} + \varepsilon_i$, $(i = 1, \ldots, n)$, with $\varepsilon_i \sim \mathrm{N}(0, 1)$. Further suppose that $y_i = 0\,(1)$ for $z_i \leq\ (>)\, 0$. Then $P(y_i = 1 \mid \boldsymbol{x}_i) = P(z_i > 0) = 1 - \Phi(-\boldsymbol{x}_i^T \boldsymbol{\beta}) = \Phi(\boldsymbol{x}_i^T \boldsymbol{\beta})$.

The existence of a latent variable suggests the use of the Gibbs sampler in combination with the DA approach to explore the posterior distribution. In particular, Albert and Chib (1993) suggested to sample alternately (1) $\boldsymbol{\beta}$ given z with (2) z given $\boldsymbol{\beta}$. In detail their Gibbs sampler works as follows:

$\boldsymbol{\beta}$ given z: Conditional on $z = \{z_1, z_2, \ldots, z_n\}$, $\boldsymbol{\beta}$ has a Gaussian distribution, i.e. $\boldsymbol{\beta} \sim \mathrm{N}(\boldsymbol{\beta}_{\mathrm{LS}}, (\boldsymbol{X}^T\boldsymbol{X})^{-1})$. This is a Bayesian regression analysis with $\sigma^2 = 1$ and $\boldsymbol{\beta}_{\mathrm{LS}} = (\boldsymbol{X}^T\boldsymbol{X})^{-1}\boldsymbol{X}^T\boldsymbol{Z}$ where $\boldsymbol{X}$ and $\boldsymbol{Z}$ are the design matrices of the covariates and the latent variables, respectively. This step involves sampling from a multivariate Gaussian distribution.

z given $\boldsymbol{\beta}$: The full conditional of z_i on $\boldsymbol{\beta}$ and y_i is proportional to (1) $\phi_{\boldsymbol{x}_i^T\boldsymbol{\beta},1}(z)I(z \leq 0)$ for $y_i = 0$ and to (2) $\phi_{\boldsymbol{x}_i^T\boldsymbol{\beta},1}(z)I(z > 0)$ for $y_i = 1$, with ϕ_{μ,σ^2} the Gaussian density with mean μ and variance σ^2 and $I(a) = 1$ if the condition a is satisfied. In this step sampling is done from truncated normals.

The above procedure shows that a small change of the model, here replacing the probit link with the logit link, can affect the choice of the preferred sampler. Indeed for the logit link the step '$\boldsymbol{\beta}$ given z' would be more complicated. □

7.6 Closing remarks

The Markov chain Monte Carlo methods are nowadays the most popular Bayesian tool to obtain posterior inference especially with complex statistical problems. However, it is recognized that MCMC methods often imply a long processing time. This asks for faster samplers or other faster approaches since a statistical modeler must be able to switch swiftly between models. Rue *et al.* (2009) suggested the use of an integrated nested Laplace approximation to directly compute accurate approximations to the posterior marginal distributions and implemented the procedure in the software INLA (see Chapter 8). The approach appears to be faster for those problems it can tackle. However, the advantage of sampling based approaches is that they may be applied to virtually each problem. Therefore, likely the MCMC procedures will remain in the Bayesian toolbox for many years to come.

Exercises

Exercise 7.1 Take extreme starting values for the parameters of the Bayesian regression analyses of Exercise 6.1, e.g. 'beta0=100,beta1=100,tau=1/0.05' and observe the initial monotone behavior of the trace plots.

Exercise 7.2 Export the Markov chains obtained in Exercise 7.1 to CODA or BOA and explore the stationarity of the chains. Let the Gibbs sampler run long enough such that, upon convergence, the MC standard error is at most 5% of the posterior standard deviation of the regression parameters.

Exercise 7.3 Import the data of the Mice Example of the *WinBUGS* document *Examples Vol I* into R. Write an R program that implements the Gibbs sampler for the model specified in the Mice Example. Then replace the Weibull distribution with a lognormal distribution. Compare the autocorrelation functions. Alternatively, use the original WinBUGS program.

Exercise 7.4 Import the data of 'osteoporosismultiple.txt' into R and perform a Bayesian probit regression analysis using the DA approach of Example VII.9 predicting *overweight* (BMI $>$ 25) from age and length. Give normal diffuse priors to the regression parameters. Assess the convergence of the Markov chains with CODA or BOA and improve their convergence rate if necessary.

Exercise 7.5 Apply thinning (=10) to the sampling algorithms of Exercise 6.1 and assess their convergence properties. Assess also their performance when centering BMI.

Exercise 7.6 Assess the convergence properties of the block Gibbs sampler of Exercise 6.6.

Exercise 7.7 Repeat the analysis of Example VII.6 for the intercrosses $AB/ab \times AB/ab$ (coupling). In this case (see Rao (1973)), the probabilities are (a) for *AB*: $(3 - 2\pi + \pi^2)/4$, (b) for *Ab*: $(2\pi - \pi^2)/4$, (c) for *aB*: $(2\pi - \pi^2)/4$ and (d) for *ab*: $(1 - 2\pi + \pi^2)/4$, where π is the recombination fraction. Derive the posterior distributions making use of the DA principle.

Exercise 7.8 Joseph *et al.* (1995) wished to estimate the prevalence of Strongyloides infection using data from a survey of all Cambodian refugees who arrived in Montreal during an 8-month period. The authors considered two diagnostic tests. For the serology diagnostic test, 125 subjects showed a positive test outcome while 37 subjects had a negative outcome. Information extracted from the literature and expert knowledge gave the 95% equal tail prior CI for the sensitivity and specificity equal to [0.65, 0.95], [0.35, 1.00], respectively. Derive the prior distributions and repeat the analysis of Example VII.7 making use of the DA approach.

Exercise 7.9 Apply the Gibbs sampler of Example VII.9 on the caries data set (caries.txt) analyzed in Example VI.9 and compare your results with the MCMC analyses of Example VI.9. You can also compare your results with those obtained from the WinBUGS program 'chapter 7 caries.odc'.

8

Software

Twenty years ago Bayesian software was basically nonexistent, but with the introduction of **B**ayesian inference **U**sing **G**ibbs **S**ampling (BUGS) and, in particular, with WinBUGS that situation changed drastically. WinBUGS together with the introduction of the MCMC techniques implied no less than a revolution in the use of Bayesian methods and is, in fact (together with its related software) still the standard Bayesian software. Apart from the WinBUGS developments, the last decade has seen a proliferation of dedicated Bayesian software written mostly in R. Even the big player on the statistical software market, SAS®, has decided to start developments in Bayesian software. Hence, the Bayesian toolbox for the practitioner is rapidly expanding. The state of art, as described in this chapter, will therefore quickly become history.

In this chapter, practical aspects of Bayesian software are discussed. We introduce WinBUGS, OpenBUGS and related software. In addition, we provide examples on the use of the recently developed Bayesian SAS procedures, and finally we briefly discuss Bayesian programs developed in the R language.

The aim of this chapter is to get the reader acquainted with the basics of Bayesian software. To this end, we will primarily use the osteoporosis regression problem as a guiding example. In the remainder of the book, additional aspects of the software will be commented upon. An additional and important source of information are the manuals of the packages. The WinBUGS manual together with Examples manuals I and II and the SAS manual SAS-STAT are both excellent sources for further details. For WinBUGS we can also recommend the books Lawson *et al.* (2003) and Ntzoufras (2009).

8.1 WinBUGS and related software

WinBUGS is the Windows version of the program BUGS. WinBUGS carries out Bayesian inference on statistical problems using MCMC methods. Its development started in 1989 in the MRC Biostatistics Unit at Cambridge with BUGS (Gilks *et al.* 1994). At the time of writing this book, there were over 30 000 registered users making WinBUGS definitely the

Bayesian Biostatistics, First Edition. Emmanuel Lesaffre and Andrew B. Lawson.

```
model
{for (i in 1:N){
     tbbmc[i] ~ dnorm(mu[i],tau)
     mu[i] <- beta0+beta1*bmi[i]}
     sigma2 <- 1/tau
     sigma <- sqrt(sigma2)
     beta0 ~ dnorm(0,1.0E-6)
     beta1 ~ dnorm(0,1.0E-6)
     tau ~ dgamma(1.0E-3,1.0E-3)}
list(tbbmc=c(1.798, 2.588, 2.325, 2.236, 1.925, 2.304, 2.183, 2.010,
 ......
1.728, 2.183, 1.703, 1.505, 1.850),
bmi=c(23.61, 30.48, 27.18, 34.68, 26.72, 25.78, 29.24, 30.76, 21.64,
 .....
37.46, 21.79, 18.99, 28.30), N=234)
list(beta0=0.4,beta1=0.025,tau=1/0.05)
```

Figure 8.1 Osteoporosis study: WinBUGS program.

most popular (but also most versatile) package for performing complex Bayesian analyses. In Lunn *et al.* (2009a), the developers of the package give an overview of the history of the program, its basic philosophy, its future, and also its limitations and dangers. The final version of WinBUGS is version 1.4.3 but its development has stopped. Its successor OpenBUGS is the open source variant of WinBUGS. But, since WinBUGS 1.4.3 is still the most popular program for Bayesian analyses, it is the preferred software in this book. Both software packages are freely available.

The applications are described in a stepwise manner. We start with the basic WinBUGS operations.

8.1.1 A first analysis

WinBUGS works with **.odc** files. These are basically text files containing the program, the data and the initial values for a MCMC run. But an .odc file can also be a compound document that contains various types of information (text, tables, formulae, plots, graphs, etc.). To access such a file, start WinBUGS, click on **File** and then on **Open...**. WinBUGS commands are written in a language that is similar but not identical to R. In Figure 8.1, (part of) the WinBUGS commands to perform a Bayesian regression analysis on the osteoporosis data are given. The WinBUGS program can be found in 'chapter 8 osteoporosis.odc'. First, we discuss the three basic components of a WinBUGS program.

Model: Within the 'for' loop the likelihood of the normal linear regression model, regressing TBBMC on BMI, is expressed. The loop runs from 1 to N, the total number of observations in the study (the value of N is part of the data). The command `tbbmc[i] ~ dnorm(mu[i],tau)` means that TBBMC of the ith subject has a normal distribution with mean `mu[i]` and precision `tau`. Note that WinBUGS expresses variability in terms of the precision (= 1/variance). Further `mu[i] <- beta0+beta1*bmi[i]` specifies that the mean is a linear function of BMI. These two commands determine the normal linear regression likelihood. The BUGS language is *declarative* which means that the order of the statements does not matter. This is an important difference with most programming languages where a variable must first be defined before it can be used in a formula. Note that WinBUGS will provide posterior information of a parameter only when it is declared in the program. For instance, if we wish to obtain posterior summary measures of the residual variance then we need to add `sigma2 <- 1/tau` to create this new parameter. If we also specify `sigma <- sqrt(sigma2)` then we can monitor both the residual variance, and standard deviation, i.e. MCMC output is also generated for these two extra defined parameters, if requested. Unfortunately, WinBUGS does not have 'if-then-else' commands. Instead, WinBUGS provides the functions 'step' whereby `step(x) = 1` if `x` $\geq$ `0` and 0 otherwise, and 'equals' whereby `equals(x1,x2) = 1` if `x1 = x2` and `0` otherwise. These two functions can be used to simulate an if-then-else condition.

The next three lines determine the prior distributions of the regression parameters. With `beta0 ~ dnorm(0,1.0E-6)` we choose a diffuse prior for the intercept, i.e. a Gaussian distribution with mean 0 and variance 10^6. The same is done for the slope. WinBUGS does not allow improper priors for most of its analyses. The only exception is in spatial modeling with the function 'dflat', which represents a uniform distribution. The prior for the precision is specified with `tau ~ dgamma(1.0E-3,1.0E-3)`, which is equivalent to assuming that the prior for σ^2 is IG(10^{-3}, 10^{-3}).

Data: After the model specification, the data are provided in a list statement. Note, we have replaced part of the data by dots to gain space. Different formats (rectangular, list, etc.) for providing data are possible in WinBUGS.

Initial values: With `list(beta0=0.4,beta1=0.025,tau=1/0.05)` the initial values for the intercept, slope and residual precision are specified.

To obtain posterior samples, one requires three WinBUGS tools: (a) the **Specification Tool**, (b) the **Sample Monitor Tool**, and (c) the **Update Tool**. The following actions need to be taken to receive the desired posterior information:

Specification Tool: Click on the **Model** option of the menu bar and choose **Specification...**. The box **Specification Tool** appears. Place the cursor anywhere in the program and then click on **check model**. When there are no syntax errors, WinBUGS sends the message 'model is syntactically correct' in the left bottom corner of the screen (where all messages from WinBUGS appear) otherwise an error message appears. A list of error messages can be found in the WinBUGS manual in the section *Tips and Troubleshooting*. To load the data, highlight the 'list' command of the data part and click on **load data**. WinBUGS sends the message 'data loaded' (or an error message) and the two buttons **check model** and **load data** are deactivated. Then click on **compile**. When the message data 'model compiled' appears, initial values can be imported by clicking on **load inits**. Note that only initial values can be given to stochastic nodes (see below for definition of stochastic node). For instance, in the regression program, one cannot give a starting value for `sigma2`, but one can give a starting value for `tau`. We can start sampling upon the message 'model is initialized'. When initial values have been given for all stochastic nodes, as here, then the buttons **load inits** and **gen inits** are switched off. Otherwise, both buttons remain switched on and by clicking on **gen inits** WinBUGS generates initial values for the remaining parameters. This is an interesting tool especially for hierarchical models where it can be quite laborious to provide starting values for all random effects. But, it is not advisable to use this option for a variance/precision parameter. For instance, when no initial value for *tau* was provided, an error message appeared when we attempted to generate the starting value. Note, it may take a prohibitively long time to ask WinBUGS to generate a large number of starting values. If all is fine, WinBUGS is

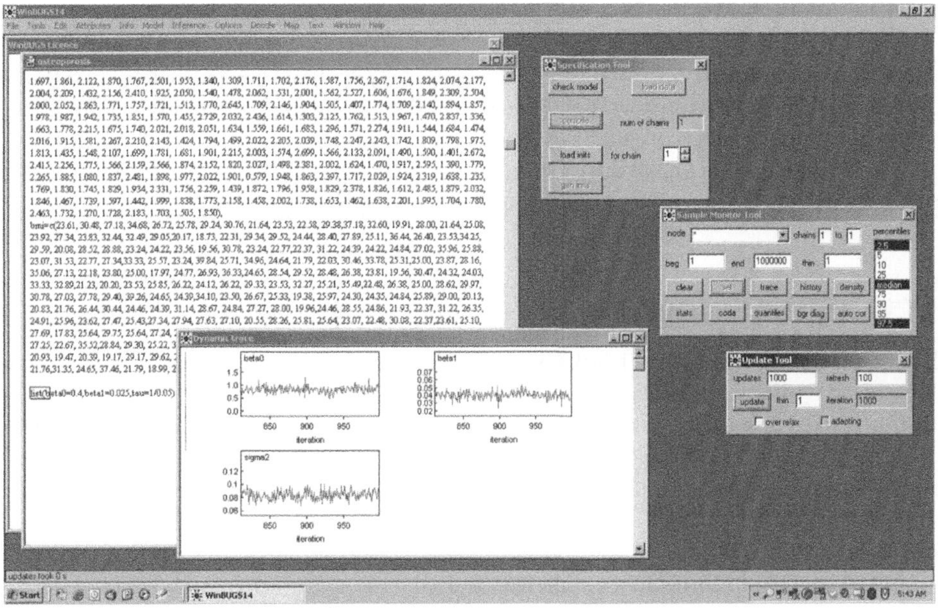

Figure 8.2 Osteoporosis study: WinBUGS screen dump after 1000 iterations.

ready to start sampling but it is not guaranteed at this stage that the MCMC sampler will work properly. Indeed, run-time errors may still occur.

Sample Monitor Tool: To prepare the sampling part of the analysis, we click on the **Inference** option of the menu bar and choose **Samples...**, which triggers the box **Sample Monitor Tool** to appear. Type next to **node** only those parameters of interest, e.g. here 'beta0' and then click on **set**. The same was done for 'beta1' and for 'sigma2'. The term 'node' is used because of the intimate connection of WinBUGS with *Directed Acyclic Graphs* (DAGs) (see Section 8.1.6). Finally, by typing in '*' and clicking on **set**, WinBUGS will monitor these three parameters while sampling. By clicking on **trace** a *dynamic trace plot* (empty at this stage) for each parameter appears on the screen.

Update Tool: To choose the number of MCMC iterations, click on option **Model** of the menu bar and choose **Update...**. The box **Update Tool** appears. Specify the number of iterations. To effectively start the sampling, click on **update** and you see some action in the dynamic trace plot. After having generated, say 1000 samples, a screen as in Figure 8.2 appears.

If extra iterations are needed, click again on **update** and specify the extra number of iterations. To ignore the first x burn-in iterations from the chain, type $x + 1$ in the box **beg** of the **Sample Monitor Tool**. Click on **density** to look at the densities and **stats** for posterior summary measures. From the **stats** box one can read off the node, the posterior mean and SD, the MC error, the 2.5%, 50%, 97.5% posterior quantiles, the start (iteration) and sample (the number iterations considered in the calculations).

A click on **auto cor** of the **Sample Monitor Tool** gives the autocorrelation function and produces a graph as in Figure 7.9. If there is high autocorrelation among the sampled values, a simple trick to reduce the dependence in the Markov chain (although with loss of information) is to apply thinning. WinBUGS allows thinning in two different ways. Suppose that you wish to retain only 10% of the sampled values then fill in '10' next to **thin** of the **Update Tool**. On the other hand, if you wish to discard 90% of the already sampled values, then fill in '10' next to **thin** of the **Sample Monitor Tool**. Note that in the first thinning operation ten times more values are sampled than requested.

This completes our first WinBUGS analysis of the osteoporosis data. This exercise was primarily meant for the reader to get acquainted with the basics of WinBUGS.

8.1.2 Information on samplers

By default WinBUGS uses the block Gibbs sampler. That blocking is in use can be verified by clicking on **Options** in the menu bar and then on **Blocking options. . . .** If in the box **Blocking Options** 'fixed effects' is switched on, WinBUGS employs the block Gibbs sampler based on the algorithm of Gamerman (1997). This method samples all regression parameters in one block. To find out the sampler for a full conditional, click on **Info** in the main menu and then on **Node Info. . . .** The box **Node Tool** appears. Fill in the node, say 'beta0' and click on **methods**. In the log file the message 'beta0 UpdaterGLM.NormalUpdater' appears specifying again that the GLM approach of Gamerman is used.

In Section 8.1.1, the blocking option was switched on. To switch off the blocking option, recompile the program. Then WinBUGS will prompt whether it is 'ok' that 'the new model will replace the old one'. Click on 'ok' and on **Options** from the menu bar, select **Blocking Options. . .** and switch off fixed effects. To sample from the posterior, continue as sketched in Section 8.1.1. With the **Node Info** option we can find out if the sampler has been changed. In the log file the message 'beta0 UpdaterNormal.StdUpdater' appears, which means that the normal sampler is used for each regression parameter separately. When the blocking option is switched off, the mixing is poor due to a multicollinearity problem (between beta0 and beta1).

The standard settings of each of the univariate samplers used in the WinBUGS program can be obtained from the **Options** menu and then by clicking on **Update Options. . . .** The **Updater options** window appears with the default options taken for each sampler. For the osteoporosis example, two samplers appear in the window: 'UpdaterGamma' (the conjugate sampler, used for σ^2) and 'UpdaterGLM' (for the regression parameters jointly when Blocking Options are switched on). Clicking on each sampler shows the default options for that sampler. For instance, in the case of 'UpdaterGLM', the overrelaxation option (see Section 7.3.2) chooses from 16 candidates to generate the subsequent value in the chain. One can change these options in the current run. However, this needs to be done with care. Here, follows an example that changing these options can have dramatic implications for the convergence of the chain.

In Chapter 12, we look for the most appropriate model to analyze the Ames mutagenic assay data. Several models were programmed in WinBUGS; see Section 12.3 for details. The WinBUGS program for the short-term toxicity model with $\theta = 1$ makes use of the Metropolis sampler. Using the Update Options as indicated above, one can check that WinBUGS needs 4000 iterations to tune the normal sampler. In Figure 8.3 (top), we show the acceptance rate of the Metropolis sampler when 20 000 iterations were completed. This graph can be obtained from the **Model** option on the main menu and then choosing **Monitor Met**. Clearly, around 4000 iterations, the acceptance rate lies between 20% and 40%. Suppose now that one reduced this tuning phase to 750 to speed up the initial sampling process. Then Figure 8.3 (bottom) shows that the acceptance rate is far from optimal. In fact, the history plot of the parameters then shows that the Markov chains do not converge (not shown).

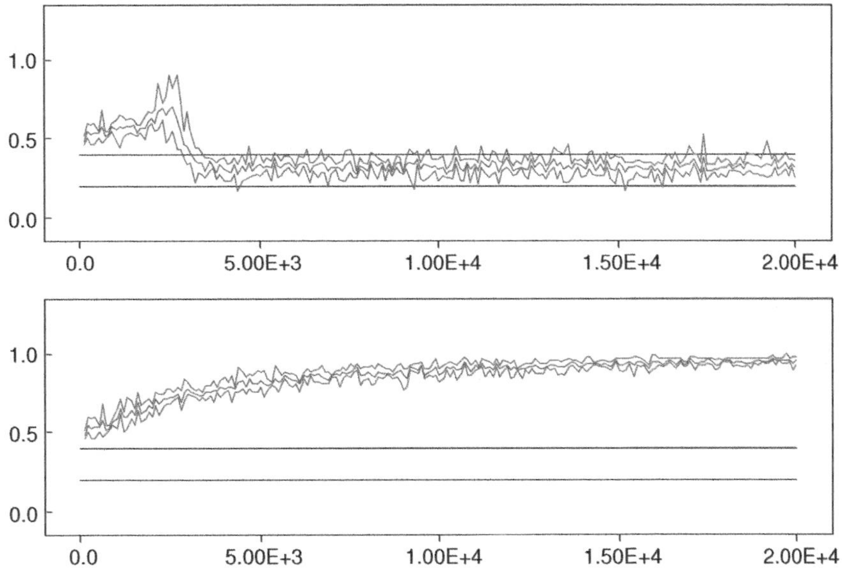

Figure 8.3 Ames assay IPCS data (Chapter Bioassay): Metropolis acceptance rate monitor in WinBUGS based on the short-term toxicity model with $\theta = 1$ obtained from 20 000 iterations, when based on (top) 4000 tuning iterations and (bottom) 750 tuning iterations.

8.1.3 Assessing and accelerating convergence

We now illustrate how convergence of the Markov chain can be tested with WinBUGS. While in the first analysis, we used only one set of starting values, now we take multiple starting values. In the WinBUGS program, eight list statements containing the starting values are given to initiate eight chains (in practice 2–4 chains are enough). The starting values were chosen in an 'overdispersed' manner (see Example VII.2). Note that before the program is compiled, you need to fill in '8' in the **Specification Tool** box. Then one is prompted eight times for starting values. The history trace plot of the slope in Figure 8.4 shows that the eight chains are mixing well but the mixing with each chain is slow. Posterior summary measures can be obtained as in the previous analysis, either based on all chains or on a subset of the chains. Chains are selected in the **Sample Monitor Tool** box. The only convergence diagnostic that can be used

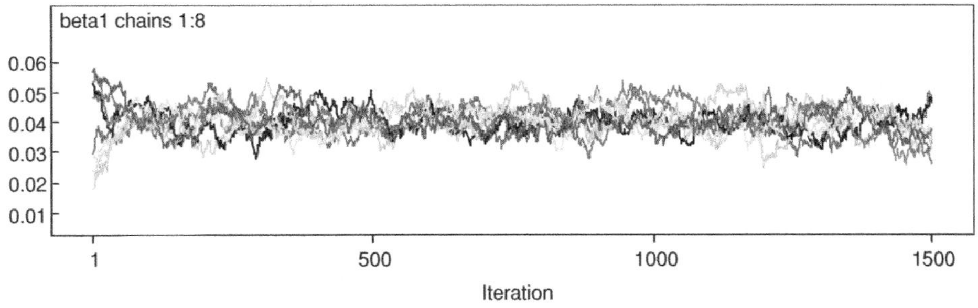

Figure 8.4 Osteoporosis study: history plot obtained from WinBUGS after 1500 iterations and based on eight overdispersed starting positions.

with WinBUGS is the Brooks–Gelman–Rubin (BGR) diagnostic. To activate this diagnostic click on **bgr diag** of the **Sample Monitor Tool**. In Figure 7.6, the BGR diagnostic based on the above eight chains was shown. Numerical values of the numerator and denominator can be obtained by double clicking with the left mouse when the cursor is in the BGR window and then clicking with the right mouse while holding the ctrl key. To obtain a formal assessment of convergence, the chains must be exported to S+ or R. This is done by clicking on button **coda**. A window 'CODA index' contains the following administrative information about the stored chain values:

```
beta0    1       1500
beta1    1501    3000
sigma2   3001    4500
```

The above three lines simply point to the positions of the parameters in the windows 'CODA for chain x', where x runs from 1 to 8. Save each window as a .txt file by clicking on **File** in the main menu and then on **Save as....** For instance, the contents in the window 'CODA index' may be saved as 'ind.txt' while the chain values in the other windows as 'out8.txt', 'out7.txt', ..., 'out1.txt'. These files can then be processed afterward with the R package CODA.

The CODA functions for assessing the convergence of the osteoporosis regression analysis can be found in the R program 'chapter 8 osteoporosis BGR-CODA.R'. Parts of the CODA output were shown in Chapter 7. A simple trick to improve convergence is to center (and standardize) the covariate(s). This can be done by replacing the mean model specification by `mu[i] <- beta0+beta1*(bmi[i]-mean(bmi[]))/sd(bmi[])`, where `mean(bmi[])` computes the average BMI and `sd(bmi[])` the standard deviation of BMI. The high posterior correlation between beta0 and beta1 can be highlighted by looking at the cross-correlations which are delivered by the **Correlation Tool** from the **Inference** option on the main menu, see Figure 8.6. Note the peculiar way of indicating that `bmi` is a vector, i.e. `bmi[]`. In more complicated settings, other tricks might be needed, e.g. overrelaxation may be invoked in WinBUGS by switching on **over relax** in the **Update Tool**.

8.1.4 Vector and matrix manipulations

In Figure 8.5, the WinBUGS program is shown to regress TBBMC on age, weight, length, BMI, and a measure of muscle strength. We look at the subgroup of 186 elderly women who have no missing values on these measurements. The file 'chapter 8 osteomultipleregression.odc' is a compound document that contains the WinBUGS commands. The purpose of this section is to introduce vector and matrix notations and manipulations in WinBUGS.

Now, all data (including constant '1') are collected in a matrix `x` with 186 rows and 6 columns. The regression coefficients are collected in the vector `beta`. The command `mu[i] <- inprod(beta[],x[i,])` computes the inner product of the regressor vector `beta[]` with the data vector `x[i,]` and gives the mean value `mu[i]` (mean of TBBMC for the *i*th individual). Further, with `for (r in 1:6) {mu.beta[r] <- 0.0}` the prior means of the regression coefficients are fixed at zero. The double 'for-loop' defines the elements of the prior precision matrix of the regression coefficients. Finally, `beta[1:6] ~ dmnorm(mu.beta[], prec.beta[,])` states that a multivariate normal prior distribution is used for the regression coefficients with mean vector and precision matrix specified as parameters.

```
model{
for (i in 1:N){
    tbbmc[i] ~dnorm(mu[i],tau)
    x[i,1]<-1; x[i,2]<-age[i]; x[i,3]<-weight[i]; x[i,4]<-length[i]
    x[i,5]<-bmi[i]; x[i,6]<- strength[i]
    mu[i] <- inprod(beta[],x[i,])
}
    sigma2 <- 1/tau
    sigma <- sqrt(sigma2)
    for (r in 1:6) { mu.beta[r] <- 0.0}
    c <- 1.0E-6
    for (r in 1:6) { for (s in 1:6){
    prec.beta[r,s] <- equals(r,s)*c
    }}
    beta[1:6] ~ dmnorm(mu.beta[], prec.beta[,])
    tau ~ dgamma(1.0E-3,1.0E-3)
  }
list(N=186)

age[]        length[]      weight[]     bmi[]      strength[]     tbbmc[]
71.00        157.00        67.00        27.18        96.25          2.325
73.00        163.00        71.00        26.72        85.25          1.925
...............................
86.00        155.00        68.00        28.30        70.25          1.850
END
list(beta = c(0,0,0,0,0,0), tau=1)
```

Figure 8.5 Osteoporosis study: regression model in vector and matrix notation.

The data section consists of two parts. The first part consists of a list statement specifying the number of patients and the second, rectangular part contains the regressor and response values. The regression data are stored in vector format. The data part ends with an END statement. Note that, to enter the data in WinBUGS, one needs to click on both parts of the data structure and each time on **load data**.

We performed the regression analysis with the blocking mode switched off. Thus, we also expected a poor convergence rate here. But this did not happen. The reason is that WinBUGS processes the regression coefficients `beta[]` as one object and automatically chooses for the block Gibbs sampler. This can be seen by clicking on **Node Info**. The message `beta[1] UpdaterMVNormal.Updater` means that the regression parameters are handled jointly. It does not imply, however, that the cross-correlations must be low among the regression parameters. Figure 8.6(a) demonstrates a high cross-correlation between the intercept and the regression coefficients of weight, length, and BMI but also that the latter regression coefficients are highly cross-correlated due to the introduction of weight and length. Despite the high cross-correlations, convergence can be good. It just depends on the choice of the sampler.

Multicollinearity causes statistical problems (badly estimated regression coefficients). An approach to deal with multicollinearity is to apply ridge regression. We know from Section 5.7 that if $\boldsymbol{\beta}$ is given a normal prior $\mathrm{N}(\mathbf{0}, \tau^2\mathrm{I})$ then this has a similar effect as applying a classical ridge regression analysis with ridge parameter $\lambda = \sigma^2/\tau^2$. Therefore, we replaced the value for c in Figure 8.5 by 5. Hereby, in fact, we applied a ridge regression analysis. The posterior median for λ was equal to 0.2 which is an acceptably small value. The matrix

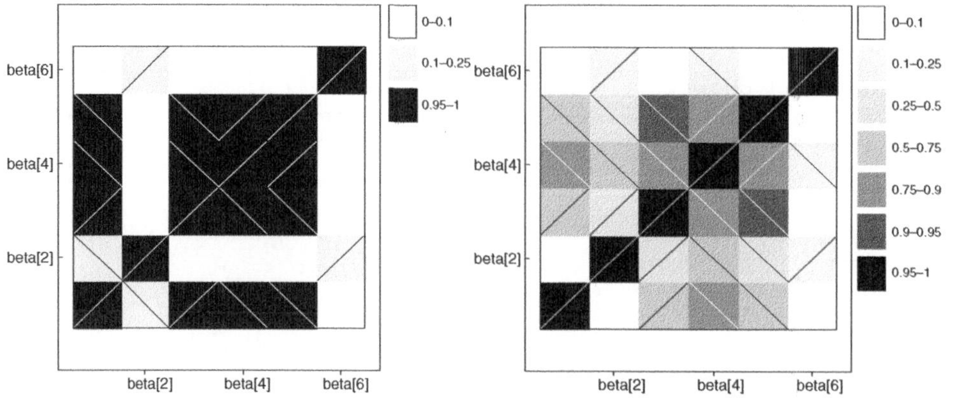

Figure 8.6 Osteoporosis study: cross-correlation matrix of regression parameters with vague normal regression prior (LHS) and ridge regression prior (RHS).

of cross-correlations in Figure 8.6(b) shows that the problem of multicollinearity has been resolved.

In Sections 5.6.1 and 11.5, the usefulness of Zellner's g-inverse prior in variable selection is illustrated. This prior is obtained by replacing the commands defining the precision matrix by those in Figure 8.7 (see 'chapter 8 osteomultiple-ginverse.odc')

8.1.5 Working in batch mode

Repeatedly running WinBUGS is laborious. However, it is possible to run WinBUGS without necessarily having to point and click your way through the commands. This is done by using WinBUGS scripts. Using this feature, WinBUGS can be called from within other programs. For instance, the program *R2WinBUGS* (Sturtz *et al.* 2005) provides an interface between R and WinBUGS. The advantage of R2WinBUGS is that it allows for an easy exchange of objects from WinBUGS to R thereby exploiting the R functionality. Details on the R2WinBUGS package are found in Sturtz *et al.* (2005) or the R2WinBUGS manual (http://cran.r-project.org/).

Figure 8.8 shows how WinBUGS is called from within R with the R2WinBUGS function **bugs** to analyze the osteoporosis regression problem. The file 'chapter 8 osteoporosis-R2WB.R' contains the commands. The parameters that are passed to WinBUGS in the **bugs** call are now described. The term **data** refers to a list object with the names of the columns of the data in the working directory, here `data <- list ("tbbmc", "bmi", "N")`, whereby `tbbmc` and `bmi` are vectors created in R. The option **inits** refers to a list object

```
c <- 1/N
for (r in 1:6) { mu.beta[r] <- 0.0}
for (r in 1:6) { for (s in 1:6){
prec.beta[r,s] <- inprod(x[,r],x[,s])*tau*c
}}
```

Figure 8.7 Osteoporosis study: WinBUGS commands to specify Zellner's precision matrix.

```
osteo.sim <- bugs(data, inits, parameters, "osteo.model.txt",
                  n.chains=8, n.iter=1500,
                  bugs.directory="c:/Program Files/WinBUGS14/",
                  working.directory=NULL, clearWD=FALSE);
print(osteo.sim)
plot(osteo.sim)
```

Figure 8.8 Osteoporosis study: call to WinBUGS using R2WinBUGS.

of initial values of the model parameters and **parameters** is a list object with names of the parameters. The file **osteo.model.txt** contains the WinBUGS syntax shown in Example VII.1. Eight chains were started up with 1500 iterations for each chain. Further, the executable WinBUGS file resides in `bugs.directory="c:/Program Files/WinBUGS14/"`. The eight coda files are located in the working directory. The option **clearWD=FALSE** indicates that these files are not deleted but can be processed afterward by CODA. With the function **print**, a table is produced containing posterior information (mean, median, etc.). The function **plot** produces the BGR diagnostic test for assessing convergence of the chains (see Figure 8.9). A WinBUGS log file is stored containing a list of the executed commands,

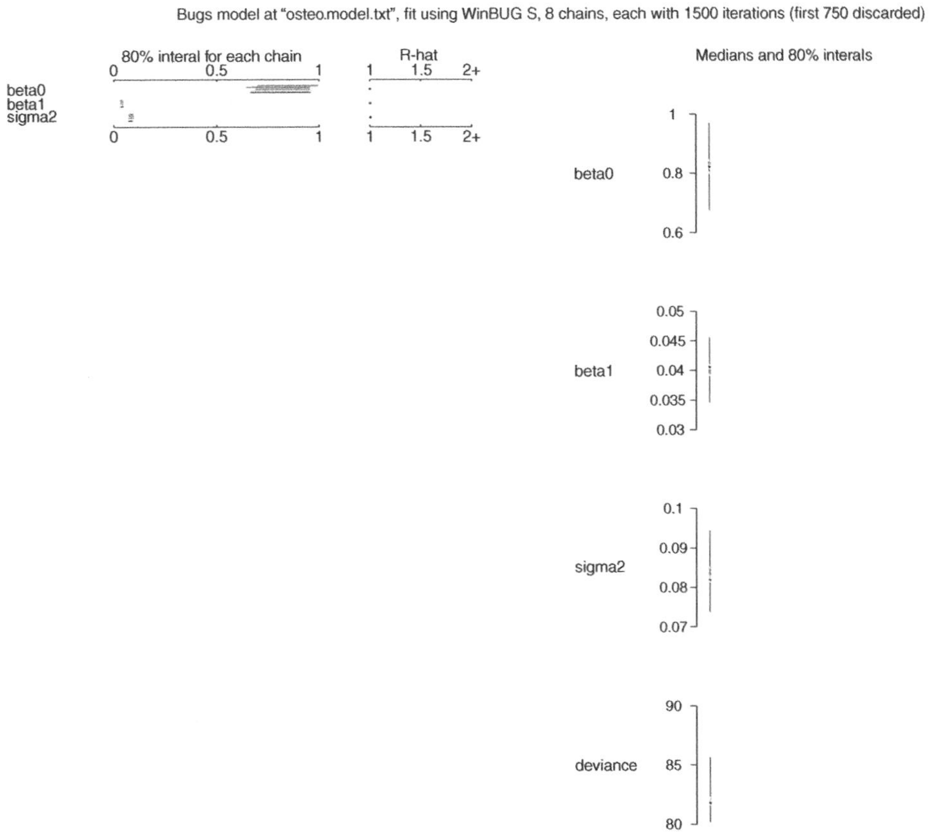

Figure 8.9 Osteoporosis study: graphical output produced by R2WinBUGS.

posterior summary statistics and a trace plot. Note that only a limited set of plots and analyses can be obtained directly from R2WinBUGS. For instance, the more formal convergence diagnostics such as Geweke diagnostic must be obtained by accessing CODA.

8.1.6 Troubleshooting

At each stage: syntax checking, data loading, compilation, providing initial values and running the sampler, errors may occur. For instance, a trap window will occur when WinBUGS has discovered a runtime error. In that case, the program stops sampling. The trap window is a dump of the status of the program when the error occurs. If this happens, try clicking the update button twice to restart the program. If this does not help, the program or the initial values need a change. Unfortunately, most of often, the trap window is cryptic and rarely helps in debugging. In the section *Tips and Troubleshooting* of the WinBUGS manual common error messages are listed. In the same section instructions are provided to resolve certain problems. For instance, it is mentioned that the 'probit' function creates often overflow problems. We encountered similarly numerical overflow problems with the function 'logit'. It sometimes helps to replace `logit(x) <- p` by `p <- exp(x)/(1+exp)`. Another solution is to combine the logit function with the functions 'min' and 'max' to constraint the value of 'x'.

8.1.7 Directed acyclic graphs

A graphical model is a pictorial representation of a statistical model in which nodes represent random variables and lines represent the dependence between the random variables. A graphical representation of a statistical model is useful to break up complex models into small (simple) parts, communicate the essence to nonstatisticians and to provide a basis for local computations.

In a *DAG*, also known as a *Bayesian network*, all links are directed, i.e. the arrows are added to lines and express that the child's node depends on the father's node, but not vice versa. In addition, no cycles are permitted which means that there is no path (while walking on the directed lines in the direction of the arrows) that brings you to your starting position. When the *directed local Markov property* or *conditional independence assumption* holds, each node v is independent of its nondescendants given its parents. For instance, suppose a probability model V involves random variables A, B, C and D. Suppose also that we represent the variables graphically in a family tree as in Figure 8.10 with D the child, C the parent

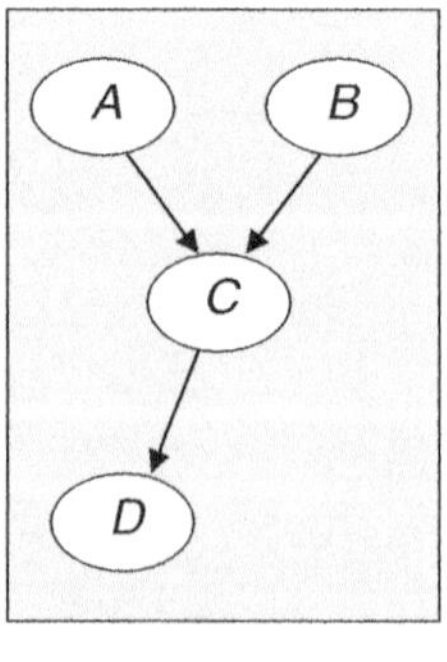

Figure 8.10 Example of a directed acyclic graph.

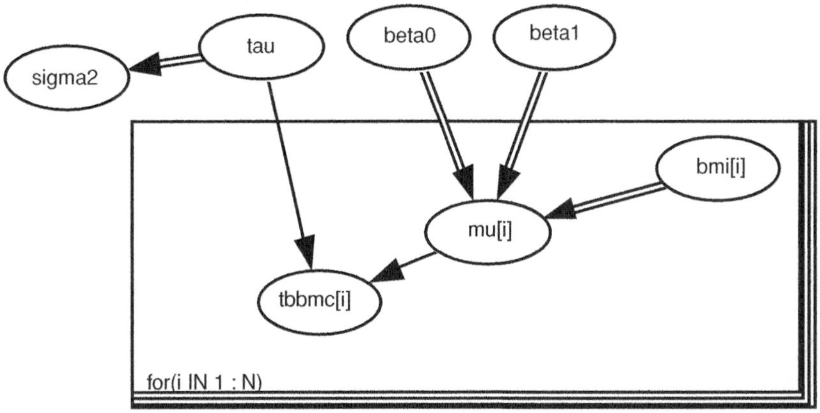

Figure 8.11 Osteoporosis study: doodle for a simple linear regression with response TBBMC and regressor BMI.

and A and B the grandparents. The graph represents conditional independence of A, B, and D given C which is written as: $A \perp D \mid C$ and $B \perp D \mid C$. This conditional independence implies that $p(A, B, C, D) = p(A)p(B)p(C \mid A, B)p(D \mid A, B)$. However, if a direct line connected A with D then the model is still a DAG but conditional independence would be lost.

For the above DAG with conditional independence, $p(V) = \prod_{v \in V} p(v \mid \text{parents}[v])$ and the full conditionals are given by

$$p(v \mid V \backslash v) = p(v \in \text{parents}[v]) \prod_{v \in \text{parents}[w]} p(w \in \text{parents}[w]).$$

It is this split in the full conditionals that makes a DAG interesting for Bayesian computations.

The *Doodle* option in WinBUGS visualizes a (Bayesian) model as a DAG and the assumed conditional independencies. In Figure 8.11, a DAG representation of the osteoporosis regression model was obtained from the Doodle option. There are three types of nodes: constants (fixed by design), stochastic nodes: variables that are given a distribution (observed = data or unobserved = parameters), logical nodes: logical functions of other nodes. The nodes `tbbmc[i]` and `beta0` are stochastic, while `sigma2` is a logical node. There are also two types of directed lines, single and double. The single lines represent stochastic relationships while the double represent logical relationships. Finally, some of these relationships are repeated over the subjects, i.e. those that are located within the rectangle(s) called *plate*(s).

What follows are some details on the nodes that are implemented in WinBUGS:

- *Stochastic nodes*: WinBUGS allows for univariate and multivariate different distributions, e.g. Bernoulli, exponential, student and multivariate normal, and can be truncated or censored. WinBUGS provides also multivariate priors.
- *Logical nodes*: WinBUGS allows for different logical expressions, e.g. abs, cos, logit, step, and equals. No 'if-then-else' statements are allowed in WinBUGS.

8.1.8 Add-on modules: GeoBUGS and PKBUGS

There are two add-on modules to WinBUGS which we briefly describe here for the sake of completeness.

GeoBUGS is an add-on module to WinBUGS which provides an interface for producing maps of the output from disease mapping and other spatial models and creating and manipulating adjacency matrices that are required as input for carrying out spatial smoothing.

PKBugs is an add-on module to WinBUGS for specifying complex population pharmacokinetic/pharmacodynamic (PK/PD) models. Due to the complexity of patients' dosing histories, the fact that each dose itself typically requires a complex nonlinear model, the presence of possibly time-varying covariates, censored observations, and outlying observations/individuals WinBUGS appears to be inefficient for such models. PKBugs aims to provide an answer to this.

8.1.9 Related software

OpenBUGS: The development of OpenBUGS started in 2004 in Helsinki. Both WinBUGS and OpenBUGS use the BUGS language which is based on component Pascal. The current version of OpenBUGS, OpenBUGS 3.2.1 (http://www.openbugs.info/w/) has a similar performance as WinBUGS. However, in particular (often difficult to convergence) cases the two programs can behave quite differently. A major difference between OpenBUGS and WinBUGS is in the way that the expert system selects the updating algorithm to use for the class of full conditional distribution of each node, i.e. WinBUGS defines one algorithm for each possible class whereas there is a greater class of algorithms available in OpenBUGS. This permits greater flexibility and extensibility from OpenBUGS as compared to WinBUGS. OpenBUGS has also improved blocking algorithms, but there is no specific blocking option.

Several new functions and distributions have been added to OpenBUGS. In addition the functionality of the different options has been extended compared to WinBUGS. For instance, in WinBUGS censoring is taken care of by the function I (lower, upper), but truncation could not be handled. In OpenBUGS censoring is allowed via C (lower, upper) and truncation via T (lower, upper). In OpenBUGS a `dloglik` distribution was added for use with the 'zero' Poisson trick for generic likelihoods and priors. OpenBUGS provides also more details about the samplers by default.

JAGS: JAGS is another software which can be used to fit Bayesian models using Markov chain Monte Carlo methods. JAGS is platform independent and is written in C++. It was developed by Martyn Plummer. Version 3.1.0 can be downloaded from http://www-fis.iarc.fr/~martyn/software/jags/allows. JAGS provides some extra functions like mexp() (matrix exponential), sort() (for sorting elements) and `%*%` (matrix multiplication). Just as with OpenBUGS, truncation and censoring are allowed. WinBUGS and OpenBUGS store data in row major order whereas JAGS stores values of an array in column major order. The main advantage of JAGS over the BUGS family is its platform independence. Therefore, it is part of many repositories of Linux distributions making it easily extendable through user-written (C++) modules.

Interface with WinBUGS, OpenBUGS and JAGS: For several popular packages an interface has been developed with WinBUGS. R2WinBUGS is an example of such software, linking R to WinBUGS. Interfaces have also been written for other packages, such as SAS,

STATA® and MATLab®. Two programs provide the link between R and OpenBUGS: BRugs and R2OpenBUGS (http://openbugs.info/w/UserContributedCode). R2jags (http://cran.r-project.org/web/packages/R2jags/index.html) is an interface between JAGS and R.

8.2 Bayesian analysis using SAS

SAS is a versatile package of programs providing tools for setting up data bases, general data handling, statistical programming, and statistical analyses. It is the standard tool for statisticians working in the pharmaceutical industry. Statistical analyses in SAS are done via procedures (abbreviated as PROC). SAS provides a broad range of statistical procedures but mainly of a frequentist nature. In SAS version 9.2 Bayesian options were added to existing frequentist procedures, i.e. in PROC GENMOD (analysis of discrete responses), PROC LIFEREG (parametric survival models), PROC MI (multiple imputation procedures), PROC MIXED (linear mixed effects models) and PROC PHREG (proportional hazards regression). In SAS version 9.2 the procedure MCMC was launched for fitting a wide range of Bayesian models, but was still experimental. In version 9.3, the MCMC procedure received the status of an established SAS procedure.

Two SAS procedures allow for a Bayesian regression analysis: PROC GENMOD and PROC MCMC. As with WinBUGS, we introduce the use of some SAS Bayesian procedures via a linear regression analysis on the osteoporosis data. The SAS programs are included in 'chapter 8 osteoporosis.sas'. We have used version 9.3 for all calculations in this section. More illustrations of the use of SAS can be found in the remainder of the book. For more details on the SAS statements and options, we refer to the SAS manuals or to the website: http://support.sas.com/documentation/.

8.2.1 Analysis using procedure GENMOD

Background: The SAS procedure GENMOD allows fitting generalized linear models (GLIMs) to univariate and correlated data. The Bayesian option in PROC GENMOD is based on Gibbs sampling and uses the ARS algorithm of Gilks and Wild (1992) for log-concave full conditionals. For other conditionals, it uses the ARMS algorithm.

Syntax: Figure 8.12 shows a typical PROC GENMOD program to perform a Bayesian linear regression analysis. The procedure is embedded in an output delivery system (ODS) environment to produce high-quality graphics. The statement `proc genmod data=osteoporosis;` instructs the procedure to search for a data set called 'osteoporosis' in its working directory. The statement `model tbbmc=bmi/dist=normal;`

```
ods graphics on;
proc genmod data=osteoporosis;
model tbbmc = bmi / dist=normal;
bayes seed =777 nbi=5000 nmc=10000 cprior=jeffreys sprior=improper
diagnostics=all plots(fringe smooth) = all outpost=osteout;
run;
ods graphics off;
```

Figure 8.12 Osteoporosis study: PROC GENMOD statements to perform a Bayesian linear regression analysis with SAS.

instructs to regress TBBMC on BMI assuming that the response has a normal distribution. The next line starts with **bayes** to invoke the Bayesian option. The option `seed=777` ensures that different runs start with the same seed. Further, `nbi=5000 nmc=10000` instructs to run 5000 burn-in iterations and 10 000 extra iterations. For the regression parameters, we have chosen a Jeffreys prior (option `cprior=jeffreys`).

PROC GENMOD offers three types of priors for regression parameters: (a) uniform, i.e. $p(\boldsymbol{\beta}) \propto c$ (`cprior=uniform`), (b) Gaussian (`cprior=normal`), i.e. $p(\boldsymbol{\beta}) \propto \mathrm{N}(\boldsymbol{\mu}, \Sigma)$ where $\boldsymbol{\mu}$ and Σ can be defined in various ways and (c) Jeffreys prior, which means that $p(\boldsymbol{\beta}) \propto \left|\phi^{-1}\,\mathrm{I}(\boldsymbol{\beta})\right|^{1/2}$ where ϕ is the dispersion parameter of the Bayesian generalized linear model (BGLIM) (see Section 4.8). One can fix this value to 1 or take the current estimate of ϕ in the chain. More details on Jeffreys prior for BGLIMs were given in Section 5.6.2. Priors for the variance part can be specified on: (a) the dispersion parameter (ϕ) (`dprior`), (b) the scale parameter ($\phi^{1/2}$) (`sprior`) and (c) the precision parameter (ϕ^{-1}) (`pprior`). With `sprior=improper` Jeffreys prior $p(\phi^{1/2}) \equiv p(\sigma) \propto \sigma^{-1}$ for the scale parameter is specified. In contrast to WinBUGS, now improper priors are allowed. The user should, therefore, check that improper posteriors are avoided.

The option `diagnostics=all` in Figure 8.12 instructs to compute the autocorrelations of lags 1, 5, 10, and 50, the effective sample size and the four formal diagnostics (Geweke, Gelman–Rubin, Heidelberger–Welch and Raftery–Lewis). For all model parameters, a trace plot, an autocorrelation plot and a kernel density plot are produced by the command `plots(fringe smooth) = all`. Specifying 'fringe' adds the density of points on the x-axis and the option 'smooth' overlays a smoothed trace plot with the actual trace plot. Furthermore, the instruction `outpost=osteout` stores the `nmc=10000` sampled values of the parameters together with the logarithm of the posterior in a user-defined file called `osteout`. This file can be processed at a later stage to produce posterior summary measures or plots not supported by PROC GENMOD. Finally, the statement `run` instructs to execute the procedure. Additional options can be specified, e.g. `thinning=10` instructs to store only 10% of the Markov chain. If a specific option is not chosen, the default choice is taken. For example, in our program thinning is taken by default equal to 1.

Output: PROC GENMOD starts with a maximum likelihood procedure, then reports on the chosen priors and the chosen initial values (output not shown). The program automatically chooses three initial values for each parameter. Further, the program reports the deviance information criterion (DIC) and p_D values (see Chapter 10) for model evaluation purposes.

Posterior summary measures including an highest posterior density (HPD) interval are given for each parameter including a posterior correlation matrix of the parameters from which we can see that the posterior cross-correlation between the intercept and the slope equals −0.987 (not shown), confirming a multicollinearity problem in the model. In Figure 8.13, the trace plot, the autocorrelation (ACF) plot and the density plot of the slope are displayed. We expected to see a high autocorrelation for the regression parameters as was obtained with the WinBUGS analyses without blocking. However, the posterior autocorrelations indicate close to independent sampling. The reason is that PROC GENMOD first centers (automatically) the covariates such that the multicollinearity problem is resolved before sampling (this is, however, not documented in the manual). For the output, the results are back-transformed to the original scale.

According to the Gelman–Rubin, Geweke and Heidelberger–Welch diagnostics convergence was not rejected (with the standard settings) but for the Raftery–Lewis diagnostic the chain was not long enough (output not shown).

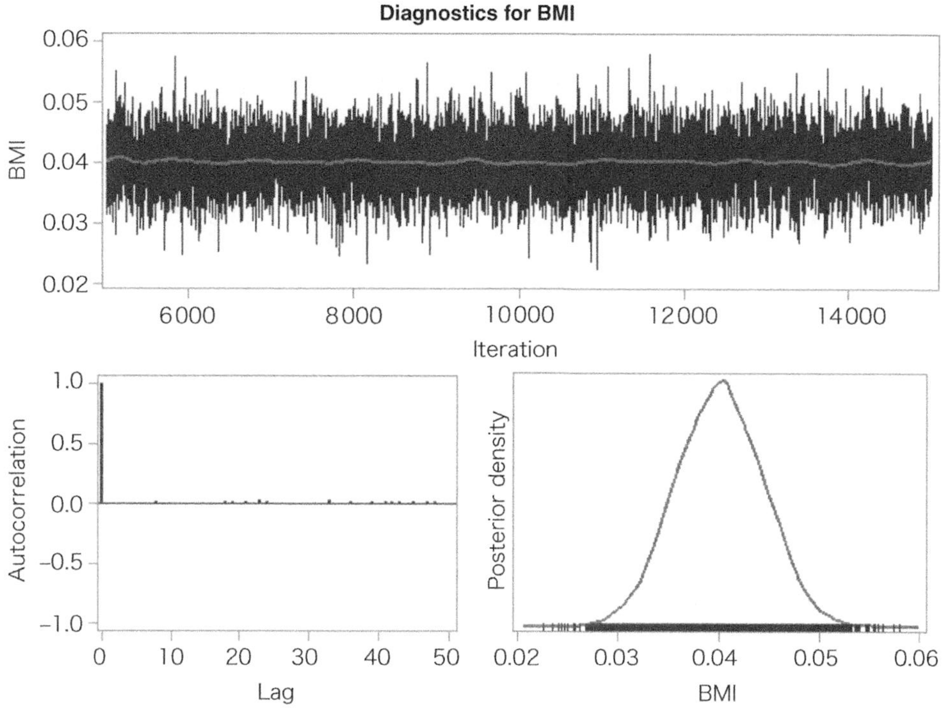

Figure 8.13 Osteoporosis study: trace plot, autocorrelation (ACF) plot, and density plot of the slope for the Bayesian regression analysis produced by PROC GENMOD.

Figure 8.14 reports that the estimated effective sample sizes (see Section 7.2.5) for the three parameters are around 10 000. This is the effect of centering BMI. The *autocorrelation time* can be thought of as the sum of significant autocorrelations in a Markov chain, with a significant autocorrelation defined as greater than 0.05. Here, none of the nontrivial autocorrelations were important and hence the autocorrelation times were all equal to 1. The efficiency is defined as the ratio of the effective sample size ESS to the Markov chain size n, i.e. ESS/n. Finally, using the Monte Carlo standard error (MCSE) equal to the standard deviation of the sampled (Monte Carlo) mean ($\text{MCSE} = \text{SD}/\sqrt{ESS}$) we can compute a classical 95% confidence interval for the true posterior mean. For example, this interval is equal to $0.0401 \pm 1.96 \times 0.000043 = [0.0400, 0.0402]$ for β_1. From the ratio MCSE/SD $\approx 1/100$ we infer that only 1% of the posterior variability is due to simulation.

Additional features: PROC GENMOD allows for different distributions such as: binomial, gamma, geometric, and different link functions such as: identity, log, logit. Since the `bayes` option is incorporated in a procedure that originally performed only frequentist statistical analyses, some (but many not) of the existing options can be combined with the Bayesian option.

8.2.2 Analysis using procedure MCMC

Background: The procedure MCMC is a versatile program for MCMC sampling suitable to fit a variety of statistical models in combination with different priors. PROC MCMC also allows

Effective sample sizes			
Parameter	**ESS**	**Autocorrelation Time**	**Efficiency**
Intercept	10322.3	0.9688	1.0322
BMI	10347.7	0.9664	1.0348
Scale	10000.0	1.0000	1.0000

Monte Carlo standard errors			
Parameter	**MCSE**	**Standard deviation**	**MCSE/SD**
Intercept	0.00115	0.1166	0.00984
BMI	0.000043	0.00437	0.00983
Scale	0.000133	0.0133	0.0100

Figure 8.14 Osteoporosis study: precision with which the parameters of the Bayesian regression analysis were estimated by PROC GENMOD.

for programming of user-defined priors, log-likelihood functions, and samplers. However, the procedure does not assume that the model is a DAG, hence there is no restriction on using a symbol (or a node) multiple times. The procedure hinges on the block Metropolis(–Hastings) sampler combined with a great variety of proposal densities. The RANDOM statement that was added to PROC MCMC in version 9.3 greatly improved the rate of convergence for fitting hierarchical models. An illustration of this novel feature is deferred to Chapter 9.

Syntax: Figure 8.15 displays the commands for a Bayesian regression analysis of the osteoporosis data using PROC MCMC. Like any other SAS procedure, there is an explicit loop over the input data set. In other words, the MODEL statement, applied to variable

```
ods graphics on;
 proc mcmc data=osteoporosis outpost=osteout nbi=10000 nmc=20000
   nthin=10
          monitor=(beta0 beta1 beta2 sigma2 sigma) init=pinit
            mchist=detailed
          diag=all plots=(TRACE AUTOCORR DENSITY) seed=7771;
     parms beta0 0 beta1 0 beta2 0 sigma2 1;
     prior beta0 beta1 beta2 ~ normal(0, var = 10000);
         prior sigma2 ~ igamma(0.0001,scale=0.0001);
         sigma =sqrt(sigma2);
     mu = beta0 + beta1*bmi + beta2*bmi2;
     model tbbmc ~ normal (mean=mu,var= sigma2);
   run;
ods graphics off;
```

Figure 8.15 Osteoporosis study: PROC MCMC commands to perform a Bayesian regression analysis.

names, is equivalent to the for-loop over N (in data) in WinBUGS. Because of this assumption there is no need to use the indexing on each variable (node) as in WinBUGS. From a statistical point of view, this is equivalent to assuming that all observations are independent which can be lifted with the PROC-level option JOINTMODEL but more programming is required then. Multiple MODEL statements are allowed and they can be used to declare either joint, or marginal+conditional, distributions on the response variables. All programming statements need to be thought as being enclosed in the for-loop over N in WinBUGS, that each is processed for every observation in the simulation. If one wishes to place them outside of the data loop, one needs to use the BEGINNODATA and ENDNODATA statements.

We now added a quadratic term (`bmi2` $\equiv \text{BMI}^2$) to the model. In addition, we divided BMI by 10 to improve the clarity of the output (to avoid too many zeroes behind the decimal point). The option `outpost=osteout` saves the `nmc=20000` sampled values of the parameters (and log of posterior) after `nbi=10000` burn-in samples. The option `nthin=10` means that only every 10th value must stored which here implies that only 2000 values of the chain were actually stored. This is in contrast to WinBUGS where 200 000 values would have been generated and 20 000 stored. The option `monitor=(beta0 beta1 beta2 sigma2 sigma)` is specified to monitor the regression parameters, the residual variance and residual standard deviation, respectively. Note that this statement can be replaced with `monitor=(_parms_ sigma)`, where `_parms_` is a shorthand for all model parameters. The proposal density is adapted in the tuning phase to achieve an optimal acceptance rate. The option `init=pinit` tabulates parameter values after the tuning phase. This option also tabulates the tuned proposal parameters used by the Metropolis algorithm. The option `mchist=detailed` produces detailed output on various aspects of the MCMC sampling procedure such as the tuning, burn-in, and sampling history tables, including scale values, acceptance probabilities and blocking information.

The option `diag=all` asks that all diagnostics (autocorrelations, effective sample sizes, Monte Carlo errors and the convergence diagnostics of Geweke, Raftery–Lewis and Heidelberger–Welch) are given. Note that PROC MCMC does not produce the Gelman–Rubin diagnostic. The option `plots=(TRACE AUTOCORR DENSITY)` asks for ODS graphs (trace plots, ACF plots and posterior density plots). The ‘parms’ instruction serves two purposes: (1) starting values are given for all parameters and (2) it defines the blocks of the block MH-Sampler except for the parameters that are sampled with a (conditional)-conjugate sampler. For instance, the statement `parms beta0 0 beta1 0 beta2 0 sigma2 1;` requests that all parameters are sampled jointly (in one block). However, by default, the variance parameter is sampled separately with the inverse gamma (conjugate) distribution as sampler. Therefore, the procedure takes two blocks: one block for all regression parameters and one block for the variance parameter. The option `sigma =sqrt(sigma2);` (combined with the monitor option) instructs to look also at the residual standard deviation. The likelihood is specified by two statements: `mu = beta0 + beta1*bmi + beta2*bmi2;` and `model tbbmc ~ normal (mean=mu,var= sigma2);`. By default, the normal sampler is used but this can be changed to a multivariate t-distribution with, say, three degrees of freedom by adding the option `propdist = t(3)` to the PROC MCMC statement. The PRIOR statement declares prior distributions, and is equivalent to the ~ in WinBUGS and is outside the for-loop over the data. Like the MODEL statement, multiple PRIOR statements can be used in declaring either a joint, or marginal+conditional, distribution over the parameters.

Proposal covariance for block 2			
Parameter	beta0	beta1	beta2
beta0	0.2720	-0.2006	0.0361
beta1	-0.2006	0.1493	-0.0271
beta2	0.0361	-0.0271	0.0050

Figure 8.16 Osteoporosis study: normal proposal density for the three regression parameters with PROC MCMC.

Output: The sampling procedure is a blocked Metropolis sampler with one block consisting of the three regression parameters and another block consisting of the variance parameter. For the first block, a three-dimensional normal proposal density was chosen and the variance parameter was sampled with an inverse gamma sampler. The proposal density is $N_3(\boldsymbol{\theta}^k \mid c^2\Sigma)$ whereby c as well as Σ were adapted in the tuning phase to achieve approximately an acceptance rate of 0.234. The covariance matrix $c^2\Sigma$ of the proposal density at the end of the tuning phase was obtained by the option `init=pinit` and is shown in Figure 8.16. The posterior autocorrelations were low for all lags. Again the trace plots showed good mixing for all parameters. Further, Geweke and Heidelberger–Welch diagnostics indicated good mixing but the chain was too small for the Raftery–Lewis diagnostic. The effective sample size was around 1600 for the regression parameters while for the variance parameter it exceeded even 2000. The MC errors were all below 5% of the posterior SD. Finally, the posterior summary measures indicated a positive regression coefficient for BMI and a negative regression coefficient for BMI^2 with credible intervals that did not encompass zero.

To illustrate the effect of blocking, we repeated the above analysis with two different `parms` statements. When the following two `parms` statements were given: `parms beta0 0 beta1 0 beta2 0; parms sigma2 1;` nothing changed, as expected. However, for the following four `parms` statements: `parms beta0; parms beta1 0; parms beta2 0; parms sigma2 1;`, sampling deteriorated. The convergence diagnostics indicated a significant deviation from convergence for the regression parameters (but convergence for the variance parameter). In addition, the effective sample size for the regression parameters dropped to about 6. This shows the importance of a good choice of the blocks (in combination with PROC MCMC).

Additional features: Missing data are allowed, as well as truncated and censored data.

8.2.3 Other Bayesian programs

Two extra SAS procedures include a Bayesian option:

1. *PROC LIFEREG*: allows for parametric survival analysis. The sampler is the same as that of PROC GENMOD and roughly similar Bayesian options are provided.

2. *PROC PHREG*: the Bayesian equivalent of the popular semiparametric Cox proportional hazards survival model. The procedure uses Gibbs sampling for the regression parameters and piecewise hazard model parameters. About the same Bayesian options as with PROC LIFREG are available.

The procedures GENMOD, LIFEREG and PHREG allow for multiple chains and the application of the Gelman–Rubin diagnostic, while the procedure MCMC is based on the single chain methodology.

Two other SAS procedures have a Bayesian option, i.e. PROC MI and PROC MIXED. The first procedure imputes missing data using MCMC techniques and assumes multivariate normality of the observations. The procedure appears to use the Gibbs sampler, but details are not provided. The second procedure is one of the most popular recent SAS statistical procedures for fitting mixed effects models to data in a frequentist manner. In SAS version 9.2 a PRIOR statement has been added to the options of PROC MIXED. This novel feature now allows for a Bayesian analysis to Gaussian hierarchical models. The procedure uses by default the independent Metropolis–Hastings algorithm (see Section 6.3.4) but offers another three sampling algorithms.

8.3 Additional Bayesian software and comparisons

8.3.1 Additional Bayesian software

First Bayes is an excellent program for classroom teaching to fresh students in Bayesian methods. The package has been developed by O'Hagan and can be downloaded from `www.firstbayes.co.uk/` and comes with a manual.

It is impossible to give a comprehensive overview of Bayesian software for the simple reason that lately we have seen an explosion of Bayesian programs primarily written in R and Matlab. For R packages one might consult the `CRAN` website (http://cran.r-project.org/). Another possibility is the website of the International Society for Bayesian Analysis (http://bayesian.org/) or just to Google the web. Below is a personal choice of some Bayesian software that might be useful for fitting models considered in this book. All these packages use MCMC techniques to arrive at the Bayesian solution:

- *MLwiN* package (http://www.bristol.ac.uk/cmm/software/mlwin/) is dedicated software for modeling hierarchical data. The package has a frequentist and a Bayesian component based on MCMC algorithms. A good source for this package is Rasbash *et al.* (2009) or Lawson *et al.* (2003).

- *MCMCglmm* (see CRAN website): R package for fitting Generalised Linear Mixed Models using MCMC methods. Most commonly used distributions are supported but also less popular ones like the zero-inflated Poisson and the multinomial. Missing values and left, right, and interval censoring are accommodated for all traits. The package allows various residual and random effect variance structures.

- *MNP* (see CRAN website): R package that fits the Bayesian multinomial probit model.

- *MCMCpack* (http://mcmcpack.wustl.edu/): R package that fits several models that are useful for social scientists such as IRT models and change-point models, also useful for biostatisticians.

- *msm* (see CRAN website): R package that fits multistate models.

- *BACC* (http://www2.cirano.qc.ca/~bacc/bacc2003/index.html): available on different platforms with R, S+, Matlab versions containing a wide range of programs used by econometricians but also useful for biostatisticians.

- *BayesX* (http://www.stat.uni-muenchen.de/~bayesx/bayesx.html): R package for estimating a variety of highly structured additive regression models, such as generalized additive models (GAMs), generalized additive mixed models (GAMM), varying coefficient models (VCM), etc.
- *BNT* (http://code.google.com/p/bnt/): Matlab package for directed graphical models. One may consult also the website http://www.cs.ubc.ca/~murphyk/Software/bnsoft.html for a great variety of programs to fit graphical models.

The approach followed in the integrated nested Laplace approximations (INLA) package (http://www.r-inla.org/home) is drastically different. INLA is based on sophisticated Laplace approximations (Rue *et al.* 2009). The package is applicable to (basically) each model that can be thought of a Gaussian model either immediately, or via a transformation or in a latent sense. Since no sampling is involved, computations appear to be much faster than with MCMC algorithms while keeping a high precision on the posterior estimates of the parameters.

A quite useful freely available software tool to access the R packages is **RStudio v0.94** (http://rstudio.org/). RStudio is available for all major platforms including Windows, Mac OS X and Linux. It divides the screen into four subscreens: an editor, a console, a screen showing the workspace and the history, and a fourth screen that shows the generated plots and allows to install, load and update R packages.

8.3.2 Comparison of Bayesian software

The programming environments of WinBUGS and SAS are clearly different. WinBUGS has an open-ended environment similar to the S+/R programming (but with more limitations), while SAS offers a more procedural environment, some of the procedures also have a programming environment. An in-depth comparison of WinBUGS and the Bayesian SAS programs needs to be done with care, since both packages can handle quite a range of statistical models and experience with the package plays a great role. We have not envisaged such a thorough comparison here, rather we wished to illustrate by some elementary examples how different the two programs operate. Nevertheless, for a particular hierarchical model, i.e. a logistic random effects model (Chapter 9), we have compared several frequentist and Bayesian statistical packages including WinBUGS 1.4.3, SAS PROC MCMC version 9.2 and MLwiN 2.13 (Li *et al.* 2011). Two conclusions are important. First, the packages differ considerably in programming environment and flexibility toward tackling statistical problems whereby WinBUGS and SAS can handle the greatest variety of problems. Second, the packages also differ greatly with respect to computational efficiency. Namely, MLwinN was clearly the winner and SAS PROC MCMC version 9.2 was hopelessly inefficient. With the introduction of the RANDOM statement in version 9.3, sampling hierarchical models is now much more efficient and often comparable to WinBUGS.

8.4 Closing remarks

In this chapter, we have focused on the facilities of primarily two Bayesian programs: WinBUGS and SAS. While at this stage, the majority of the Bayesian analyses are done using WinBUGS and with dedicated R packages, it is conceivable that the Bayesian SAS procedures will gain in popularity definitely among SAS users but likely also among a more general class of applied statisticians.

Exercises

Exercise 8.1 Perform the analysis of Exercises 7.1 and 7.2 in WinBUGS with blocking options both switched on and off.

Exercise 8.2 Apply some acceleration techniques to improve the convergence rate in Exercise 8.1 of the WinBUGS sampler when the blocking options are switched off.

Exercise 8.3 Perform the analysis of Exercises 7.1 and 7.2 in SAS using PROC GENMOD and PROC MCMC.

Exercise 8.4 Run the Mice Example of the WinBUGS document 'Examples Vol I' with WinBUGS and replace the Weibull distribution with a lognormal distribution. Produce the autocorrelation function in both cases. Try out also some acceleration techniques.

Exercise 8.5 Run the Mice Example of the WinBUGS document 'Examples Vol I' in SAS using the Bayesian option in PROC LIFEREG and PROC MCMC. Try out different MH samplers with PROC MCMC. Compare the convergence rates and posterior summary measures between the SAS procedures but also to that of WinBUGS. Then replace the Weibull distribution with a lognormal distribution and evaluate again the performance of samplers.

Exercise 8.6 Perform the analysis of Exercise 7.7 using WinBUGS. Repeat the analyses with PROC MCMC.

Exercise 8.7 Perform the analysis of Exercise 7.8 in SAS using PROC MCMC.

Exercise 8.8 Analyze the caries data of Example VII.9 with PROC GENMOD and PROC MCMC. Try out different MH samplers with PROC MCMC. Compare the convergence rates and posterior summary measures between the SAS procedures but also to that of WinBUGS.

Exercise 8.9 Take the Kidney Example of the WinBUGS document 'Examples Vol I'. Look only at the first event (i.e. change the model and the data structure). Run the WinBUGS program and explore whether the convergence rate can be improved.

Exercise 8.10 Analyze the first event in the Kidney Example of the WinBUGS document 'Examples Vol I' with the Bayesian option in the SAS procedure LIFEREG and procedure MCMC.

Exercise 8.11 Analyze the interval-censored data (contained in file 'chapter 7 interval censoring.R') with WinBUGS and PROC MCMC.

Exercise 8.12 Take the Dugongs Example of the WinBUGS document 'Examples Vol II' and observe what happens when centering the covariate age. What is your conclusion?

Exercise 8.13 Take the Dugongs Example of the WinBUGS document 'Examples Vol II' and observe what happens when the prior distribution for γ is changed into (a) Beta(1, 3) and (b) Beta(3, 1).

Part II

BAYESIAN TOOLS FOR STATISTICAL MODELING

9

Hierarchical models

9.1 Introduction

In this chapter, we introduce *Bayesian hierarchical models* (BHMs). A BHM is a Bayesian statistical model for data that have an hierarchical structure. Such data are also referred to as *clustered*. Clustered data are abundant in the medical literature. Examples are measurements taken repeatedly over time on the same subject, data that exhibit a spatial hierarchy such as surfaces on teeth and teeth in a mouth, multi-center clinical data with patients within centers, cluster randomized trials where centers are randomized to interventions, meta-analyses, etc.

A proper statistical analysis of clustered data must take the correlation in the data into account. Different frequentist approaches have been proposed to handle correlated data. The generalized estimating equations (GEEs) technique introduced by Liang and Zeger (1986) is a popular approach that relies on minimal distributional assumptions treating the correlation structure among the repeated measures as nuisance. If one is willing to make some distributional assumptions, insight can be obtained in the correlation structure of the data. A class of frequentist parametric models that explicitly models the association consists of the *mixed effects models* also called *multilevel models* or *(frequentist) hierarchical models*. In these models, one distinguishes *fixed* from *random effects*. A fixed effect is a constant parameter that pertains to a population of subjects and expresses a *population* effect of the regressor. On the other hand, random effects are parameters that vary across subjects and express the subject-specific effects. The alternative term 'multilevel model' reflects that for hierarchical data the subjects are clustered in several levels.

The BHM is a hierarchical model whereby all parameters are given a prior distribution. It seems unnecessary for a BHM to distinguish between fixed and random effects, since in a Bayesian context, all parameters are random. Nevertheless, this distinction appears to be useful and we stick to it here. Many of the properties attributed to the frequentist hierarchical model also apply to the BHM, but a BHM might offer more to the statistical practitioner. First, the Bayesian approach takes automatically into account all uncertainty in the model parameters. Second, the MCMC algorithms offer a great flexibility in relaxing the strong parametric assumptions prevalent in most frequentist hierarchical models.

Bayesian Biostatistics, First Edition. Emmanuel Lesaffre and Andrew B. Lawson.

We introduce the BHM via two simple examples, i.e. the Poisson-gamma model and the Gaussian hierarchical model. Both models have the advantage that (to some extent) analytical results can be presented, which gives insight in how parameters are estimated. We also contrast the *full Bayesian approach* with the frequentist *Empirical Bayesian approach*. The general class of Bayesian mixed models governing the *Bayesian linear mixed model* (BLMM) with the Gaussian hierarchical model as a particular case, is the next topic. The *Bayesian generalized linear mixed model* (BGLMM) constitutes a larger class of BHMs. Further extensions of the BGLMM have been suggested but, unfortunately, cannot be treated here because of space limitations. Ensuring that a noninformative BGHLM prior yields a proper posterior may not be easy. A particular case is the choice of the NI prior for the level-2 variance in a BHM. This problem has raised quite some interest and is treated in this chapter. Further, we review and illustrate dedicated techniques that assess and accelerate the convergence of the Markov chain in an hierarchical context. Finally, we contrast the performance of frequentist and Bayesian hierarchical modeling approaches.

Most analyses were performed with WinBUGS 1.4.3 and OpenBUGS 3.2.1. For some examples, we also used the Bayesian SAS® procedure MCMC version (primarily) 9.3. Details on the syntax of the programs are largely ignored in this chapter, but we rather refer to the programs at the website of the book. To check convergence of the Markov chain, we visually inspected the trace plots. We often initiated multiple chains and applied the Brooks–Gelman–Rubin (BGR) convergence test. In many cases also, the whole battery of convergence diagnostics was applied (as an ultimate check). Finally, we let the chain run until the MCerror is less than 5% of the posterior SD.

9.2 The Poisson-gamma hierarchical model

9.2.1 Introduction

A gentle introduction to the BHM is provided by the Poisson-gamma model. We start with a model without covariates.

Example IX.1: Lip cancer study: Description
Spatial risk assessment is nowadays one of the major foci in public health. The geographical distribution of the prevalence and incidence of a disease plays an important role in understanding its etiology. An example of such a geographical, also called spatial, epidemiological study is the study on mortality from lip cancer among males in the former German Democratic Republic including Berlin (GDR). This area has been under surveillance since 1961 (Möhner *et al.* 1994). In 1989, 2342 deaths were recorded from lip cancer among males in 195 regions of GDR. For each region, the observed frequency of deaths, i.e. y_i, $(i = 1, \ldots, n = 195)$, was recorded and an expected count, e_i was calculated as follows. A reference population, in this case the whole of GDR, was split-up into age deciles. In each decile, the observed overall prevalence of lip cancer mortality among males was computed. The overall prevalence in each age decile was then multiplied with the population size of each region in the respective age decile. The sum of the products, i.e. e_i, is an estimate of the true count in that region if the risk of dying from lip cancer for a male were equal across all regions in GDR. The ratio $\text{SMR}_i = y_i/e_i$ is called the *standardized mortality rate* or *morbidity rate* in case the prevalence of a disease is examined. SMR_i is an estimate of the *true relative risk (RR)*, i.e. θ_i for mortality (or morbidity) in the ith region. In Figure 9.1(a), the histogram is shown of the standardized

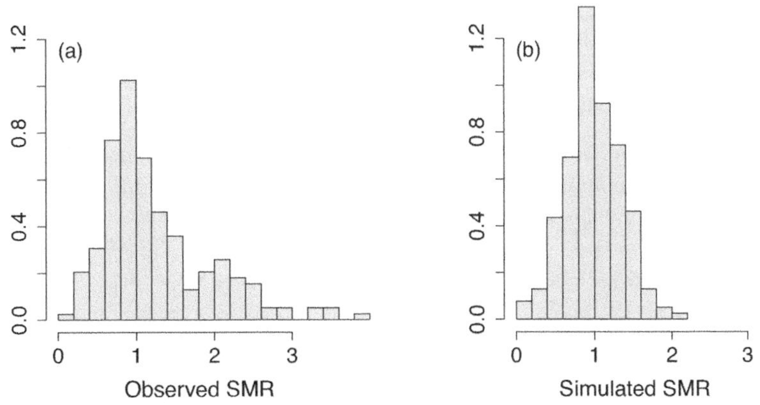

Figure 9.1 Lip cancer study: histogram of (a) observed SMRs and (b) simulated SMRs assuming that the 195 regions of GDR have the same risk.

mortality rate for lip cancer among males in GDR across the 195 regions. Since the reference population is internal (GDR), a region with $\theta_i > 1$ exhibits an increased risk for dying from lip cancer (compared to the overall GDR risk), while regions with $\theta_i \leq 1$ show no increased or even a decreased risk. Banuro (1999) applied a variety of spatial Bayesian models to these data. Here, we consider a simple BHM. □

SMRs could be displayed on a (geographical) map, called a *disease map*, to visually pinpoint regions with an increased risk for mortality (or morbidity). However, SMR_i is an unreliable estimate of θ_i for a relatively sparsely populated region and it is recommended to use a more stable estimate of θ_i for constructing the disease map. This robust estimate is based on a BHM, as will be seen now.

9.2.2 Model specification

The lip cancer-mortality data are clustered, i.e. the male subjects are clustered in the regions of GDR. What assumptions should we make on the regions? More specifically what is reasonable to assume about y_i and θ_i?

Example IX.2: Lip cancer study: Basic assumptions
The first level data are the mortality counts y_i. We assume that $y_i \sim \text{Poisson}(\theta_i\, e_i)$, $(i = 1, \ldots, n)$ and that given θ_i the y_i are independent. This implies that the males in each of the regions contribute independently to the observed counts. This is often a reasonable assumption but can be relaxed easily in a Bayesian context as will be seen in Section 9.5.

We can make (at least) three assumptions about the second level (latent) data, i.e. the regions and hence the θ_is:

A1: The n regions are unique, not related to each other. Under this assumption, information from region j on θ_j $(j \neq i)$ does not provide any information on θ_i implying that the maximum likelihood estimate (MLE) of θ_i is equal to SMR_i with asymptotic variance θ_i/e_i. In that case, SMR_i shows a high variability for a sparsely populated region (with small e_i) and the (Bayesian) estimate of θ_i depends only on y_i.

A2: The counts $y_1, y_2, \ldots, y_n$ are a simple random sample of GDR (or a super population) and hence each SMR_i estimates the same risk θ. Since the reference region (GDR) is internal, this means here that $\theta_1 = \ldots = \theta_n = \theta = 1$. For an external reference region, i.e. when $\theta \neq 1$, and under the Poisson assumption, the MLE of θ is $\sum_i y_i / \sum_i e_i$.

A3: The regions share some common environmental conditions, especially when they are close together geographically. For instance, climatological conditions, air pollution and life style do not change drastically when crossing the border of a region. This implies that the θ_is are related. To express this we assume that $\{\theta_1, \ldots, \theta_n\}$ is a random sample from $p(\theta \mid \cdot)$, which is called the prior distribution of θ_i.

The choice between assumptions A1 and A3 largely depends on subjective arguments. For instance, one could always argue that each region is unique. But, then one ignores that regions share the same climatological conditions, undergo to a large extent the same industrial pollution, and has inhabitants who exhibit roughly the same dietary behavior.

Assumption A2 can be tested statistically. Here, we verified this assumption informally using a simple simulation exercise. Namely, to verify assumption A2 for the lip cancer–mortality data we sampled counts using $y_i \sim \text{Poisson}(e_i)$ and plotted the sampled SMRs in Figure 9.1(b). A simple graphical inspection demonstrates that the observed SMRs show considerably more variation than the sampled ones, suggesting heterogeneity in the true RRs. Assumption A3 appears thus quite reasonable and will be made here. □

Assumption A3 is a compromise between A1 and A2 and implies that $\theta_1, \ldots, \theta_n$ have a common distribution $p(\theta \mid \boldsymbol{\psi})$, with $\boldsymbol{\psi}$ a vector of hyperparameters. Under this assumption the set $\boldsymbol{\theta} = \{\theta_1, \ldots, \theta_n\}$ is called exchangeable in the sense of Section 3.5. Further, subjects within regions are exchangeable but not between regions. Thus exchangeability is applied here on the two levels of the hierarchy. An implication of exchangeability is that θ_i are estimated using information from all regions. This phenomenon is called 'borrowing strength (from the other regions)'.

Having chosen assumption A3, which prior $p(\theta \mid \boldsymbol{\psi})$ should we take? A computationally convenient choice is the conjugate for the Poisson distribution, i.e. to assume that the θ_i are i.i.d. according to $\text{Gamma}(\alpha, \beta)$ $(i = 1, \ldots, n)$. Then the a priori mean and variance of the θ_is is α/β and α/β^2, respectively.

Without specifying a prior distribution for the hyperparameters α and β, the above model is a frequentist hierarchical model. In general, the choice of the hyperprior $p(\alpha, \beta)$ depends on our prior belief about the hyperparameters. Occasionally, historical data are available allowing to specify an informative prior, but often one chooses a vague prior. Upon the choice of the hyperprior the specification of the BHM is complete. The hierarchical structure of the model (and data) is shown in Figure 9.2. Note that the level-1 observations (y_i) are observed, while the level-2 (θ_i) observations are latent and thus unobserved. The Poisson-gamma model is a two-level hierarchical model with following levels:

- Level 1: $y_i \mid \theta_i \sim \text{Poisson}(\theta_i\, e_i)$ for $i = 1, \ldots, n$
- Level 2: $\theta_i \mid \alpha, \beta \sim \text{Gamma}(\alpha, \beta)$ for $i = 1, \ldots, n$
- Prior: $(\alpha, \beta) \sim p(\alpha, \beta)$

The distribution of θ_i is often referred to as a prior in the Bayesian literature, since in the paradigm there is no difference between parameters and latent random variables. However,

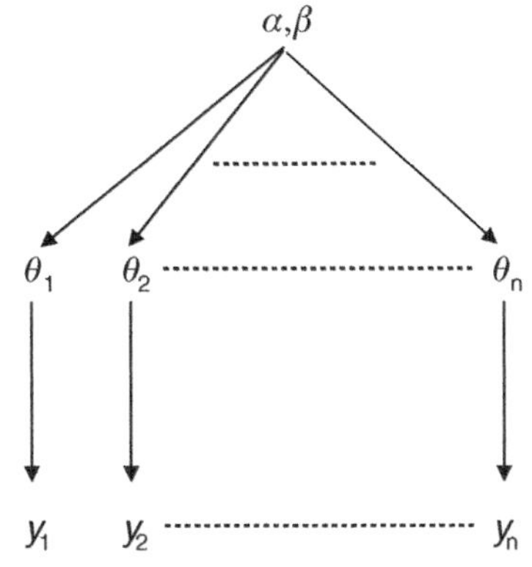

Figure 9.2 Lip cancer study: hierarchical structure in the data.

to emphasize the hierarchical structure of the data, we have put here (and will do so in the remainder of the book) this distribution as part of the model description.

The above Poisson-gamma model is inspired by the lip cancer study. In a more general setting, we may have m_i counts y_{ij} for each θ_i. In that case, the first level of the above two-level hierarchical model becomes

- Level 1: $y_{ij} \mid \theta_i \sim \text{Poisson}(\theta_i\, e_i)$ for $j = 1, \ldots, m_i;\ \ i = 1, \ldots, n$.

9.2.3 Posterior distributions

Based on the distributional assumptions made above, the posterior distribution can be derived. Let $\boldsymbol{y}$ represent the set of observed counts $\{y_1, \ldots, y_n\}$, then the joint posterior distribution is

$$p(\alpha, \beta, \boldsymbol{\theta} \mid \boldsymbol{y}) \propto \prod_{i=1}^{n} p(y_i \mid \theta_i, \alpha, \beta) \prod_{i=1}^{n} p(\theta_i \mid \alpha, \beta)\; p(\alpha, \beta).$$

By assuming that $y_i \sim \text{Poisson}(\theta_i\, e_i)$, we implicitly assume hierarchical independence for the counts, and thus,

$$p(\alpha, \beta, \boldsymbol{\theta} \mid \boldsymbol{y}) \propto \prod_{i=1}^{n} \frac{(\theta_i e_i)^{y_i}}{y_i!} \exp\left(-\theta_i e_i\right) \prod_{i=1}^{n} \frac{\beta^{\alpha}}{\Gamma(\alpha)} \theta_i^{\alpha-1}\, e^{-\beta\theta_i}\; p(\alpha, \beta). \tag{9.1}$$

A Gibbs sampling approach requires the determination of the full conditionals. In the following example, we chose independent exponential priors for the hyperparameters: $p(\alpha) = \lambda_\alpha \exp(-\lambda_\alpha \alpha)$ and $p(\beta) = \lambda_\beta \exp(-\lambda_\beta \beta)$. For this choice, the full conditionals are:

$$p(\theta_i \mid \boldsymbol{\theta}_{(i)}, \alpha, \beta, \boldsymbol{y}) \propto \theta_i^{y_i+\alpha-1} \exp\left[-(e_i + \beta)\theta_i\right] \;\; (i = 1, \ldots, n),$$

$$p(\alpha \mid \boldsymbol{\theta}, \beta, \boldsymbol{y}) \propto \frac{\left(\beta^n \prod \theta_i\right)^{\alpha-1}}{\Gamma(\alpha)^n} \exp(-\lambda_\alpha \alpha),$$

$$p(\beta \mid \boldsymbol{\theta}, \alpha, \boldsymbol{y}) \propto \beta^{n\alpha} \exp\left[-\left(\sum \theta_i + \lambda_\beta\right)\beta\right],$$

with $\boldsymbol{\theta}_{(i)}$ is equal to $\boldsymbol{\theta}$ without θ_i. The DAG of the Poisson-gamma model is given in Figure 9.4.

The first and third full conditionals are gamma distributions. The first gamma distribution follows from the fact that the gamma distribution is a conditional conjugate to the Poisson distribution. Clearly, $p(\theta_i \mid \boldsymbol{\theta}_{(i)}, \alpha, \beta, \mathbf{y}) \equiv p(\theta_i \mid \alpha, \beta, y_i)$ and hence, given the hyperparameters each such full conditional depends only on the count and the RR of the ith region. Note that also $p(\alpha \mid \boldsymbol{\theta}, \beta, \mathbf{y}) \equiv p(\alpha \mid \boldsymbol{\theta}, \beta)$ and $p(\beta \mid \boldsymbol{\theta}, \alpha, \mathbf{y}) \equiv p(\beta \mid \boldsymbol{\theta}, \alpha)$.

Instead of sampling from the full conditionals, a block sampling approach could also be implemented, alternating between (1) $\boldsymbol{\theta} \mid \alpha, \beta, \mathbf{y}$ and (2) $\alpha, \beta \mid \boldsymbol{\theta}, \mathbf{y}$. The conditional distribution of $\boldsymbol{\theta}$ is the product of n independent gamma distributions, so here sampling should be no problem. Sampling from $p(\alpha, \beta \mid \boldsymbol{\theta}, \mathbf{y})$ cannot be done with standard sampling algorithms, but a Gibbs sampler helps here (Exercise 9.3).

9.2.4 Estimating the parameters

Since α, β and $\boldsymbol{\theta}$ are estimated here using an MCMC approach, there is in principle no need to look for analytical expressions of the parameter estimates. Nevertheless, if such relationships exist they may give insight in the obtained MCMC estimates. For the Poisson-gamma model, some results can be derived:

- Since $p(\theta_i \mid \alpha, \beta, y_i) = \text{Gamma}(\alpha + y_i, \beta + e_i)$, the posterior mean of θ_i (given α and β) is equal to $E(\theta_i \mid \alpha, \beta, y_i) = (\alpha + y_i)/(\beta + e_i)$. It follows immediately that

$$\frac{\alpha + y_i}{\beta + e_i} = B_i \frac{\alpha}{\beta} + (1 - B_i)\frac{y_i}{e_i}, \tag{9.2}$$

  with $B_i = \beta/(\beta + e_i)$ a shrinkage factor that indicates how much the observed SMR_i is shrunk toward the overall mean by taking the posterior mean instead. This phenomenon is similar to what we have seen in Chapter 2.

- The marginal posterior distribution of θ_i is

$$p(\theta_i \mid \mathbf{y}) = \int p(\theta_i \mid \alpha, \beta, y_i) p(\alpha, \beta \mid \mathbf{y}) \, d\alpha \, d\beta, \tag{9.3}$$

  with $p(\alpha, \beta \mid \mathbf{y})$ given in expression (9.4). The shrinkage seen in (9.2) for a given α and β also applies marginalized over the posterior of these parameters. Hence, $\overline{\theta}_i$ is less extreme than the observed SMR_i and we say that there is *shrinkage* toward the overall mean.

- The marginal posterior distribution of α and β is

$$p(\alpha, \beta \mid \mathbf{y}) \propto \prod_{i=1}^{n} \frac{\Gamma(y_i + \alpha)}{\Gamma(\alpha) y_i!} \left(\frac{\beta}{\beta + e_i}\right)^{\alpha} \left(\frac{e_i}{\beta + e_i}\right)^{y_i} p(\alpha, \beta). \tag{9.4}$$

Note that only the posterior distribution $p(\theta_i \mid \alpha, \beta, y_i)$ can be determined analytically. The other posterior distributions and posterior summary measures must be calculated numerically. Besides MCMC techniques, other numerical approaches are possible here. For instance, Gelman *et al.* (2004) combined calculations on a grid for α and β with the Method of Composition for θ_i.

```
model
   {
   for( i in 1 : n ) {
 # Poisson likelihood for observed counts
   observe[i]~dpois(lambda[i]) ;  lambda[i] <- theta[i]*expect[i]
   smr[i] <- observe[i]/expect[i]
   theta[i] ~dgamma(alpha,beta)
 # Shrinkage factor
   B[i] <- beta/(beta +  expect[i])
 # Distribution of future observed counts from region i
   predict[i]  ~ dpois(lambda[i])
   }
 # Distribution of future observed counts for a particular
expected count  100
   theta.new  ~dgamma(alpha,beta); lambda.new <- theta.new*100
   predict.new  ~ dpois(lambda.new)
 # Prior distributions for "population" parameters
   alpha ~ dexp(0.1); beta ~  dexp(0.1)
 # Population mean and population variance
   mtheta <- alpha/beta; vartheta <- alpha/pow(beta,2);
sdtheta <- sqrt(vartheta)
   }
```

Figure 9.3 Lip cancer study: WinBUGS program.

Example IX.3: Lip cancer study: A WinBUGS analysis

In Figure 9.3, we show part of the WinBUGS program for analyzing the lip cancer mortality data corresponding to the model developed above; see the file 'chapter 9 lip cancer PG.odc'. The vague prior for the hyperparameters was taken as a product of two exponential distributions, namely, $p(\alpha, \beta) = 0.1 \exp(-0.1\alpha) \times 0.1 \exp(-0.1\beta)$. One can verify that WinBUGS employs the gamma sampler for the θ_i and β nodes, while adaptive rejection sampling is used for the α node (see Section 8.1.2).

Three chains of size 10 000 iterations were initiated. The BGR plots in WinBUGS showed quick convergence despite that the autocorrelation for the hyperparameters α and β was around 0.5 for lag 20. The θ_is were sampled basically in an independent manner. Exporting the chains to CODA allowed to apply a battery of convergence diagnostics. The overall Geweke test was significant for chain 1. For all chains the dynamic Geweke plot showed several excursions outside the boundaries of -2 and 2. On the other hand, Heidelberger–Welch tests were passed for all chains and for both α as well as β. As an extra check we ran a further 10 000 iterations but the parameter estimates remained basically the same.

The posterior summary measures shown in Table 9.1 were based on iterations 5001–10 000. The average of the θ_is was estimated as 1.19, accurately determined (Monte Carlo error = 7.557E−4). The estimated standard deviation of the θ_is is about 0.5 indicating the variability of the true risks. Highest posterior density (HPD) intervals were computed in CODA and we obtained for α [4.275, 7.692] as 95% HPD interval and [4.373, 7.814] as 95% equal tail interval.

A disease map based on the posterior mean $\overline{\theta}_i$ yields a less ragged graph than a disease map based on SMR_i. WinBUGS computes the posterior summary measures of the node θ if

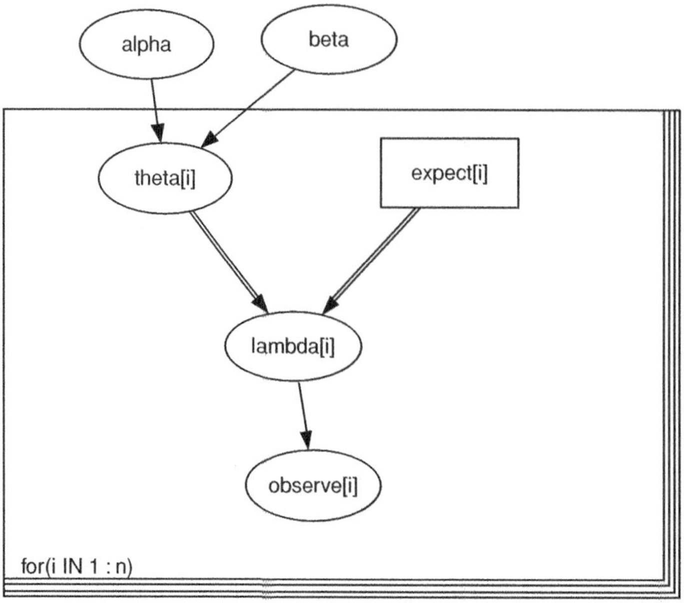

Figure 9.4 Lip cancer study: DAG for the Poisson-gamma model created by the Doodle option in WinBUGS; see Figure 9.3 for an explanation of the nodes.

monitored (via 'Sample Monitor Tool'). WinBUGS also allows a graphical inspection of the θ_is, using a box plot or a caterpillar plot (Option 'Inference > Comparison Tool'). In Figure 9.5, a caterpillar plot is shown of $\overline{\theta}_1, \ldots, \overline{\theta}_{30}$ together with the respective 95% equal-tail CIs. One could also plot the posterior estimates in a disease map of GDR. This can be done using the option **Map** but only when the map of GDR has been imported in WinBUGS. More on spatial models can be found in Chapter 16.

To illustrate the shrinkage effect we show in Figure 9.6(a) a scatterplot of $\overline{\theta}_i$ versus SMR_i. Clearly, the $\overline{\theta}_i$s show less variability and are shrunk toward the overall posterior mean. The shrinkage factor B_i is obtained from `B[i] <- beta/(beta+expect[i])`. The plot of the posterior mean of B_i versus $\log(e_i)$ is shown in Figure 9.6(b). This graph shows that there is more shrinkage when the expected count is low. In that case, the estimate of the risk very much depends on the global average and thus on all other regions. This is the meaning of 'borrowing strength'.

Table 9.1 Lip cancer study: posterior summary measures obtained from an analysis based on the WinBUGS program of Figure 9.3.

Node	Mean	sd	MC error	2.5%	Median	97.5%	Start	sample
Alpha	5.844	0.8656	0.04197	4.325	5.786	7.712	5001	15000
Beta	4.91	0.7728	0.03763	3.563	4.861	6.573	5001	15000
mtheta	1.193	0.04556	7.557E-4	1.107	1.191	1.287	5001	15000
sdtheta	0.4976	0.04384	0.002051	0.4194	0.4951	0.5906	5001	15000
vartheta	0.2496	0.04443	0.002071	0.1759	0.2451	0.3488	5001	15000

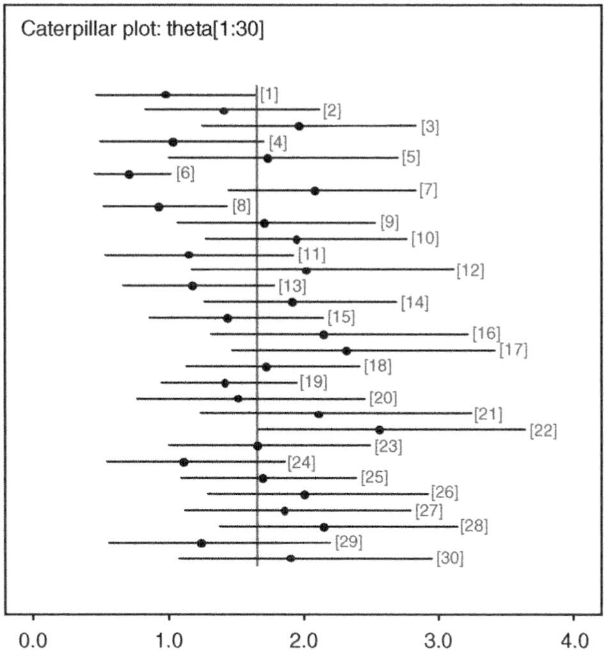

Figure 9.5 Lip cancer study: posterior estimates of $\theta_1, \ldots, \theta_{30}$ (caterpillar plot) obtained from the WinBUGS program of Figure 9.3.

In Section 9.5.7, we explain that care is needed in choosing the hyperprior for the variance parameter of a Gaussian hierarchical model. Therefore, we have taken here two alternative hyperpriors as a sensitivity analysis. Namely, we have also considered (1) independent uniform priors on the interval [0,100] for α and β and (2) the product of a N(0, 10^3) prior for the mean α/β and an IG(10^{-3}, 10^{-3}) prior for the variance α/β^2 of the θ_is. No material differences were observed, though.

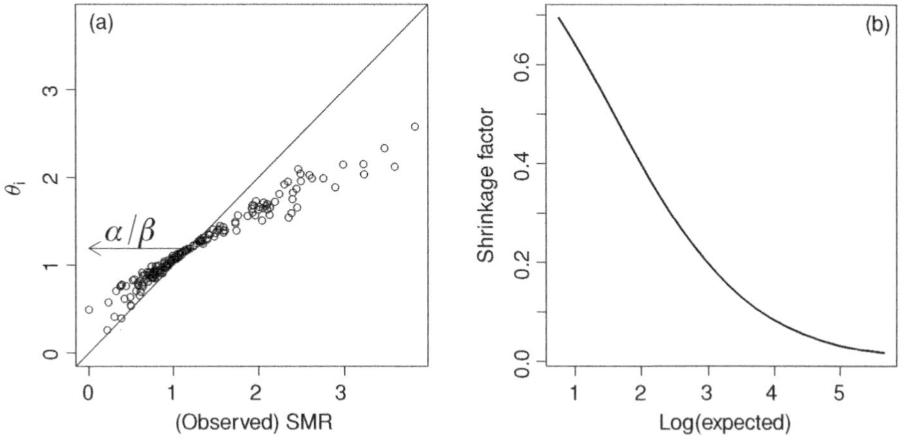

Figure 9.6 Lip cancer study: (a) posterior mean of θ_i versus SMR$_i$, marginal mean = posterior mean of α/β, and (b) shrinkage factor versus the logarithm of the expected counts.

We now look at the Bayesian solutions under assumptions A1 and A2. To analyze the lip cancer data in WinBUGS under assumption A1, we need to express that all regions are unique. This can be accomplished by replacing the distributional assumption on the θ_is by `theta[i] ~ dunif(0,100)` and removing the commands that pertain to the hyperparameters α and β. The posterior means of the θ_is were close to the observed SMRs, a reflection that there is no 'borrowing of strength'. Under assumption A2, the RRs of the different regions estimate a common θ equal to one since the expected counts are based on the whole of former East Germany. The WinBUGS program under A2 requires two changes, i.e. `lambda[i] <- theta*expect[i]` and the prior for θ, i.e. `theta ~ dunif(0,100)` is specified outside the inner loop. We obtained 0.95 as posterior mean for θ. □

The lip cancer data were also analyzed with SAS procedure MCMC version 9.3. Some of the commands and options were explained and illustrated in Chapter 8 except for the RANDOM statement. The RANDOM statement declares a symbol as the random effect, but internally, PROC MCMC generates a vector of random-effects parameters, whose names are created by concatenating the symbol and values in the SUBJECT = variable. However, as the symbol appears in the program, PROC MCMC knows which of the random-effects parameters that it should use and replaces it accordingly. Further, the RANDOM statement declares distributions on the random effects parameters and it is equivalent to a for-loop in WinBUGS over an array of random effects parameters. With the RANDOM statement there is no need for the user to figure out the levels of the clustering (which is handled by the SUBJECT= field) and the cluster membership does not need to be indexed numerically (from 1 to N) as required in WinBUGS. Once the symbol (in the RANDOM statement) enters the program, the symbol is automatically associated with the correct random effects parameter according to the clustering-membership. This is equivalent to the `u[index[i]]` business in WinBUGS, where `u[]` is the array that holds all random effects parameters (declared outside of the data for-loop), `index` is a data set variable that declares cluster membership and `i` is used in the data-level loop.

Example IX.4: Lip cancer study: A SAS analysis

Figure 9.7 contains the program to analyze the lip cancer mortality data with SAS procedure MCMC version 9.3. The option `subject=index` specifies the variable that indexes the random effect, here `theta`. The option `monitor=(theta_1 - theta_10)` asks for posterior summary and diagnostics (in addition to the plots) for the first ten θ-values. This

```
proc mcmc data=lipcancer outpost=lipout nmc=15000 nbi=15000 seed=7;
parms alpha beta;
random theta ~ gamma(shape=alpha,iscale=beta) subject=index
monitor=(theta_1 - theta_10);
prior alpha beta: ~ expon(iscale=0.1);
mu = e * theta;
model o ~ poisson(mu);
run;
/* the CATER autocall macro produces caterpillar plot */
%cater(data=lipout, var=theta_:);
```

Figure 9.7 Lip cancer study: SAS procedure MCMC version 9.3.

output is automatically generated for the parameters α and β. Finally, the built-in macro `%cater` generates a caterpillar plot for θ. The statement `theta_` in the `%cater` macro is a shorthand notation for all variable(s names) that start with `theta_` in the DATA= data set (which is `lipout`). The program can be found in 'chapter 9 lipcancer PG.sas'.

PROC MCMC does not allow for multiple chains. To be compatible with the previous WinBUGS run, we therefore initiated one run of 30 000 iterations of which 15 000 iterations served as burn-in. The parameters α and β were sampled in one block using a Normal Metropolis updater. The random effects were sampled with a univariate Normal Metropolis sampler. For α and β the Geweke diagnostic was significant. So we increased `nmc` to 30 000 to achieve convergence. The posterior mean (SD) for α and β were 5.84 (0.89) and 4.91 (0.79), respectively. The 95% equal tail and HPD intervals are automatically provided by PROC MCMC. They are equal to [4.2462, 7.7176] and [4.1104, 7.5102] for α, while for β they are [3.4930, 6.6245] and [3.3268, 6.4110]. For all monitored parameters the MCerror was smaller than 5% of the posterior SD. Due to the relative high autocorrelation for both hyperparameters (around 0.5 for lag = 10) the relative efficiency was relatively low (around 700) for both parameters.

Finally, we note that the 9.2 version of procedure MCMC was hopelessly inefficient for hierarchical models. Indeed, the previous version of PROC MCMC did not distinguish fixed from random effects and hence did not capitalize on the conditional independence in the Poisson-gamma model. This is a nice illustration of the importance of (not) exploiting the specific characteristics in the data and the consequences this may have on the performance of the algorithm. □

9.2.5 Posterior predictive distributions

We now wish to predict future counts from a Poisson-gamma model in the light of the observed counts $\mathbf{y}$. We consider two cases. In the first case, our interest is to predict the future count of males dying from lip cancer in one of the 195 regions. In the second case, we wish to predict lip cancer mortality for new regions not considered before. In both cases some kind of exchangeability is assumed of the future counts with the observed counts. The basic theory of Bayesian prediction has been introduced in Section 3.4.2.

Example IX.5: Lip cancer study: Posterior predictive distributions
Suppose we wish to predict the number of males dying from lip cancer in the ith ($1 \le i \le 195$) region with expected count $\widetilde{e}_i$. For this calculation, we assume that the future count $\widetilde{y}_i$ is exchangeable with the current y_i given the expected count. This prediction involves the computation of $p(\widetilde{y}_i \mid \mathbf{y})$, which is the posterior predictive distribution (PPD) for the ith response. By applying hierarchical independence, the PPD is equal to

$$p(\widetilde{y}_i \mid \mathbf{y}) = \int_\alpha \int_\beta \int_{\theta_i} p(\widetilde{y}_i \mid \theta_i)\, p(\theta_i \mid \alpha, \beta, \mathbf{y})\, p(\alpha, \beta \mid \mathbf{y})\, d\theta_i\, d\alpha\, d\beta, \tag{9.5}$$

with $p(\widetilde{y}_i \mid \theta_i) = \text{Poisson}(\widetilde{y}_i \mid \theta_i \widetilde{e}_i)$, $p(\theta_i \mid \alpha, \beta, \mathbf{y}) = \text{Gamma}(\theta_i \mid \alpha + y_i, \beta + \widetilde{e}_i)$ and $p(\alpha, \beta \mid \mathbf{y})$ given by expression (9.4). There is no analytical solution to the above integral but sampling can help here. For instance, we could sample from $p(\widetilde{y}_i, \theta_i, \alpha, \beta \mid \mathbf{y})$ and retain only the sampled $\widetilde{y}_i$s. This can be done as in Section 4.6 using independent sampling algorithms, i.e. sample first from $p(\alpha, \beta \mid \mathbf{y})$, then sample from $p(\theta_i \mid \alpha, \beta, \mathbf{y})$ and finally sample from $p(\widetilde{y}_i \mid \theta_i)$. The last two sampling exercises involve standard distributions.

Sampling α and β could be done from a discrete approximation on a grid as in Gelman *et al.* (2004).

Sampling the PPD with expression (9.5) is done here using WinBUGS. The PPD for the ith region is obtained from the command `predict[i] ~ dpois(lambda[i])`. This results for region 1 ($y_1 = 5, e_1 = 6$) in a posterior mean (SD) for $\tilde{y}_1$ of 6.0 (3.0), while for region 195 ($y_{195} = 110, e_{195} = 288$), we obtained 114.0 (15.4) or $\tilde{y}_{195}$. In both cases, the predicted count appears close to the observed count, but a different story emerges when looking at the differences in a relative manner. Namely, the regions with the smallest expected counts have the largest relative differences with a maximal value for region 184 with an observed count of 0 and a predicted count of 3.5. Note that the comparison of $\widetilde{y}_i$ with y_i ($i = 1, \ldots, n$) delivers a goodness-of-fit test for the model (see also Section 10.3.4).

For the second case of prediction, imagine that we wish to predict male lip cancer mortality in regions of former West Germany. Hereby, we need to assume that the regions of the two parts of Germany are exchangeable. In that case, we assume that the RR of the new region belongs to the same (gamma) distribution as that of the 195 original regions. The PPD for $\widetilde{y}$ with expected count $\widetilde{e}$ becomes

$$p(\widetilde{y} \mid \mathbf{y}) = \int_{\alpha} \int_{\beta} \int_{\widetilde{\theta}} p(\widetilde{y} \mid \widetilde{\theta})\, p(\widetilde{\theta} \mid \alpha, \beta)\, p(\alpha, \beta \mid \mathbf{y})\, \mathrm{d}\widetilde{\theta}\, \mathrm{d}\alpha\, \mathrm{d}\beta, \tag{9.6}$$

with now $p(\widetilde{y} \mid \widetilde{\theta}) = \text{Poisson}(\widetilde{y} \mid \widetilde{\theta}\, \widetilde{e})$, $p(\widetilde{\theta} \mid \alpha, \beta, \mathbf{y}) = \text{Gamma}(\widetilde{\theta} \mid \alpha, \beta)$ and $p(\alpha, \beta \mid \mathbf{y})$ again given by expression (9.4). Note that the distribution of $\widetilde{\theta}$ depends indirectly on the past data via the marginal posterior of α and β.

Sampling PPD (9.6) can again be done using the Method of Composition, but we chose here for WinBUGS since it involves only the addition of three extra statements:

```
theta.new ~ dgamma(alpha,beta)
lambda.new <- theta.new*100
predict.new ~ dpois(lambda.new)
```

For $\widetilde{e} = 100$, we obtained for $\widetilde{y}$ as posterior mean (SD) 118.8 (50.7) and posterior median 111. □

Also in SAS, only one statement needs to be added to obtain predicted values based on the PPD. With `preddist outpred=lout;` one requests the predicted values and store these in a work file called 'lout'; see file 'chapter 9 lipcancer PG.sas'.

9.3 Full versus empirical Bayesian approach

The Bayesian analysis in Section 9.2 is sometimes referred to as a *Full Bayesian (FB) analysis* to contrast it with an *Empirical Bayesian (EB) analysis*. EB estimation is a classical frequentist approach to estimate (functions of) the 'random effects' (level-2 observations) in a hierarchical context; see Carlin and Louis (2009) for an extensive treatment of the EB approach. Here, we exemplify its use in the Poisson-gamma case with the lip cancer data and show the difference with the FB approach.

An Empirical Bayesian analysis of the lip cancer mortality data requires the marginal maximum likelihood estimate of α and β, which is obtained by integrating out the θ_is from the likelihood. The marginal likelihood is expression (9.4) with a flat prior distribution for α and β, i.e. $p(\alpha, \beta) \propto c$. The value of (α, β) that maximizes (9.4) denoted $(\overline{\alpha}_{EB}, \overline{\beta}_{EB})$ is called a *marginal maximum likelihood estimate* (MMLE). In a second step, $\overline{\alpha}_{EB}$ and $\overline{\beta}_{EB}$ are plugged-in the expression of the posterior distribution for the RRs of the regions. Then $p(\theta_i \mid \overline{\alpha}_{EB}, \overline{\beta}_{EB}, y_i) = \text{Gamma}(\overline{\alpha}_{EB} + y_i, \overline{\beta}_{EB} + e_i)$ delivers all posterior summary measures for θ_i $(i = 1, \ldots, n)$. The parameters α and β of the gamma distribution are thus in the EB approach fixed to $\overline{\alpha}_{EB}$ and $\overline{\beta}_{EB}$, respectively. Since the hyperparameters are estimated from the empirical results (data), these posterior summary measures are called *Empirical Bayes* estimates. Bayesians' criticism to the Empirical Bayesian approach is that the hyperparameters are estimated from the data. Fixing the hyperparameters to their MMLEs in the subsequent calculations implies that a part of the uncertainty in the parameter estimation is ignored. We now contrast the FB and EB estimates of θ_i and their 95% credible intervals for the lip cancer data.

Example IX.6: Lip cancer study: Empirical Bayes analysis
We obtained $\overline{\alpha}_{EB} = 5.66$ and $\overline{\beta}_{EB} = 4.81$ giving an EB estimate for the mean of the θ_is equal to 1.18, which is close to the FB estimate of 1.19 (Table 9.1). The FB (posterior mean) and EB estimates of the individual θ_is (point and interval estimates) differ only slightly here. We then restricted the analysis to the first 30 regions. To better compare the FB results with the EB results, we used a flat prior on [0, 100] for α and β (then MLE $\approx$ posterior mode). The posterior mean (median) for α and β were 9.74 (8.67) and 4.87 (4.30) which are now somewhat greater than the corresponding EB estimates equal to 7.30 and 3.62, respectively. The point and interval estimates for the FB and the EB estimates are shown in Figure 9.8. While, the FB and EB 95% CIs are not too different, the FB posterior SDs were all larger than the corresponding EB posterior SDs. □

Note that bootstrapping is the frequentist approach of taking into account the sampling variability of the MMLE (Biggeri *et al.* 1993). But the Bayesian way of incorporating the

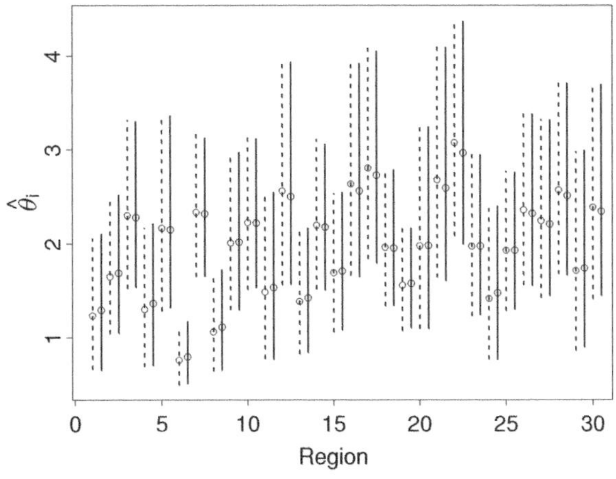

Figure 9.8 Lip cancer study: comparison of Full Bayesian posterior median with Empirical Bayesian estimate of θ_i and 95% credible interval based on analyzing first 30 regions (solid line = FB and dashed line = EB).

parameter uncertainty is more natural and immediately available as a byproduct of the sampling algorithm.

The main reason for choosing the Poisson-gamma model was that it gives insight into the estimation of the model parameters. However, in practice this is not sufficient as a motivation. In Section 9.5.5, other priors for the θ_is than the gamma are considered. But these priors are still not sufficient to adequately model the mortality data, since they do not model the spatial correlation among the θ_is. This means that the correlation among the θs which correspond to regions closer in distance should be greater than for θs further away. We address extensions of the Poisson-gamma model in Section 9.5.5, but spatial models are deferred to Chapter 16.

9.4 Gaussian hierarchical models

9.4.1 Introduction

A Gaussian hierarchical model is a hierarchical model whereby the distribution at each level is Gaussian. We examine here the case of a *variance component model*, also called a *random effects model*, i.e. when no covariates are involved. When fixed effects (covariates) are also involved, one speaks of a *linear mixed model*.

The Bayesian version of the Gaussian hierarchical model is known as the *Bayesian linear model*. The seminal papers by Lindley and Smith (Lindley (1971), Lindley and Smith (1972), Smith (1973b) and Smith (1973a)) are the basis of the current Bayesian Gaussian hierarchical approach. In fact, expression (9.8) was first derived by Lindley (1971) and generalized in subsequent papers. We illustrate the derivations on this class of hierarchical models using the dietary Inter-regional Belgian Bank Employee Nutrition Study (IBBENS) introduced in Section 2.7.

9.4.2 The Gaussian hierarchical model

The two-level Bayesian Gaussian hierarchical model makes the following distributional assumptions:

- Level 1: $y_{ij} \mid \theta_i, \sigma^2 \sim \mathrm{N}(\theta_i, \sigma^2)$ for $j = 1, \ldots, m_i$; $i = 1, \ldots, n$
- Level 2: $\theta_i \mid \mu, \sigma_\theta^2 \sim \mathrm{N}(\mu, \sigma_\theta^2)$ for $i = 1, \ldots, n$
- Priors: $\sigma^2 \sim p(\sigma^2)$ and $(\mu, \sigma_\theta^2) \sim p(\mu, \sigma_\theta^2)$

The hyperparameters μ and σ_θ^2 are usually taken independent a priori, such that $p(\mu, \sigma_\theta^2) = p(\mu)p(\sigma_\theta^2)$. An alternative model formulation is $\theta_i = \mu + \alpha_i$, with $\alpha_i \sim \mathrm{N}(0, \sigma_\theta^2)$. Note that we need to specify a prior for σ^2 too. The choice of the hyperprior $p(\mu, \sigma_\theta^2)$ will be addressed later. Suppose $\boldsymbol{y} = \{y_{ij}, j = 1, \ldots, m_i; i = 1, \ldots, n\}$ and $\boldsymbol{\theta} = \{\theta_1, \ldots, \theta_n\}$ then, based on the above distributional assumptions, the joint posterior distribution is

$$p(\boldsymbol{\theta}, \sigma^2, \mu, \sigma_\theta^2 \mid \boldsymbol{y}) \propto \prod_{i=1}^{n} \prod_{j=1}^{m_i} \mathrm{N}(y_{ij} \mid \theta_i, \sigma^2) \prod_{i=1}^{n} \mathrm{N}(\theta_i \mid \mu, \sigma_\theta^2)\; p(\sigma^2)\; p(\mu, \sigma_\theta^2). \tag{9.7}$$

Hierarchical independence of the y_{ij} and the hyperparameters is again assumed which means that, given θ_i and σ^2, the distribution of y_{ij} does not depend on μ and σ_θ^2.

9.4.3 Estimating the parameters

As for the Poisson-gamma model, it is insightful to know how the θ_i and the hyperparameters are estimated from the data and how shrinkage applies here. To this end, we fixed σ^2, which allows to relate the results obtained here with the results of Section 2.7, i.e. with expression (2.13). In addition, when fixing σ^2, the joint posterior depends on the observed data only via the n sample means $\overline{y}_i$ of y_{ij} ($j = 1, \ldots, m_i$). Let $\sigma_i^2 = \sigma^2/m_i$ denote the variance of the ith sample mean, then using a similar approach as in Section 2.7 the posterior of θ_i given μ and σ_θ^2 (and also σ^2 and the data) is $\mathrm{N}(\overline{\theta}_i, \overline{\sigma}_{\theta_i}^2)$ with

$$\overline{\theta}_i = \frac{\frac{1}{\sigma_\theta^2}\mu + \frac{1}{\sigma_i^2}\overline{y}_i}{\frac{1}{\sigma_\theta^2} + \frac{1}{\sigma_i^2}} \quad \text{and} \quad \overline{\sigma}_{\theta_i}^2 = \frac{1}{\frac{1}{\sigma_\theta^2} + \frac{1}{\sigma_i^2}}. \tag{9.8}$$

The above result shows that $\overline{\theta}_i = B_i\mu + (1 - B_i)\overline{y}_i$, with B_i a shrinkage factor equal to $B_i = \frac{1}{\sigma_\theta^2} / \left(\frac{1}{\sigma_\theta^2} + \frac{1}{\sigma_i^2}\right)$. Shrinkage is, therefore, large for the ith cluster when m_i is relatively small. In that case the posterior uncertainty for θ_i measured by $\overline{\sigma}_{\theta_i}$ is much smaller than when based on only the data of the ith cluster alone. Moreover, when $\sigma_\theta \to \infty$ then $\overline{\theta}_i \to \overline{y}_i$. The shrinkage factor is also related to the *intraclass correlation* defined as $ICC = \frac{\sigma_\theta^2}{\sigma_\theta^2 + \sigma^2}$. Because $B_i = \sigma^2/(\sigma^2 + m_i\sigma_\theta^2)$ shrinkage will be relatively large for a low ICC especially when m_i is small.

For a flat prior on μ and conditional on σ_θ^2 and σ^2, it can be shown (Gelman *et al.*, 2004) that the posterior of μ marginalized over the distribution of the θ_is is $\mathrm{N}(\overline{\mu}, \overline{\sigma}_\mu^2)$ with

$$\overline{\mu} = \frac{\sum_{i=1}^n \frac{1}{\sigma_i^2 + \sigma_\theta^2}\overline{y}_i}{\sum_{i=1}^n \frac{1}{\sigma_i^2 + \sigma_\theta^2}} \quad \text{and} \quad \overline{\sigma}_\mu^2 = \sum_{i=1}^n \frac{1}{\sigma_i^2 + \sigma_\theta^2},$$

which shows that the posterior mean $\overline{\mu}$ is dominated by the large clusters.

Example IX.7: Dietary study: A comparison of cholesterol intake between subsidiaries with WinBUGS

One of the aims of the IBBENS was to examine the variability in food habits between employees of the eight subsidiaries and to relate this to mortality rates of the corresponding regions. Here, we contrast the variability of cholesterol intake (*chol*) in mg/day between the subsidiaries to the variability within the subsidiaries. There was some deviation from normality for *chol* in each subsidiary (significant Shapiro–Wilk normality test), but the normal probability plots were fairly straight and hence we worked under the assumption of normality. In Table 9.2, the observed means of *chol* per subsidiary are given.

We fitted a Bayesian–Gaussian hierarchical model to the cholesterol-intake data of the 8 subsidiaries using the WinBUGS program 'chapter 9 dietary study chol.odc'. Figure 9.9 shows the DAG of the model from which the assumption of hierarchical independence can be inferred. The following priors were chosen: $\mu \sim \mathrm{N}(0, 10^6)$, $\sigma^2 \sim \mathrm{IG}(10^{-3}, 10^{-3})$ and $\sigma_\theta \sim \mathrm{U}(0, 100)$. For a motivation of the variance priors, consult Section 9.5.7. We initiated three chains each of size 10 000. The BGR diagnostic in WinBUGS indicated convergence almost instantly. We then exported the chain values to CODA and applied the whole battery of tests. There were numerical problems in computing the Geweke test (often happened in

Table 9.2 Dietary study: observed mean (SE) and standard deviation (SD) of cholesterol intake per sub(sidiary).

Sub	m_i	Mean (SE)	SD	FBW (SD)	FBS (SD)	EML (SE)	EREML (SE)
1	82	301.5 (10.2)	92.1	311.8 (12.6)	312.0 (12.0)	313.8 (10.3)	312.2 (11.3)
2	51	324.7 (17.1)	122.1	326.4 (12.7)	326.6 (12.7)	327.0 (11.7)	326.7 (12.3)
3	71	342.3 (13.6)	114.5	336.8 (11.7)	336.6 (11.7)	335.6 (10.7)	336.4 (11.6)
4	71	332.5 (13.5)	113.9	330.8 (11.6)	330.9 (11.5)	330.6 (10.7)	330.8 (11.6)
5	62	351.5 (19.0)	150.0	341.2 (12.8)	341.3 (12.6)	339.5 (11.1)	340.9 (11.8)
6	69	292.8 (12.8)	106.4	307.3 (14.2)	307.8 (13.5)	310.7 (10.8)	308.4 (11.6)
7	74	337.7 (14.1)	121.3	334.1 (11.4)	334.2 (11.2)	333.4 (10.6)	333.9 (11.5)
8	83	347.1 (14.5)	132.2	340.0 (11.4)	340.0 (11.4)	338.8 (10.2)	340.0 (11.2)

Notes: FBW (SD), FBS (SD) is the posterior mean (posterior SD) obtained from a Full Bayesian analysis using WinBUGS, SAS® Proc MIXED, respectively. EML (SE) is the posterior mean (standard error) calculated using a maximum likelihood Empirical Bayesian approach. EREML (SE) is the posterior mean (standard error) calculated using a restricted maximum likelihood Empirical Bayesian approach.

other examples too). But for all other tests convergence was confirmed. Therefore, we based the posterior summary measures on the last 5000 iterations.

The posterior mean of μ is equal to 328.3 with posterior SD = 9.44. The posterior median of σ is 119.5 and for σ_θ we obtained 18.26. The posterior means of θ_i for $(i = 1, \ldots, 8)$ are shown in Table 9.2. From these values, one can infer that the group means do not vary much

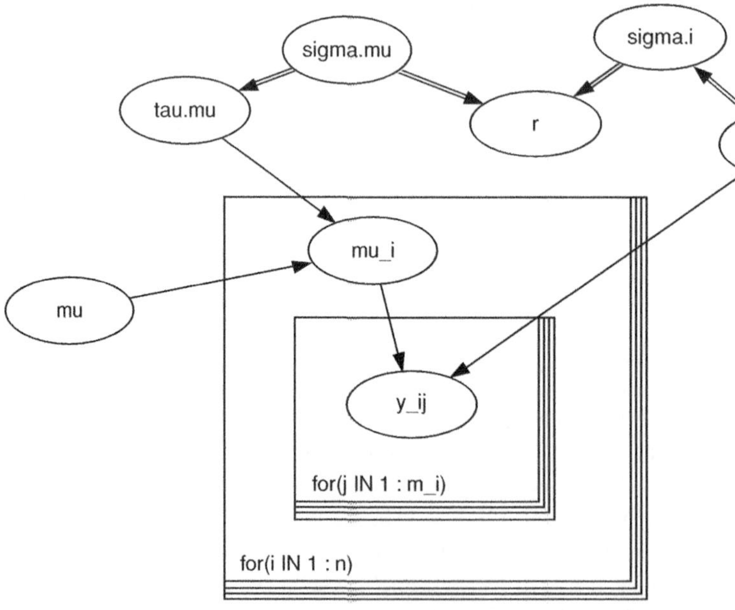

Figure 9.9 Dietary study: DAG for the Bayesian Gaussian hierarchical model created by the Doodle option in WinBUGS. The nodes theta.i, sigma.i, sigma.mu, tau.mu, and r correspond to θ_i, σ, $1/\sigma_\theta^2$, σ_θ and ICC, respectively.

```
proc mixed data=d.dietary;
class subsidiary;
model chol = / s;
random intercept/subject=subsidiary s;
prior jeffreys / nsample=30000  seed=34875770 out=sample;
run;
```

Figure 9.10 Dietary study: SAS PROC MIXED program.

relative to the within-subsidiary variability. Consequently, the ICC is rather low, with posterior median 0.022. Finally, the posterior medians of B_i $(i = 1, \ldots, 8)$ vary between 0.33 and 0.45 showing a relatively uniform and moderate shrinkage toward the overall mean, primarily because all m_i are relatively large. □

The analysis in Example IX.7 is based on assumption A3. We leave it to the reader to perform the Bayesian analysis under assumptions A1 and A2 (Exercise 9.5).

While the SAS procedure MIXED is primarily used for maximum likelihood estimation in a frequentist context, recently it also allows for a Bayesian approach. We applied the Bayesian option on the dietary study.

Example IX.8: Dietary study: A comparison of cholesterol intake between subsidiaries with SAS

The SAS procedure MIXED has an option PRIOR that requests for a Bayesian analysis of the data. In Figure 9.10 (chapter 9 dietary study chol.sas), we show the statements to perform a Bayesian Gaussian hierarchical analysis on the cholesterol data. The default prior for the variance parameters is Jeffreys but can be explicitly requested by adding the option 'Jeffreys'. Other priors are 'flat' corresponding to a uniform distribution, or 'data= ' when the prior is determined from historical data. Different sampling algorithms (importance sampling, rejection sampling and random walk) are available, but the default sampler is the independent Metropolis–Hastings algorithm with a proposal density matched to the posterior. Various options are available. In Figure 9.10, we request a chain of size 30 000 and export the sampled values to the file 'sample'. In Table 9.2, we provide the posterior mean (SD) of the subsidiary means. Clearly, the two Bayesian programs (WinBUGS and MIXED) yield similar results. Note that the acceptance rate was 0.98 as desired (see Section 6.3.4). □

9.4.4 Posterior predictive distributions

We now determine the distribution of cholesterol intake of a future bank employee. As for the Poisson-gamma model, we consider two cases: (1) the bank employee works in one of the eight subsidiaries or (2) the bank employee works in a new subsidiary from the same bank. In both cases, the PPD is required and similar computations as in expressions (9.5) and (9.6) are required (Exercise 9.6). No closed expressions are available and hence we used MCMC techniques to establish the PPDs.

Example IX.9: Dietary study: Posterior predictive distributions using WinBUGS

There are extra commands needed to produce (1) the PPD of an individual new value as well as the average of 82 new observations from the first subsidiary and (2) the PPD of observations from a new subsidiary (both individual values as well as average of (nnew=) 82 observations). These commands are found in the WinBUGS file mentioned above. The posterior predictive mean (SD) of the average of the 1st subsidiary is 312.2 (18) while for the average of 82 observations from a new subsidiary it is 328.6 (27.39). Clearly, the predictive means are close to the posterior means (which should be the case) but they have a considerable higher SD. □

9.4.5 Comparison of FB and EB approach

For the EB approach, we first determined the marginal likelihood in μ and σ_θ^2 and then computed the MMLEs. Given the MMLEs the estimates of $\overline{\theta}_i$ are established as posterior means. When fixing σ^2, we have seen above that analytical expressions are available that express the $\overline{\theta}_i$ as a weighted sum of the overall mean and the sample means. For σ^2 unknown, no explicit expressions are available. We have used the SAS procedure MIXED in Example IX.10 to estimate the $\overline{\theta}_i$ using an EB approach. In the frequentist literature, the estimates are referred to as *EBLUP estimates*, where EBLUP stands for Empirical Best Linear Unbiased Prediction (Carlin and Louis 2009).

Example IX.10: Dietary study: An EB analysis with SAS PROC MIXED
The SAS procedure MIXED delivers maximum likelihood (ML) and restricted maximum likelihood (REML) estimates for Gaussian hierarchical models. The estimated random effects are EBLUP estimates either based on ML or on REML. In Table 9.2, we can see that the frequentist and Bayesian estimates of $\overline{\theta}_i$ are close, but also that the Bayesian posterior SDs obtained exceed the corresponding EB posterior SDs. We return to the comparison of the frequentist and the Bayesian solution in Example IX.22. □

9.5 Mixed models

9.5.1 Introduction

In this section, we explore a variety of Bayesian mixed models. First we show that the Bayesian–Gaussian hierarchical model is a special case of the *BLMM*. An important and rich class of BHMs is given by the *Bayesian generalized linear mixed models (BGLMMs)*. The extension is based on the generalized linear model (GLIM) introduced in Section 4.8. We illustrate the BGLMM for binary and count responses. However, the Poisson-gamma model is a particular case of another extension of GLIM to hierarchical data, which will be illustrated here. Finally, we end this section with a further generalization, namely, the *Bayesian nonlinear mixed model*.

9.5.2 The linear mixed model

The Gaussian hierarchical model is a particular case of the (Gaussian) linear mixed model (LMM). The LMM for the jth observation on the ith subject is given by

$$y_{ij} = \boldsymbol{x}_{ij}^T\boldsymbol{\beta} + \boldsymbol{z}_{ij}^T\boldsymbol{b}_i + \varepsilon_{ij},\ (j = 1, \ldots, m_i; i = 1, \ldots, n), \tag{9.9}$$

which gives in vector notation

$$\boldsymbol{y}_i = \boldsymbol{X}_i\boldsymbol{\beta} + \boldsymbol{Z}_i\boldsymbol{b}_i + \boldsymbol{\varepsilon}_i,\ (i = 1, \ldots, n) \tag{9.10}$$

where $\boldsymbol{y}_i = (y_{i1}, \ldots, y_{im_i})^T$ is a $m_i \times 1$ vector of responses, $\boldsymbol{X}_i = (\boldsymbol{x}_{i1}^T, \ldots, \boldsymbol{x}_{im_i}^T)^T$ the $(m_i \times (d+1))$ design matrix, $\boldsymbol{\beta} = (\beta_0, \beta_1, \ldots, \beta_d)^T$ a $(d+1) \times 1$ vector of regression coefficients also called the *fixed effects*, $\boldsymbol{Z}_i = (z_{i1}^T, \ldots, z_{im_i}^T)^T$ the $(m_i \times q)$ design matrix of the ith $q \times 1$ vector of *random effects* $\boldsymbol{b}_i$ and $\boldsymbol{\varepsilon}_i = (\varepsilon_{i1}, \ldots, \varepsilon_{im_i})^T$ a $m_i \times 1$ vector of measurement errors.

Typically, one makes the following distributional assumptions: $\boldsymbol{b}_i \sim \mathrm{N}_q(\boldsymbol{0}, \mathrm{G})$ with G a $(q \times q)$ covariance matrix. To highlight that G is related to random effects, its (j, k)th element, with $j \neq k$, is denoted as σ_{b_j,b_k} and for $j = k$ as $\sigma_{b_j}^2$. Further, $\boldsymbol{\varepsilon}_i \sim \mathrm{N}_{m_i}(\boldsymbol{0}, \mathrm{R}_i)$ with R_i a $(m_i \times m_i)$ covariance matrix. Often, R_i is taken equal to $\sigma^2 \mathrm{I}_{m_i}$ and $\boldsymbol{b}_i$ is assumed statistically independent of $\boldsymbol{\varepsilon}_i$ $(i = 1, \ldots, n)$. These assumptions imply that

$$\boldsymbol{y}_i \mid \boldsymbol{b}_i \sim \mathrm{N}_{m_i}(\boldsymbol{X}_i\boldsymbol{\beta} + \boldsymbol{Z}_i\boldsymbol{b}_i, \mathrm{R}_i), \tag{9.11}$$

$$\boldsymbol{y}_i \sim \mathrm{N}_{m_i}(\boldsymbol{X}_i\boldsymbol{\beta}, \boldsymbol{Z}_i\mathrm{G}\boldsymbol{Z}_i^T + \mathrm{R}_i). \tag{9.12}$$

The LMM is popular for analyzing longitudinal studies with irregular time points and a Gaussian response. In that case, $\boldsymbol{y}_i$ represents the m_i responses taken repeatedly at time points $t_{i1}, t_{i2}, \ldots, t_{im_i}$. The jth row of $\boldsymbol{X}_i$ is typically given by $\boldsymbol{x}_{ij} = (1, x_{ij1}, x_{ij2}, \ldots)^T$ where $x_{ij1}, x_{ij2}, \ldots$ can be time-independent covariates such as gender, age at baseline and/or time-dependent covariates such as the time at which the jth measurement is taken, i.e. t_{ij}, or any other covariate that changes with time. Suppose $\boldsymbol{x}_{ij} = (1, t_{ij})^T$, then the jth element of $\boldsymbol{X}_i\boldsymbol{\beta}$ is equal to $\beta_0 + \beta_1 t_{ij}$, which represents the average linear evolution of the response of the population from which the subjects were sampled. Further, if the jth row of $\boldsymbol{Z}_i$ is given by $z_{ij} = (1, t_{ij})^T$, then the jth element of $\boldsymbol{Z}_i\boldsymbol{b}_i$ is equal to $b_{0i} + b_{1i}t_{ij}$ and represents the linear deviation of the evolution of the response of the ith subject from the average evolution. Then the LMM is called the *random intercept and slope model*. Leaving out b_{1i} leads to a *random intercept model*. By providing all parameters of the LMM, a prior distribution a *BLMM* is obtained. Summarized, a BLMM with the classical normal distributional assumptions is given by (we have suppressed the dependence of the distributions on the covariates) the following:

- Level 1: $y_{ij} \mid \boldsymbol{\beta}, \boldsymbol{b}_i, \sigma^2 \sim \mathrm{N}(\boldsymbol{x}_{ij}^T\boldsymbol{\beta} + z_{ij}^T\boldsymbol{b}_i, \sigma^2)$ $(j = 1, \ldots, m_i;\ i = 1, \ldots, n)$
- Level 2: $\boldsymbol{b}_i \mid \mathrm{G} \sim \mathrm{N}_q(\boldsymbol{0}, \mathrm{G})$ $(i = 1, \ldots, n)$
- Priors: $\sigma^2 \sim p(\sigma^2)$, $\boldsymbol{\beta} \sim p(\boldsymbol{\beta})$ and $\mathrm{G} \sim p(\mathrm{G})$

The joint posterior distribution for the BLMM is then given by

$$p(\boldsymbol{\beta}, \mathrm{G}, \sigma^2, \boldsymbol{b}_1, \ldots, \boldsymbol{b}_n \mid \boldsymbol{y}_1, \ldots, \boldsymbol{y}_n) \propto \prod_{i=1}^{n}\prod_{j=1}^{m_i} p(y_{ij} \mid \boldsymbol{b}_i, \sigma^2, \boldsymbol{\beta}) \prod_{i=1}^{n} p(\boldsymbol{b}_i \mid \mathrm{G}) p(\boldsymbol{\beta}) p(\mathrm{G}) p(\sigma^2). \tag{9.13}$$

Lindley and Smith (1972) and Fearn (1975) showed analytically that for known variances, the random effects and the fixed effects have a posteriori a normal distribution. When the variances are unknown no explicit solutions can be given and one has to rely on numerical procedures. The full conditionals for the fixed effects $\boldsymbol{\beta}$, the random effects $\boldsymbol{b}_i$ and the variance components G and σ^2 take simple forms and this is exploited by Gibbs sampling. In a frequentist approach, the random effects are integrated out giving closed expressions for the LMM. The marginal likelihood is then maximized to find the MLEs. In the Bayesian approach, the random effects are sampled together with the fixed-effects parameters. Marginal inference on the fixed-effects parameters is obtained by 'forgetting' the sampled random effects parameters (see also Section 9.8). It is easy to see that the Gaussian hierarchical model of Section 9.4.2 is a particular case of the BLMM.

We now illustrate the BLMM with two examples. First, we include covariates in the dietary example. The second example is a longitudinal study.

Example IX.11: Dietary study: A comparison of cholesterol intake between subsidiaries corrected for age and gender

We question here how much of the subsidiary variability in cholesterol intake can be explained by age and gender. We assume the following model:

$$y_{ij} = \beta_0 + \beta_1 \,\text{age}_{ij} + \beta_2 \,\text{gender}_{ij} + b_{0i} + \varepsilon_{ij},$$

with y_{ij} the cholesterol intake of the ith subject in the jth subsidiary and gender $= 0$ for a female employee. Further, assume $b_{0i} \sim \text{N}(0, \sigma_{b_0}^2)$ and $\varepsilon_{ij} \sim \text{N}(0, \sigma^2)$. Vague priors were given for all parameters. The WinBUGS program is found in 'chapter 9 dietary study chol age gender.odc'. Three chains were initiated each was run for 10 000 iterations achieving convergence almost instantly. After removal of 5000 burn-in values, the posterior means (SD) were $-0.69(0.57)$ for β_1 and $-62.67(10.67)$ for β_2 demonstrating that age had no major impact on cholesterol intake in contrast to gender with female employees having an important lower cholesterol intake than men. Based on the current model, the posterior median for σ and σ_{b_0} is 116.3, 14.16, respectively, while the model without covariates (Example IX.7) gave 119.5 and 18.3, respectively. Thus the covariates have reduced the between-subsidiary variability but kept the within-subsidiary variability constant. The posterior mean of the intraclass correlation decreased to 0.015. □

The second example is a clinical trial in dermatology that we briefly introduced in Example I.1. In that example we only compared a particular response at the end of the study. However, the randomized controlled clinical trial (RCT) is an example of a longitudinal study. We now analyze the study results using a Bayesian random intercept and slope model.

Example IX.12: Toenail RCT: Fitting a Bayesian linear mixed model

In this double-blinded multicentric RCT (36 centers) sportsmen and elderly people were treated for toenail dermatophyte onychomycosis with either of two oral medications: Itraconazol 250 mg daily (treat $= 0$) or Lamisil 250 mg daily (treat $= 1$). The patients received treatment for 12 weeks and were evaluated at 0, 1, 2, 3, 6, 9 and 12 months (De Backer *et al.* 1996). As response, we have taken the unaffected nail length for the big toenail of a subgroup of 298 patients. Figure 9.11 shows the individual profiles of the unaffected nail length split up according to treatment. Looking at the profiles the treatments seem to work on average. The increase of SD (from about 2.5 to 5 mm) over time suggests a random intercept and slope model (Verbeke and Molenberghs 2000).

The following random intercept and slope mixed model

$$y_{ij} = \beta_0 + \beta_1 t_{ij} + \beta_2 t_{ij} \times \text{treat}_i + b_{0i} + b_{1i} t_{ij} + \varepsilon_{ij}$$

was fitted with WinBUGS (chapter 9 toenail LMM.odc) with y_{ij} the unaffected toenail length, time $t_{ij} = 0, 1, 2, 3, 6, 9$ or 12 months and treatment $treat_i$. No main effect for treatment was included in the model since at baseline the effect of treatment must be zero given the randomized character of the study. The directed acyclic graph (DAG) of the model is shown in Figure 9.12.

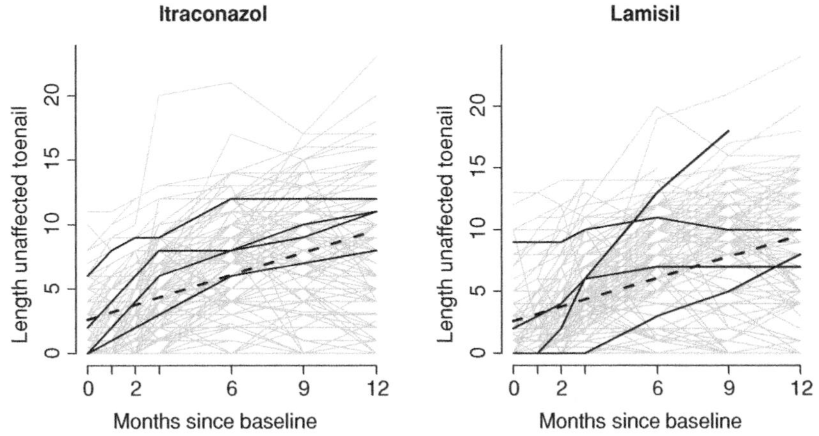

Figure 9.11 Toenail RCT: profiles of unaffected nail length according to treatment (with some individual profiles highlighted). The straight (dashed) lines are the average evolutions in the treatment groups obtained from the posterior means of the fixed effects.

We assumed normal distributions for the random components of the model, as specified before. The fixed effects parameters were given vague normal priors. The covariance matrix of the random intercept and slope was given a vague Inverse-Wishart prior with two degrees of freedom, i.e. IW(D, 2) with D = diag(0.1, 0.1).

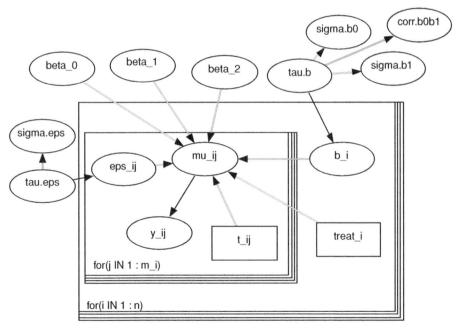

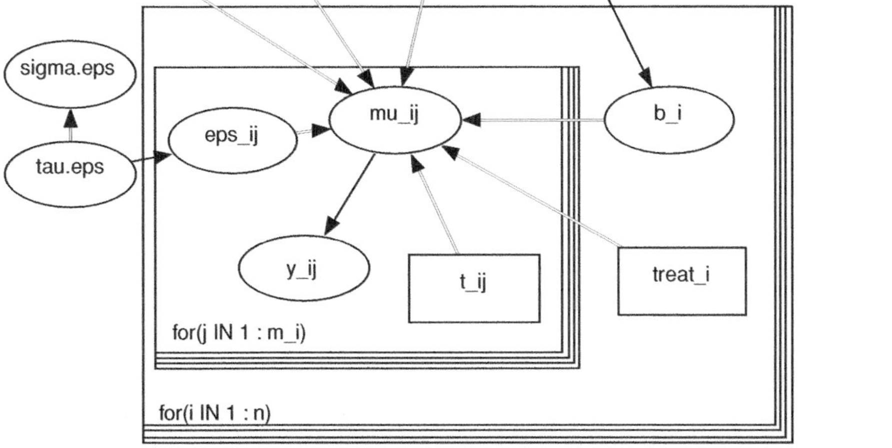

Figure 9.12 Toenail RCT: DAG corresponding to the BLMM of unaffected nail length, created by the Doodle option in WinBUGS.

Three chains were initiated each of size 10 000. The mixing rate was immediately good and the posterior measures were based on the last 5000 iterations. The following posterior means (SD) for the fixed effects were obtained: $\beta_1 : 0.58(0.043)$ and $\beta_2 : 0.057(0.058)$. For the variance parameters we obtained as posterior medians: $\sigma_{b_0} : 2.71$, $\sigma_{b_1} : 0.48$, $\text{corr}(b_0, b_1) = -0.39$ and $\sigma : 1.78$. Thus we conclude that over time the average unaffected nail length increases but that the two treatments have no different effect. A frequentist analysis using the SAS procedure MIXED yielded MLEs close to the Bayesian estimates. □

For the above two examples the frequentist analysis gives basically the same numerical results as the Bayesian analysis. So, it is not immediately clear what an applied statistician might gain from a Bayesian approach (apart from the change in philosophy). However, the generality of the MCMC approach in combination with the WinBUGS package allows for choosing other distributions for the random effects in the model (see Section 9.5.5).

9.5.3 The generalized linear mixed model

We assume again that the data exhibit a two-level hierarchy, i.e. there are m_i subjects in n clusters with responses y_{ij}. According to Section 4.8, y_{ij} ($j = 1, \ldots, m_i$; $i = 1, \ldots, n$) satisfy the assumptions of a GLIM when

$$p(y_{ij} \mid \theta_{ij}; \phi_{ij}) = \exp\left[\frac{y_{ij}\theta_{ij} - b(\theta_{ij})}{a(\phi_{ij})} + c(y_{ij}; \phi_{ij})\right], \tag{9.14}$$

with $a(\phi_{ij}) > 0$ a known scale function and θ_{ij} unknown canonical parameters. In the ordinary GLIM, $\mu_{ij} = E(y_{ij} \mid \theta_{ij})$ is expressed as a function of the covariates $\boldsymbol{x}_{ij}$ via a known link function g, i.e. $g(\mu_{ij}) = \boldsymbol{x}_{ij}^T\boldsymbol{\beta}$. For a BGLIM, all parameters are assumed to have prior distributions. However, the problem with this model is that it ignores the clustering in the data.

A natural extension of the BLMM is obtained by generalizing the linear model to a GLIM. Using the notation of Section 9.5.2, the BGLMM is defined as

$$g(\mu_{ij}) = \boldsymbol{x}_{ij}^T\boldsymbol{\beta} + \boldsymbol{z}_{ij}^T\boldsymbol{b}_i \; (j = 1, \ldots, m_i;\; i = 1, \ldots, n). \tag{9.15}$$

In general, $\boldsymbol{b}_i$ ($i = 1, \ldots, n$) are i.i.d., have a distribution $F_{\boldsymbol{b}}$, and determine the distribution of θ_{ij}. It is often assumed that the random effects have a normal distribution, say $\text{N}_q(\boldsymbol{0}, \text{G})$ (Molenberghs and Verbeke 2005), then with the canonical link function, $\theta_{ij} \sim \text{N}(\boldsymbol{x}_{ij}^T\boldsymbol{\beta}, \boldsymbol{z}_{ij}^T\text{G}\boldsymbol{z}_{ij})$. Thus, the BGLMM is given by the following:

- Level 1: $y_{ij} \mid \theta_{ij}, \phi_{ij} \sim \exp\left[\frac{y_{ij}\theta_{ij} - b(\theta_{ij})}{a(\phi_{ij})} + c(y_{ij}; \phi_{ij})\right]$, $(j = 1, \ldots, m_i;\; i = 1, \ldots, n)$
- Level 2: $g(\mu_{ij}) = \boldsymbol{x}_{ij}^T\boldsymbol{\beta} + \boldsymbol{z}_{ij}^T\boldsymbol{b}_i$ with i.i.d. $\boldsymbol{b}_i \sim \text{N}_q(\boldsymbol{0}, \text{G})$ $(i = 1, \ldots, n)$
- Priors: $\boldsymbol{\beta} \sim p(\boldsymbol{\beta})$ and $\text{G} \sim p(\text{G})$

with G a $q \times q$-covariance matrix.

An example of a BGLMM is the logistic-normal-binomial model whereby $\text{logit}(\pi_{ij}) = \boldsymbol{x}_{ij}^T\boldsymbol{\beta} + b_{0i}$ with π_{ij} the probability of success for the ith subject at time t_{ij} and b_{0i} a random intercept typically used to model repeated binary responses. This model implies that $E\left[\text{logit}(\pi_{ij})\right] = \boldsymbol{x}_{ij}^T\boldsymbol{\beta}$. Note that the regression coefficients have a *subject-specific* interpretation. Namely, β_j expresses the increase in $g(\mu_{ij})$ when covariate x_{ij} is increased with one unit conditional on b_{0i}. Another interpretation is that $\text{expit}(\boldsymbol{x}_{ij}^T\boldsymbol{\beta})$ represents the median relationship of the probability of 'success' and $\boldsymbol{x}_{ij}^T\boldsymbol{\beta}$. Full conditionals often take simple forms, such that the posterior distributions can be obtained relatively easily, especially with the WinBUGS software.

We illustrate the BGLMM on the lip cancer mortality study with log(RR) modeled as a linear function of AFF which is the percentage of the population engaged in agriculture, forestry and fisheries. This variable is included to capture the effect of exposure to sunlight on the prevalence of the disease. In addition, we include a random intercept representing unknown covariates characterizing each of the regions.

Example IX.13: Lip cancer study: A Poisson-lognormal model correcting for AFF
We question how much of the spatial variability in lip cancer mortality can be attributed to AFF. Assume that the mortality counts y_i satisfy $y_i \mid \mu_i \sim \text{Poisson}(\mu_i)$, with $\mu_i = \theta_i\, e_i$. We assume that the μ_i related to AFF_i as follows:

$$\log(\mu_i/e_i) = \beta_0 + \beta_1\,\text{AFF}_i + b_{0i},$$

with AFF_i centered around its mean and $b_{0i} \sim \text{N}(0, \sigma_{b_0}^2)$ a random intercept governing the correlation among the responses of the different regions. This model can be easily implemented in WinBUGS (chapter 9 lip cancer PLNT with AFF.odc).

The regression coefficients were given independent vague normal priors and σ_{b_0} a uniform prior in [0,100]. Based on three chains of each 20 000 iterations and removing in total 30 000 burn-in iterations, we obtained as posterior mean (SD) for β_1: 2.23 (0.33) with 95% equal tail CI [1.55, 2.93]. The posterior median for σ_{b_0} is equal to 0.38. The conclusion is that AFF is an important predictor for lip cancer mortality. Further, the model without AFF resulted in a posterior median for σ_{b_0} equal to 0.44. This shows that AFF 'explains' about 25% of the variability of the random intercept. □

In the second example, we analyzed the longitudinal toenail data introduced in Example IX.12 but now with a binary outcome. A logistic random intercept and slope model seems logical to fit with the random intercept expressing the subject-specific latent level of each of the patients throughout the study and the random slope the subject-specific evolution of the disease process. This analysis turned out to be quite challenging. Therefore, we first illustrate the use of a logistic random intercept model.

Example IX.14: Toenail RCT: A Bayesian logistic random intercept model
One of the secondary endpoints was the degree of separation of the nail plate from the nail bed (onycholysis) due to the toenail infection. For 294 (out of 298) patients, this response was measured. We binarized the response: 0 = none or mild, 1 = moderate or severe for the purpose of our analysis. In Figure 9.13, it is shown that under both treatments, an important drop of patients with onycholysis is seen, with a somewhat greater effect under Lamisil. The question is whether this extra decrease in percentage is a genuine effect or random fluctuation. To answer this question, we fitted the logistic random intercept model given by

$$\text{logit}(\pi_{ij}) = \beta_0 + \beta_1\, t_{ij} + \beta_2\, t_{ij} \times \text{treat}_i + b_{0i},$$

with π_{ij} the probability of showing onycholysis for the ith subject at time t_{ij} and b_{0i} the random intercept of the ith subject. The standard deviation of b_{0i} was given a U(0,100) vague prior and

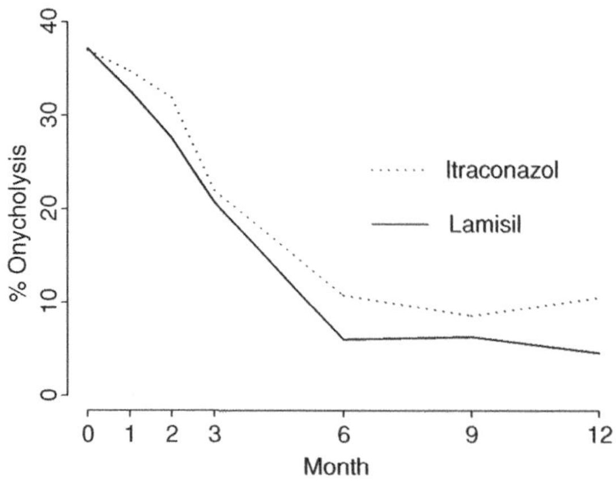

Figure 9.13 Toenail RCT: percentages of patients with onycholysis treated with Itraconazol or Lamisil during the study period.

vague normal independent priors were given to the regression coefficients. The WinBUGS program can be found in 'chapter 9 toenail RI BGLMM.odc'.

Three chains were initiated with 10 000 iterations each. The last 5000 iterations were kept to compute the posterior summary measures. As posterior means (SD) for the fixed effects we obtained: $\beta_0 : -1.74(0.34)$, $\beta_1 : -0.41(0.045)$, $\beta_2 : -0.17(0.069)$. The posterior median of $\sigma^2_{b_0}$ was 17.44. The intracluster correlation coefficient (ICC) for the logistic random intercept model ICC $= \sigma^2_{b_0}/(\sigma^2_{b_0} + \pi^2/3)$ (Hedeker and Gibbons 1994) was quite high (0.84) showing that there was a pronounced tracking in the response. With respect to the clinical results, it appears that Lamisil induces a greater decrease in disease activity than Itraconazol.

A frequentist analysis using SAS procedure GLIMMIX gave very similar numerical results as obtained above. The program can be found in 'chapter 9 toenail binary GLIMMIX and MCMC.sas'. The file contains also MCMC commands version 9.2. It is illustrative to run this program and to realize that this sampling approach is quite inefficient for this model. For the version 9.3 of the SAS program, we refer to the next example. □

It was more difficult to fit a logistic random intercept and slope model to the above binary responses. This is exemplified in the next example.

Example IX.15: Toenail RCT: A Bayesian logistic random intercept and slope model
A potentially more plausible model is the logistic random intercept and slope model whereby the random slope expresses that the subject-specific evolution is different for each individual. Using the above notation, this model is given by

$$\text{logit}(\pi_{ij}) = \beta_0 + \beta_1 t_{ij} + \beta_2 t_{ij} \times \text{treat}_i + b_{0i} + b_{1i} t_{ij},$$

with b_{1i} the random slope of the ith subject. We considered two cases: independent and dependent random effects. In the first case the standard deviations of random intercept and slope were given initially independent U(0, 100) priors, while in the second case we used the same prior as in Example IX.12. Both WinBUGS programs can be found in 'chapter 9 toenail RI+RS BGLMM.odc'.

It was quite problematic to get started with WinBUGS. We first ran a likelihood based analysis using SAS PROC GLIMMIX to generate starting positions. Our first WinBUGS run was based on the MLE of the model parameters. Promptly the error message 'undefined real result' appeared, which means numeric overflow. Reducing the starting values in absolute values did not help. The problem was reduced but not solved when we replaced `logit(p[iobs]) <- beta[1] + beta[2]*time[iobs] + ...` with `p[iobs] <- exp(beta[1] + beta[2]*time[iobs] + ...`. With the functions '`min`' and '`max`' we could prevent numerical overflow.

For both the independent and dependent cases, three starting positions were taken and the chains were run for 10 000 iterations with thinning=10 (thus in fact 100 000 iterations per chain). We now report only the dependent case. The BGR plot in WinBUGS showed for β_2 relative quick convergence. The posterior summary measures on the last 3×5000 iterations. We obtained -0.38 (0.19) as posterior mean (SD) for β_2 and a 95% CI equal to $[-0.78, -0.039]$ with MCerror $= 0.0054$. Hence we could conclude that the two treatments seem to differ somewhat in effect. The random intercept and slope were negatively correlated (posterior median $= -0.58$, 95% CI $= [-0.74, -0.33]$), the posterior median (95% CI) of the variance of the random intercept and slope were 73.61 ([42.93, 127.1]) and 1.18 ([0.62, 2.02]), respectively. Exporting the chains to CODA delivers additional information as seen above. The autocorrelations were relatively high for the variance parameters but for β_2 they were equal to 0.28 and 0.01 at lags 10 and 50, respectively. Geweke diagnostic for β_2 was not significant and the dynamic version only occasionally exceeded the boundaries, but this was not the case for all other parameters although overall convergence was not clearly rejected. Further, β_2 passed both Heidelberger–Welch tests.

A SAS analysis using procedure MCMC was also initiated, for the program see 'chapter 9 toenail RI+RS BGLMM.sas'. Since the procedure MCMC does not allow multiple chains and to be compatible with the WinBUGS run, we initiated one chain of length 300 000 but applied thinning=10 (recall the different implication of thinning in SAS versus WinBUGS). No computational problems were encountered (such as numerical overflow). Again, we left out half of the chain to compute the posterior summary measures. Now, the autocorrelations for β_2 were 0.93 and 0.70 (even after thinning) at lags 10 and 50, respectively, and thus quite high. However, all parameters passed the Geweke test and all parameters passed the first of the two Heidelberger–Welch tests, however, β_2 did not pass the second Heidelberger–Welch test. The posterior mean (SD) of β_2 was equal to -0.0110 (0.0227) with equal tail 95% CI $=$ $[-0.055, 0.036]$ indicating no effect of treatment. Since β_2 was estimated with low precision (effective sample size $= 51$), we concluded that to obtain a robust result on the effect of treatment, the SAS procedure needs a longer chain.

The reason why WinBUGS and SAS differ considerably in convergence performance on this data set is not immediately clear since the programs use the same sampler. □

An immediate generalization of the BGLMM is to add a residual term (Sun *et al.* 2000) by taking

$$g(\mu_{ij}) = \boldsymbol{x}_{ij}^T\boldsymbol{\beta} + \boldsymbol{z}_{ij}^T\boldsymbol{b}_i + \varepsilon_{ij},\ (j = 1, \ldots, m_i; i = 1, \ldots, n),$$

with $E(\varepsilon_{ij}) = 0$ or $E[\exp(\varepsilon_{ij})] = 1$ and $\boldsymbol{b}_i$ independent from ε_{ij}. These residual terms are included to account for lack of fit when there is extra (possibly unexplained) variation and outliers.

In case there are no level-1 covariates another modeling approach was suggested by Albert (1988). In his proposal, the canonical parameters θ_i have independent distributions belonging to the exponential family

$$p(\theta_i \mid \zeta_i, \lambda) = \exp\{\lambda[\theta_i\, \zeta_i - b(\theta_i)] + k(\zeta_i; \lambda)\}, \tag{9.16}$$

with $E(\mu_i) = E\left[\frac{d\,b(\theta_i)}{d\theta_i}\right] = \zeta_i$ and λ a dispersion parameter. Replacing λ by $1/\lambda$ in the above expression gives the classical expression of a GLIM, but working with (9.16) has analytical advantages (Albert 1988). ζ_i is the prior mean of the sampling mean μ_i. Further, distribution (9.16) is conjugate to the family defined by (9.14) whereby the subindex j is removed in θ and ϕ (Exercise 5.16). Albert (1988) suggested to let ζ_i, instead of μ_i, depend on covariates with

$$g(\zeta_i) = \boldsymbol{x}_i^T \boldsymbol{\beta}, \ \ (i = 1, \ldots, n). \tag{9.17}$$

Summarized, the two-level BHM suggested by Albert (1988) assumes the following:

- Level 1: $y_{ij} \mid \theta_i, \phi_i \sim \exp\left[\frac{y_{ij}\,\theta_{ij} - b(\theta_i)}{a(\phi_i)} + c(y_{ij}; \phi_i)\right]$, $(j = 1, \ldots, m_i; i = 1, \ldots, n)$
- Level 2: $\theta_i \mid \zeta_i, \lambda \sim \exp\{\lambda[\theta_i\, \zeta_i - b(\theta_i)] + k(\zeta_i; \lambda)\}$ & $g(\zeta_i) = \boldsymbol{x}_i^T \boldsymbol{\beta}$, $(i = 1, \ldots, n)$
- Prior: $(\boldsymbol{\beta}, \lambda) \sim p(\boldsymbol{\beta}, \lambda)$

Albert's model expresses the means of the random effects θ_i as a function of covariates, which gives the regression coefficients a *population-averaged* meaning. That is, β_j expresses the increase in ζ_i (up to the link function) in the population of subjects when covariate x_i is increased with one unit. For this reason, Albert's model is called (in the frequentist literature) a *marginal model* (Molenberghs and Verbeke 2005).

Kahn and Raftery (1996) used a specific case of Albert's model to relate covariates $\boldsymbol{x}_i$ of the ith hospital to its discharge probability π_i of Medicare stroke patients to skilled nursing facilities and called it the *beta binomial-logit model*. An advantage of this model is that the covariates express a marginal effect on the probability π_i namely $\text{logit}\,[E(\pi_i)] = \boldsymbol{x}_i^T \boldsymbol{\beta}$, whereas in the above BGLMM case the covariates express a conditional effect since for the BGLMM $E\left[\text{logit}(\pi_i)\right] = \boldsymbol{x}_i^T \boldsymbol{\beta}$. Unfortunately it is not clear how to extend Albert's model in the presence of subject-specific covariates. Below, we illustrate Albert's model on the lip cancer mortality data.

Example IX.16: Lip cancer study: Correcting for AFF with Albert's model

We have applied Albert's Bayesian hierarchical GLIM to the lip cancer–mortality data with (a centered) AFF as covariate to explain part of the heterogeneity of the log(RR)s. In the notation introduced earlier, we assumed that the counts y_i satisfy $y_i \mid \mu_i \sim \text{Poisson}(\mu_i)$ with $\mu_i = \theta_i\, e_i$. Here $\theta_i \mid \zeta_i, \lambda \sim \text{Gamma}(\zeta_i\lambda, \lambda)$, with λ a dispersion parameter (variance of gamma distribution is here ζ_i/λ). Finally, we let

$$\log(\zeta_i) = \beta_0 + \beta_1\, \text{AFF}_i.$$

The WinBUGS program is given in 'chapter 9 lip cancer PG Albert with AFF.odc'. We used vague normal independent priors for the regression coefficients and a U(0,100) prior for $1/\sqrt{\lambda}$ inspired by the results of Section 9.5.7. To check the impact of this prior, alternative vague priors for λ were also considered. Based on three chains of size 10 000 iterations, the trace plots showed high mixing and the BGR diagnostic plot confirmed quick convergence. Therefore, we based the posterior summary measures on the last 5000 iterations. We obtained as posterior mean (SD) for β_0: 0.162 (0.035) and for β_1: 1.92 (0.31) (95% equal tail CI: [1.29,2.51]). The posterior median of the scale parameter λ was equal to 6.05 (95% equal tail CI: [4.35, 8.53]). We checked that the results were robust for other reasonable priors of λ.

Our analysis thus showed again a strong effect of AFF but now on log(mean RR). Note that the estimate of the slope is smaller for Albert's model than what was obtained in Example IX.13. Part of the difference has to do with the choice of the model. But from the frequentist literature we also know that in absolute value the population-average slope is smaller than the subject-specific slope, which seems to be the case also here. □

In practice, the models need to be more flexible than those described above. For instance, the assumption of a normal random effects distribution in the classical BGLMM might be limiting. Some of these extensions can be covered by existing software. For instance, we show below that the normality assumption of the random effect in the Poisson-lognormal model can easily be relaxed with WinBUGS. When no software exists for the problem at hand then dedicated routines need to be developed, but we have seen that the MCMC machinery is of great help here.

Example IX.17: Lip cancer study: Relaxing the normal distribution in the lognormal model

Above, we have assumed that on the logarithmic scale the random intercept has a normal distribution. In most frequentist software this is the only allowable random effects distribution. With WinBUGS (file 'chapter 9 lip cancer PLNT with AFF.odc') it involves changing just one command to replace the normal distribution with a t_3-distribution. Based on this model and three chains of size 20 000 (burn-in 10 000), the posterior mean (SD) for the regression coefficients β_0, β_1 was 0.11 (0.035), 2.20 (0.36), respectively. The posterior median of $\sigma_{b_{0i}} =$ 0.26 must be multiplied with $\sqrt{3}$ (SD of standard t_3-distribution) to obtain the standard deviation of the random intercept resulting in $\sqrt{3} \times 0.257 = 0.44$.

A further generalization of the considered models could consist in letting WinBUGS determine the degrees of freedom (k) of the t-distribution. For this extension, we assumed a uniform distribution of k on discrete set of values. The WinBUGS program can be found in the same file, but basically the same results were found. However, it was difficult to establish the best value of k since its posterior was rather diffuse (see also Exercise 9.9). □

Also other, non-standard distributions distributions for the random effects and/or measurement error are easy to fit in a Bayesian context for instance with WinBUGS (see Arellano-Valle *et al.* 2007).

9.5.4 Nonlinear mixed models

Another generalization of the BLMM is the Bayesian nonlinear mixed model for repeated measurements. In this model, one assumes for the jth observation on the ith subject (using the notation of previous sections) that

$$y_{ij} = f(\boldsymbol{\phi}_i, \boldsymbol{x}_{ij}) + \varepsilon_{ij}, \;\; (j = 1, \ldots, m_i; i = 1, \ldots, n), \tag{9.18}$$

with f a nonlinear function of the covariate vector $\boldsymbol{x}_{ij}$ and a parameter vector $\boldsymbol{\phi}_i$ of length r. It is classically assumed that the measurement error term ε_{ij} has a normal distribution $\mathrm{N}(0, \sigma^2)$. The parameter vector $\boldsymbol{\phi}_i$ depends on the subject. A popular way to describe this dependence is as follows:

$$\boldsymbol{\phi}_i = \boldsymbol{W}_i\boldsymbol{\beta} + \boldsymbol{Z}_i\boldsymbol{b}_i, \tag{9.19}$$

where $\boldsymbol{W}_i$ is a $r \times (d+1)$ design matrix, $\boldsymbol{\beta}$ a $(d+1) \times 1$ vector of regression coefficients, $\boldsymbol{Z}_i$ a $(r \times q)$ design matrix of the ith $q \times 1$ vector of random effects $\boldsymbol{b}_i$. It is classically assumed that $\boldsymbol{b}_i \sim \mathrm{N}(\boldsymbol{0}, \mathrm{G})$. Note that the design matrix $\boldsymbol{W}_i$ is typically used for specifying group structures in the parameters and is not necessarily the same as the design matrix $\boldsymbol{X}_i$ which pertains to subject-specific covariates. Model (9.18) is more general than the BGLMM, since the link function g is more restrictive than the function f with the former a function of one variable (score $\boldsymbol{x}_i^T\boldsymbol{\beta}$) and the latter a general function.

The nonlinear mixed model has received much attention in the statistical research community especially after the publication of the seminal paper of Lindstrom and Bates (1990). Nonlinear mixed models have found their way in a variety of applications. An important application area is *pharmacokinetics*. The aim in pharmacokinetics is to understand the intrasubject processes of drug absorption, distribution and elimination governing achieved concentrations. Further, it is of interest to explore how these processes vary across subjects. In HIV research one uses nonlinear mixed models to characterize the mechanisms underlying the interaction between the HIV virus and the immune system by describing the decay and rebound of virus levels following HIV treatment. Other application areas are dairy research, wildlife research, fisheries research, growth curves, etc. For an up-to-date reference of this class of models, we refer to Davidian and Giltinan (2003).

The *Bayesian nonlinear mixed model (BNLMM)* combines a nonlinear mixed model with priors for all its parameters and is specified as

- level 1: $y_{ij} \mid \boldsymbol{\phi}_i, \boldsymbol{x}_{ij}, \sigma^2 \sim \mathrm{N}[f(\boldsymbol{\phi}_i, \boldsymbol{x}_{ij}), \sigma^2]$, $(j = 1, \ldots, m_i;\ i = 1, \ldots, n)$
- level 2: $\boldsymbol{\phi}_i \mid \boldsymbol{W}_i, \boldsymbol{Z}_i, \boldsymbol{\beta} \sim \mathrm{N}(\boldsymbol{W}_i\boldsymbol{\beta}, \boldsymbol{Z}_i\mathrm{G}\boldsymbol{Z}_i^T)$ $(i = 1, \ldots, n)$
- priors: $\boldsymbol{\beta} \sim p(\boldsymbol{\beta})$, $\sigma^2 \sim p(\sigma^2)$ and $\mathrm{G} \sim p(\mathrm{G})$

Since the function f can be quite general, it might be sometimes a challenge to fit this model with WinBUGS, as pointed out by Davidian and Giltinan (2003). However, for certain standard pharmacokinetics analyses, a WinBUGS interface, PKBugs, is available. We will illustrate the BNLMM with an experimental study on mice in arteriolosclerosis.

Example IX.18: Arteriosclerosis study: Reperfusion models after femoral artery occlusion

Collateral artery development is crucial for prevention and recovery of tissue ischemia caused by arterial occlusive diseases. Since immune responses play a crucial role in arteriogenesis, van Weel *et al.* (2007) examined the cellular components of the immune system and their effects on arteriogenesis.

In van Weel *et al.* (2007) different genetically modified mice underwent a surgical procedure that blocked one of the main leg arteries. The effect of the surgical induced ischemia was measured at days 0, 3, 7, 14, 21 and 28. At each of these days, the perfusion in the affected leg was compared to the perfusion in the unaffected leg resulting in an ischemic/nonischemic perfusion ratio (IPR) over time. Here we re-analyzed two groups: the C57BL/6 mice and the

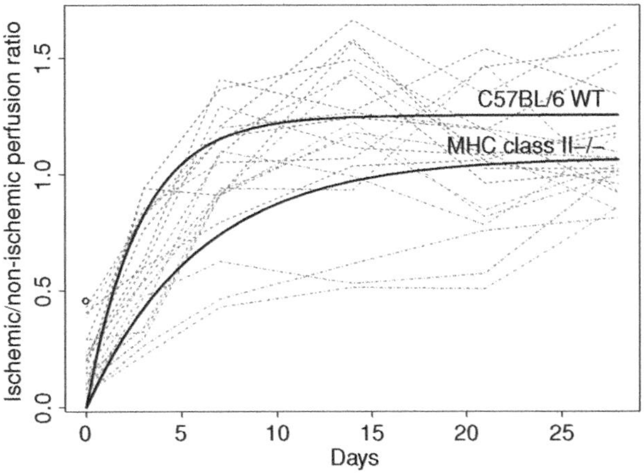

Figure 9.14 Arteriosclerosis study: individual profiles of the perfusion ratio of ischemic to nonischemic limbs in two groups of mice. The bold lines are obtained from the fixed effects predictions from the BNLMM, the dotted (dashed) lines correspond to the C57BL/6 WT (MHC class II−/−) mice.

MHC class II−/− mice. The C57BL/6 mice are the most widely used lab mouse strain as a model for human diseases, while the mice of the second group were genetically modified inducing a deficiency of MHC cells of class II. The individual profiles of IPR in the two groups are shown in Figure 9.14. van Weel *et al.* (2007) proposed the following nonlinear mixed model for the response y_{ij} (IPR):

$$y_{ij} = \phi_{1i}\left\{1 - \exp\left[-\exp(\phi_{2i}t_j)\right] + \varepsilon_{ij}\right\}, \ (j = 1, \ldots, 6;\ i = 1, \ldots, n), \qquad (9.20)$$

with $t_j = 0, 3, 7, 14, 21, 28$, $\phi_{1i} = \beta_1$ and $\phi_{1i} = \beta_2$ for mice from the first and second group, respectively, $\phi_{2i} = \beta_3 + b_i$ when the ith mouse belongs to the first group or $\phi_{2i} = \beta_4 + b_i$ when it belongs to the second group. The first parameter (ϕ_1) expresses the ultimate IPR as time evolves, while the second parameter (ϕ_2) expresses the rate at which the final ratio is attained. We assumed heterogeneity in ϕ_2 but not in ϕ_1. Interest lies in the difference between $\beta_3 - \beta_4 = \delta$.

In matrix notation, the model implies for the ith mouse of the first group

$$\boldsymbol{\phi}_i = \boldsymbol{W}_i\boldsymbol{\beta} + \boldsymbol{b}_i = \begin{pmatrix} 1 & 0 & 0 & 0 \\ 0 & 0 & 1 & 0 \end{pmatrix} \begin{pmatrix} \beta_1 \\ \beta_2 \\ \beta_3 \\ \beta_4 \end{pmatrix} + \begin{pmatrix} 0 \\ b_i \end{pmatrix},$$

with $\boldsymbol{\phi}_i \equiv (\phi_{1i}, \phi_{2i})^T$. For a mouse of the second group the row vectors of $\boldsymbol{W}_i$ should select the second and fourth β-parameters. Finally, it was assumed that $\varepsilon_{ij} \sim \mathrm{N}(0, \sigma^2)$ and $b_i \sim \mathrm{N}(0, \sigma_b^2)$.

We have taken independent vague normal priors for the β-parameters and uniform priors on [0,100] for σ and σ_b. The WinBUGS program can be found in 'chapter 9 arterio study.odc'. Three chains were started up with 10 000 iterations. The mixing was good and based on the classical diagnostics we could take the posterior measures on the last 5000 iterations (see also Exercise 9.17). The posterior mean (SD) of δ is 0.70 (0.37) (95% equal tail: [−0.002, 1.47]) and so we conclude that there is no clear evidence of a difference between the two types of mice. □

9.5.5 Some further extensions

In practice we need many more models than discussed up to now. For instance, the ordinal logistic random effects model would be needed in the toenail study if we had not discretized the response. For a Bayesian ordinal random effects model with a flexible random effects distribution, see Mansourian *et al.* (2012). When more than one outcome is recorded in a longitudinal study, we need an extension to a multivariate repeated measurements model (see Wilks *et al.* 1993). An important other example constitutes frailty models, which are survival models with additional random effects. These models are treated in Chapters 14 and 15.

9.5.6 Estimation of the random effects and posterior predictive distributions

Estimating the random effects in a Bayesian approach is similar to estimating the fixed effects as both are considered stochastic. In longitudinal studies it is often of interest to estimate/predict the individual curves. This involves the estimation of linear combinations of fixed and random effects, i.e.

$$\boldsymbol{\lambda}_{\beta}^{T}\widehat{\boldsymbol{\beta}} + \boldsymbol{\lambda}_{b}^{T}\widehat{\boldsymbol{b}_i},$$

with $\widehat{\boldsymbol{\beta}}$ and $\widehat{\boldsymbol{b}_i}$ taken as the posterior mean, median or mode of the respective parameters. The exploration of the random effects is also useful to highlight whether the assumed distribution is valid or whether there are outliers in the data.

The PPD for the Poisson-gamma model is found in expressions (9.5) and (9.6). These expressions carry over to the BGLMM with θ_i replaced by $\boldsymbol{b}_i$. The new observation will now represent all measurements of a new individual or some future observations of an already included subject. Fearn (1975) derived explicit expressions for the PPD of a BLMM when the variance parameters are known. With the availability of the MCMC machinery and software such as WinBUGS determining the PPD of future observations is easy.

In the next example we explore the random effects in the toenail data for the continuous response. We checked the normality assumption of the random effects and performed individual predictions.

Example IX.19: Toenail RCT: Exploring the random effects in the Bayesian linear mixed model

The posterior means of the random intercepts and slopes of the BLMM in Example IX.12 are shown in Figure 9.15. The histogram of the random intercepts is right skewed casting doubt on the normality assumption for the random intercept. Deviation from normality may be due to various reasons, e.g. because an important covariate was omitted. Verbeke and Lesaffre (1996) showed that the estimated random effects are shrunk, which makes it hard to detect non-normality. Hence, if non-normality is found in the estimated random effects then this is a sign that the true random intercept distribution is probably not normal.

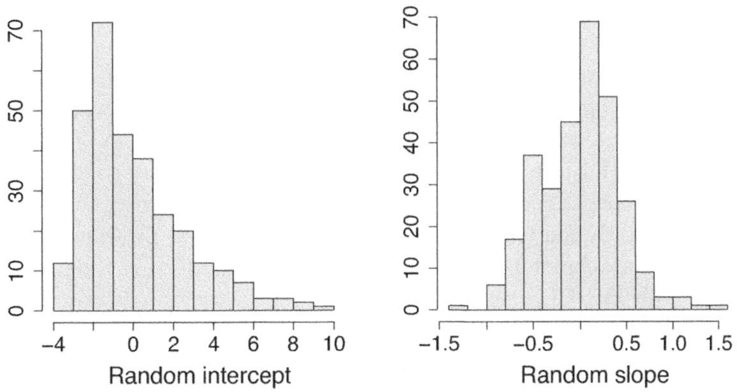

Figure 9.15 Toenail RCT: histograms of estimated random intercept and slope obtained from BLM.

In the case of a BLMM, the predicted evolution for the ith subject is the linear combination, i.e. $\boldsymbol{x}_{ij}^T\widehat{\boldsymbol{\beta}} + z_{ij}^T\widehat{\boldsymbol{b}}_i$ $(j = 1, \ldots, m_i)$. The predicted profiles for the individuals are obtained simply from the stats table in WinBUGS, which gives also 95% boundaries of the predicted curves. This stats table can be exported to R to produce the graphs. However, it is more efficient to use R2WinBUGS, which allows processing of WinBUGS within R.

To obtain the PPD of future observations of patient, extra lines of coding are needed. For instance, for the distribution of a future observation from subject `id[iobs]` we added the command `newresp[iobs] ~ dnorm(mean[iobs], tau.eps)`. On the other hand, to obtain the distribution of profiles from new patients, a different route needs to be followed since the random effect needs to be sampled directly from its normal prior (similar to predicting the mortality from new regions in Example IX.5). In Figure 9.16, we plotted the

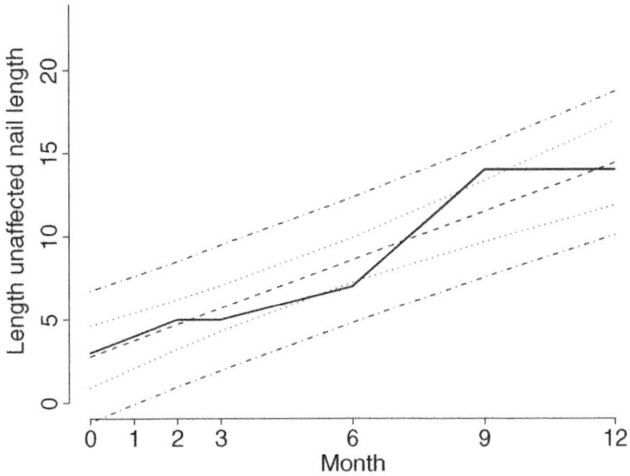

Figure 9.16 Toenail RCT: observed profile (solid line), predicted profile (dashed line) and 95% boundary lines (dotted lines) for the predicted mean and 95% boundary lines (dot-dashed lines) for new responses coming from Itraconazole patient 3 as obtained from the BLM developed in Example IX.5.

mean of the future profiles of Itraconazol patient 3 and corresponding 95% boundary profiles for the individual profiles.

As a final illustration, we predicted the future response $y_{i,j+1}$ of the ith subject with covariate vectors $\boldsymbol{x}_{i,j+1}$ and $z_{i,j+1}$ given the past responses $y_{m1}, \ldots, y_{mj}$ with covariate vectors $\boldsymbol{x}_{m1}, \ldots, \boldsymbol{x}_{mj}$ and $z_{m1}, \ldots, z_{mj}$ for $m = 1, \ldots, n$. This is easily done with WinBUGS. Suppose that we wish to predict the response at month 12 (which is now missing) of the first Itraconazol patient. To perform the prediction, we augment the vector of responses for that subject with a missing value 'NA'. Namely, we enlarge the vector (4, 6, 7, 9, 13, 0) to (4, 6, 7, 9, 13, 0, NA) and augment the vectors of covariates appropriately. In this way, we obtained 6.073 as posterior mean with 95% CI equal to [0.92, 11.28].

Note that the correct prediction of individual curves (and hence also the PPD) depends on the distributional assumptions of the model. The fact that the random intercepts do not have a Gaussian distribution might affect the correctness of the results. □

9.5.7 Choice of the level-2 variance prior

For the Bayesian normal linear regression model, Jeffreys prior $p(\sigma^2) \propto 1/\sigma^2$ is the classical choice to express no prior information on the variance parameter. For Gaussian hierarchical models an appropriate vague prior for the level-2 variance is not immediately clear. Hill (1965) and Tiao and Tan (1965) proved already more than 40 years ago that Jeffreys prior for the level-2 variance σ_θ^2 in a Gaussian hierarchical model results in an improper posterior. Gelman (2006) gave an intuitive explanation why this happens. Namely, with prior $1/\sigma_\theta^2$, the marginal $p(\boldsymbol{y} \mid \sigma_\theta)$ approaches a finite nonzero value as σ_θ approaches zero, but $1/\sigma_\theta^2$ attains an infinite mass near zero such that the posterior has infinite mass around zero. In addition, one can never rule out a zero variance for the latent variable in an hierarchical model, especially when the number of level-2 observations is low and provide only little information on σ_θ.

To avoid impropriety of the posterior, WinBUGS only allows the proper approximation to Jeffreys prior, i.e. IG(ε, ε), with ε small. However, replacing Jeffreys prior by IG(ε, ε) is not a solution since the posterior distribution of the parameters depends heavily on the choice of ε (Spiegelhalter *et al.* 2004). The strong impact of Jeffreys prior (and its approximation) can be seen in the bimodal shape of the posterior distribution of σ_θ. Triggered by the poor behavior of Jeffreys prior in this context (and its proper approximation), a variety of suggestions for an appropriate vague prior $p(\sigma_\theta)$ appeared in the literature; see Seltzer (1993), Seltzer *et al.* (1996) and Browne and Draper (2006). Liu and Hodges (2003) pointed out that bi-modality of a posterior is always the result of a conflict between the prior and the data. Spiegelhalter *et al.* (2004) explored several proper 'noninformative' priors and concluded that the U(0,c) prior for σ_θ can be recommended, which was also the conclusion of Gelman (2006).

We now illustrate the problems when using the IG(ε, ε) prior for σ_θ^2 and compare its performance with the uniform U(0,c) prior on σ_θ. We also illustrate the performance of the 'parameter expanded' model suggested by Gelman (2006). Our computations are based on the IBBENS dietary data which were modified to exemplify better the dependence of the posterior on the prior.

Example IX.20: Dietary study: Choosing a vague proper prior for the level-2 variance
We have modified the IBBENS dietary cholesterol intake data by adding a normal random variable with mean = 0 and SD = 20 to the subsidiary means, see 'chapter 9 dietary study

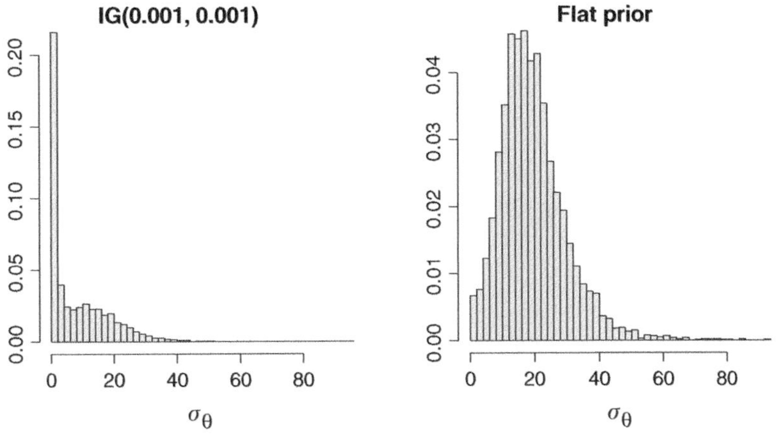

Figure 9.17 (Modified) Dietary study: posterior distribution of σ_θ using IG(10^{-3}, 10^{-3})-prior for σ_θ^2 and U(0, 100) prior for σ_θ.

chol2.odc'. In Figure 9.17, we show the posterior of σ_θ under the IG(10^{-3}, 10^{-3})-prior for σ_θ^2 and the uniform prior U(0, 100) for σ_θ. The first prior shrinks the posterior of σ_θ toward zero and hence the prior demonstrates a strong effect on the posterior of σ_θ.

We also examined the dependence of the other parameter estimates on the prior for σ_θ. The trace plots in Figure 9.18 of the overall mean of the θ_is summarize the results. Overall the sampling of μ is acceptable under the flat prior, but under the inverse gamma prior the chain regularly got stuck at zero. Note that also the chain under the flat prior occasionally got

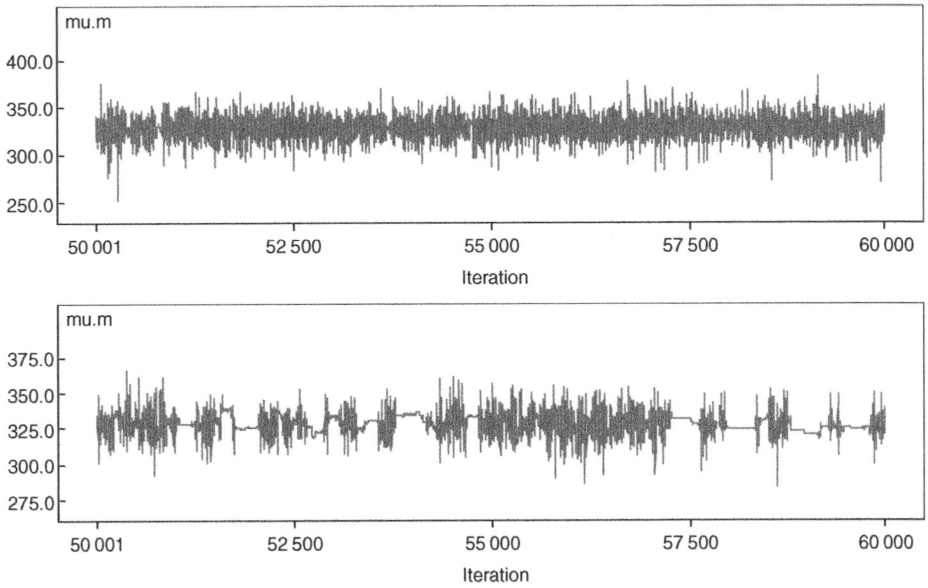

Figure 9.18 (Modified) Dietary study: trace plots of posterior distribution of μ (mu.m) using top: U(0, 100) prior for σ_θ and bottom: IG(10^{-4}, 10^{-4})-prior for σ_θ^2.

stuck at zero. In addition, the prior of σ_θ had a great impact on the estimates of the individual θ_i values.

Finally, we applied the prior suggested by Gelman (2006), which is explained in Section 9.7 (see that section for details). The WinBUGS program based on this approach is found in 'chapter 9 dietary study chol2 fold.odc'. The parameter ξ was given a normal prior with variance 10^2, while for σ_η^2 an IG(0.5, 0.5)-prior was chosen. This trick produced basically the same results as with the uniform prior. Note that the posterior mean of μ was largely unaffected by the choice of the variance prior, as was also concluded from a simulation study by Browne and Draper (2006). □

The above discussion dealt only with the variance of a random intercept. But what if we have a random intercept and slope? In this context, Natarajan and Kass (2000) reported on a simulation study and found that taking 'default' priors for the variance components (inverse gamma or inverse Wishart) can lead to misleading inferences. Thus, the vague priors that we have taken for the random intercept + slope in the previous examples might be problematic. We have chosen these priors since these are still the standard choice. An appropriate proper vague prior for a covariance matrix for the higher level observations in an hierarchical model is needed. But for dimension 2, i.e. with random intercept and slope, one might take a uniform prior for the standard deviation of the intercept and the slope and combine it with a uniform prior on the correlation (see Exercise 9.15). The conclusion of the exercise was that, when the diagonal elements of the scale matrix D in the inverse Wishart IW(D, 2) prior for random intercept and slope were taken small, then all parameter estimates of the model were close to the frequentist results and close to the results obtained from uniform priors on the standard deviations and the correlation of the random effects. However, for large diagonal elements the estimates of the covariance matrix of the random effects could be quite different. These results confirm the assertion in Section 5.3.3. A drawback of using the uniform priors (with WinBUGS) is that sampling from the posterior distribution requires considerably longer time than with the inverse Wishart prior, which is easily explained since the latter is a conditional conjugate for Gaussian models. Finally, Gelman *et al.* (2008) suggested for the general case to use parameter expansion extending his suggestion of Gelman (2006).

9.6 Propriety of the posterior

The impact of improper priors on the propriety of the posterior has been examined in the literature in several theoretical papers. These results are important for users of the SAS procedure MCMC since it allows improper priors. But, even if the prior for σ_θ is proper we need to take care that it is not influencing the posterior unduly, as seen in Section 9.5.7. While proving propriety of the posterior for a general (hierarchical) model is impossible, restricting to a particular class of hierarchical models allows to derive necessary and sufficient propriety conditions. Hobert and Casella (1996) derived conditions for the priors of a Gaussian BLMM, a flat prior for the fixed effects and $(\sigma^2)^{-(a+1)}$ priors for variance parameters. They also noticed that an improper posterior can yield proper full conditionals and 'well-behaved' Markov chains. This is quite disturbing since classical convergence diagnostics will not detect this problem. Sun *et al.* (2001) generalized these conditions to correlated random effects. Ghosh *et al.* (1998), Gelfand and Sahu (1999) and Natarajan and Kass (2000) looked at the propriety of a BGLMM posterior with improper priors. For logistic or probit random effects models, the propriety conditions are relatively easy to verify and relate to the conditions for separability derived by Albert and Anderson (1984) and Lesaffre and Albert (1989).

9.7 Assessing and accelerating convergence

In principle, checking the convergence of Markov chains obtained from hierarchical models is similar to checking convergence in any other model. The only problem is that the introduction of random effects implies a large number of parameters to monitor and to check for convergence. This may become quickly impractical, and therefore, it is suggested to select a handful of random effects ($\boldsymbol{b}_i$s) and to check convergence of the Markov chain only on this limited set.

There are, however, some specific tricks to accelerate the convergence of a Markov chain which apply only for BHMs. We restrict ourselves to those techniques that can be applied with software such as WinBUGS and SAS. First, note that the tricks seen in Chapter 7, e.g. centering and standardizing the covariates and overrelaxation, may also be helpful here. Acceleration tricks that are specific for BHMs are: *hierarchical centering*, *reparameterization by sweeping* and *parameter expansion*.

(a) Hierarchical centering: In the frequentist GLMM literature (and software) the random effects are most often centered for convenience around zero, but whether centering is applied or not is not really important. This is different in the Bayesian case. When the random effects are centered around zero one refers to an *uncentered* BHM. It has been shown by Gelfand *et al.* (1995) for the BLMM and generalized to the BGLMM by Gelfand *et al.* (1996) that centering around zero may seriously deteriorate the rate of mixing.

The uncentered Gaussian hierarchical model is given by

$$\begin{aligned} y_{ij} &= \mu + \alpha_i + \varepsilon_{ij}, \\ \alpha_i &\sim \mathrm{N}(0, \sigma_\alpha^2), \end{aligned} \tag{9.21}$$

with $j = 1, \ldots, m_i$; $i = 1, \ldots, n$ and $\varepsilon_{ij} \sim \mathrm{N}(0, \sigma^2)$.

Assume that the variances $\sigma^2, \sigma_\alpha^2$ are known and take a flat prior for μ. Then Gelfand *et al.* (1995) derived the posterior correlations involving the level-2 observations (random effects α_i) for $m_i = m$, namely,

$$\rho_{\mu,\alpha_i} = -\left(\frac{\sigma_\alpha^2/n}{\sigma_\alpha^2/n + \sigma^2/m}\right)^{\frac{1}{2}}, \tag{9.22}$$

$$\rho_{\alpha_i,\alpha_j} = -\left(\frac{\sigma_\alpha^2/n}{\sigma_\alpha^2/n + \sigma^2/m}\right), \tag{9.23}$$

with $i \neq j$. Under *hierarchical centering*, it is understood that the Gaussian hierarchical model is expressed as in Section 9.4.2, which is

$$\begin{aligned} y_{ij} &= \theta_i + \varepsilon_{ij}, \\ \theta_i &\sim \mathrm{N}(\mu, \sigma_\alpha^2), \end{aligned} \tag{9.24}$$

and $\varepsilon_{ij} \sim \mathrm{N}(0, \sigma^2)$. In that case, Gelfand *et al.* (1995) showed that the posterior correlations are given by

$$\rho_{\mu,\theta_i} = \left(\frac{\sigma^2}{\sigma^2 + mn\,\sigma_\alpha^2}\right)^{\frac{1}{2}}, \tag{9.25}$$

$$\rho_{\theta_i,\theta_j} = \left(\frac{\sigma^2}{\sigma^2 + mn\,\sigma_\alpha^2}\right), \tag{9.26}$$

for $i \neq j$. It can be easily verified that the posterior correlations are lower under hierarchical centering when $\sigma_\alpha^2 > \sigma^2/m$. But since the results in Gelfand *et al.* (1995) were derived under known model variances, explorative computations are needed to determine whether $\sigma_\alpha^2 > \sigma^2/m$ holds. The conclusion of whether centering is needed might therefore change once the final estimates of the variances are known. Gelfand *et al.* (1995) showed that hierarchical centering might also be beneficial in the multi-level case and for a BLMM. In Gelfand *et al.* (1996) they extended their arguments to the BGLMM.

In practice, one estimates the variances using, say, a least-squares technique, and decides for one of the two centering approaches.

(b) Reparameterization by sweeping: Vines *et al.* (1996) proposed another method for reparameterizing Bayesian mixed models. The motivation for their approach is the observation that model (9.21) is essentially overparameterized since a constant a could be added to μ and subtracted from each α_i without altering the likelihood of the data. With $\overline{\alpha} = \frac{1}{n}\sum_i \alpha_i$, they suggested a reparameterization with $\phi_i = \alpha_i - \overline{\alpha}$, $\nu = \mu + \overline{\alpha}$ and $\delta = \mu - \overline{\alpha}$. The method is called *sweeping* since the mean is swept from the random effects onto μ. Further, the identifiability problem is resolved since $\sum_i \phi_i = 0$. The following reparameterization was suggested:

$$\begin{aligned} y_{ij} &= \nu + \phi_i + \varepsilon_{ij}, \\ \phi_{-n} &\sim \mathrm{N}_{n-1}(0, \sigma_\alpha^2 \mathrm{K}_{n-1}), \\ \phi_n &= -\sum_{i=1}^{n-1} \phi_i, \end{aligned} \tag{9.27}$$

with $\phi_{-n} = (\phi_1, \phi_2, \ldots, \phi_{n-1})^T$ and K_{n-1} a $(n-1) \times (n-1)$ matrix with $1 - \frac{1}{n}$ on the main diagonal and $-\frac{1}{n}$ elsewhere. The sweeping operator gives as posterior correlations

$$\rho_{\nu,\phi_i} = 0, \quad \rho_{\phi_i,\phi_j} = -\frac{1}{n},$$

for $i \neq j$. One can check that the correlations are small for $n \geq 10$, which then can improve the mixing of the chains.

Our experience with this method is that it effectively improves the mixing rate of the chain but at the cost of speed (each iteration takes more time) and sometimes considerable extra programming.

(c) Parameter expansion techniques: Gelman (2006) suggested to reformulate model (9.21) as

$$y_{ij} \sim \mathrm{N}(\theta_i, \sigma^2),$$

with $\theta_i = \mu + \alpha_i = \mu + \xi\,\eta_i$ and $\eta_i \sim \mathrm{N}(\theta_i, \sigma_\eta^2)$. The parameter ξ is given a diffuse normal prior. Gelman suggested an IG(0.5, 0.5)-prior for σ_η^2. The method is called *parameter expansion* since the random effects α_i are split up into a parameter ξ and a random effect η_i. The overparameterization reduces the dependence among the parameters in a hierarchical model and it improves MCMC convergence. The method is based on earlier work of Liu *et al.* (1998), Liu and Wu (1999) and van Dyk and Meng (2001).

Example IX.21: Dietary study: Improving convergence
In all cases below, we ran a single chain of 10 000 iterations and based the estimates on the last 5000 iterations.

(a) *Hierarchical centering*: A simple inspection of the data showed that the within-subsidiary variance $\sigma^2 \approx 14\,500$ and the between-subsidiary variance $\sigma_\alpha^2 \approx 450$. With an average subsidiary size around 70, $\sigma_\alpha^2 > \sigma^2/70 \approx 210$ and lower posterior correlations are to be expected with hierarchical centering. Both an uncentered and a hierarchical centered analysis were performed on the cholesterol intakes of the IBBENS study. Upon convergence, the estimated values for ρ_{μ,α_i} and ρ_{α_i,α_j} were for the uncentered case −0.48 and 0.26, respectively, and for the hierarchically centered case 0.35 and 0.081, respectively. In addition, hierarchical centering lowered the MCerror for μ: MCerror-uncentered = 0.32, MCerror-centered = 0.23.

(b) *Reparameterization by sweeping*: We applied the sweeping approach of Vines *et al.* (1996) and upon convergence obtained a MCerror for μ of 0.15 which represents a great improvement. The MCerror for ν was even lower and equal to 0.078. However, the price to pay is that the program needs about 15 times more computation time.

(c) *Parameter expansion techniques*: The model was specified above and the priors were specified in Example IX.10. With the same size of the Markov chain, the MCerror for μ was equal to 0.22, about half of the MCerror for the uncentered case. □

9.8 Comparison of Bayesian and frequentist hierarchical models

At several instances in this chapter we have compared the estimated parameters by Bayesian and frequentist techniques. In this section we review some analytical and simulation results that compares the two approaches for Gaussian hierarchical models.

9.8.1 Estimating the level-2 variance

Estimating σ_θ^2 can be problematic when the true value is small. This has been noticed in the frequentist literature, especially when the method of moments (MINVQUE) is used. With this approach a negative estimate of σ_θ^2 may be obtained when the level-2 observations exhibit low variation. In that case, the ML estimate and the REML estimate may result in a zero estimate of the variance. This creates difficulties in hypothesis testing and the calculation of confidence intervals. Hill (1965), Tiao and Tan (1965), Box and Tiao (1973) derived analytically the marginal posterior distributions of the random effects ANOVA parameters based on noninformative priors. They concluded that in the Bayesian context, $\sigma_\theta^2 \ll \sigma^2$ does not create problems whenever the posterior distribution is proper. Indeed, even when the Bayesian estimate, say mode, is zero the posterior distribution is still well defined and can easily deliver credible intervals. The downside of the Bayesian procedure is, however, that the (95%) credible interval for the variance parameter never includes the true value if it is actually zero. Finally, Browne and Draper (2006) concluded from a large simulation study, that the posterior mode and median of the variance parameters are preferable in terms of the Mean-Squared-Error (see also Lambert 2006).

9.8.2 ML and REML estimates compared with Bayesian estimates

When the parameters are given flat priors, the MLE of variance parameters can be obtained from the mode of a joint posterior. In addition, Harville (1974) proved for the BLMM with normality of the measurement errors that the REML estimator for the variance components must be equal to the mode of their marginal posterior distribution when the regression parameters are integrated out. Thus, if the posterior of the variance parameters is roughly symmetric then the mean of the marginal posterior of the variance parameter approximates the REML solution. This correspondence is only proven for flat priors and a linear model. But, in a Bayesian exercise the marginal posterior estimates are always obtained by integrating out the other parameters. Thus, one might expect that the Bayesian approach also delivers REML-like solutions for other mixed models. There is also a close connection of the frequentist with the Bayesian estimates of the random effects. In Section 9.3, it is seen that the BLUP estimator is in fact a particular case of a Bayesian estimator whereby the marginal estimates of the model parameters are imputed into the model.

Here follows an illustration of some of the correspondences between the frequentist and Bayesian estimates of variance parameters. For this we use again the cholesterol intake data of Example IX.13.

Example IX.22: Dietary study: Comparison with frequentist estimation
We now have a closer look at the correspondence between the ML and REML estimates and the Bayesian estimators of the variance components. Using SAS PROC MIXED the MLE of σ is 119.4 and the MLE of $\sigma_\theta = 14.4$, while for the REML estimates we obtained $\sigma = 119.4$ and $\sigma_\theta = 16.3$. The Bayesian analysis upon which the values in Table 9.2 were based, has a vague prior for μ, a uniform prior for σ_θ and an IG(10^{-3}, 10^{-3}) prior for σ^2. According to the estimated θ_i-values in Table 9.2, we conclude that the ML and REML estimates for σ_θ must be quite different from the Bayesian estimates. In fact, the posterior median of σ_θ was 18.26. However, this does not invalidate the above assertion on the equivalence between ML and REML estimators and the Bayesian estimators, since this result is based on flat priors for all parameters and on posterior modes. Changing the prior for σ to a uniform on [0, 1000] confirmed this relationship by graphically determining the posterior mode from a smoothed density of the sampled values. □

From the above one might conclude that, apart from the different philosophical background of the two approaches, it does not matter too much which approach is taken to analyze hierarchical models. This is only partly true. First, we have seen that the Bayesian allows easier to relax distributional assumptions than the classical approach. Second, in the frequentist approach, the standard errors of the estimated fixed effects in linear and generalized LMMs do not take into account that the sampling variability of the matrices G and R. Moreover, it is quite hard to take this sampling variability into account. For this reason, the SAS procedures MIXED and GLIMMIX address this problem and use estimated degrees of freedom in their t and F-statistics. As seen repeatedly, the Bayesian approach takes into account all uncertainty on the parameters and that without an extra effort. In addition, the frequentist coverage of the Bayesian $100(1-\alpha)\%$ CIs based on NI priors is often close to $100(1-\alpha)\%$.

9.9 Closing remarks

This chapter served as an introduction to Bayesian hierarchical/mixed models. This is an exciting area and there is much more can be done than what is treated here both in practical as well as in theoretical terms. The reader may consult the book of Dey *et al.* (2000) to explore further developments. Furthermore, all considered models are (necessarily) likelihood-based and then the Bayesian estimation procedure is robust against missing at random mechanisms (Daniels and Hogan, 2008). We elaborate on missing data mechanisms in Chapter 15 where we also show an analysis that allows for a particular missing-not-at random mechanism.

Exercises

Exercise 9.1 Show that the MLE of θ under assumption A2 in Section 9.2.2 is given by $\sum_i y_i / \sum_i e_i$. Derive also the posterior summary measures for different priors on θ, (1) flat prior, (2) Jeffreys prior, and (3) a normal prior with mean 1 and variance 10^2.

Exercise 9.2 Write a R function to Gibbs sample from the Poisson-gamma hierarchical model based on GDR lip cancer data.

Exercise 9.3 Determine the WinBUGS samplers for the nodes μ, θ_i, σ^2 and σ_θ^2 in the WinBUGS program 'chapter 9 dietary study chol.odc'.

Exercise 9.4 Perform a WinBUGS analysis of the dietary cholesterol data under assumptions A1 and A2.

Exercise 9.5 Compare the Bayesian analysis of Example IX.8 to a frequentist analysis and verify that the results are quite similar.

Exercise 9.6 Compare the analysis of Example IX.12 with an analysis where treatment is included as main effect.

Exercise 9.7 Example IX.17: In Gelman and Meng (1996, p. 193) it is argued that a uniform prior on the degrees of freedom (ν) essentially puts all of its mass on infinity. As an alternative, the authors suggest to take as prior $p(\nu) \propto 1/\nu^2$. Implement this suggestion into a WinBUGS program and evaluate the change in posterior estimates of the parameters. Do you agree with their statement?

Exercise 9.8 Compare the analysis of Example IX.14 with an analysis where treatment is included as main effect.

Exercise 9.9 Show that the random intercept of the logistic random intercept model of Example IX.14 has a bimodal distribution, with one mode around −2.4. Show also that the subjects with an estimated random intercept around −2.4 correspond to those cases with zeros as response over the whole study period.

Exercise 9.10 Determine the predicted profiles and the distribution of future observations for the BNLMM of Example IX.18. Estimate the one missing response in the data.

Exercise 9.11 Use the WinBUGS program 'chapter 9 dietary study chol2.odc' to examine the dependence of the posterior of σ_θ on the choice of ε in the inverse gamma 'noninformative' prior $\text{IG}(\varepsilon, \varepsilon)$.

Exercise 9.12 In the WinBUGS program 'chapter 9 generated.odc' a Bayesian–Gaussian hierarchical model is given using fictive data from Tiao and Tan (1965). The data were generated such that the frequentist estimate of σ_θ^2 is negative. Check that this is indeed the case. Further, apply the Bayesian approach to estimate σ_θ^2.

Exercise 9.13 Example IX.12: Check the impact of choosing an Inverse Wishart prior for the covariance matrix of the random intercept and slope on the estimation of the model parameters, by varying the parameters of the prior. Compare this solution with the solution obtained from taking a product of three uniform priors on the standard deviation of the random intercept and slope, and the correlation, respectively. Use 'chapter 9 toenail LMM.odc'.

Exercise 9.14 Gelman (2006) suggested to reformulate the Gaussian hierarchical model as

$$\begin{aligned} y_{ij} &\sim \text{N}(\mu + \xi\, \eta_i, \sigma^2) \\ \xi &\sim \text{N}(0, \sigma_\eta^2). \end{aligned}$$

In WinBUGS program 'chapter 9 dietary study chol folded.odc' the original IBBENS data are analyzed according to the above model with a half-Cauchy prior with scale parameter 25 for σ_θ using a $\text{N}(0, 5^2)$ prior on ξ and an $\text{IG}(0.5, 0.5)$-prior for σ_η^2. Replay the analysis and vary the parameters of the priors to examine their impact on the posterior $p(\sigma_\theta \mid \mathbf{y})$. In Gelman (2006), it is claimed that the above reformulation of the Gaussian hierarchical model reduces the autocorrelation of the sampled parameters. Verify this on the behavior of σ_θ.

Exercise 9.15 Example IX.18: Although in the first 10 000 iterations the trace plots behaved well, when running the chains further it became apparent that the variance parameter σ got stuck at zero for one chain and that for quite some iterations. Apply the parameter expansion technique of Section 9.7 (adapt the program 'chapter 9 arterio study.odc') to improve convergence of this parameter. Does this change in the program alter your clinical conclusions?

Exercise 9.16 The R program 'chapter 9 dietary study-R2WB.R' uses the R2WinBUGS program for the analysis of dietary study. Run this program and produce your own trace plots, histograms, scatter plots, etc.

10

Model building and assessment

10.1 Introduction

We now explore Bayesian procedures for model building and model criticism. We assume that there are just a few good candidate models from which we wish to select. Therefore, the criteria for model selection that are reviewed in this chapter essentially compare the models two by two. Model and variable selection techniques involving a large number of candidate models are the subject of Chapter 11.

Statistical models are typically built by either a top-down approach (from theory to data when there is a well-developed theory such as in biological and economic research) or by a bottom-up approach (from data to model what often occurs in medical and epidemiologic research). However, a recipe to come up with the best statistical model does not exist. It is even not realistic to assume that the true model will ever be found as Box once argued: 'all models are wrong but some are useful'. In a statistical analysis, the final model is the result of variable selection, model choice and model criticism. Models are tested for their performance in inference and prediction. In this chapter, we focus on the model building and criticism aspects of the modeling exercise. The issues and problems in statistical modeling in frequentist methods are similar to those in the Bayesian approach, except for two aspects: (1) a Bayesian model is the combination of the likelihood and a prior, and therefore modeling involves now two choices, and (2) Bayesian inference is (nowadays) based on MCMC techniques in contrast to frequentist approaches where asymptotic inference is most common.

To build the ultimate statistical model, substantive arguments are combined with modeling activities such as variable selection, variable transformations, checking the goodness of fit (GOF) of the model, etc. In addition, and perhaps most importantly, the choice of the final model depends on who is doing the analysis and for what purposes.

In this chapter, we review criteria to select from a handful of statistical models. The Bayes factor, introduced in Chapter 3, is an obvious candidate for this task but theoretical and practical obstacles render its use not straightforward. Nevertheless, it is an indispensable tool for variable selection (see Chapter 11). Here, we treat two approximations to the Bayes factor: the pseudo-Bayes factor and the Bayesian Information Criterion (BIC). Together with

Bayesian Biostatistics, First Edition. Emmanuel Lesaffre and Andrew B. Lawson.

Akaike's Information Criterion (AIC), the BIC is the most often used frequentist information theoretic criterion. The AIC is introduced at length to serve as an introduction to the Deviance Information Criterion (DIC). This criterion is a popular tool for Bayesian model selection but produces occasionally peculiar results and caused a lot of discussion on the WinBUGS forum. We also review Bayesian GOF techniques, such as the posterior predictive check, and methods to locate outliers and influential observations. Finally, we explore GOF procedures that are based on expanding the model. Summarized, we look in this chapter for explorative tools that check and improve the fitted model.

10.2 Measures for model selection

In this section, we review and illustrate the use of Bayesian criteria for choosing the most appropriate model from a handful of candidates, but essentially we will look only at the comparison of two models.

10.2.1 The Bayes factor

10.2.1.1 Use in model selection

The Bayes factor was introduced in Section 3.8.2 as a Bayesian tool for hypothesis testing and that for both nested and non-nested models. Here, we illustrate its use in model selection. Suppose that there are two candidate (classes of) models for the data $\boldsymbol{y}$: M_1 with parameters $\boldsymbol{\theta}_1$ and M_2 with parameters $\boldsymbol{\theta}_2$. To choose the most appropriate model for the data at hand, one needs the marginal (averaged) likelihood under each model since the actual values of $\boldsymbol{\theta}_1$ and $\boldsymbol{\theta}_2$ are never known. For model M_m one computes

$$p(\boldsymbol{y} \mid M_m) = \int p(\boldsymbol{y} \mid \boldsymbol{\theta}_m, M_m)\, p(\boldsymbol{\theta}_m \mid M_m)\, \mathrm{d}\boldsymbol{\theta}_m, \quad (m = 1, 2),$$

which is also the prior predictive distribution for model M_m (Section 3.4.2). The posterior probability for model M_m

$$p(M_m \mid \boldsymbol{y}) = \frac{p(\boldsymbol{y} \mid M_m)\, p(M_m)}{p(\boldsymbol{y})} = \frac{p(\boldsymbol{y} \mid M_m)\, p(M_m)}{p(\boldsymbol{y} \mid M_1)\, p(M_1) + p(\boldsymbol{y} \mid M_2)\, p(M_2)}, \quad (m = 1, 2)$$

tells us which of the two models is most supported by the data. Further, the Bayes factor

$$BF_{12}(\boldsymbol{y}) = p(\boldsymbol{y} \mid M_1)/p(\boldsymbol{y} \mid M_2)$$

summarizes the evidence in the data for model M_1 compared to model M_2 irrespective of the prior probabilities $p(M_1)$ and $p(M_2)$. (Note that we have changed the notation of the Bayes factor from that in Chapter 3 to indicate which models are compared.) When $BF_{12}(\boldsymbol{y})$ is greater than one, then the posterior odds for M_1 is increased compared to the prior odds. For equal prior probabilities, model choice based on the Bayes factor is the same as model choice based on the above model posterior probabilities.

In the following example, we compute the Bayes factor to choose between two models for the dmft-index in the Signal-Tandmobiel® study of Example II.3.

Example X.1: Caries study: Choosing between a Poisson and a binomial distribution for the dmft index

Suppose, we wish to check which of the following two models fits best the distribution of the dmft index: (a) model M_1: Poisson(θ_1) where θ_1 represents the average dmft-index, or (b) model M_2: Bin(20, θ_2) with θ_2 the probability of caries experience for deciduous teeth in the mouth. To calculate the averaged likelihoods, we need to choose prior distributions for θ_1 and θ_2. Suppose, it is justified to take a gamma distribution for θ_1 and a beta distribution for θ_2. Then the averaged likelihoods for the sample of $n = 4351$ children are, respectively,

- $p(\mathbf{y} \mid M_1) = \prod_{i=1}^{n} \int \text{Poisson}(y_i \mid \theta_1) \, \text{Gamma}(\theta_1 \mid \alpha_{1,0}, \beta_{1,0}) \, d\theta_1$,
- $p(\mathbf{y} \mid M_2) = \prod_{i=1}^{n} \int \text{Bin}(y_i \mid 20, \theta_2) \, \text{Beta}(\theta_2 \mid \alpha_{2,0}, \beta_{2,0}) \, d\theta_2$.

For the two models, the integrations can be performed analytically. For model M_1, the contribution of the ith child with response y_i is $\text{NB}(y_i \mid \alpha_{1,0}, \beta_{1,0})$ while for model M_2 it is $\text{BB}(y_i \mid 20, \alpha_{2,0}, \beta_{2,0})$. The values $\alpha_{1,0}, \beta_{1,0}, \alpha_{2,0}$ and $\beta_{2,0}$ are supplied by the user. For the Poisson likelihood, we assume $\theta_1 \sim \text{Gamma}(3, 1)$ (as in Example II.3) to reflect the prior knowledge of an average dmft-index around 3 with 95% prior uncertainty ranging from 0.62 to 7.2. For the Poisson distribution, it is assumed that the dmft-values are sums of independent caries events. In that case $\theta_1/20$ should approximately correspond to θ_2, the probability that a tooth shows caries experience. A matching beta prior for θ_2 is the Beta(2.9, 16.5) distribution which overlaps the Gamma(3,1) distribution almost completely on the θ_2 scale. Thus, $p(\mathbf{y} \mid M_1)$ is the product of NB(3, 1) likelihoods and $p(\mathbf{y} \mid M_2)$ is the product of BB(20, 2.9, 16.5) likelihoods. With the averaged likelihood under the Poisson model denoted as L_1 and for the binomial model as L_2, we obtained $\log L_1 = -9781.793$ and $\log L_2 = -10065.36$. This shows that the Poisson model is 'very strongly' preferred over the binomial model with $\log BF_{12}(\mathbf{y}) = 283.57$.

That the Bayes factor favors the Poisson distribution does not imply that the Poisson model is appropriate which we can see in Figure 10.1. In addition, the fit of the Poisson distribution is only marginally better than the binomial fit, despite the strong preference for the Poisson model. □

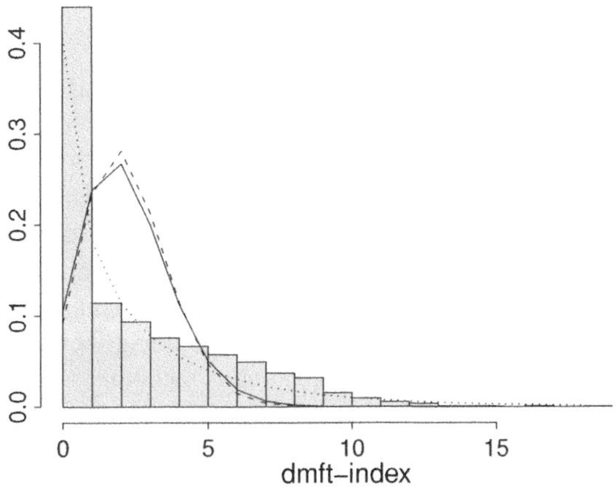

Figure 10.1 Caries study: histogram of dmft index and fitted Poisson (solid line), binomial (dashed line) and negative binomial (dotted line) distributions.

Occasionally, the Bayes factor can be determined analytically, but in general, it requires a numerical algorithm. An illustration of a naive numerical computation is given in next example.

Example X.2: Caries study: Choosing between three distributions for the dmft index with the Bayes factor
We now consider a third candidate model M_3 for y_i, i.e. the negative binomial distribution $\text{NB}(y_i|\alpha, \beta)$ given by expression (3.15). Based on ML, we obtained NB(0.56, 0.25) as best fitting negative binomial distribution, shown in Figure 10.1. Given the better fit of the negative binomial distribution, we expect that the Bayes factor favors model M_3 over models M_1 and M_2. Recall that in Example VI.10, the negative binomial distribution was preferred over the Poisson distribution using the RJMCMC approach.

Two parameters are involved with model M_3, i.e. $(\theta_3, \theta_4) \equiv (\alpha, \beta)$ and thus we need a bivariate prior distribution. For this exercise, we have taken flat priors for all three models, i.e. (a) model M_1: $\theta_1 \sim \text{U}(0, 20)$, (b) model M_2: $\theta_2 \sim \text{U}(0, 1)$, and (c) model M_3: $\theta_3 \sim \text{U}(0, 1)$ independently of $\theta_4 \sim \text{U}(0, 1)$. No analytical expressions are available now, hence we need to rely on numerical approximations. A brute force method, that only works in low-dimensional problems, is to randomly sample values $\boldsymbol{\theta}_m^1, \ldots, \boldsymbol{\theta}_m^K$ from the prior $p(\boldsymbol{\theta}_m \mid M_m)$ and to approximate the integral as follows:

$$p(\mathbf{y} \mid M_m) = \int p(\mathbf{y} \mid \boldsymbol{\theta}_m, M_m)\, p(\boldsymbol{\theta}_m \mid M_m)\, \text{d}\boldsymbol{\theta}_m \approx \frac{1}{K} \sum_{k=1}^{K} p(\mathbf{y} \mid \boldsymbol{\theta}_m^k, M_m). \tag{10.1}$$

Based on (10.1), we obtained $\log L_1 = -13040.75$, $\log L_2 = -13246.82$ and $\log L_3 = -10499.42$. Again, the Poisson model is preferred over the binomial model, but the uniform priors produced a different Bayes factor, i.e. $\log BF_{12}(\mathbf{y}) = 206.07$. On the other hand, $\log BF_{31}(\mathbf{y}) = 2541.33$ and $\log BF_{32}(\mathbf{y}) = 2747.40$ reveal a strong evidence for model M_3.

Finally, to further illustrate the dependence of the Bayes factor on the choice of the prior, we based the marginal likelihood for model M_3 on uniform priors on [0,10] for θ_3 and θ_4. For this prior $\log L_3 = -15186.84$ and apparently now model M_3 appears to be the worst of all three models. □

10.2.1.2 Computing the Bayes factor

The Bayes factor requires the calculation of the marginal likelihood which most often involves a computational procedure. Various approaches for calculating the Bayes factor in a direct manner have been reviewed in Kass and Raftery (1995). Ntzoufras (2009) provides WinBUGS programs for some of the simplest algorithms. However, the most promising algorithms are computationally involved perhaps even more involved than the MCMC algorithms for estimating the parameters. In Chapter 11, we will see that the Bayes factor can also be obtained from an indirect computation, namely as a by-product of the MCMC algorithm. We now briefly review some of these direct approaches. First, there are the general purpose numerical integration techniques such as the quadrature techniques of Section 3.7.1. They can achieve good performance up to dimensions 5–10. The second approach is sampling either from the prior or from the posterior. Sampling from the prior was done in Example X.2, but since the prior has often a much larger spread than the posterior, sampling from the prior implies that many sampled $\boldsymbol{\theta}$-values do not contribute much to the sum in equation (10.1) since their likelihood contribution is close to zero. Sampling from the posterior allows us to restrict to primarily realistic values of $\boldsymbol{\theta}$. Using the equality

$$\frac{1}{p(\mathbf{y} \mid M_m)} = \int \frac{1}{p(\mathbf{y} \mid \boldsymbol{\theta}_m, M_m)} \frac{p(\mathbf{y} \mid \boldsymbol{\theta}_m, M_m) p(\boldsymbol{\theta}_m \mid M_m)}{p(\mathbf{y} \mid M_m)} \, \mathrm{d}\boldsymbol{\theta}_m,$$

$$= \int \frac{1}{p(\mathbf{y} \mid \boldsymbol{\theta}_m, M_m)} p(\boldsymbol{\theta}_m \mid \mathbf{y}, M_m) \, \mathrm{d}\boldsymbol{\theta}_m,$$

Newton and Raftery (1994) suggested as estimate for the marginal likelihood the *harmonic mean of likelihoods* given by

$$\left(\frac{1}{K} \sum_{k=1}^{K} \frac{1}{p(\mathbf{y} \mid \boldsymbol{\theta}_m^k, M_m)} \right)^{-1}.$$

However, the estimator has a wild behavior and improvements have been suggested (Ntzoufras 2009). Yet other sampling techniques such as importance sampling, bridge sampling and MCMC sampling have been proposed; see Ntzoufras (2009) and references therein.

10.2.1.3 Pros and cons of the Bayes factor

The Bayes factor is based on the marginal likelihood of the data whereby the likelihood for $\boldsymbol{\theta}$ is averaged over its uncertainty given by the prior $p(\boldsymbol{\theta})$. Interestingly, the marginal likelihood does not require fitting the model to the data. This is in sharp contrast to the frequentist approach where estimation and testing procedures are closely linked. Indeed, while the Bayes factor is the natural Bayesian equivalent of the frequentist likelihood ratio test for model testing, it cannot be obtained from a Bayesian modeling exercise whereby two models are fit to the data. It is, though, a formally correct solution to model choice with, however, a number of practical limitations. In their review paper, Kass and Raftery (1995) summed up the pros and cons of the Bayes factor, some of which were already illustrated in Examples X.1 and X.2 two examples.

Arguments in favor of the Bayes factor are (1) the Bayes factor offers a way of evaluating evidence in favor of H_0, as seen in Chapter 3; (2) external information can be incorporated; (3) nonstandard models and non-nested models are allowed for, and (4) invariance to parameter transformation (in contrast to the information-theoretic approaches mentioned later). However, the use of the Bayes factor in practice is not straightforward because of the difficulty in choosing an appropriate prior $p(\boldsymbol{\theta})$. As an illustration, see the effect of the change in priors in Example X.2. The important drop in marginal likelihood for model M_3 was caused by the prior $p(\theta_3, \theta_4) \propto \mathrm{U}(0, 10) \times \mathrm{U}(0, 10)$ which averages the negative binomial likelihood over many unrealistic $\boldsymbol{\theta}$-values. We have seen in Section 3.8.3 that this causes the Bartlett–Lindley's paradox for nested models. The dependence of the Bayes factor on the choice of prior does not decrease with increasing sample size as with the posterior distribution. In addition, when comparing models with a different number of parameters or a different kind of parameters, it is not immediately clear how to choose matching priors as illustrated in Example X.2. For another example, consider choosing between a gamma distribution and a Box-Cox transformation model, i.e. $(y^\lambda - 1)/\lambda \sim \mathrm{N}(\mu, \sigma^2)$, for a positive random variable y. The first model has two parameters while the second model has three parameters but of a different nature. Even more problematic is that the Bayes factor cannot be used with improper priors. Indeed, while an improper prior may lead to a proper posterior, an improper prior always results in an improper marginal distribution (see Section 5.4.4). In that case, the Bayes factor becomes undetermined. A simple example that illustrates this indeterminacy now follows. Suppose that a Gaussian distribution (M_1) and a t_3-distribution (M_2), both with an unknown location parameter μ and a known scale parameter, are compared using the Bayes factor. Assume improper flat priors for μ, then with equal prior probabilities for the two models:

$$\frac{p(M_1 \mid \mathbf{y})}{p(M_2 \mid \mathbf{y})} = \frac{p(\mathbf{y} \mid M_1)}{p(\mathbf{y} \mid M_2)} \frac{p(M_1)}{p(M_2)} = \frac{\int p(\mathbf{y} \mid \mu, M_1) p(\mu \mid M_1)\, \mathrm{d}\mu}{\int p(\mathbf{y} \mid \mu, M_2) p(\mu \mid M_2)\, \mathrm{d}\mu} = \frac{\int p(\mathbf{y} \mid \mu, M_1) c_1\, \mathrm{d}\mu}{\int p(\mathbf{y} \mid \mu, M_2) c_2\, \mathrm{d}\mu} \propto \frac{c_1}{c_2}.$$

For the improper priors, it does not matter which constants c_1 and c_2 are taken. Given the arbitrariness of the choice of constants, the Bayes factor is not defined for such priors. Moreover, O'Hagan and Forster (2004, p. 179) showed that the Bayes factor is even sensitive to the choice of the prior when the prior is not particularly weak and the data are strong.

Finally as seen earlier, numerical computation of the Bayes factor is far from trivial.

Therefore, it should not come as a surprise that Bayesians are divided about the value of the Bayes factor as a tool for model selection. Gelfand (Gilks *et al.* 1996, p. 149) writes '... use of Bayes factors often seem inappropriate in real applications'. Gelman *et al.* (2004) hardly spent two pages on the Bayes factor in their book, giving an example where the Bayes factor could be considered useful and another example where it causes confusion. O'Hagan (2006), on the other hand, argued that 'Bayes factors are an important part of the applied Bayesian statistician's toolkit'. Notwithstanding the problems, Albert (1999) provided an elegant illustration of the use of the Bayes factor in model building and criticism with a Poisson-gamma hierarchical model.

Two approximations of the Bayes factor are frequently used in practice: the BIC and the *pseudo-Bayes factor*. We first discuss the pseudo-Bayes factor.

10.2.1.4 A variation on the Bayes factor: The pseudo-Bayes factor

A major difficulty with the Bayes factor is that it cannot be used with improper priors. Various suggestions were made in the literature to bypass this obstacle. One approach is to use part of the data to update the (improper) prior to a proper posterior and then base the Bayes factor on this posterior. This goes as follows (Gelfand and Dey 1994): Suppose that the data $\mathbf{y} = \{y_1, \ldots, y_n\}$ are split up into a learning part $\mathbf{y}_L = \{y_i\ (i \in L)\}$ and a testing part $\mathbf{y}_T = \{y_i\ (i \in T)\}$, with L and T nonoverlapping parts of $\{1, \ldots, n\}$. Further, for a subset S of $\{1, \ldots, n\}$ let

$$L\left(\boldsymbol{\theta}_m \mid \mathbf{y}_S, M_m\right) = \prod_{i \in S} p(y_i \mid \boldsymbol{\theta}_m, M_m),$$

and define the conditional density as

$$\begin{aligned} p(\mathbf{y}_T \mid \mathbf{y}_L, M_m) &= \int L\left(\boldsymbol{\theta}_m \mid \mathbf{y}_T, M_m\right) p(\boldsymbol{\theta}_m \mid \mathbf{y}_L, M_m)\, \mathrm{d}\boldsymbol{\theta}_m \\ &= \frac{\int L\left(\boldsymbol{\theta}_m \mid \mathbf{y}_T, M_m\right) L\left(\boldsymbol{\theta}_m \mid \mathbf{y}_L, M_m\right) p(\boldsymbol{\theta}_m \mid M_m)\, \mathrm{d}\boldsymbol{\theta}_m}{\int L\left(\boldsymbol{\theta}_m \mid \mathbf{y}_L, M_m\right) p(\boldsymbol{\theta}_m \mid M_m)\, \mathrm{d}\boldsymbol{\theta}_m}. \end{aligned} \qquad (10.2)$$

Expression (10.2) defines a predictive density which averages the joint density of $\mathbf{y}_T$ over the prior for $\boldsymbol{\theta}_m$ updated by $\mathbf{y}_L$. When $p(\mathbf{y} \mid M_m)$ is replaced by $p(\mathbf{y}_T \mid \mathbf{y}_L, M_m)$ a variant of the Bayes factor is obtained

$$BF_{12}^*(\mathbf{y}) = p(\mathbf{y}_T \mid \mathbf{y}_L, M_1)/p(\mathbf{y}_T \mid \mathbf{y}_L, M_2), \tag{10.3}$$

where the Bayes factor evidently depends on the choice of the learning part. Particular choices of L and T produce some well-known variations of the Bayes factor, such as the *intrinsic Bayes factor* and the *posterior Bayes factor* (Gelfand and Dey 1994). The advantage of $BF_{12}^*(\mathbf{y})$ over $BF_{12}(\mathbf{y})$ is that it can be computed with improper priors (as long as the posterior is proper) but it requires setting apart a learning set and its choice is to a great extent arbitrary.

With the choice of $T_i = \{i\}$ and $L_i = \{1, \ldots, i-1, i+1, \ldots, n\}$ $(1 \le i \le n)$, we obtain n learning and testing sets, i.e. $\mathbf{y}_{L_i} \equiv \mathbf{y}_{(i)} = \{y_1, \ldots, y_{i-1}, y_{i+1}, \ldots, y_n\}$ and $\mathbf{y}_{T_i} \equiv y_i$. This yields the cross-validation density $p(y_i \mid \mathbf{y}_{(i)}, M_m)$ introduced by Geisser (1980), also called the *conditional predictive ordinate* (CPO$_i$). Geisser and Eddy (1979) defined the pseudo-Bayes factor (PSBF) for comparing models M_1 and M_2 as

$$\text{PSBF}_{12} = \frac{\prod_i p(y_i \mid \mathbf{y}_{(i)}, M_1)}{\prod_i p(y_i \mid \mathbf{y}_{(i)}, M_2)} = \frac{\prod_i \text{CPO}_i(M_1)}{\prod_i \text{CPO}_i(M_2)}. \tag{10.4}$$

It can be noticed that PSBF$_{12}$ differs from expression (10.3) in that the marginal likelihood (conditional on $\mathbf{y}_L$) in (10.3) is replaced by a product of conditional densities. This follows from a suggestion of Geisser and Eddy (1979) who used $\prod_i p(y_i \mid \mathbf{y}_{(i)}, M_m)$ as a surrogate for $p(\mathbf{y} \mid M_m)$. Gelfand and Dey (1994) showed that the pseudo-Bayes factor is asymptotically related to AIC and does not suffer from Lindley's paradox.

For the computation of PSBF$_{12}$, we need $p(y_i \mid \mathbf{y}_{(i)}, M_m)$ and compute CPO$_i(M_m)$. How this can be done in combination with MCMC sampling is shown in Section 10.3 where we also show that WinBUGS (or R2WinBUGS) can be used for this. Here, we assume that CPO$_i(M_m)$ can be computed and denote its estimate as $\widehat{\text{CPO}}_i(M_m)$. PSBF$_{12}$ is computed by multiplication of $\widehat{\text{CPO}}_i(M_m)$ over the n observations for $m = 1, 2$ and taking the ratio. In practice, one reports log(PSBF$_{12}$). We now illustrate the use of the PSBF to choose between the three discrete distributions for the dmft index in the Signal-Tandmobiel study.

Example X.3: Caries study: Choosing between three distributions for the dmft index with the pseudo-Bayes factor

Under the settings of Example X.2, we compute the PSBF to choose between a Poisson (M_1), binomial (M_2) and negative binomial (M_3) model. In 'chapter 10 PSBF dmft index.odc' we computed $1/\widehat{\text{CPO}}_i(M_m)$ $(i = 1, \ldots, n)$ for the three count models. The program 'chapter 10 PSBF dmft index.R' computes the pseudo-Bayes factor based on the generated output. This results in $\sum_i \log[\widehat{\text{CPO}}_i(M_1)] = -2.64$, $\sum_i \log[\widehat{\text{CPO}}_i(M_2)] = -2.81$, $\sum_i \log[\widehat{\text{CPO}}_i(M_1)] = -1.97$ and therefore $\widehat{\text{PSBF}}_{12} = 1.19$, $\widehat{\text{PSBF}}_{13} = 0.51$ and $\widehat{\text{PSBF}}_{23} = 0.43$. The conclusion is the same as with the ordinary Bayes factors, namely, that the negative binomial distribution is to be preferred. □

The CPO, and in general predictive distributions, are also useful for outlier detection in a Bayesian manner. We return to that in Section 10.3.

10.2.2 Information theoretic measures for model selection

The two most popular frequentist information criteria to choose between models are: AIC and BIC. However, strictly speaking BIC is not based on information-theoretic concepts (Anderson and Burnham 1999) but is rather a special case of the Bayes factor. That BIC is treated here and not in Section 1.2.1, has to do with the fact AIC and BIC are often reviewed together in the literature. Note that, despite BIC is a Bayesian concept, it is more popular in frequentist applications.

AIC and BIC balance model fit with model complexity defined as the number of free model parameters also called *effective degrees of freedom*. The effective degrees of freedom often coincides with the number of freely varying parameters (p) in the model. In models involving smoothing and in hierarchical models, the degrees of freedom are less than p. It will be shown in this section that model complexity also depends on the focus of the model which determines on its turn the choice of the information criterion. We start with introducing AIC to serve as background for the Deviance Information Criterion (DIC), which is the most popular Bayesian criterion in model selection and the Bayesian generalization of AIC.

10.2.2.1 AIC and BIC

The most popular frequentist measure for model selection is AIC developed by Hirotsugu Akaike who called it 'another information criterion' (Akaike 1974). AIC is a measure of model fit penalized for model complexity and is especially useful to select among non-nested statistical models. The basis for AIC is the *Kullback-Leibler (K-L) distance* between two densities f and g defined as

$$I(f,g) = \int \log\left[\frac{f(x)}{g(x)}\right] f(x)\,dx. \tag{10.5}$$

The K-L-distance between the true density p^t of the distribution of $\boldsymbol{y}$ and $p_\theta(\boldsymbol{y}) \equiv p(\boldsymbol{y} \mid \boldsymbol{\theta})$, which is the proposed model for fitting $\boldsymbol{y}$ parameterized by a p-dimensional parameter vector $\boldsymbol{\theta} \in \Theta$ is

$$I(p^t, p_{\boldsymbol{\theta}}) = E^t\left[\log p^t(\boldsymbol{y})\right] - E^t\left[\log p_{\boldsymbol{\theta}}(\boldsymbol{y})\right] \geq 0.$$

E^t signifies that the expectation is taken with respect to p^t. Define $\boldsymbol{\theta}^t$ as the value that minimizes $I(p^t, p_{\boldsymbol{\theta}})$. The K-L distance is zero only when p^t can be written exactly as $p(\boldsymbol{y} \mid \boldsymbol{\theta}^t)$.

$I(p^t, p_{\boldsymbol{\theta}^t})$ measures how well the class of models $\Im = \{p_{\boldsymbol{\theta}} \mid \boldsymbol{\theta} \in \Theta\}$ can fit the data. For two classes $\Im_1$, $\Im_2$ with respective K-L distances I_1, I_2 the one with the smallest value is to be preferred. Note that when comparing I_1 with I_2, only the second term in the expression of the K-L distance is needed. In practice $\boldsymbol{\theta}^t$ is not known, but nevertheless, we wish to know which model fits best the (future) data. One could estimate $E^t[\log p(\boldsymbol{y} \mid \boldsymbol{\theta}^t)]$ by $\log p(\boldsymbol{y} \mid \widehat{\boldsymbol{\theta}}(\boldsymbol{y}))$ with $\widehat{\boldsymbol{\theta}}(\boldsymbol{y})$ the maximum likelihood estimate (MLE) of $\boldsymbol{\theta}$ based on the data $\boldsymbol{y}$. Since under general regularity conditions $\widehat{\boldsymbol{\theta}}(\boldsymbol{y}) \to \boldsymbol{\theta}^t$ for $n \to \infty$, one might hope for a good performance of this measure. However, in $\log p(\boldsymbol{y} \mid \widehat{\boldsymbol{\theta}}(\boldsymbol{y}))$ the data are doubly used: (1) once to estimate $\boldsymbol{\theta}$ and (2) another time to evaluate the predictive performance of the fitted model. Hence, this is not the way to estimate the performance of the model on new data. In fact, we need $E^t E^{t*}[\log p(\boldsymbol{y}^* \mid \widehat{\boldsymbol{\theta}}(\boldsymbol{y}))]$, with E^{t*} the expectation over new data $\boldsymbol{y}^*$ independent of $\boldsymbol{y}$ but having the same distribution p^t. The negative bias induced by taking $\log p(\boldsymbol{y} \mid \widehat{\boldsymbol{\theta}}(\boldsymbol{y}))$ is the expected value (under true model) of

$$\log p(y \mid \theta^t) - \log p(y \mid \widehat{\theta}(y)).$$

To express the bias of the fitted model we define

$$d\left[y, \theta^t, \widehat{\theta}(y)\right] = -2 \log p\left(y \mid \theta^t\right) + 2 \log p(y \mid \widehat{\theta}(y)). \tag{10.6}$$

It can be shown that the expected value of $d[y, \theta^t, \widehat{\theta}(y)]$ under the true model is equal to

$$E^t \left\{d\left[y, \theta^t, \widehat{\theta}(y)\right]\right\} \approx \rho = \mathrm{tr}\left[\mathfrak{K}(\theta^t)\mathfrak{I}(\theta^t)^{-1}\right], \tag{10.7}$$

with $\mathfrak{I}(\theta^t) = -E^t[\frac{\partial^2 \log p(y|\theta^t)}{\partial \theta^2}]$ and $\mathfrak{K}(\theta^t) = E^t[\frac{\partial \log p(y|\theta^t)}{\partial \theta} \frac{\partial \log p(y|\theta^t)}{\partial \theta}^T]$.

When $p^t(y) = p(y \mid \theta^t)$, then $\rho = p$ and $-2\, E^t E^{t*}[\log p(y^* \mid \widehat{\theta}(y))]$ (the factor -2 is classically included in the literature) is estimated by

$$\mathrm{AIC} = -2 \log p(y \mid \widehat{\theta}(y)) + 2p = -2 \log \mathrm{L}(\widehat{\theta}(y) \mid y) + 2p. \tag{10.8}$$

AIC is called a *penalized model selection criterion* since it penalizes the maximized −2(log-likelihood) with the penalty term $2p$ for overfitting the data. The model with the lowest AIC among a set of candidate models is to be preferred. The penalty term is also referred to as 'model complexity', since the more parameters are involved the more complex the model is. In addition, since AIC estimates $-2\, E^t E^{t*}[\log p(y^* \mid \widehat{\theta}(y))]$ it measures the predictive ability of the model.

The penalty increases with the number of parameters in the model. In fact, it is simply a reflection that a complex model has a higher power to provide a good fit to the data than a simple model. But this fit is specific for the data at hand and most likely the quality of fit cannot be achieved in future data.

Example X.4: Theoretical example: AIC for a linear regression model
For a Gaussian regression model with $(d + 1)$ regressors (including constant), $AIC = n \log(\widehat{\sigma}^2) + 2p + C$, where $\widehat{\sigma}^2 = \sum \widehat{\varepsilon}_i^2/n$ with $\widehat{\varepsilon}_i$ the estimated residual of the ith individual. Here $p = d + 2$, representing the regression coefficients and the residual variance. The constant $C = n \log(2\pi) + n$ is reported here for use in Example X.5, but is not important in practice since AIC is only used for comparing models. □

Approximation (10.8) is good when the sample size is large and the proposed model is not too different from the true model. For a small sample, one uses the corrected AIC_c obtained from AIC by replacing p by $p(\frac{n}{n-p-1})$. When the class $\mathfrak{I}$ does not contain the true distribution, the penalty term is equal to $2\mathrm{tr}[\mathfrak{K}(\theta)\mathfrak{I}(\theta)^{-1}]$ and Takeuchi's Information Criterion (TIC) is obtained.

The BIC, suggested by Schwarz (1978), is another popular penalized model selection criterion. The formula for BIC is

$$\mathrm{BIC} = -2 \log \mathrm{L}(\widehat{\theta}(y) \mid y) + p \log(n). \tag{10.9}$$

As for AIC, models with a smaller value of BIC are preferred. BIC is popular in frequentist statistics but is in fact a Bayesian measure. We now sketch the proof given by Raftery (1995) and Kuha (2004) that BIC is obtained from a Laplace approximation of the marginal likelihood. This derivation is useful for the understanding of some variable selection techniques in Chapter 11. For notational simplicity, we omit the subindex m. The expression $g(\boldsymbol{\theta}) = \log[p(\mathbf{y} \mid \boldsymbol{\theta}, M)p(\boldsymbol{\theta} \mid M)]$ for model M can be expanded around the p-dimensional posterior mode $\boldsymbol{\theta}_M$, as follows:

$$\log p(\mathbf{y} \mid M) = \log p(\mathbf{y} \mid \boldsymbol{\theta}_M, M) + \log p(\boldsymbol{\theta}_M \mid M) + (p/2)\log(2\pi) - (1/2)\log \mid A \mid + O(n^{-1}),$$

with $A = -\ddot{g}(\boldsymbol{\theta}_M)$ whereby $\ddot{g}$ denotes a second derivative with respect to its parameters. $O(n^{-1})$ represents a term that goes as fast to zero as $1/n$ for $n \to \infty$.

For a large sample, $\boldsymbol{\theta}_M \approx \widehat{\boldsymbol{\theta}}$, the MLE and $A = \Im(\widehat{\boldsymbol{\theta}})$. This yields $\log p(\mathbf{y} \mid M) = \log p(\mathbf{y} \mid \widehat{\boldsymbol{\theta}}, M) - (p/2)\log n + O(1)$, with $O(1)$ a term that does not vanish when $n \to \infty$. A better approximation (of $O(n^{-1/2})$) is obtained when the prior $p(\boldsymbol{\theta}|M)$ is equal to the *unit information prior* given by

$$\mathrm{N}\left(\boldsymbol{\theta} \mid \widehat{\boldsymbol{\theta}}, n\widehat{V}\right), \tag{10.10}$$

with $\widehat{V} = \Im(\widehat{\boldsymbol{\theta}})^{-1}$ (or replaced by the observed Fisher information matrix). This prior distribution contains the same amount of information as (on average) a single observation. Then $\log p(\mathbf{y} \mid M) = \log p(\mathbf{y} \mid \widehat{\boldsymbol{\theta}}, M) - (p/2)\log n + O(n^{-1/2})$ and $-2\log BF_{12}(\mathbf{y}) = -2\{\log p(\mathbf{y} \mid M_1) - \log p(\mathbf{y} \mid M_2)\} \approx -2\{\log p(\mathbf{y} \mid \widehat{\boldsymbol{\theta}}_1, M_1) - \log p(\mathbf{y} \mid \widehat{\boldsymbol{\theta}}_2, M_2)\} + (p_1 - p_2)\log n + O(n^{-1/2})$ which is approximately $\mathrm{BIC}_1 - \mathrm{BIC}_2$. Summarized: BIC with a particular prior is a large sample version of a Bayes factor. Raftery (1995, 1999) advocated the unit information prior in model and variable selection. Note that AIC can also be seen as a special case of a Bayes factor, but with a prior comparable to that of the likelihood (Kass and Raftery 1995).

AIC and BIC are derived from two different principles, but both adhere *Occam's Razor principle* derived from a well-known statement of the English logician William Occam (1285–1347) that 'entities must not be multiplied beyond necessity' (see also Forster 2000). This translates here as: if two models describe the observations equally well, we should choose the simpler one. In practice, both measures provide only a rough indication of which model to choose. Classically, only a difference of more than 5 is considered as substantive evidence for the model with the smallest AIC or BIC, while a difference of more than 10 represents strong evidence. From expressions (10.8) and (10.9), we infer that BIC favors simpler models than AIC for larger values of n (when $n \geq 8$). The performance of AIC and BIC has been compared in a variety of application areas by means of analyses on real data sets and simulations (see Kuha 2004; Lin and Dayton 1997; Ward 2008 and references therein). The conclusion from these papers is mixed in the sense that there is no clear winner, but all indicate that BIC has a tendency to select simpler models than AIC especially for large sample sizes. Why there is a greater preference for simpler models (hence conservatism) with BIC is seen from the fact that BIC is an approximation to the Bayes factor with the unit information prior, which might be too widespread (and thus does not represent the actual knowledge one has on the model) such that BIC may suffer from Lindley's paradox.

For hierarchical models, we need to be careful when determining the effective degrees of freedom for the computation of AIC. Indeed, in a hierarchical model, there are fixed effects and random effects, the latter not varying freely. Hence, the effective number of parameters in a hierarchical model must be less than the total number of parameters. Further, for a hierarchical model one may choose between the conditional likelihood (given the random effects) or the marginal likelihood (integrated over the random effects) as basis for computing AIC. We illustrate these issues with a Gaussian hierarchical model in the next example.

Example X.5: Theoretical example: Conditional and marginal likelihood of a linear mixed model
We now look at the Gaussian hierarchical model of Example IX.7 in a frequentist context. Using the assumptions made in that example and with the same notation, the conditional likelihood given the random effects is $L_C(\boldsymbol{\theta}, \sigma \mid \mathbf{y}) = \prod_i^n \prod_j^{m_i} \mathrm{N}(y_{ij} \mid \theta_i, \sigma^2)$. Integrating the conditional likelihood over the random effects produces the marginal likelihood L_M. The marginal distribution is determined by: $y_{ij} \sim \mathrm{N}(\mu, \sigma^2 + \sigma_\theta^2)$, $(j = 1, \ldots, m_i;$ $i = 1, \ldots, n)$ and $\mathrm{corr}(y_{ij}, y_{i'j'}) = \sigma^2$ if $j \neq j'$, $i = i'$ and 0 if $i \neq i'$. For the Gaussian hierarchical model, the penalty term in AIC is equal to the number of freely varying parameters. In the marginal model, this number is 3. In the conditional model, there are $n + 2$ parameters with n parameters pertaining to the random effects. When $\sigma_\theta = 0$, their contribution reduces to one while for $\sigma_\theta = \infty$ all clusters are considered to be unrelated and the random effects imply n free parameters. □

Hodges (1998) and Hodges and Sargent (2001) defined the effective number of parameters in a Gaussian linear mixed model, denoted ρ, as the trace of a (nonorthogonal) projection matrix. In this way, ρ becomes the effective dimension of the predicted response corresponding to the traditional interpretation of the effective degrees of freedom. Lu *et al.* (2007) extended their proposal to generalized linear mixed models.

Example X.6: Theoretical example: Effective degrees of freedom of a linear mixed model
For the Gaussian hierarchical model in Example X.5 with $m_i = m$ $(i = 1, \ldots, n)$, Hodges and Sargent (2001) obtained for the conditional model $\rho = 1 + (n - 1)m/(m + \psi)$ with $\psi = \sigma^2/\sigma_\theta^2$. Hence, ρ depends on the ratio of the within- to between-cluster variability. When $\psi \to 0$, i.e. when the between-cluster variation is large to the within-cluster variation, $\rho \to n$. We interpret this limiting case as that the n different θ_is have no common distribution (there will be no shrinkage in the EB estimates). When $\psi \to \infty$, the within-cluster variation (σ^2) is large compared to the between-cluster variation (σ_θ^2) and the fitted θ_i shrink to μ together with $\rho \to 1$. □

Next, we need to consider the choice of the likelihood in the computation of the hierarchical version of AIC. A key question is whether we should take the conditional or the marginal likelihood for the calculation of AIC. This question turns out to be also relevant for DIC. Note that this choice reflects our focus with the statistical model. To see this, recall that AIC is a measure of predictive ability of the statistical model. In the case of a Gaussian hierarchical model, the marginal likelihood involves only $\mu, \sigma_\theta^2, \sigma^2$ without explicit reference to the included clusters. Therefore, AIC based on the marginal likelihood evaluates the predictive ability of the model when observations from future clusters of the $\mathrm{N}(\mu, \sigma_\theta^2)$ distribution are taken. On the other hand, since the conditional likelihood involves θ_i $(i = 1, \ldots, n)$, AIC based on the conditional likelihood evaluates prediction of observations from the current clusters. In Example IX.9, we predicted the cholesterol intake of future individuals of the same subsidiaries as in the dietary study. To evaluate the predictive ability of the model in this case, we must use the conditional likelihood. When the cholesterol intake of individuals from other subsidiaries (that could have been sampled originally) is of interest, then we base AIC on the marginal likelihood. Thus, the choice between the conditional and marginal model for the computation of AIC depends on the focus of the model: here predicting either future observations from existing clusters or from future clusters (i.e. the population of clusters). Vaida and Blanchard (2005) provided other illustrations of the inappropriateness of the classical AIC when the focus is on cluster level. They also derived the conditional AIC for a Gaussian linear mixed model.

10.2.2.2 Deviance Information Criterion

We now turn to the Bayesian case and treat the DIC proposed by Spiegelhalter *et al.* (2002) as a tool for model selection in a Bayesian context. A key question is how to define the effective number of parameters in a Bayesian context, especially for complex models.

To define the complexity of the model in a Bayesian context, Spiegelhalter *et al.* (2002) suggested to replace $\boldsymbol{\theta}^t$ in expression (10.6) by a random variable $\boldsymbol{\theta}$ and to take the expectation of expression (10.6) over the posterior $p(\boldsymbol{\theta} \mid \mathbf{y})$. This produces p_D, a Bayesian measure of complexity. More specifically,

$$p_D = E_{\boldsymbol{\theta}|\mathbf{y}}\left\{\mathrm{d}\left[\mathbf{y}, \boldsymbol{\theta}, \overline{\boldsymbol{\theta}}(\mathbf{y})\right]\right\} = E_{\boldsymbol{\theta}|\mathbf{y}}\left[-2\log p(\mathbf{y} \mid \boldsymbol{\theta}) + 2\log p(\mathbf{y} \mid \overline{\boldsymbol{\theta}}(\mathbf{y}))\right], \qquad (10.11)$$

with $\overline{\boldsymbol{\theta}}(\mathbf{y})$ the posterior mean. p_D can also be written as

$$p_D = \overline{D(\boldsymbol{\theta})} - D(\overline{\boldsymbol{\theta}}), \qquad (10.12)$$

with $D(\boldsymbol{\theta}) = -2\log p(\mathbf{y} \mid \boldsymbol{\theta}) + 2\log f(\mathbf{y})$ called the *Bayesian deviance*. $\overline{D(\boldsymbol{\theta})}$ is the posterior mean of $D(\boldsymbol{\theta})$, while $D(\overline{\boldsymbol{\theta}})$ is equal to $D(\boldsymbol{\theta})$ evaluated in the posterior mean of the parameters. The term $f(\mathbf{y})$ is independent of parameters and is introduced to compute DIC. For instance, for the exponential family with $E(\mathbf{y}) = \boldsymbol{\mu}(\boldsymbol{\theta})$ the authors propose $f(\mathbf{y}) = p(\mathbf{y} \mid \boldsymbol{\mu}(\boldsymbol{\theta}) = \mathbf{y})$. However, the term $f(\mathbf{y})$ cancels out from the expression of p_D. Note that in WinBUGS the term $f(\mathbf{y})$ is not computed.

Much of p_D's credibility comes from the fact that it coincides with frequentist measures of complexity for a normal likelihood combined with a flat prior for the mean parameter and fixed variance parameters. The analogy with ρ in the development of AIC follows from comparing expressions (10.7) and (10.11). In fact the frequentist expectation over the true model is replaced here by a Bayesian expectation over the posterior distribution. In the general case p_D and ρ may differ considerably (Lu *et al.* 2007).

Spiegelhalter *et al.* (2002) proposed DIC as a Bayesian model selection criterion, defined as

$$DIC = D(\overline{\boldsymbol{\theta}}) + 2p_D = \overline{D(\boldsymbol{\theta})} + p_D. \qquad (10.13)$$

While $f(\mathbf{y})$ is included in the computation of DIC (but not in WinBUGS), it plays no role in model choice. An attractive aspect of p_D and DIC is that both can readily be calculated from an MCMC run by monitoring $\boldsymbol{\theta}$ and $D(\boldsymbol{\theta})$. Let $\boldsymbol{\theta}^1, \ldots, \boldsymbol{\theta}^K$ represent a converged Markov chain, then $\overline{D(\boldsymbol{\theta})}$ can be approximated by $\frac{1}{K}\sum_{k=1}^K D(\boldsymbol{\theta}^k)$ and $D(\overline{\boldsymbol{\theta}})$ by $D(\frac{1}{K}\sum_{k=1}^K \boldsymbol{\theta}^k)$. The implementation of p_D and DIC in WinBUGS has encouraged greatly its use.

The rule of thumb for using DIC in model selection is roughly the same as for AIC and BIC, namely, a difference in DIC of more than 10 rules out the model with the higher DIC while with a difference of less than 5 there is no clear winner. Note that DIC is subject to sampling variability since it is based on the output of an MCMC procedure.

By means of several examples we now illustrate the use (and) pitfalls of p_D and DIC in choosing the best fitting model. Some of these limitations were already mentioned in the discussion part of Spiegelhalter *et al.* (2002). They caused considerable confusion among WinBUGS users. Especially for novel users we hope that these illustrations are illuminating. Further explanation and examples can be found at the WinBUGS website. We also illustrate some theoretical results on the relationship between AIC and DIC, such as the asymptotic equivalence of AIC and DIC for nonhierarchical models proved by Zhu and Carlin (2000).

Example X.7: Osteoporosis study: p_D and DIC compared to p and AIC

The regression model of Example IV.7 with TBBMC regressed on BMI is an example of a nonhierarchical model. A frequentist regression analysis yields AIC $= 85.6$, AIC$_c = 85.7$ and BIC $= 95.4$ since $n = 234$, $p = 3$ and $\widehat{\sigma}^2 = 0.082$. To obtain p_D and DIC with WinBUGS the chain must have converged. Then one clicks on option **Inference** of the menu bar and chooses **DIC**. The window **DIC Tool** appears. A click on **set** prepares WinBUGS for monitoring p_D and DIC. Based on 1000 additional iterations and upon clicking on DIC, WinBUGS showed a window **DIC** containing Dbar $(\overline{D(\boldsymbol{\theta})}) = 82.619$, Dhat $(D(\overline{\boldsymbol{\theta}})) = 79.582$, $p_D = 3.038$ and DIC $= 85.657$. These results provide a numerical illustration of the asymptotic relationship (Zhu and Carlin 2000) between AIC and DIC for nonhierarchical models.

One can also verify that Dhat is the posterior mean of the deviance. For instance, by monitoring the built-in logical node 'deviance' (equal to $D(\boldsymbol{\theta})$). □

The next example is a more extensive application of p_D and DIC on a Bayesian linear mixed model.

Example X.8: Potthoff & Roy growth-curve study: Model selection using p_D and DIC

We consider here the well-known data set first analyzed by Potthoff and Roy (1964). Dental growth measurements of the distance (mm) from the center of the pituitary gland to the pteryomaxillary fissure were obtained on 11 girls and 16 boys at ages (years) 8, 10, 12 and 14. The variables are gender (1 = female, 0 = male) and age; see Figure 10.2 for the individual profiles as a function of age.

We fitted several (Gaussian) linear mixed models to the longitudinal profiles. The different WinBUGS programs can be found in 'chapter 10 Potthoff–Roy growthcurves.odc'. The following models were explored:

- *Model* M_1: $y_{ij} = \beta_0 + \beta_1\,\text{age}_j + \beta_2\,\text{gender}_i + \beta_3\,\text{gender}_i \times \text{age}_j + b_{0i} + b_{1i}\,\text{age}_j + \varepsilon_{ij}$, with y_{ij} the distance measurement for the ith subject at age $2(j+3)$ $(j = 1, 2, 3, 4)$, $\boldsymbol{b}_i = (b_{0i}, b_{1i})^T$ random intercept and slope with distribution $\text{N}((0,0)^T, \text{G})$, $\text{G} = \begin{pmatrix} \sigma_{b0}^2 & \rho\sigma_{b0}\sigma_{b1} \\ \rho\sigma_{b0}\sigma_{b1} & \sigma_{b1}^2 \end{pmatrix}$, $\varepsilon_{ij} \sim \text{N}(0, \sigma_0^2)$ for males and $\varepsilon_{ij} \sim \text{N}(0, \sigma_1^2)$ for females;
- *Model* M_2: model M_1, but assuming $\rho = 0$;
- *Model* M_3: model M_2, but assuming $\sigma_0 = \sigma_1$;
- *Model* M_4: model M_1, but assuming $\sigma_0 = \sigma_1$;

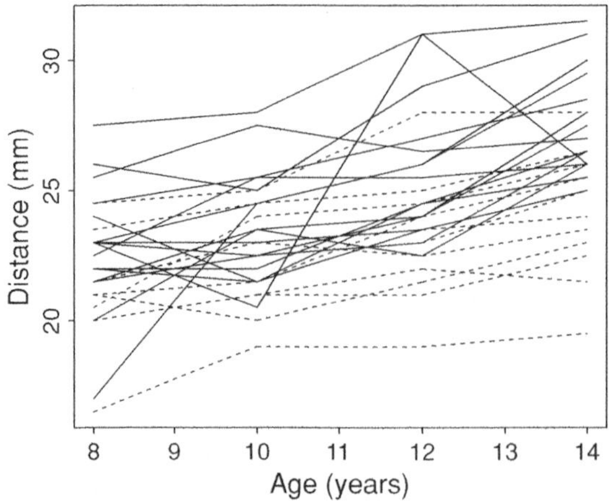

Figure 10.2 Potthoff & Roy growth curve study: Profiles of the distance from the center of the pituitary gland to the pteryomaxillary fissure as a function of age split up according to gender (solid line = boys, dashed line = girls).

- *Model* M_5: model M_1, but the random effects have a bivariate scaled t_3-distribution and measurement error distributions are scaled t_3-distributions;
- *Model* M_6: model M_1, but only the measurement error distributions are scaled t_3-distributions;
- *Model* M_7: model M_1, but the random effects have a bivariate scaled t_3-distribution.

The nested model comparisons involve: (a) models M_1, M_2, M_3; (b) models M_1, M_2, M_4, and (c) models M_5, M_6, M_7. The other model comparisons are not nested. The total number of parameters for model M_1 is 63 which is equal to the sum of 4 fixed effects parameters, 54 random effects parameters, 3 variance parameters for the random effects and 2 variance parameters for measurement error.

For all parameters, we considered vague priors, namely, for the regression coefficients we have taken $N(0, 10^6)$ and $IG(10^{-3}, 10^{-3})$ was taken for the measurement error variance(s). In model M_1, we tested three choices for the inverse Wishart prior of G. In addition, we assumed uniform priors for the standard deviation of the random intercept, slope and correlation, i.e. $\sigma_{b0}, \sigma_{b1} \sim U(0, 100)$ and $\rho \sim U(-1, 1)$. Based on our findings in Exercise 10.2 and the simulation results of Natarajan and Kass (2000), we opted for the uniform priors for all models considered in this example.

For all models, we initiated three chains with 20 000 iterations for each chain. The Brooks–Gelman–Rubin (BGR) diagnostics implemented in WinBUGS suggested to remove 10 000 burn-in iterations. DIC and p_D were calculated on the last 10 000 iterations. Occasionally, we let the chains run longer (e.g. model M_5) to verify the stability of the results.

In Table 10.1, we can observe that for model M_1 the effective number of parameters is approximately 34 showing the restrictions among the random effects. Comparing model M_1 with M_2 shows that there is not much evidence for correlated random effects. This is also seen from the 95% CI for $\rho = [-0.829, 0.931]$. From the posterior summary measures of models M_1 to M_4, it appeared that boys and girls have a different variance for the measurement error.

Table 10.1 Potthoff and Roy growth curve study: output WinBUGS for the evaluation of linear mixed models (see the text for a description) using p_D and DIC.

Model	Dbar	Dhat	p_D	DIC
M_1	343.443	308.887	34.556	377.999
M_2	344.670	312.216	32.454	377.124
M_3	376.519	347.129	29.390	405.909
M_4	374.065	342.789	31.276	405.341
M_5	328.201	290.650	37.552	365.753
M_6	343.834	309.506	34.327	378.161
M_7	326.542	288.046	38.047	364.949

This can also observed from Figure 10.1 where we can see that there is one boy with an unusual profile.

The next question is whether the default normal distribution for the random effects and measurement error is justified. To explore this, models M_5 to M_7 were fitted to the data. From Table 10.1, we observe that a scaled t_3-distribution seems more appropriate especially for the measurement error. It is known that the t-distribution with low degrees of freedom provides a more robust error distribution in the sense that it accommodates better outlying observations (see Lange *et al.* 1989). There is not much difference in DIC between models M_5 and M_7. Why p_D is different between models M_5 to M_7 is treated in Example X.7. In Table 10.2, the posterior summary measures of models M_1 and M_5 are shown. The choice of the t-distribution appears to affect the posterior estimates of fixed effects, but even more so the variance parameters.

Finally, we observed, e.g. in model M_7 often the random effects variance parameters got stuck at zero. To remedy this problem, we applied the parameter expansion approach of Section 9.7; see model M_{7b} in the WinBUGS file. While this trick accelerated convergence, it did not alter the posterior summary measures. □

Table 10.2 Potthoff and Roy growth curve study: parameter estimates of models M_1 and M_5 obtained from WinBUGS.

	Model M_1				Model M_5			
Node	Mean	SD	2.5%	97.5%	Mean	SD	2.5%	97.5%
β_0	16.290	1.183	14.010	18.680	17.040	0.987	15.050	18.970
β_1	0.789	0.103	0.589	0.989	0.694	0.086	0.526	0.867
β_2	1.078	1.453	−1.844	3.883	0.698	1.235	−1.716	3.154
β_3	−0.309	0.126	−0.549	−0.058	−0.243	0.106	−0.454	−0.035
σ_{b0}	1.786	0.734	0.385	3.381	1.312	0.541	0.341	2.502
σ_{b1}	0.139	0.065	0.021	0.280	0.095	0.052	0.007	0.209
ρ	−0.143	0.500	−0.829	0.931	−0.001	0.503	−0.792	0.942
σ_0	1.674	0.183	1.362	2.074	1.032	0.154	0.764	1.365
σ_1	0.726	0.111	0.540	0.976	0.546	0.101	0.382	0.783

The above models can also be fitted using SAS® procedure MCMC (see Exercise 10.4). With the same data we now illustrate the meaning of 'focus' of a statistical analysis and its impact on p_D and DIC. We also compare p_D and DIC to their frequentist counterparts p and AIC.

Example X.9: Potthoff & Roy growth curve study: Conditional and marginal DIC
All models in Example X.8 were specified conditionally. For instance, for model M_4

$$y_{ij} \mid \boldsymbol{b}_i \sim \mathrm{N}(\mu_{ij}, \sigma^2) \; (j = 1, \ldots, 4; i = 1, \ldots, 27)$$

with

$$\mu_{ij} = \beta_0 + \beta_1 \, \mathrm{age}_j + \beta_2 \, \mathrm{gender}_i + \beta_3 \, \mathrm{gender}_i \times \mathrm{age}_j + b_{0i} + b_{1i} \, \mathrm{age}_j.$$

This is a conditional model with deviance

$$D_C(\boldsymbol{\mu}, \sigma^2) \equiv D_C(\boldsymbol{\beta}, \boldsymbol{b}, \sigma^2) = -2 \sum_i \sum_j \log \mathrm{N}(y_{ij} \mid \mu_{ij}, \sigma^2),$$

where $\boldsymbol{\mu}$ is the vector of all μ_{ij}, $\boldsymbol{\beta} = (\beta_0, \beta_1\, \beta_2, \beta_3)^T$ and $\boldsymbol{b}$ the stacked vector of all $\boldsymbol{b}_i$. In this model interest lies in the current 27 $\boldsymbol{b}_i$'s, hence we need a *conditional DIC*, which is the DIC reported by WinBUGS. Recall that we obtained $p_D = 31.282$ and DIC $= 405.444$ for this model.

If we wish a marginal DIC then we first need to marginalize the conditional models over the distribution of the random effects $\boldsymbol{b}_i$. The marginalized M_4 is given by

$$\boldsymbol{y}_i \sim \mathrm{N}_4 \left(\boldsymbol{X}_i \boldsymbol{\beta}, \mathbf{Z}\mathrm{G}\mathbf{Z}^T + \mathrm{R}\right), \; (i = 1, \ldots, 27), \tag{10.14}$$

with $\boldsymbol{y}_i = (y_{i1}, y_{i2}, y_{i3}, y_{i4})^T$ and

$$\boldsymbol{X}_i = \begin{pmatrix} 1 & 8 & \mathrm{gender}_i & 8 \times \mathrm{gender}_i \\ 1 & 10 & \mathrm{gender}_i & 10 \times \mathrm{gender}_i \\ 1 & 12 & \mathrm{gender}_i & 12 \times \mathrm{gender}_i \\ 1 & 14 & \mathrm{gender}_i & 14 \times \mathrm{gender}_i \end{pmatrix}, \boldsymbol{Z} = \begin{pmatrix} 1 & 8 \\ 1 & 10 \\ 1 & 12 \\ 1 & 14 \end{pmatrix}, \mathrm{R} = \sigma^2 \mathrm{I}_4.$$

The corresponding deviance to this marginal(ized) model is

$$D_M(\boldsymbol{\beta}, \sigma^2, G) = -2 \sum_i \log \mathrm{N}_4 \left(\boldsymbol{y}_i \mid \boldsymbol{X}_i \boldsymbol{\beta}, \mathbf{Z}\mathrm{G}\mathbf{Z}^T + \mathrm{R}\right). \tag{10.15}$$

In the marginal model the $\boldsymbol{b}_i$'s only serve to model the covariance structure, but there is no interest in the current $\boldsymbol{b}_i$'s. This *marginal DIC* can also be obtained from WinBUGS provided the marginal model (10.14) is used. We obtained $p_D = 7.072$ and DIC $= 442.572$. The difference between the conditional and the marginal output highlights the difference in focus: in the marginal model the focus is on the fixed effects and prediction pertains to the future children while in the conditional (hierarchical) model the focus is on the random effects with prediction pertaining to the 27 children involved in this study.

Finally, a frequentist mixed model analysis with SAS procedure MIXED (see 'chapter 10 Potthoff-Roy growthcurves.sas') produced AIC = 443.8 with $p = 8$ demonstrating again the correspondence between AIC and DIC for nonhierarchical models. Recall that AIC and DIC are exactly equal only for noninformative priors, known variance parameters and a large sample size. □

In the previous example, we illustrated the assertion of (Spiegelhalter *et al.* 2002) that the use of DIC for selecting a model depends on the focus of the statistical analysis. Millar (2009) provides another example. Namely, for overdispersed counts one could choose a Poisson-gamma model. But, averaged over the gamma random effects, this model is just a negative binomial distribution. This implies that if one chooses in WinBUGS for a Poisson-gamma model the conditional DIC is obtained, while working with the negative binomial distribution provides a marginal DIC. Thus, although the fit of the two models to the data is identical, p_D and DIC will be quite different for the two implementations (Exercise 10.5). It is, therefore, inappropriate to compare the DIC of a Poisson-gamma with that of a negative binomial distribution (see also Exercise 10.8).

The next example illustrates the dependence of p_D on the variability of the random effects. We also illustrate that, as for AIC, DIC depends on the scale of the response.

Example X.10: Dietary study: Impact of variability of random effects and scale of response on p_D and DIC

The analysis of Example IX.8 yields the first row of Table 10.3 and shows that, while the total number of parameters is 11, the total effective number of parameters is around 7. The difference of 4 quantifies the constraints that tie the random effects together. We then fixed $\log(\sigma_\theta)$ to prespecified values decreasing from 5 to -1 in steps of one. From Table 10.3, we see that the ultimate p_D must be around 2 what happens when $\log(\sigma_\theta) = -1$ forcing all $\overline{\theta_i}$ to be equal to $\overline{\mu} = 327.3$. The WinBUGS programs are provided in 'chapter 9 dietary study chol DIC sigmas.odc'.

On the original scale (assuming *chol* has a normal distribution) $p_D = 6.928$ and DIC = 6991.30. However, the distribution of *chol* is right skewed. A lognormal distribution may be fitted to *chol* in WinBUGS by specifying that it has a lognormal distribution or that log(*chol*) has a normal distribution. While irrelevant for statistical modeling, the choice matters for DIC. In the first case, DIC is based on the likelihood of *chol*, while in the second case DIC

Table 10.3 Dietary study: dependence of p_D and DIC on the variability of the random effects.

$\log(\sigma_\theta)$	Dbar	Dhat	p_D	DIC
Estimated	6984.150	6977.250	6.902	6991.060
5	6983.430	6974.500	8.937	6992.370
4	6983.100	6974.550	8.546	6991.640
3	6982.860	6976.230	6.632	6989.490
2	6987.900	6984.440	3.459	6991.360
1	6991.780	6989.530	2.248	6994.030
0	6992.530	6990.510	2.018	6994.550
−1	6992.560	6990.680	1.880	6994.440

is based on the likelihood of log(*chol*). In the first case, WinBUGS reported $p_D = 6.285$ and DIC $= 6909.670$, while in the second case $p_D = 6.285$ and DIC $= 457.525$ was obtained. Clearly p_D is invariant to the implementation but DIC was much affected (as well as AIC). But a correction is needed to make DIC comparable to the DIC obtained on the original scale. The corrected DIC is obtained from expression (10.34). With this correction, we obtained the same DIC as in the first case. Thus, we can conclude that a Gaussian hierarchical model with a log-transformed response provides a better fit to the dietary data (see also Exercise 10.6). □

Both p_D and DIC seem to do their job properly. Namely, p_D is higher for a more complex model and DIC appears to select the correct model. The measures are quite popular among WinBUGS users but also caused a lot of confusion. In Spiegelhalter *et al.* (2002) and at the WinBUGS website, the authors documented on some potential difficulties with their proposal:

- p_D and DIC depend on the parameterization of the model. That is, when $\boldsymbol{\theta}$ is transformed to $\boldsymbol{\psi} = h(\boldsymbol{\theta})$ with h a nonlinear monotonic transformation then p_D and DIC will change (Spiegelhalter *et al.* 2002). Note, however, that the deviance (and hence 'Dbar') is invariant to parameter transformation.
- From (10.12) and Jensen's inequality it follows that if the likelihood is log-concave in $\boldsymbol{\theta}$ and evaluated in $\overline{\boldsymbol{\theta}}$ then $p_D \geq 0$. A negative p_D may occur with a nonlog-concave likelihood (Example X.11) and when the prior is in conflict with the data (Exercise 10.9). But when the posterior mean is a good summary measure, i.e. when the posterior is roughly symmetric and unimodal, then a positive p_D will likely occur. Suppose that this occurs on a particular scale, say $\boldsymbol{\psi} = h(\boldsymbol{\theta})$, then $\boldsymbol{\psi}$ might be taken as stochastic node in WinBUGS. If this is not feasible, then the Markov chain based on $\boldsymbol{\theta}$ could be exported to compute 'Dhat' on the posterior mean of $\boldsymbol{\psi}$.
- p_D and DIC are not defined for discrete $\boldsymbol{\theta}$ since $\overline{\boldsymbol{\theta}}$ usually fails to take one of these values. When one of the stochastic nodes is discrete, e.g. when a mixture model is fitted to the data, DIC is greyed out in WinBUGS; see Exercise 10.7 for an example.

We illustrate the dependence of p_D and DIC on the parameterization in the model with the well-known genetic linkage example analyzed in Rao (1973, pp. 368–369). We further demonstrate that p_D can be negative. This example is inspired by the slides on DIC at the WinBUGS website.

Example X.11: Linkage study in genetics: Negative p_D's
When two factors are linked with a recombination fraction θ, the intercrosses $AB/ab \times AB/ab$ (coupling) have expected proportions for *AB*: $(3 - 2\theta + \theta^2)/4$, *Ab*: $(2\theta - \theta^2)/4$, *aB*: $(2\theta - \theta^2)/4$, *ab*: $(1 - 2\theta + \theta^2)/4$. With observed frequencies 125, 18, 20 and 34 the multinomial log-likelihood is a log-concave function of θ but not for $\psi = \theta^\alpha$ ($\alpha \geq 4$). For prior $\theta \sim \text{Beta}(1, 1)$ the prior of $\psi = \theta^\alpha$ is Beta$(1/\alpha, 1)$. For each value of α, we then let ψ be the stochastic node and ran WinBUGS on this parameterization. Table 10.4 shows the dependence of p_D and DIC on α and hence on the stochastic node. For α large, $p_D < 0$ which is clearly noninterpretable (see also Exercise 10.10). □

Table 10.4 Linkage study in genetics: p_D and DIC as a function of the power of θ.

Power	p_D	DIC
1	0.963	17.043
5	0.798	16.816
10	0.436	16.494
20	0.047	15.948
30	−0.470	15.752

10.2.2.3 Evaluation of information criteria for model selection and recent developments

In several papers, the performance of the information criteria for model selection were compared, both theoretically as well as with simulation studies. Zhu and Carlin (2000) proved the asymptotic equivalence of AIC and marginal DIC for nonhierarchical models, while Vaida and Blanchard (2005) proved the equivalence of the AIC and DIC for a linear mixed effects model with known variances. In `http://www.mrc-bsu.cam.ac.uk/bugs/winbugs/DIC-slides.pdf`, Spiegelhalter makes use of the correspondence of AIC and DIC to suggest the use of AIC in a Bayesian context if the interest lies in the marginal model and thus in predicting the response of future subjects belonging to the same level-2 distributions. Simulation studies can be found in Lin and Dayton (1997), Burnham and Anderson (2002), some discussants of Spiegelhalter *et al.* (2002), Ando (2007) and Ward (2008). These authors concluded that: (a) AIC and DIC tend to choose too complex models in comparison to BIC and (b) DIC often makes a reasonable model choice but its theoretical foundations remain puzzling. Ward (2008) experienced that the Bayes factor appeared to select often the appropriate model and claimed that the Bayes factor penalizes in a natural way too complex models. This was already mentioned by Dawid (2002) who argued that the penalization comes from the fact that the marginal likelihood integrates over all uncertainty in the model which is greater when the model is complex.

Robert and Titterington (2002), Richardson (2002), Ando (2007) and Plummer (2008) raised concerns on the optimistic nature of DIC caused by making use twice of the observed data: once to construct the posterior distribution and once to compute the expected log-likelihood. To remedy this problem, Pourahmadi and Daniels (2002) suggested a BIC variant of DIC, i.e. DIC $= D(\overline{\theta}) + p_D \log(n)$ with n the number of subjects. Ando (2007) worked from first principles and showed that his Bayesian predictive information criterion (BPIC) takes the double use of the data into account. Plummer (2008) suggested penalized loss functions for Bayesian model comparison. With the expected deviance as loss function he reduced the optimism by making use of a penalized expected deviance (PED). Namely, the first part in p_D, i.e.

$$D^e \equiv E_{\boldsymbol{\theta}|\mathbf{y}}\left[-2\log p(\mathbf{y} \mid \boldsymbol{\theta})\right] = -2\sum_{i=1}^{n} D_i^e(y_i \mid \mathbf{y}) = -2\sum_{i=1}^{n}\int \log p(y_i \mid \boldsymbol{\theta})p(\boldsymbol{\theta} \mid \mathbf{y})\mathrm{d}\boldsymbol{\theta},$$

is overoptimistic (too small). A better estimate is given by

$$D_{CV}^e = -2\sum_{i=1}^{n} D_{CV,i}^e(y_i \mid \mathbf{y}_{(i)}) = -2\sum_{i=1}^{n}\int \log p(y_i \mid \boldsymbol{\theta})p(\boldsymbol{\theta} \mid \mathbf{y}_{(i)})\mathrm{d}\boldsymbol{\theta}.$$

The difference $D^e - D^e_{CV} = p_{\text{opt}} = \sum_{i=1}^n p_{\text{opt},i}$ expresses the optimism by using the data twice. The penalized expected deviance is then PED $= D^e + p_{\text{opt}}$. Since p_{opt} can be split up according to the n observations, one estimate of p_{opt} could be obtained from n separate MCMC chains, with a single observation deleted in each run. Since this procedure is quite time consuming, Plummer suggested an alternative approach using importance sampling. This criterion has been recently implemented into R2jags.

Another criticism to DIC is that it lacks theoretical foundation outside the generalized linear models (GLIMs). To address this problem, Celeux *et al.* (2006) suggested seven versions of DIC for use in models with missing data, e.g. random effects models and mixture models. Plummer (2008) showed that for $p_D \ll n$, DIC can be seen as an approximation to a loss function based on the deviance. In a series of papers, Hodges and colleagues focused on the effective degrees of freedom and defined it as the dimension of fitted values. Lu *et al.* (2007) illustrated that a poorly fitting model affects p_D, so that a given model may give identically smooth fitted values when fit to two data sets but gives a different p_D when the model fits one of the data sets poorly. Consequently, p_D cannot be interpreted as the dimensionality of the fitted space, which is also our experience. Cui *et al.* (2010) summed up additional difficulties of p_D as measure for model complexity. They also argued that model complexity and model comparison should be treated separately (see also Plummer 2008).

Recently, Aitkin (2010) suggested to look at the whole posterior distribution of the difference in deviances for model comparison. For comparing models M_1 and M_2, he suggested to compute $\{D_j^k = -2\log \text{L}(\boldsymbol{\theta}_j^k),\ k = 1, \ldots, K\}$ with $\boldsymbol{\theta}_j^k$ $(j = 1, 2)$ a sample from the posterior distribution $p(\boldsymbol{\theta} \mid \boldsymbol{y}, M_j)$. This gives a sample from the posterior distribution of deviances under model M_j. Then $\{D_{1,2}^k = D_1^k - D_2^k,\ k = 1, \ldots, K\}$ is a sample from the posterior distribution of the difference in deviances. The median of this sample estimates the posterior probability that model M_1 is better than model M_2. The 95% CI for $D_{1,2}^k$ indicates that model M_1 is 'significantly better' than model M_2 if this credible interval lies left to 0.

Finally, note that R2WinBUGS reports a different value for DIC than WinBUGS; see the vignette of R2WinBUGS for further details and Example X.12 for a comparison with the DIC as reported from WinBUGS.

10.2.3 Model selection based on predictive loss functions

AIC and DIC are measures of predictive ability of the model based on the Kullback-Leibler measure. There are many other approaches to GOF that compare the observed outcome with its fitted/predicted value. Suppose that for outcome y_i its 'fitted' value under a given model is $\widehat{y}_i$, then a simple and quite general approach to model comparison is to construct a distance measure between y_i and $\widehat{y}_i$ and to average this over the observations. One example that is used frequently in non-Bayesian approaches is the *mean squared error (MSE)* which is given for n observations by

$$\text{MSE} = \frac{1}{n}\sum_{i=1}^{n}(y_i - \widehat{y}_i)^2,$$

and is just the average squared residual. Within an MCMC analysis, this could be employed but the posterior variability in $\widehat{y}_i$ needs to be addressed. For example, we could choose the posterior mean value of $\widehat{y}_i$ to represent the model fits. Hence, in a Bayesian context the model MSE could be defined as

$$\text{MSE} = \frac{1}{n}\sum_{i=1}^{n}(y_i - \bar{\widehat{y}}_i)^2,$$

with $\bar{\widehat{y}}_i = \sum_{k=1}^{K} \widehat{y}_i^k / K$ and where $\widehat{y}_i^k$ is the predicted value of y_i obtained from a converged Markov chain $(\boldsymbol{\theta}^k)_k$. An alternative approach is to assess the disparity at each iteration:

$$\text{MSE} = \frac{1}{K}\frac{1}{n}\sum_{k=1}^{K}\sum_{i=1}^{n}(y_i - \widehat{y}_i^k)^2 = \frac{1}{K}\sum_{k=1}^{K}\text{MSE}_k,$$

where $\widehat{y}_i^k$ is the fit at the kth iteration, and MSE_k is the MSE at the kth iteration.

An alternative measure that is used within a Bayesian approach is based on the posterior predictive distribution (PPD). The *posterior predictive loss* (*PPL*) and *mean-square predictive error* (*MSPE*) were proposed by Laud and Ibrahim (1995) and Gelfand and Ghosh (1998). In essence, a loss function (squared error or otherwise) could be set up between an observation and its predicted value. To obtain this predicted value, a simulation from the fitted model is used, in fact from the PPD, generating $\widetilde{y}_i$. This value is compared to the observed value via the PPL function. For squared error loss we have

$$\text{MSPE} = \frac{1}{n}\sum_{i=1}^{n}(y_i - \widetilde{y}_i)^2, \tag{10.16}$$

while for an absolute value loss we have

$$\text{MAPE} = \frac{1}{n}\sum_{i=1}^{n}|y_i - \widetilde{y}_i|.$$

As in the case of the MSE, in an MCMC context a decision must be made as to how to estimate the predictive value. Usually a measure is computed at each iteration of the sampler and then averaged over the sample. Hence, the final form would be in that case

$$\text{MSPE} = \frac{1}{K}\sum_{k=1}^{K}\text{MSPE}_k, \tag{10.17}$$

with MSPE_k calculated using (10.16) at the kth iteration of the MCMC process. Gelfand and Ghosh (1998) extended their measure to other classes of models such as survival models and generalized linear (mixed) models.

It is straightforward to generate in WinBUGS a predictive distribution value as it is just a simulated value from the data distribution given the current parameters sampled. For example, for a normal data distribution this would lead to the WinBUGS code:

```
y[i] ~ dnorm(mu[i],tauy); ytilde[i] ~ dnorm(mu[i],tauy)
```

with `ytilde[i]` the ith element of an n-dimensional unobserved parameter vector which will be filled with predictive values of `y[i]` at each iteration.

Note that MSPE is always available as a measure and does not suffer from the negative p_D problem of DIC. However, MSPE does not compensate for model complexity. This was already alluded to in Spiegelhalter *et al.* (2002). Banerjee (unpublished note) demonstrated this for a normal linear regression model when marginalized over the model parameters. Hence, MSPE is more equivalent to the deviance than the DIC. But as for DIC, MSPE depends on the scale of the response. Finally, note that MSPE is different from a posterior predictive check introduced in Section 10.3.4. We now compute MSPE for the osteoporosis data set.

Example X.12: Osteoporosis study: Predictive evaluation of models
In 'chapter 10 osteo multiple regression.R', TBBMC is regressed on age, BMI, weight, length, caint (calcium intake), creat (serum creatinine), DBP (diastolic blood pressure), menost (number of years since start of menopause) and igfi (IGF-1 which is a hormone similar in molecular structure to insulin). Using R2WinBUGS, we fitted four models, model M_1: all regressors, model M_2: length and weight removed, model M_3: creat and menost removed in addition and model M_4: only BMI included. For each of the models DIC, p_D and MSPE is recorded. Each time we ran a single chain analysis of 15 000 iterations and removed the first 7500 iterations. The following results were obtained for the four respective models: DIC (399.02, 395.14, 393.27, 1206.48), p_D (12.14, 10.09, 8.07, 3.10) and MSPE (205.06, 202.82, 202.96, 30647.71). We also used WinBUGS to estimate the parameters for model M_1 and obtained DIC = 397.27 and p_D = 11.24, both close to the values obtained from R2WinBUGS.

According to DIC, model M_3 is best (although not decisively) while according to MSPE there is no clear preference between models M_2 and M_3 illustrating that with MSPE there is (less) penalty for model complexity. Both measures though agree that the model with only BMI is worst. □

Another example of a comparison of MSPE with DIC can be found in Song *et al.* (2010).

10.3 Model checking

10.3.1 Introduction

The criteria introduced in Section 10.2 help us to choose the best model among a set of candidate models. However, the selected model is not necessarily sensible nor does it guarantees a good fit to the data. Statistical model evaluation typically requires a lot of exploration such as (i) checking that inference from the chosen model is reasonable, (ii) verifying that the model can reproduce the data, (iii) sensitivity analyses by varying certain aspects of the model. These activities apply to a Bayesian and a frequentist approach, but in the Bayesian approach also the prior needs attention and Bayesian model checking techniques are primarily based on sampling techniques. We now briefly sketch the Bayesian model checking activities. These topics will be elaborated on in this section.

(i) Verifying that the model is reasonable is a critical inspection of the posterior output making use of background knowledge. For instance, we hope that the prior is not in conflict with the data. In addition, in a Bayesian analysis, it is supposed that we learn from the data. The first problem can be spotted by checking whether prior and posterior distributions differ much in location (in view of prior SD). The second problem is diagnosed when the posterior variance of the parameter is close to the prior variance indicating an identifiability problem and no learning from the data.

(ii) Adequate prediction of the data at hand is expected for a good probability model. Stern and Sinharay (2005) call this a self-consistency check. Contrasting the observed data with the expected data under the considered model for individual observations is akin to outlier detection techniques. While the early Bayesian approaches to outlier detection are based on the exact posterior distributions of residuals, the recent procedures are based on the output of MCMC techniques. In addition, we may be interested in contrasting observed summary measures with those predicted from the model. This leads to posterior predictive checks which extend frequentist GOF significance tests and are based on frequentist sampling ideas.

(iii) In a Bayesian sensitivity analysis the prior distribution and the likelihood are perturbed to see how much this affects inference. A sensitivity analysis was done in Example IX.17 where we examined the dependence of the parameter estimates on the distribution of the random effects. Evaluating the impact of varying the link function in a Bayesian generalized linear model (BGLIM) is another example of a sensitivity analysis. One can also explore the sensitivity of the parameter estimates when observations are removed or perturbed. This involves the search for influential observations. Influence diagnostics have been developed for a variety of models in a frequentist context. For some models, analytical results and good first order approximations allow for a quick exploration. Unfortunately, this is not the case in the Bayesian context, where already for the linear case, the computations can become involved. Importance sampling techniques introduced in Section 3.7.2 are of help here. Finally, model expansion, i.e. embedding the current model in a larger class of models, is another tool for model sensitivity.

For many of the model checking tools past-processing of the MCMC output is necessary. Then it becomes advantageous to perform the analyses in a richer programming environment than WinBUGS. This can be done by calling WinBUGS from within R using the R2WinBUGS package or using the Bayesian SAS procedures. We first briefly review frequentist GOF techniques in linear regression models since they have been the topic of statistical research for many decades. We then look at various Bayesian techniques for model checking. Examples are primarily analyzed with WinBUGS and R2WinBUGS, but attention is also paid to SAS procedures.

10.3.2 Model-checking procedures

10.3.2.1 Frequentist model checking

The classical normal linear regression model assumes (1) a linear relationship of the response with the covariates, (2) normality of the error term, and (3) equality of variance of the error terms. Textbooks, such as Myers (1998) and Cook and Weisberg (1982), describe a variety of formal and graphical techniques to check the appropriateness of these structural (e.g. linearity in covariates) and distributional (e.g. normality responses) assumptions. For instance, residual plots may identify the subjects for which their response is badly predicted by the model. The normality assumption may be checked by formal tests such as the Kolmogorov–Smirnov test or graphical procedures such as the normal probability plot (NPP). For checking the structural assumption of linearity in the covariates various graphics have been suggested, such as: partial regression plots, partial residual plots, augmented partial residual plots, etc. Influential observations, i.e. observations that have a high impact on the parameter estimation when deleted or perturbed, may be detected by influence measures such as Cook's distance (Cook 1977).

For GLIMs testing structural assumptions additionally involves verifying the link function (and sometimes the variance function). The Pearson and the deviance residuals are used to check distributional assumptions. Their finite sample distribution is often not tractable and sampling techniques, such as bootstrapping, may be needed to deliver confidence envelopes around NPPs. For binary regression models, even simple graphical checks do not work well (Albert and Chib 1995). For the exploration of influential observations one-step diagnostics have been proposed by Pregibon (1981). Finally, for nonlinear models (Seber and Wild 1989) and models for correlated and multilevel data (Verbeke and Molenberghs 2000), things become more complex.

10.3.2.2 Bayesian detection of outlying observations

Checking the fit of a model at each subject in a Bayesian context can be done by exploring the posterior distribution of the residuals. A subject with a large residual, i.e. an outlier, indicates that the model falls short in predicting its response properly. Several Bayesian approaches for outlier detection are available. We start with some early analytical approaches to highlight the difference between the Bayesian and the frequentist distributional theory.

(i) Bayesian residual analysis: The residual $\varepsilon_i = y_i - \mu_i$ measures the deviation of the observed response y_i from the predicted response μ_i. In practice, μ_i is unknown and in a Bayesian context, we derive its posterior expectation. It is preferable to compute this expectation by making use of an auxiliary data set, say z and take $\mathrm{E}(y_i \mid z)$ for μ_i. But additional data are rarely available. As an alternative, one may take $\mathrm{E}(y_i \mid \boldsymbol{y})$ and define as a Bayesian residual

$$\varepsilon_i = y_i - \mathrm{E}(y_i \mid \boldsymbol{y}).$$

For the linear regression model of Section 4.7.1 with Jeffreys prior, $\mathrm{E}(y_i \mid \boldsymbol{y}) = \boldsymbol{x}_i^T \widehat{\boldsymbol{\beta}}$ with $\widehat{\boldsymbol{\beta}}$ the LSE of $\boldsymbol{\beta}$. If r_i is large, then the model fits the ith observation poorly. The decision to flag the ith subject as an outlier depends on the posterior distribution of $\varepsilon_i = y_i - \boldsymbol{x}_i^T \boldsymbol{\beta}$. With a priori $\varepsilon_i \sim \mathrm{N}(0, \sigma^2)$, Chaloner and Brant (1988) computed the posterior probability $p(|\varepsilon_i| > k\sigma \mid \boldsymbol{y})$ with k chosen such that the prior probability of no outliers (in the sample) is large. An observation will then be flagged as outlier when this probability exceeds the corresponding prior probability.

Zellner (1975) and Chaloner and Brant (1988) derived that the posterior of ε_i is a noncentral t_{n-d-1}-distribution with (posterior) mean $\widehat{\varepsilon_i} = y_i - \boldsymbol{x}_i^T \widehat{\boldsymbol{\beta}}$ and squared scale parameter $s^2 h_{ii}$, with s^2, the classical residual variance and $h_{ii} = \boldsymbol{x}_i^T (\boldsymbol{X}^T \boldsymbol{X})^{-1} \boldsymbol{x}_i$, the classical measure of leverage. One may note the difference between the sampling distribution of ε_i and the posterior distribution of ε_i. The former is the distribution of the residual under repeated sampling of the data (whereby $\boldsymbol{y}$ and $\widehat{\boldsymbol{\beta}}$ have a sampling distribution) while the latter is the posterior of the residual (via the posterior of $\boldsymbol{\beta}$ given $\boldsymbol{y}$). For instance, for a good fitting model, $\widehat{\varepsilon_i}/s_{(i)}\sqrt{1 - h_{ii}}$, with $s_{(i)}$ the SD based on the sample without ith observation, has a t_{n-d-1}-sampling distribution. Further, Chaloner and Brant (1988) showed that the joint posterior distribution of $\boldsymbol{\varepsilon} = (\varepsilon_1, \ldots, \varepsilon_n)^T$ has $(d + 1)$ dimensions since it depends on the posterior of the $(d + 1)$-dimensional parameter vector $\boldsymbol{\beta}$, whereas the sampling distribution of $\widehat{\boldsymbol{\varepsilon}}$ has $(n - d - 1)$ dimensions. Other analytical outlier detection methods were derived by Box and Tiao (1968) and Abraham and Box (1978).

In practice the decision to flag an outlier is often based on less stringent criteria (inspired by frequentist arguments) and is decided when the standardized residual

$$t_i = \frac{y_i - \mathrm{E}(y_i \mid \boldsymbol{y})}{\sqrt{\mathrm{Var}(y_i \mid \boldsymbol{y})}} \tag{10.18}$$

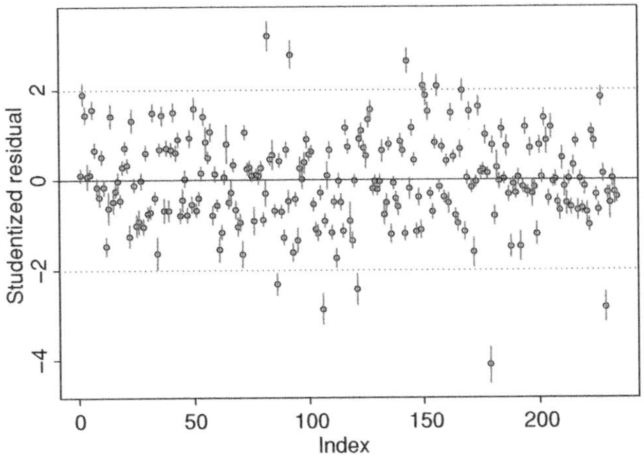

Figure 10.3 Osteoporosis study: index plot of posterior mean and 95% CI of $t_i = (y_i - \boldsymbol{x}_i^T \boldsymbol{\beta})/(\sigma\sqrt{1-h_{ii}})$.

exceeds in absolute value, say 2. For a linear regression problem, we might use σ or $\sigma\sqrt{1-h_{ii}}$ for the denominator in expression (10.18). We now illustrate these results using the osteoporosis data.

Example X.13: Osteoporosis study: Detection of outliers
We have computed Bayesian ordinary residuals for the regression model analyzed in Example VI.5 using R2WinBUGS. The program can be found in 'chapter 10 osteo study-outliers.R'. The MCMC results of the posterior mean of ε_i $(i = 1, \ldots, n)$ and the 95% CI are basically equal to the analytical results of Zellner (1975) and Chaloner and Brant (1988). In Figure 10.3, we show the posterior distributions of the studentized residuals $t_i = (y_i - \boldsymbol{x}_i^T \boldsymbol{\beta})/(\sigma\sqrt{1-h_{ii}})$ in an index plot. Roughly 5% of the observations are beyond |2| with the largest residual corresponding to subject 179 (subject with BMI = 23.23 and TBBMC = 0.579). Some graphs may be obtained also from within WinBUGS. For instance, index plots of the posterior means of the ordinary and standardized residuals may be obtained in WinBUGS using the option 'caterpillar' from the menu option **Compare**. However, to produce the studentized residuals within WinBUGS requires the h_{ii} values and thus an initial classical regression analysis; see 'chapter 10 osteo study-outliers.odc' for an illustration. □

In the discrete (binary) case, neither the sampling nor the posterior distribution of the Pearson and deviance residuals is known. While analytical results are lacking, MCMC computations are still feasible. Albert and Chib (1995) proposed to use a MCMC algorithm to determine the outliers. Let y_i $(i = 1, \ldots, n)$ represent the n binary responses and $\pi_i = p(y_i = 1) = F(\boldsymbol{x}_i^T \boldsymbol{\beta})$ their probability of success with $F(\cdot)$ a known cdf. Suppose a converged Markov chain $\boldsymbol{\beta}^1, \ldots, \boldsymbol{\beta}^K$ from $p(\boldsymbol{\beta} \mid \boldsymbol{y})$ is available then the posterior distribution of $\varepsilon_i^k = y_i - \pi_i^k$ with $\pi_i^k = F(\boldsymbol{x}_i^T \boldsymbol{\beta}^k)$ is readily obtained. Plotting the quantiles of ε_i^k versus the posterior mean of π_i may highlight outlying observations (Exercise 10.12).

In the computation of t_i, the observed data $\boldsymbol{y}$ are used twice. Independent data $\boldsymbol{z}$ to compute $\mathrm{E}(y_i \mid \boldsymbol{z})$ in expression (10.18) are, however, often not available. An alternative is then to use a cross-validation approach, i.e. compute $r_i^* = y_i - \text{E}(y_i \mid \boldsymbol{y}_{(i)})$, with $\text{E}(y_i \mid \boldsymbol{y}_{(i)})$ the expected value of the ith response based on the posterior from all observations except the ith. Similarly, the standardized residuals then become $t_i^* = [y_i - \text{E}(y_i \mid \boldsymbol{y})]/\sqrt{\text{var}(y_i \mid \boldsymbol{y}_{(i)})}$. In a classical regression, cross-validation residuals are computed fast. However, this simple case is already computationally demanding in a Bayesian context. For simple models, a trick may allow WinBUGS to do the job in a reasonable amount of time, but we would not advice to use this technique in other models or for large data sets.

Example X.14: Osteoporosis study: Cross-validated residuals using WinBUGS
In 'chapter 10 osteo study-cross validation.odc', we computed the cross-validation residuals. First, all data were analyzed. Then a trick was used for parallel processing 234 Markov chains. These chains correspond to leaving out each observation at a time which is done by creating an indicator variable for each observation and adding this variable to the linear structure. In this way, 234 linear regression models are fit in parallel. In addition, 234 copies of the data are produced within the WinBUGS program. As expected, the cross-validation residuals were (up to sampling variability) always larger in absolute value than the ordinary residuals (results not shown). □

(ii) Predictive approaches to outlier detection: The PPD (3.9) evaluated in y_i is called the *posterior predictive ordinate* (PPO_i). That is

$$\text{PPO}_i = p(y_i \mid \boldsymbol{y}) = \int p(y_i \mid \boldsymbol{\theta}) p(\boldsymbol{\theta} \mid \boldsymbol{y})\, d\boldsymbol{\theta} \tag{10.19}$$

is the value of the PPD at y_i. For a low value of PPO_i the ith observation is in the tail area of the density and if judged too low, the ith observation is flagged as an outlier. The PPO_i values cannot easily be calibrated which means that it is difficult to say what is 'small'. A simple standardization like $\text{rPPO}_i = \text{PPO}_i/\max\{\text{PPO}_i\}$ might help to spot outlying observations. The ith PPO can be estimated from an MCMC run by

$$\widehat{\text{PPO}}_i = \widehat{p}(y_i \mid \boldsymbol{y}) = \frac{1}{K} \sum_{k=1}^{K} p(y_i \mid \boldsymbol{\theta}^k), \tag{10.20}$$

with $\{\boldsymbol{\theta}^1, \ldots, \boldsymbol{\theta}^K\}$ a converged Markov chain from $p(\boldsymbol{\theta} \mid \boldsymbol{y})$.

The PPO makes use of the data $\boldsymbol{y}$ twice: first in determining the posterior distribution and second in evaluating the density at y_i. To remedy the double use of the observed data, Geisser (1980) suggested the *CPO*. It is a cross-validatory measure of extremeness of y_i whereby the density is evaluated in y_i with the posterior based on $\boldsymbol{y}_{(i)}$ (sample without y_i). That is, $\text{CPO}_i = p(y_i \mid \boldsymbol{y}_{(i)}) = \int p(y_i \mid \boldsymbol{\theta}) p(\boldsymbol{\theta} \mid \boldsymbol{y}_{(i)}) d\boldsymbol{\theta}$. The CPO was used in Section 10.2.1 to construct the pseudo-Bayes factor, here it is used to highlight surprising observations. Geisser (1985) called the procedure of setting aside a part of the data to estimate the parameters and evaluating the fitted model on the remaining part of the data, the *predictive approach to outlier detection*. The analytical properties of CPO were explored by Pettitt (1990) (see also references therein) especially for the normal distribution. Weiss (1996) showed that CPO_i can be expressed as a Bayes factor (see Equation (10.23b)) while others developed the CPO for sets of observations (Pettitt 1990).

Here, we are interested in computing the CPO using MCMC output. A simple derivation shows how to compute CPO_i:

$$\frac{1}{p(y_i \mid \boldsymbol{y}_{(i)})} = \frac{p(\boldsymbol{y}_{(i)})}{p(\boldsymbol{y})} = \int \frac{p(\boldsymbol{y}_{(i)} \mid \boldsymbol{\theta})p(\boldsymbol{\theta})}{p(\boldsymbol{y})} d\boldsymbol{\theta} = \int \frac{1}{p(y_i \mid \boldsymbol{\theta})} p(\boldsymbol{\theta} \mid \boldsymbol{y}) d\boldsymbol{\theta} = \text{E}_{\boldsymbol{\theta}|\boldsymbol{y}}\left(\frac{1}{p(y_i \mid \boldsymbol{\theta})}\right).$$

This derivation makes use of the conditional independence of the y_i given $\boldsymbol{\theta}$. This result shows that CPO_i can be estimated as an harmonic mean, i.e.

$$\widehat{\text{CPO}}_i = \left(\frac{1}{K}\sum_k \frac{1}{p(y_i \mid \boldsymbol{\theta}^k)}\right)^{-1}. \tag{10.21}$$

CPO_i can be estimated in WinBUGS (Ntzoufras 2009, pp. 359, 375) by monitoring the stochastic node $1/p(y_i \mid \boldsymbol{\theta}^k)$ for each i, but the final computation needs post-processing. Pettit and Smith (1985) and Weiss (1996) suggested to calibrate CPO_i. However, if only used to spot outlying observations, calibration may not be necessary. Indeed $1/\widehat{\text{CPO}}_i$ will be small for an outlying observation and easily spotted in an index plot. A problem with the harmonic estimate (10.21) is that its variance could become infinite which makes it an unreliable estimate of CPO_i. This happens with seriously outlying observations since $p(y_i \mid \boldsymbol{\theta}^k)$ is in the denominator. For a reliable estimate of CPO_i genuine cross-validation, i.e. effectively removing the ith observation and evaluating the density $p(z \mid \boldsymbol{y}_{(i)})$ at $z = y_i$, might be required.

Example X.15: Caries study: Application of posterior predictive ordinate to detect outliers

The R program 'chapter 10 caries with residuals.R' uses R2WinBUGS to fit a Poisson model to the dmft index of 500 children. The covariates in the model are described in Exercise 10.12. To compute the PPO_is, the command

```
ppo[i] <- exp(-lambda[i] + dmft[i]* log(lambda[i]) - logfact(dmft[i]))
```

was added to the WinBUGS program. The posterior mean of ppo[i] was imported into R and additional R commands produced Figure 10.4(a). No particularly outlying subject was

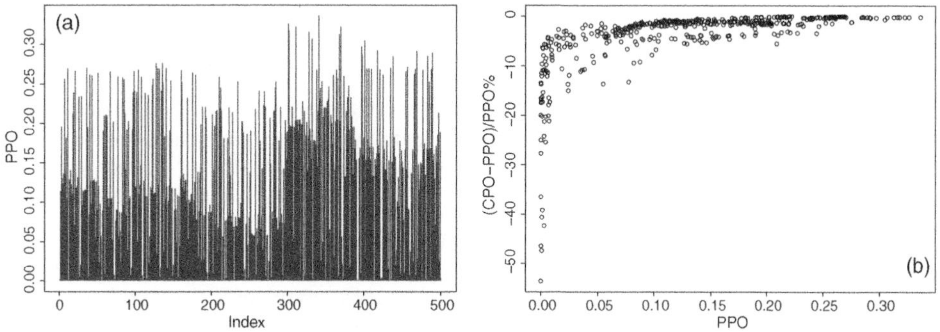

Figure 10.4 Caries study: (a) index plot of PPO and (b) relative difference of CPO versus PPO.

spotted, but many subjects appear to have a relatively low PPO-value possibly indicating a bad fitting model. The standardized version rPPO_i was also computed but did not add any more insight. With command *icpo[i]* $< -1/ppo[i]$ the inverse of CPO_i was estimated using its posterior mean and was then exported to R to compute the estimate (10.21). In Figure 10.4(b), it is demonstrated that CPO_i is always smaller than PPO_i especially for outlying observations. □

(iii) DIC diagnostics: Spiegelhalter *et al.* (2002) suggested to decompose DIC and p_D into n individual components. The deviance of the sample, i.e. $D(\boldsymbol{\theta}) = -2\log p(\boldsymbol{y} \mid \boldsymbol{\theta}) + 2\log f(\boldsymbol{y})$ can be split up into the contributions of the n subjects as follows:

$$D(\boldsymbol{\theta}) = \sum_{i=1}^{n} D_i(\boldsymbol{\theta}), \tag{10.22}$$

with $D_i(\boldsymbol{\theta}) = -2\log p(y_i \mid \boldsymbol{\theta}) + 2\log f(y_i)$. Similarly, DIC and p_D can be split up as $\text{DIC} = \sum_{i=1}^{n} \text{DIC}_i$ and $p_D = \sum_{i=1}^{n} p_{Di}$, respectively, with $\text{DIC}_i = \overline{D_i(\boldsymbol{\theta})} + p_{Di}$ and $p_{Di} = \overline{D_i(\boldsymbol{\theta})} - D_i(\overline{\boldsymbol{\theta}})$. DIC is used as an overall model fit diagnostic, with a relatively large value indicating a bad fit. Hence, if DIC_i is large then the model is not fitting well for the ith observation. In addition, p_{Di} can tell us about the leverage of the ith observation. This can be seen for the normal linear regression model since $p_D = \sum_i p_{Di} = tr(H)$, with H the 'hat' matrix (Spiegelhalter *et al.* 2002, p. 592). $\overline{D_i(\boldsymbol{\theta})}$ can also indicate outlying observations, but rather $dr_i = \pm\sqrt{\overline{D_i(\boldsymbol{\theta})}_i}$ is used with the sign depending on the sign of $y_i - E(y_i \mid \overline{\boldsymbol{\theta}})$. Wheeler *et al.* (2010) used the DIC-based diagnostics to explore several (disease mapping) models on an HIV data set. Below, we apply the diagnostics to the lip cancer study of Example IX.1.

Example X.16: Lip cancer study: Searching for outliers with PPO, CPO and DIC diagnostics

In Example IX.13, we fitted a Poisson-lognormal distribution to the lip cancer data. The Poisson-lognormal model is now explored to detect outlying values using various outlier diagnostics. To illustrate the use of SAS for computing PPO and CPO, we have provided the program 'chapter 10 lipcancer P lognormal.sas'. This program contains the MCMC statements for fitting the model and the SAS commands for pastprocessing the output. The index plots for PPO, CPO and ICPO are quite the same as obtained from WinBUGS (e.g. Figure 10.5(a)).

While DIC and p_D are available in WinBUGS, their individual components are not. By making use of R2WinBUGS we computed the DIC_i, dr_i and p_{Di} diagnostics; see 'chapter 10 lip cancer with residuals.R'. Again three chains were initiated with each 20 000 iterations and leaving out half of it for the burn-in part. In Figure 10.5, three diagnostics are shown and the posterior means of the random intercept. The index plot of $1/\widehat{\text{CPO}}_i$ clearly points to two outlying regions, i.e. 118 and 169. Regions 118, 169 have an observed count of 10, 22 and an expected count of 33.49, 102.16, respectively. These two regions are also outstanding in the index plot of estimated random intercepts, i.e. $\widehat{b}_{0i}$. The index plots DIC_i and dr_i confirm the outlying character of these regions but to a lesser extent, they point also to other outlying regions. Nevertheless the DIC diagnostics and the CPO values are highly correlated (Spearman correlation = 0.95). Finally, neither of the above two regions have a high leverage according to the p_{Di} values (plot not shown). □

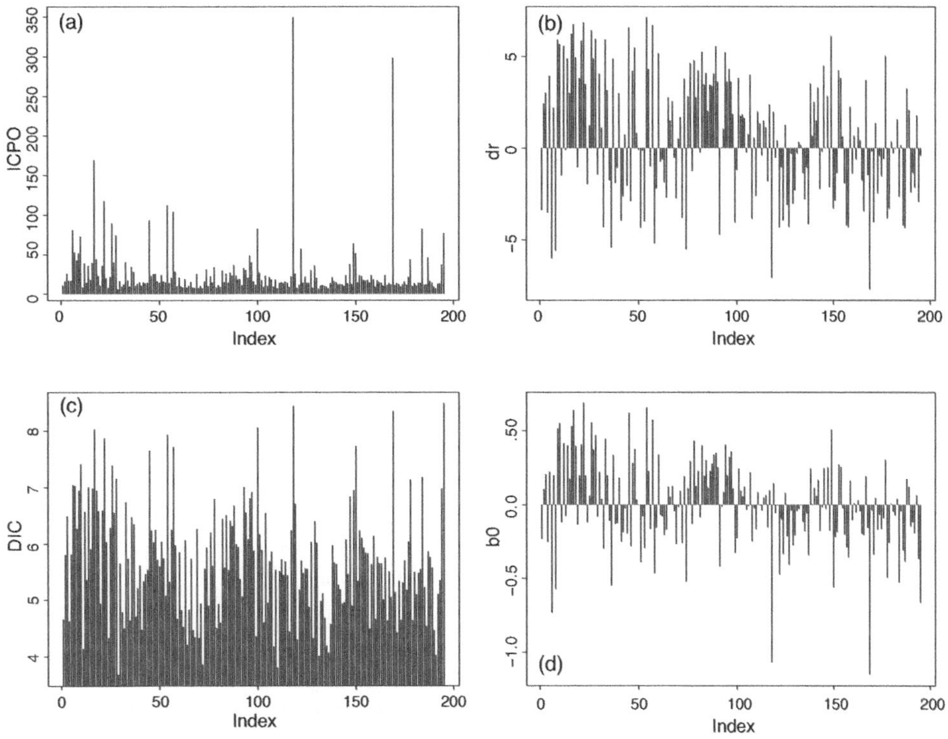

Figure 10.5 Lip cancer study: index plot of (a) $1/\widehat{\mathrm{CPO}}_i$, (b) $\mathrm{d}r_i$, (c) DIC_i and (d) $\widehat{b}_{0i}$.

10.3.3 Sensitivity analysis

The aim of a sensitivity analysis is to check how much the conclusions of a statistical analysis change when one deviates from the original statistical model. In a Bayesian context, this means that the likelihood as well as the prior are perturbed and their effect is evaluated. Various perturbations may be envisaged. One could change the distributional aspects of the model. For instance, in a mixed effects model (BLMM or BGLMM) one might vary the distribution of random effects or of the measurement error. In a BGLMM, one might explore the effect of choosing different link functions. One might also be interested in measuring the effect of slightly perturbing the responses or certain covariate values, or of deleting single or sets of subjects. When only a few alternative models are considered, then it is probably easiest just to replay the Bayesian analysis with the changed settings as was done in Example X.8 and in examples in previous chapters. Another possibility to obtain posterior summary measures from the perturbed model is to reuse the Markov chain by sampling from this chain, as was illustrated in Section 3.7.2. This approach is also useful when case-deletion diagnostics are needed.

While a sensitivity analysis should be part of any (Bayesian) statistical analysis, it must be feasible without too much extra computing efforts and the job should be accomplished fairly quickly. However, this might not be trivial in a Bayesian context. A variety of computational procedures have been suggested which will be reviewed now. In all of these procedures, it is important to combine the basic MCMC software with general statistical software.

We now outline how importance sampling and importance sampling-resampling can be applied to perform a sensitivity analysis. Afterward, we treat the detection of influential observations which makes use of these techniques.

(i) Bayesian sensitivity analysis via perturbation functions: Let the initial model M_0 consist of a sampling density $p_0(y \mid \boldsymbol{\theta}, \boldsymbol{x})$ and a prior $p_0(\boldsymbol{\theta})$. Assume a sample y_i $(i = 1, \ldots, n)$ with covariate vectors $\boldsymbol{x}_i$ $(i = 1, \ldots, n)$ is available, then the posterior is

$$p_0(\boldsymbol{\theta} \mid \boldsymbol{y}, \boldsymbol{X}) \propto \prod_{i=1}^{n} p_0 y_i \mid \boldsymbol{\theta}, \boldsymbol{x}_i) p_0(\boldsymbol{\theta}),$$

with $\boldsymbol{X}$ the matrix of covariate values. A Bayesian sensitivity analysis involves assessing the change in posterior distribution when model M_0 is perturbed. A formal approach to this assessment was suggested by Kass *et al.* (1989) who proposed the use of *perturbation functions*. Different choices of the perturbation function lead to different sensitivity analyses. The perturbation function $h(\boldsymbol{\theta}) \equiv h(\boldsymbol{\theta}, \boldsymbol{y}, \boldsymbol{X})$ multiplies $p_0(\boldsymbol{\theta} \mid \boldsymbol{y}, \boldsymbol{X})$ and thereby produces model M_1 and posterior $p_1(\boldsymbol{\theta} \mid \boldsymbol{y}, \boldsymbol{X})$. Weiss (1996) considered several perturbation functions. For example, $h_{1i}(\boldsymbol{\theta}) \propto 1/p_0(y_i \mid \boldsymbol{\theta}, \boldsymbol{x}_i)$ corresponds to leaving out the ith observation from the likelihood. Other examples are: (1) $h_2(\boldsymbol{\theta}) \propto q(\boldsymbol{\theta})/p_0(\boldsymbol{\theta})$ which corresponds to changing the prior from $p_0(\boldsymbol{\theta})$ to $q(\boldsymbol{\theta})$, (2) the sensitivity to y_i-values can be assessed by $h_{3i}(\boldsymbol{\theta}, \delta) \propto p_0(y_i + \delta \mid \boldsymbol{\theta}, \boldsymbol{x}_i)/p_0(y_i \mid \boldsymbol{\theta}, \boldsymbol{x}_i)$ and (3) for the sensitivity to $\boldsymbol{x}_i$ one could take $h_{4i}(\boldsymbol{\theta}, \boldsymbol{\delta}) \propto p_0(y_i \mid \boldsymbol{\theta}, \boldsymbol{x}_i + \boldsymbol{\delta})/p_0(y_i \mid \boldsymbol{\theta}, \boldsymbol{x}_i)$. To simplify the notation, we omit from now on the dependence on covariates. It is readily seen that the perturbed posterior is equal to

$$p_1(\boldsymbol{\theta} \mid \boldsymbol{y}) = p_0(\boldsymbol{\theta} \mid \boldsymbol{y}) h(\boldsymbol{\theta}) / E_0 \left[h(\boldsymbol{\theta}) \mid \boldsymbol{y} \right], \tag{10.23a}$$

with $E_0[h(\boldsymbol{\theta}) \mid \boldsymbol{y}]$ the posterior expectation of $h(\boldsymbol{\theta})$ under $p_0(\boldsymbol{\theta} \mid \boldsymbol{y})$. Weiss (1996) called equation (10.23) the Bayes theorem for perturbations. Further, Weiss showed that

$$B(M_0, M_1) = \frac{p(\boldsymbol{y} \mid M_0)}{p(\boldsymbol{y} \mid M_1)} = \frac{\int p_0(\boldsymbol{y} \mid \boldsymbol{\theta}) p_0(\boldsymbol{\theta}) \mathrm{d}\boldsymbol{\theta}}{\int p_0(\boldsymbol{y} \mid \boldsymbol{\theta}) p_0(\boldsymbol{\theta}) h(\boldsymbol{\theta}) \mathrm{d}\boldsymbol{\theta}} = \frac{1}{E_0 \left[h(\boldsymbol{\theta}) \mid \boldsymbol{y} \right]}, \tag{10.23b}$$

which relates $E_0[h(\boldsymbol{\theta}) \mid \boldsymbol{y}]$ to a Bayes factor. In addition, for $h_{1i}(\boldsymbol{\theta})$, $B(M_0, M_1) = p_0(\boldsymbol{y})/p_0(\boldsymbol{y}_{(i)})$ which shows that CPO_i is a Bayes factor.

The impact of the perturbation can be assessed by a divergence measure between the two posteriors. A popular choice for such a divergence measure is the Kullback–Leibler (K-L) distance defined by expression (10.5). The K-L distance $I(p_0(\boldsymbol{\theta} \mid \boldsymbol{y}), p_1(\boldsymbol{\theta} \mid \boldsymbol{y})) \equiv I_{0,1}(\boldsymbol{\theta})$ measures the impact of the perturbation on all parameters while $I_{0,1}(\boldsymbol{\tau}(\boldsymbol{\theta})) = I(p_0(\boldsymbol{\tau}(\boldsymbol{\theta}) \mid \boldsymbol{y}), p_1(\boldsymbol{\tau}(\boldsymbol{\theta}) \mid \boldsymbol{y}))$ evaluates the impact of the perturbation on $\boldsymbol{\tau}(\boldsymbol{\theta})$, a part or a function of the parameter vector. Weiss (1996) showed that $I_{0,1}(\boldsymbol{\tau}(\boldsymbol{\theta})) \leq I_{0,1}(\boldsymbol{\theta})$ which means that the global influence of a perturbation is always greater than the effect of the perturbation on a part of the parameters. For the normal linear model, $I_{0,1}(\boldsymbol{\theta})$ can be written in terms of the classical leverage, residual quantities and influence measures such as Cook's distance (see Geisser 1985; Guttman and Peña 1993; Johnson and Geisser 1983). However, interpreting $I_{0,1}(\boldsymbol{\theta})$ in an absolute sense is difficult. Alternatively, one could use the L_1-distance or a χ^2-divergence as influence measures (Weiss 1996).

(ii) Computation of influence measures: As illustrated below, the sensitivity analysis using the perturbation approach can become computationally involved. A practical, though ad hoc, approach to avoid these extra computations could be to use classical influence diagnostics to pinpoint influential observations. For the linear model, Cook (1977) provided closed expressions to express the influence of individual subjects on the regression estimates while for GLIMs Pregibon (1981) suggested one-step influence diagnostics. Both types of diagnostics are available in standard software and could be used to assess the impact of observations on the likelihood. Of course from a Bayesian viewpoint, this strategy does not appear elegant, moreover these diagnostics ignore the role of the prior. More importantly, this strategy would break down for more complex models some of which we do not dare to propose with ML procedures.

From the Bayes theorem for case deletion (equation (10.23) applied to $h_{1i}(\boldsymbol{\theta})$) one can easily show that

$$\frac{p(\boldsymbol{\theta} \mid \mathbf{y})}{p(\boldsymbol{\theta} \mid \mathbf{y}_{(i)})} = \frac{\text{CPO}_i}{p(y_i \mid \boldsymbol{\theta})} = h_{1i}(\boldsymbol{\theta}).$$

Further, the divergence measure $I_{0,1}(\boldsymbol{\theta})$ for $p(\boldsymbol{\theta} \mid \mathbf{y})$ and $p(\boldsymbol{\theta} \mid \mathbf{y}_{(i)})$ based on a converged Markov chain $\boldsymbol{\theta}^1, \ldots, \boldsymbol{\theta}^K$ is estimated by $\widehat{I}_i(h_1) = \frac{1}{K}\sum_{k=1}^{K} \log h_{1i}(\boldsymbol{\theta}^k)$. This method can identify globally influential cases, i.e. those that have a great impact on $\boldsymbol{\theta}$. The inequality $I_{0,1}(\boldsymbol{\tau}(\boldsymbol{\theta})) \leq I_{0,1}(\boldsymbol{\theta})$, shows that we need to explore only globally influential cases. For other perturbation schemes a similar strategy can be taken.

Diagnostic $\widehat{I}_i(h_1)$ depends on $\widehat{\text{CPO}}_i$ which can be quite unstable especially with highly influential cases, as illustrated below in Example X.17. Importance sampling is an alternative approach to detect influential cases in combination with MCMC techniques (Hastings 1970). Suppose $\boldsymbol{\theta}^1, \ldots, \boldsymbol{\theta}^K$ is a (dependent) sample from $p(\boldsymbol{\theta} \mid \mathbf{y})$, then the importance weights for deleting the ith observation at iteration k are $w_i^{*k} \equiv h_{1i}(\boldsymbol{\theta}^k)$ and the normalized weights are $w_i^k = w_i^{*k} / \sum_{l=1}^{K} w_i^{*l}$. The posterior mean of the summary measure $t(\boldsymbol{\theta})$ after deletion of case i is estimated by the weighted sample mean

$$\widehat{t(\boldsymbol{\theta})}_i = \sum_{k=1}^{K} w_i^k t(\boldsymbol{\theta}^k). \tag{10.24}$$

Obviously when CPO_i is badly estimated then this must apply also to these weights. In fact, this was already mentioned in Section 3.7.2. Sufficient (general) conditions were derived by Doss (1994) for having finite importance weights based on Markov chains. Peruggia (1997) provided simple to verify conditions for the Bayesian linear model and showed that for high leverage points the variance of the weights becomes infinite. Epifani *et al.* (2008) considered sufficient conditions for yet some other models.

When the variance of the weights is large, it is likely that a few of the weights w_i^k will dominate $\widehat{t(\boldsymbol{\theta})}_i$. Gelman *et al.* (2004, p. 316) suggested the use of the weighted sampling-resampling (SIR) algorithm but with resampling without replacement. That is, once a $\boldsymbol{\theta}^k$ has been selected it is removed from the set in the second sampling stage of the SIR algorithm. In this way, the impact of a large weight is greatly diminished. Note that all these procedures benefit greatly from Markov chains with a low autocorrelation, which can be obtained by thinning. For hierarchical models, Bradlow and Zaslavsky (1997) exploited (the often made assumption of) conditional independence to suggest alternative weighting schemes and to choose the weighting scheme with stable importance weights. In addition, they explored case-deletion at the different levels of the hierarchy.

We conclude that the detection of influence observations in a Bayesian context is an active research area (see Millar and Stewart 2007; Peruggia 2007) but also that the procedures are computational involved which is a burden for their every-day use. We now search for influential cases in the osteoporosis study.

Example X.17: Osteoporosis study: Detection of influential observations
To better illustrate the Bayesian techniques for detecting influential observations, we have increased the response (TBBMC) of subject 197 by a value of 2. This subject has a relatively high leverage of $h_{197,197} = 0.02$ (the maximal value of h_{ii} in the sample is 0.05) which in combination with a (fabricated) huge residual ends up in a large Cook's distance. In Figure 10.6(a) the scatterplot of BMI versus TBBMC is shown together with the two fitted regression lines (with and without subject 197). All computations were based on a single chain of size 1500 leaving out 750 burn-in iterations. The R program is given in 'chapter 10 osteo-study influence.R'.

First we computed $\widehat{I_i}(h_1)$ $(i = 1, \ldots, 234)$ to evaluate the global influence of each case. Clearly subject 197 is identified in Figure 10.6(b) as a high influential case. Figure 10.6(c) shows that the variance of the importance weights for that subject (across the values of the Markov chain) is the greatest which might imply that $\widehat{I_{197}}(h_1)$ was not well determined. In Figure 10.6(d), we see that a handful of importance weights dominate the importance sampling estimate of the posterior summary measures for subject 197. In Figures 10.6(e) and (f), the standardized changes of the intercept β_0 and slope β_1 are shown by leaving out each observation, i.e. for the slope we computed $\widehat{\text{DFBETA}}_{1i} = (\overline{\beta}_{1,(i)} - \overline{\beta}_1)/\overline{\sigma}_{\beta_1}$ where $\overline{\beta}_1$ is the estimated posterior mean of the slope based on the total sample, $\overline{\beta}_{1,(i)}$ the estimated posterior mean of β_1 when the ith observation is omitted from the sample and $\overline{\sigma}_{\beta_1}$ the estimated posterior standard deviation of β_1 based on the total sample. Note that $\overline{\beta}_{1,(i)}$ is computed using expression (10.24). Again subject 197 stands out. Finally, we compared the estimated change from importance sampling to the exact change by physically removing each observation with the trick used in Example X.14. Despite the imbalance in the weights we observed that both computations produced basically the same estimated changes in regression coefficients (plot not shown). □

Now, we search for influential observations in the arteriosclerosis study. These data have an hierarchical structure and we should now look for influential subjects and influential observations (per subject).

Example X.18: Arteriosclerosis study: Detection of influential observations
We might be concerned that the analysis of the nonlinear mixed effects model (9.20), in Example IX.18, is too much dependent on a single observation. For this reason, it is useful to check the stability of the model under case deletion. In particular, we are interested in the sensitivity of estimating δ (see Example IX.18 for an interpretation of δ). Case deletion has now two meanings. A case can be a whole subject, then one speaks of *subject diagnostics* while *observation diagnostics* measure the effect of deleting single observations. For the subject diagnostics, CPO and importance weights relate to the whole subject (20 subjects each with maximally six repeated measures), while the observation diagnostics measure the impact of removing individual observations ($120 - 1 = 119$ observations since one subject

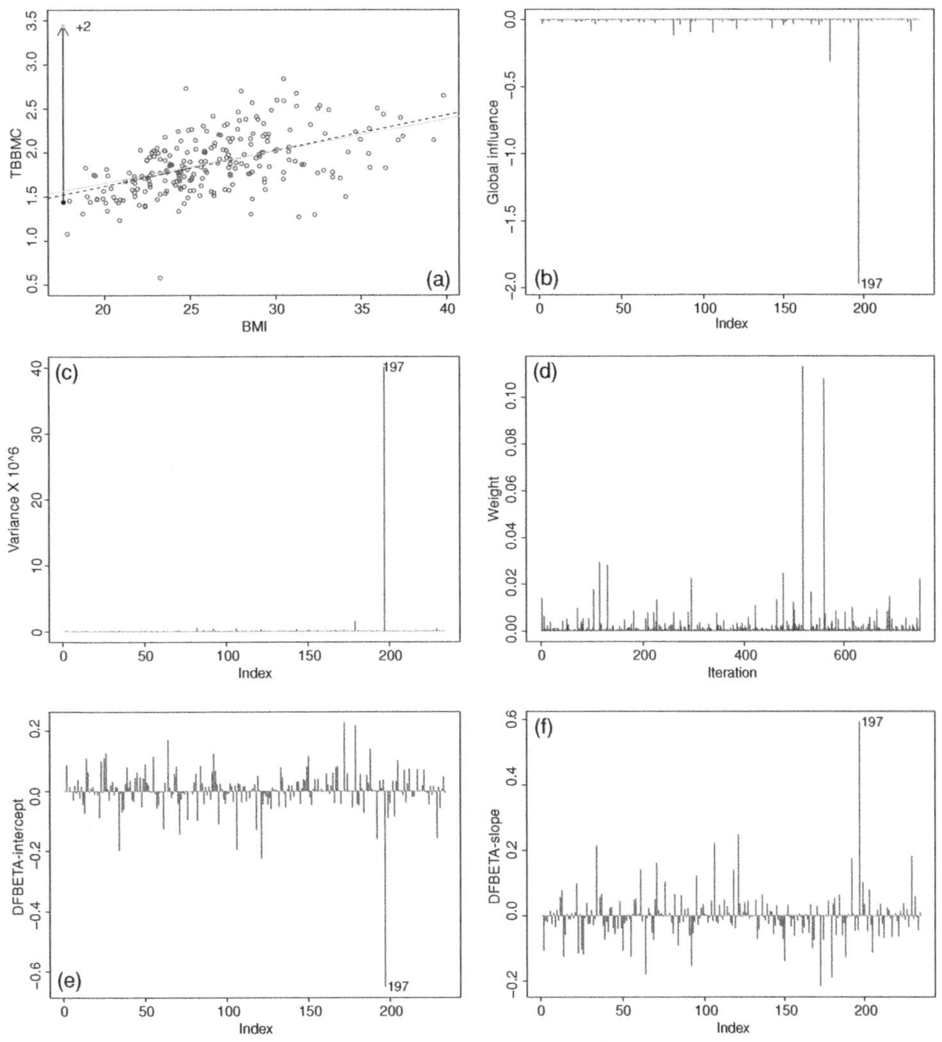

Figure 10.6 Osteoporosis study: (a) scatter plot of BMI versus TBBMC together with the regression line including subject 197 (solid line) and excluding that subject (dashed line), (b) index plot of $\widehat{I_i}(h_1)$, (c) index plot of var(w_i), (d) index plot of importance weights w^k_{197}, (e) index plot of $\widehat{\text{DFBETA}}_0$ and (f) index plot of $\widehat{\text{DFBETA}}_1$ (both obtained from importance sampling).

has a missing value). The R commands are found in 'chapter 10 arterior study-influence.R'. While convergence was relatively fast (see also Exercise 9.17) more iterations were needed for a reliable estimate of the PPO and CPO diagnostics. We ran $3 \times 1\,000\,000$ iterations with thinning of 100 and retained the last half for processing the necessary information.

The influence diagnostics on the original data set did not highlight any particular subject or observation that is highly influential. Of course, it might be that all subjects/observations have a high influence, which would not be surprising in a small data set. To illustrate better the diagnostic procedures we distorted, as in the previous example, one observation. Namely,

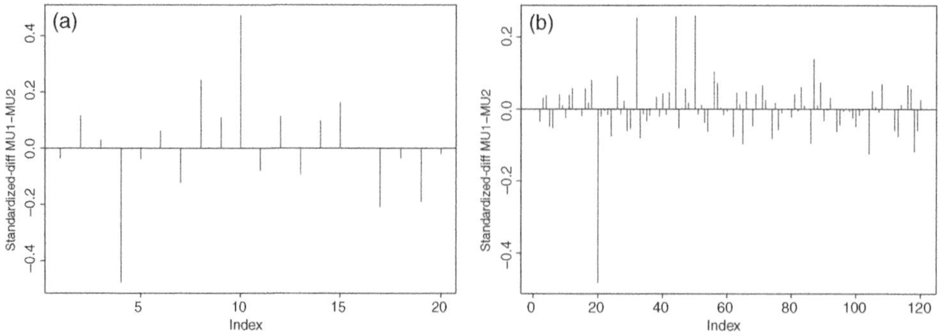

Figure 10.7 Arteriosclerosis study: index plots that show impact on δ by omitting (a) subjects ($\overline{\text{DFBETA}}_i$) and by omitting, and (b) observations ($\overline{\text{DFBETA}}_{ij}$).

we increased the 2nd measurement of the 4th subject (observation 20) from 0.76 to 1.76. The global influence diagnostic correctly indicates the fourth subject as influential and even more so the 20th observation. The variability of the weights for observation 20 was quite high, but was not that extreme for the fourth subject. The impact on δ on subject and observation level can be read off in Figure 10.7. Note that, compared to the original analysis, the distortion of observation 20 implies an increase of the estimated δ of about half of its standard error, which is quite appreciable.

We then compared the standardized impact of each subject and observation on δ by (1) importance sampling, (2) SIR algorithm with replacement, and (3) SIR algorithm without replacement. For the SIR algorithms, we sampled each time 1000 values from the original chain. Importance sampling and the SIR algorithm with replacement gave similar results and indicated the influential character of observation 20, in contrast to the SIR algorithm without replacement from which no such message could be obtained. No general conclusions can be drawn from this analysis, but it seems wise to apply the SIR algorithm both with and without replacement. □

(iii) Sensitivity to prior: We focused here on detecting model inadequacy and neglected that a lack of model fit can be partly due to the wrong choice of the prior. Gelman *et al.* (1996) argued that for a reasonably sized study with not a too strong prior the sensitivity of the conclusions to the choice of prior is likely to be minimal. Nevertheless, since it is not always clear whether certain choices of a vague prior are indeed noninformative, it is advisable to vary the prior distributions before making final conclusions.

10.3.4 Posterior predictive checks

We now look at global measures of GOF. Suppose that under the hypothesis H_0 we postulate model M_0: $p(y \mid \boldsymbol{\theta})$ for a sample $\boldsymbol{y} = \{y_1, \ldots, y_n\}$ whereby the parameters $\boldsymbol{\theta} \in \Theta_0$ must be estimated from the data. In a frequentist context, H_0 is tested with a GOF test statistic $T(\boldsymbol{y})$. Let a large value of $T(\boldsymbol{y})$ indicate a poor model fit and suppose that, under H_0, Θ_0 takes just one value, i.e. $\Theta_0 \equiv \boldsymbol{\theta}_0$. In the frequentist case, the GOF test consists of determining the sampling distribution of $T(\boldsymbol{y})$ under H_0 and computing

$$p_C(\boldsymbol{y}, \boldsymbol{\theta}_0) = P(T(\tilde{\boldsymbol{y}}) \geq T(\boldsymbol{y}) \mid \Theta_0, H_0), \tag{10.25}$$

with $\tilde{\mathbf{y}} = \{\tilde{y}_1, \ldots, \tilde{y}_n\}$ a random sample taken from M_0. For p_C small, H_0 will be rejected. The calculation of p_C is often done by making use of (asymptotic) probabilistic theory. But a simulation experiment generating $\tilde{\mathbf{y}}$ under H_0 thereby determining the proportion of times $T(\tilde{\mathbf{y}})$ exceeds $T(\mathbf{y})$ is also possible. However, when Θ_0 contains nuisance parameters then it is not immediately clear how the simulation should be done (what values of the nuisance parameters should be taken?) and we rely again on asymptotic arguments to determine p_C. For a pivotal statistic $T(\mathbf{y})$ the sampling distribution of $T(\mathbf{y})$ does not depend on the nuisance parameters and p_C can be again determined (via simulations or using probability theory). For example, suppose y_i $(i = 1, \ldots, n)$ are counts with a multinomial distribution Mult$(k, \boldsymbol{\eta})$, where $\sum_i y_i = k$ and $\boldsymbol{\eta}$ represents the n class probabilities. Suppose one is interested in verifying that $\boldsymbol{\eta}$ belongs to a lower than n-dimensional space, say $\boldsymbol{\eta} = t(\boldsymbol{\theta})$ with $\dim(\boldsymbol{\theta}) = d < \dim(\boldsymbol{\eta}) = n$. A popular GOF test to verify this assumption consists of computing the following χ^2-test statistic:

$$X^2(\mathbf{y}, \boldsymbol{\theta}) = \sum_{i=1}^{n} \frac{[y_i - \mathrm{E}(y_i \mid \boldsymbol{\theta})]^2}{\mathrm{var}(y_i \mid \boldsymbol{\theta})}. \tag{10.26}$$

When $\boldsymbol{\theta}$ is estimated via maximum likelihood then $X^2(\mathbf{y}, \boldsymbol{\theta})$ has asymptotically a $\chi^2(n-d)$-distribution. Thus, $X^2(\mathbf{y}, \boldsymbol{\theta})$ is asymptotically a pivotal statistic. Similarly, the log-likelihood ratio test statistic LLR$(\mathbf{y})$ for testing two nested models is under H_0 asymptotically pivotal since for large n LLR$(\mathbf{y})$ has a χ^2-distribution for nuisance parameters estimated by maximum likelihood. When the (asymptotic) distribution of the GOF test statistic is hard to derive, bootstrapping may be of help.

In this section, we focus on the question of how to test GOF in a Bayesian context. To fix ideas, suppose that we wish to test the above hypothesis, then we could evaluate

$$\int X^2(\mathbf{y}, \boldsymbol{\theta}) p(\boldsymbol{\theta} \mid \mathbf{y})\, \mathrm{d}\boldsymbol{\theta}, \tag{10.27}$$

whereby the χ^2-test statistic is averaged over the uncertainty of the parameters. Although this is a valid Bayesian procedure, the problem with this approach is that a benchmark is difficult to establish. An alternative approach is to sample from the assumed model and to compare the extremeness of the observed X^2 value to the sampled values under the assumed model. This is the basic idea behind the so-called *posterior predictive P-value (PPP-value)* and the *posterior predictive check (PPC)*.

(i) The predictive approach to testing goodness of fit: The predictive approach to GOF testing is to contrast $T(\mathbf{y})$ with $T(\tilde{\mathbf{y}})$ whereby $\tilde{\mathbf{y}}$ is an i.i.d. sample drawn from the PDD $p(\tilde{y} \mid \mathbf{y})$ and to evaluate its extremeness. A preliminary version of this idea is due to Guttman (1967), but it was Rubin (1984) who formalized the concept of the PPC. Meng (1994) and Gelman *et al.* (1996) further developed this proposal into a practical procedure.

A more formal definition of a PPC goes as follows. Assume that $T(\mathbf{y})$ is a classical GOF test statistic that depends only on the data, for example $T_{\min} = \min(\mathbf{y})$ and $T_{\max} = \max(\mathbf{y})$ measure how well the model fits remote values. Further, let the data at hand $\mathbf{y}$ be generated from the distribution $p(y \mid \boldsymbol{\theta}^*)$ with $\boldsymbol{\theta}^* \in \Theta_0$ a fixed but unknown parameter vector. Suppose that the future data $\tilde{\mathbf{y}}$, also called *replicated data*, have been sampled from the same distribution.

For the PPC one evaluates the posterior predictive P-value defined by

$$\begin{aligned} p_T &= P(T(\tilde{\mathbf{y}}) \geq T(\mathbf{y}) \mid \mathbf{y}, H_0) \\ &= \int I[T(\tilde{\mathbf{y}}) \geq T(\mathbf{y})]p(\tilde{\mathbf{y}} \mid \mathbf{y})\, d\tilde{\mathbf{y}} \\ &= \int\int I[T(\tilde{\mathbf{y}}) \geq T(\mathbf{y})]p(\tilde{\mathbf{y}} \mid \boldsymbol{\theta})p(\boldsymbol{\theta} \mid \mathbf{y})\, d\tilde{\mathbf{y}}\, d\boldsymbol{\theta} \\ &= \int p_C(\mathbf{y}, \boldsymbol{\theta})p(\boldsymbol{\theta} \mid \mathbf{y})\, d\boldsymbol{\theta}, \end{aligned} \tag{10.28}$$

with I the indicator function. A small value of p_T is an indication of a bad fit of the model to the data. In the last line of the previous derivation, we made use of expression (10.25) since if the true parameter is $\boldsymbol{\theta}$ then the above evaluation boils down to computing p_C. It is also readily seen that if the posterior distribution is concentrated at $\boldsymbol{\theta}_0$, then $p_T \approx p_C$ and then the PPC reduces to a classical GOF test.

If the GOF test statistic depends on nuisance parameters then the previous approach needs to be adapted. In a Bayesian context, maximization is replaced by integration. Meng (1994) suggested this approach to extend the PPC to a *discrepancy measure* $D(\mathbf{y}, \boldsymbol{\theta})$ which is a function of both data and parameters. The PPP-value is now computed as follows:

$$\begin{aligned} p_D &= P(D(\tilde{\mathbf{y}}, \boldsymbol{\theta}) \geq D(\mathbf{y}, \boldsymbol{\theta}) \mid \mathbf{y}, H_0) \\ &= \int\int I[D(\tilde{\mathbf{y}}, \boldsymbol{\theta}) \geq D(\mathbf{y}, \boldsymbol{\theta})]p(\tilde{\mathbf{y}} \mid \boldsymbol{\theta})p(\boldsymbol{\theta} \mid \mathbf{y})\, d\tilde{\mathbf{y}}\, d\boldsymbol{\theta}. \end{aligned} \tag{10.29}$$

The χ^2-discrepancy measure defined by expression (10.26) for multinomially distributed y_i $(i = 1, \ldots, n)$ is an example of such a discrepancy measure. Applying expression (10.29) to this measure yields as PPP-value

$$\begin{aligned} p_{X^2} &= \int\int I[X^2(\tilde{\mathbf{y}}, \boldsymbol{\theta}) \geq X^2(\mathbf{y}, \boldsymbol{\theta})]p(\tilde{\mathbf{y}} \mid \boldsymbol{\theta})p(\boldsymbol{\theta} \mid \mathbf{y})\, d\tilde{\mathbf{y}}\, d\boldsymbol{\theta} \\ &\approx \int P\left[X^2 \geq X^2(\mathbf{y}, \boldsymbol{\theta})\right] p(\boldsymbol{\theta} \mid \mathbf{y})\, d\boldsymbol{\theta}, \end{aligned} \tag{10.30}$$

with X^2 representing a random variable with a $\chi^2(n - \mathrm{d})$-distribution. Expression (10.30) is obtained by integrating over $\tilde{\mathbf{y}}$ and the fact that $X^2(\tilde{\mathbf{y}}, \boldsymbol{\theta})$ has approximately a $\chi^2(n - \mathrm{d})$-distribution under H_0. Comparing expression (10.30) with (10.27) shows that defining a benchmark for the fit of the model to the data is easier with the PPC approach.

The generalization of the PPC to any discrepancy measure allows one to choose test quantities primarily based on substantive arguments, i.e. we do not have to restrict to pivotal test statistics as with classical GOF tests. In addition, the PPC allows to fix some aspects of the data when drawing replicates. For example, in a hierarchical model the replicates could be restricted to a particular cluster to check the distributional assumptions in that cluster. One could even fix certain parameters to the estimates obtained from the observed data such as in the normal distribution where mean and standard deviation are taken from the sample. In that case, the replicates are not drawn anymore from the posterior distribution.

A variant of the PPC is the *prior predictive check* (Box 1980) yielding prior predictive P-value and used to check a data-prior conflict. This approach is not popular as a GOF procedure since the prior is in many applications too vague causing the discrepancy averaging over many unrealistic parameter values. However, if the prior is better tuned to the data, then this approach may be useful (see below for the calibration of the PPP-value by a double simulation scheme).

We note that the PPC has gained much popularity because of its flexibility to test any model deviation of interest and its ease in implementing it with MCMC techniques. The approach has been widely applied.

(ii) Computation of the PPC: The computation of the PPP-value for a discrepancy measure $D(\boldsymbol{y}, \boldsymbol{\theta})$ (and for a test statistic $T(\boldsymbol{y})$) goes as follows:

1. Let $\boldsymbol{\theta}^1, \ldots, \boldsymbol{\theta}^K$ be a converged Markov chain from $p(\boldsymbol{\theta} \mid \boldsymbol{y})$.
2. Compute $D(\boldsymbol{y}, \boldsymbol{\theta}^k)$ $(k = 1, \ldots, K)$ (for $T(\boldsymbol{y})$ this needs to be done only once).
3. Sample replicated data $\tilde{\boldsymbol{y}}^k$ from $p(y \mid \boldsymbol{\theta}^k)$ (each of size n).
4. Compute $D(\tilde{\boldsymbol{y}}^k, \boldsymbol{\theta}^k)$ $(k = 1, \ldots, K)$.
5. Estimate p_D by $\overline{p}_D = \frac{1}{K}\sum_{i=1}^{K} I[D(\tilde{\boldsymbol{y}}^k, \boldsymbol{\theta}^k) \geq D(\boldsymbol{y}, \boldsymbol{\theta}^k)]$.

If $\overline{p}_D$ is small then this is an indication that the model might not fit the data well, as measured by $D(\boldsymbol{y}, \boldsymbol{\theta})$. 'Small' might be again taken as $\overline{p}_D \leq 0.05$ as in classical frequentist statistics, but the choice of 0.05 is only indicative. Gelman promotes the use of graphical output to evaluate the outcome of a PPC (see Gelman and Meng 1996; Gelman 2003; Gelman 2004). For a test statistic $T(\boldsymbol{y})$, a histogram of the replicated values $T(\tilde{\boldsymbol{y}}^k)$ can be displayed with the observed $T(\boldsymbol{y})$ superimposed. A badly fitting model is immediately recognized by the extremeness of the observed $T(\boldsymbol{y})$ on the graph. For a discrepancy measure such a plot is not possible and a X–Y-plot is suggested augmented with the 45° line. The proportion of points above the 45° line estimates p_D.

We now illustrate the use of PPC with the osteoporosis example.

Example X.19: Osteoporosis study: Checking distributional assumptions with the PPC
We illustrate the difference between a test statistic and a discrepancy measure in checking the normality of TBBMC. In 'chapter 10 osteo study-PPC.R' six PPCs have been programmed. We focus here on checking the skewness and kurtosis of the data. By fixing the mean and variance parameters to the sample mean $\overline{y}$ and variance s^2, respectively, two test statistics appear:

$$T_{\text{skew}}(\boldsymbol{y}) = \frac{1}{n}\sum_{i=1}^{n}\left(\frac{y_i - \overline{y}}{s}\right)^3 \text{ and } T_{\text{kurt}}(\boldsymbol{y}) = \frac{1}{n}\sum_{i=1}^{n}\left(\frac{y_i - \overline{y}}{s}\right)^4 - 3.$$

Discrepancy measures are obtained when the mean and variance are parameters (and thus random variables in a Bayesian context), i.e.

$$D_{\text{skew}}(\boldsymbol{y}, \boldsymbol{\theta}) = \frac{1}{n}\sum_{i=1}^{n}\left(\frac{y_i - \mu}{\sigma}\right)^3 \text{ and } D_{\text{kurt}}(\boldsymbol{y}, \boldsymbol{\theta}) = \frac{1}{n}\sum_{i=1}^{n}\left(\frac{y_i - \mu}{\sigma}\right)^4 - 3,$$

with $\boldsymbol{\theta} = (\mu, \sigma)^T$.

For each of these measures is the proportion of times the replicated data give a more extreme value than the observed data was recorded. The observed skewness and kurtosis were 0.19 and 0.49. For the PPCs we obtained $\overline{p}_{T_{\text{skew}}} = 0.13$, $\overline{p}_{T_{\text{kurt}}} = 0.055$, $\overline{p}_{D_{\text{skew}}} = 0.27$

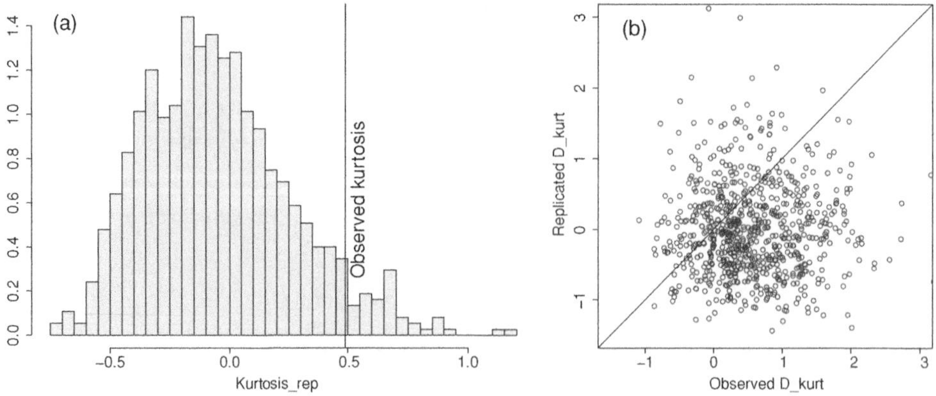

Figure 10.8 Osteoporosis study: (a) histogram of $T_{kurt}(\tilde{\mathbf{y}})$ with vertical line at observed kurtosis, and (b) scatterplot of $D_{kurt}(\mathbf{y}, \tilde{\boldsymbol{\theta}})$ versus $D_{kurt}(\tilde{\mathbf{y}}, \tilde{\boldsymbol{\theta}})$.

and $\overline{p}_{D_{\text{kurt}}} = 0.26$. Only T_{kurt} indicated non-normality but this was not confirmed by D_{kurt}. The discrepancy measures $D_{\text{skew}}, D_{\text{kurt}}$ appear more conservative than $T_{\text{skew}}, T_{\text{kurt}}$, which was also observed by Ntzoufras (2009, p. 367). This conservatism is caused by the posterior uncertainty of μ and σ which results in a greater variability of the discrepancy measures. In Figure 10.8(a), we show the histogram of $T_{\text{kurt}}(\tilde{\mathbf{y}})$ with the observed kurtosis indicated and in Figure 10.8(b) we show the scatterplot of $D_{\text{kurt}}(\tilde{\mathbf{y}}, \tilde{\boldsymbol{\theta}})$ versus $D_{\text{kurt}}(\mathbf{y}, \tilde{\boldsymbol{\theta}})$ with the 45° line, with $\tilde{\boldsymbol{\theta}}$ any of the generated $\boldsymbol{\theta}^1, \ldots, \boldsymbol{\theta}^K$ and $\tilde{\mathbf{y}}$ the corresponding replicated data.

To explore the normality assumption of the residuals from a normal linear regression regression of TBBMC on covariates, the same discrepancy measures can be applied on standardized residuals $r_i = (y_i - \widehat{y}_i)/\sigma$. In addition, Ntzoufras (2009) suggested the Kolmogorov–Smirnov discrepancy measure

$$D_{KS}(\mathbf{y}, \boldsymbol{\theta}) = \max_{i \in \{1,\ldots,n\}} \left[\Phi(y_i \mid \mu, \sigma) - (i-1)/n, i/n - \Phi(y_i \mid \mu, \sigma) \right],$$

with $\Phi(\cdot \mid 0, 1)$ the standard normal cdf and the gap discrepancy measure

$$D_{\text{gap}}(\mathbf{y}, \boldsymbol{\theta}) = \max_{i \in \{1,\ldots,(n-1)\}} (y_{(i+1)} - y_{(i)}),$$

with $y_{(i)}$ the ith ordered value of $\mathbf{y}$. A simple discrepancy measure is $D_{0.05}(\mathbf{y}, \boldsymbol{\theta}) = \sum_{i=1}^{n} \text{I}(|y_i| > 2)$, which measures the proportion of residuals greater than 2 in absolute value. With the commands in 'chapter 10 osteo study2-PPC.R', one can apply these measures on the regression analysis of Example X.12. We also searched for outliers using procedures described in Ntzoufras (2009, pp. 363–364). However, none of the procedures indicated non-normality of the residuals. □

In the next example, we apply PPCs to the lip cancer data.

Example X.20: Lip cancer study: Posterior predictive checking of the Poisson(-gamma) model

In Figure 9.1, we verified whether the $\text{SMR}_i = y_i/e_i$ $(i = 1, \ldots, n)$ were generated from a Poisson distribution for y_i with mean $\mu_i = \theta\, e_i$. This was done by sampling counts $y_i \sim \text{Poisson}(\theta\, e_i)$ and comparing the histogram of one sample of replicates with the observed histogram. Under the assumption of $\theta = 1$ this exercise was a kind of PPC although done in an ad hoc way. Now, we perform a genuine PPC and for this we estimate θ. In 'chapter 10 lip cancer PGM PPC.odc', we have programmed four PPCs to test the appropriateness of a single Poisson distribution (with offset e_i on the log scale for the mean). It is left as an exercise to the reader to incorporate this program into a R program that calls WinBUGS from R. First we checked for overdispersion by $T_{1,var}(\mathbf{y}) = \text{Var(SMR)}$ and $D_{2,var}(\mathbf{y}, \theta) = \sum_{i=1}^{n}(y_i - \mu_i)^2/\mu_i$. The latter measure represents a Pearson test which would be evaluated against a $\chi^2(n-1)$-distribution in a frequentist context. Next, we used discrepancy measures based on the deviance: (1) $D_{1,dev}(\mathbf{y}, \theta) = -2\sum_{i=1}^{n}[\mu_i + y_i \log(\mu_i)]$ which is $-2\log L$ evaluated in the observed data for the sampled values of θ and (2) $D_{2,dev}(\mathbf{y}, \theta) = -2\sum_{i=1}^{n}[(y_i - \mu_i) + y_i \log(\mu_i/y_i)]$ which consists of the deviance residuals comparing the fitted model with the saturated model. To compute $D_{2,dev}$, zero observed/replicated counts must be augmented with a small value. Finally, we compared the observed variance of SMR_i to the theoretical value equal to $\sum_{i=1}^{n}\mu_i/e_i$.

The simple Poisson model was strongly rejected for all PPCs (all PPP-values were basically zero). In a second step (see same .odc file), we verified whether the hierarchical Poisson-gamma model assuming $\theta_i \mid \alpha, \beta \sim \text{Gamma}(\alpha, \beta)$ for $i = 1, \ldots, n$ is valid. The discrepancy measures were adapted for this, i.e. we replaced θ by $\boldsymbol{\eta} = (\theta_1, \ldots, \theta_n, \alpha, \beta)^T$. For instance, $D_{1,\text{dev}}(\mathbf{y}, \theta)$ is equal to $D_{1,\text{dev}}(\mathbf{y}, \boldsymbol{\eta})$ with $\mu_i = \theta_i e_i$. For the Poisson-gamma model the PPP-values of $D_{1,dev}$ and $D_{2,dev}$ ranged between 0.14 and 0.51, providing no evidence against this model. Of course, this is not a proof that the Poisson-gamma model is appropriate, but the Poisson-gamma model appears to address the overdispersion appropriately. □

The discrepancy measures in examples X.19 and X.20 were inspired by frequentist test statistics, but PPCs can be defined using any discrepancy measure. Although some measures are not appropriate. For example, sufficient statistics, such as the mean and standard deviation in a normal model, are a wrong choice because the model fits such a measure exactly. General guidelines on how to choose the best discrepancy measure, are useful but not available.

(iii) Posterior predictive checks in hierarchical models: The PPCs in the lip cancer example evaluate whether the observed data (level-1 data) fit the hierarchical model well. But in a hierarchical model distributional assumptions are made at each level of the hierarchy and need dedicated discrepancy measures. For instance, in Example X.20, we may check the gamma distribution of the level-2 latent observations by a PPC based on a Kolmogorov–Smirnov discrepancy measure $D(\boldsymbol{\theta}, \boldsymbol{\phi})$ with now $\boldsymbol{\theta} = (\theta_1, \ldots, \theta_n)^T$ and $\boldsymbol{\phi} = (\alpha, \beta)^T$ (see Exercise 10.24). For a normal hierarchical model, Sinharay and Stern (2003) suggested $D_{SS}(\mathbf{y}, \boldsymbol{\theta}, \boldsymbol{\phi}) = |\theta_{\text{max}} - \theta_{\text{med}}| - |\theta_{\text{min}} - \theta_{\text{med}}|$ to test the symmetry of the assumed Gaussian distribution of the θs. Among other tests, this discrepancy measure was used in the next example.

Example X.21: Lip cancer study: Posterior predictive checking of the Poisson-lognormal model

In Example IX.13, we assumed $\log(\mu_i/e_i) = \beta_0 + \beta_1 \,\text{AFF}_i + b_{0i}$, with $b_{0i} \sim \text{N}(0, \sigma_{b_0}^2)$ playing the role of θ_i. Here, we wish to check the normality assumption of the random intercept. We applied the discrepancy measures $D_{\text{skew}}(\boldsymbol{\theta}, \boldsymbol{\phi})$, $D_{\text{kurt}}(\boldsymbol{\theta}, \boldsymbol{\phi})$, $D_{KS}(\boldsymbol{\theta}, \boldsymbol{\phi})$, $D_{\text{gap}}(\boldsymbol{\theta}, \boldsymbol{\phi})$ and $D_{SS}(\boldsymbol{\theta}, \boldsymbol{\phi})$ on b_{0i}. Now $\boldsymbol{\theta} = (b_{01}, \ldots, b_{0n})^T$ and $\boldsymbol{\phi} = (\beta_0, \beta_1, \sigma_{b_0}^2)^T$. We omitted the dependence on $\mathbf{y}$ for notational simplicity, but also because here the PPCs depend only indirectly on $\mathbf{y}$. In each case we computed the PPP-value as follows: (1) sample $\boldsymbol{\phi}$

from its posterior distribution and $\widetilde{\boldsymbol{\theta}}$ given $\widetilde{\boldsymbol{\phi}}$, then compute $D(\tilde{\boldsymbol{\theta}}, \tilde{\boldsymbol{\phi}})$; (2) sample $\widetilde{\widetilde{b}}_{0i}$ from $\mathrm{N}(0, \tilde{\sigma}_{b_0}^2)$ resulting in $D(\widetilde{\tilde{\boldsymbol{\theta}}}, \tilde{\boldsymbol{\phi}})$ and (3) compute the proportion of times $D(\tilde{\boldsymbol{\theta}}, \tilde{\boldsymbol{\phi}})$ is greater than $D(\widetilde{\tilde{\boldsymbol{\theta}}}, \tilde{\boldsymbol{\phi}})$. The PPCs were implemented in 'chapter 10 lip cancer PLN PPC.odc'. None of the PPP -values indicated non-normality (results not shown).

To test the power of the PPC for latent variables, we created an artificial data set for which we simulated b_{0i} from a location-scale $\chi^2(2)$-distribution with skewness equal to 1.4 and kurtosis equal to 1.7 and imputed these in the model for $\log(\mu_i/e_i)$ (look for 'simulated data' in previous odc file). To our surprise, none of the discrepancy measures indicated deviation from normality. □

The PPP-values applied to a hierarchical model in the previous example were first suggested by Gelman *et al.* (2005) and were called *extended PPP-values* by Steinbakk and Storvik (2009). Sinharay and Stern (2003) suggested a different extension of the classical PPC to the hierarchical setting in combination with their discrepancy measure D_{SS}. That is, for each sampled value of $\boldsymbol{\phi}$ they computed the posterior expectation of $D_{SS}(\mathbf{y}, \boldsymbol{\theta}, \boldsymbol{\phi})$ and obtained $D^m(\mathbf{y}, \boldsymbol{\phi}) = E[D_{SS}(\mathbf{y}, \boldsymbol{\theta}, \boldsymbol{\phi}) \mid \mathbf{y}]$. In a second step, they based the PPP-value on $D^m(\mathbf{y}, \boldsymbol{\phi})$, i.e. using a classical (nonhierarchical) PPC and obtained the *marginalized PPP-value* according to Steinbakk and Storvik (2009). In this way, the latent level-2 observations are removed from the final computation. This approach is computationally quite demanding since it involves a double sampling scheme: first sampling $\boldsymbol{\phi}$ and for each sampled value sampling $\boldsymbol{\theta}$ and establishing its posterior mean. More importantly, also Sinharay and Stern (2003) found in their example and simulations that the power of $D^m(\mathbf{y}, \boldsymbol{\phi})$ to detect non-normality is extremely low. Dey *et al.* (1998) noted that this power was low because in the example of Sinharay and Stern (2003) there is only one observed response y_i for each b_{0i}.

The next example is an hierarchical model with multiple observations per level-2 observations. Again, we wish to test the normality assumption of the random effect.

Example X.22: Toenail RCT: Checking normality of the random intercept in a logistic random intercept model

We tested the normality assumption of the random intercept of the toenail model of Example IX.14 using the discrepancy measures defined in previous example. In 'chapter 10 toenail study-PPC.R', we used R2WinBUGS and R functions to compute the discrepancy measures. None of the discrepancy measures indicated non-normality. This is surprising in view of the clear non-normality shown in the NPP (of the posterior mean) of the random intercepts in Figure 10.9(a). In Figure 10.9(b), the NPP is shown of the posterior mean of the simulated random intercept assuming normality (together with pointwise 95% CIs). As expected, there is no deviation from normality. However, there is a huge variability in the sampled random intercepts, which is explained by the fact that the posterior mean of σ_{b_0} is about 4. Due to this high fluctuation, the PPC did not detect deviations from normality in the data. □

From Examples X.21 and X.22 it appears that the PPCs may be grossly underpowered for level-2 observations. We now look at this problem more closely.

(iv) The interpretation of the PPP-value: The classical P-value p_C has a uniform distribution under H_0 by construction which implies that for a continuous test statistic $P(p_C \leq \alpha) = \alpha$ for any $0 \leq \alpha \leq 1$ and that $p_C \leq \alpha$ occurs in α% of hypothetical studies under H_0. In the literature, the PPP-value is also often interpreted as a classical P-value, in fact, it is

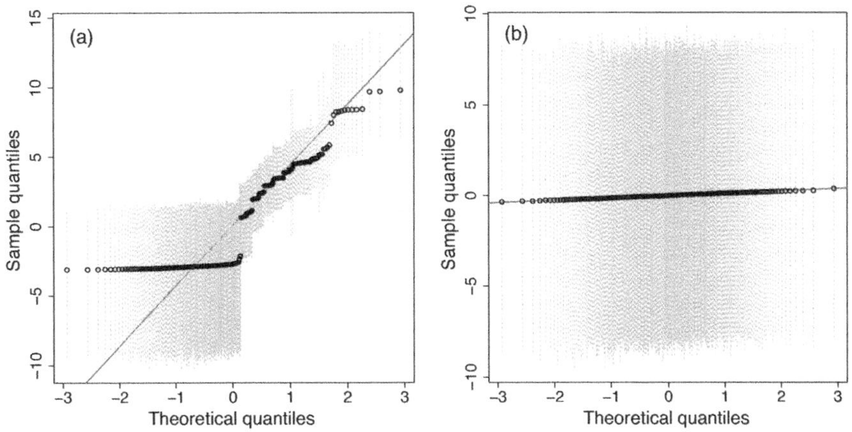

Figure 10.9 Toenail study: (a) normal probability plot of posterior mean of random intercept, and (b) normal probability plot of simulated random intercept.

referred to as a *Bayesian P-value*. But this may be not justified. Instead, the PPP-value is an average of classical P-values over the posterior uncertainty of $\boldsymbol{\theta}$ as was illustrated in (10.31). For a prior predictive P-value, Meng (1994) showed that the distribution of p_D is not uniform. Also the PPP-value does not have a uniform distribution (Robins *et al.* 2000) which makes it difficult to calibrate. Steinbakk and Storvik (2009) concluded the same for the extensions of the PPP-value to an hierarchical setting. A second problem with the PPC is its lack of power since it makes double use of the data. This was demonstrated in several studies by Steinbakk and Storvik (2009) who also derived some analytical results in a particular setting. To calibrate the PPP-value, Steinbakk and Storvik (2009) proposed a double simulation scheme which produces a Bayesian P-value that has a uniform distribution with a greater power to detect deviations from the distributional assumptions of the random effects. Their approach goes as follows:

- Compute the classical PPP-value $\overline{p}_D$, which we refer to as the 'observed p_D' to distinguish it from the simulated p_D's below;
- Sample from a so-called *null–null* model. That is, sample $\boldsymbol{\phi}^*$ from the prior $p(\boldsymbol{\phi})$, $\boldsymbol{\theta}^*$ from $p(\boldsymbol{\theta} \mid \boldsymbol{\phi}^*)$ and $\mathbf{y}^*$ from $p(\mathbf{y} \mid \boldsymbol{\theta}^*)$;
- On each simulated data set compute $\overline{p}_D$ as before and call it p^*. Repeat this S times yielding $p_1^*, \ldots, p_S^*$;
- Compute $p_S = \frac{1}{S}\sum_{s=1}^{S} I(p_s^* < \overline{p}_D)$.

This approach requires a reasonably wide but proper hyperprior $p(\boldsymbol{\phi})$ covering realistic values of the hyperparameters. Although the proposed approach is quite promising, the next example shows that the necessary computing effort is formidable.

Example X.23: Toenail RCT: Illustration of approach of Steinbakk and Storvik (2009)
We used a R2jags program to implement the approach of Steinbakk and Storvik. Recall that none of the classical discrepancy measures indicated violation of the normality assumption.

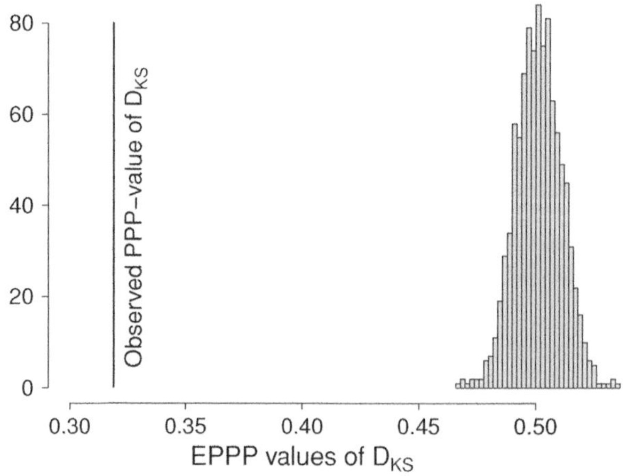

Figure 10.10 Toenail study: histogram of simulated PPP-values together with $\overline{p}_D = 0.32$.

Here, we looked only at the Kolmogorov–Smirnov discrepancy measure. The 'observed p_D' is equal to 0.32.

We first sampled $\boldsymbol{\phi}_1^*, \ldots, \boldsymbol{\phi}_S^*$, with $\boldsymbol{\phi}_s^* = (\beta_{0s}^*, \beta_{1s}^*, \beta_{2s}^*, \beta_{3s}^*, \sigma_{0s}^{*2})^T$ with S = 1000. The prior for $\boldsymbol{\phi}_s^*$ is a product of independent normal priors for the regression coefficients with mean = 0 and variance = 10^4 and a uniform prior on [0,100] for σ_{0s}^*. The other simulated values follow from the specified logistic random intercept model. Namely, we additionally simulated $\boldsymbol{\theta}_1^*, \ldots, \boldsymbol{\theta}_S^*$ with $\boldsymbol{\theta}_s^* = (b_{01s}^*, \ldots, b_{0ns}^*)^T$ and $\boldsymbol{y}_1^*, \ldots, \boldsymbol{y}_S^*$ with $\boldsymbol{y}_s^*$ the sth simulated response. For the sth generated data set, we applied the Kolmogorov–Smirnov discrepancy measure $D_{KS}(\boldsymbol{\theta}_s^*, \boldsymbol{\phi}_s^*)$ to yield the PPP-value p_s^*. Each of such analyses was based on 2000 iterations omitting 1000 burn-in iterations. In Figure 10.10, the histogram of $p_1^*, \ldots, p_S^*$ together with 'observed p_D' is shown. Under the null–null model, the p_Ds are concentrated around 0.50 quite remote from 0.32 thereby highlighting the strong deviation from normality of the random intercept.

We note that the computation of the simulated PPP-values was quite time consuming and took about 24 hours in a cluster-computing environment. □

Given the formidable computing power that is needed to calibrate the Bayesian *P*-value, the original PPC remains the method of choice in many practical applications. In hierarchical models, one may also produce diagnostic plots based on the posterior estimates of the random effects. Alternatively, other simulation-based approaches could be explored (see Marshall and Spiegelhalter 2007 and Green *et al.* 2009).

10.3.5 Model expansion

10.3.5.1 Introduction

Enlarging the model with extra parameters or equivalently embedding the current model in a larger class of models is called *model expansion*. Model expansion is a way to build a model but is also a way to test the GOF of a model. In a regression context, examples of model expansion are: (1) embedding the assumed distribution of the response in a general class of distributions, (2) relaxing the linearity assumption of the covariates by adding polynomial and/or interaction terms to the systematic part or introducing splines in the model, (3) relaxing the link function, etc. Clearly, the number of ways to expand upon a current model is infinite. We are only limited by our imagination and the computational power, but of course the final model must make sense from a substantive point of view.

10.3.5.2 Generalizing the distributional assumption

The distributional assumptions in the model can be relaxed by embedding the distribution into a larger class of distributions. For example, for a positive random variable y the normal distribution could be embedded in the modified power transformation family, suggested by Box and Cox (1964). This implies that we assume that there exists a λ for which

$$y^{(\lambda)} = (y^{\lambda} - 1)/\lambda \tag{10.31}$$

has a $\mathrm{N}(\mu, \sigma^2)$ distribution. In that case, we say that y has a *Box–Cox distribution*. The transformation parameter λ needs to be estimated from the data and hence becomes a random variable often taking a value between -2 and 2. Normality of y corresponds to $\lambda = 1$ and a lognormal distribution for y is obtained when $\lambda = 0$. Other transformation families have been suggested in the literature, e.g. Bickel and Doksum (1981) suggested the transformation $(|y|^{\lambda}\mathrm{sgn}(y) - 1)/\lambda$ with $\lambda > 0$ for a possibly negative y. Estimating λ together with the other (regression) parameters reflects better what happens in practice if one is uncertain about the scale to work on.

The Box–Cox distribution is not supported by WinBUGS nor by SAS. When the distribution is not standard, one can try the *zeros trick* or the *ones trick* in WinBUGS. The zeros trick uses the following decomposition of the total likelihood:

$$\mathrm{L} = \prod_{i=1}^{n} \mathrm{L}_i = \prod_{i=1}^{n} \exp\left[\log(\mathrm{L}_i)\right] = \prod_{i=1}^{n} \frac{\exp - \left[-\log(\mathrm{L}_i)\right]\left[-\log(\mathrm{L}_i)\right]^0}{0!}, \tag{10.32}$$

which can be seen as the likelihood of a sample of Poisson distributed random variables with mean $-\log(\mathrm{L}_i)$ and observed values all zero. Alternatively, one could apply the ones trick. Namely,

$$\mathrm{L} = \prod_{i=1}^{n} \mathrm{L}_i = \prod_{i=1}^{n} \mathrm{L}_i^{z_i}(1 - \mathrm{L}_i)^{(1-z_i)}, \tag{10.33}$$

with $z_i = 1$ for all i. Now, the likelihood resembles that of a Bernoulli distribution. In both cases, the sample consists of pseudorandom variables, but the tricks may help to let WinBUGS do the job. It may be necessary to add a large positive constant to ensure for the zeros trick that all L_i are positive. For the ones trick, one may need to divide by a large positive constant.

Another, more simplistic, approach to determine the best λ is to perform several Bayesian analyses with powers chosen from the set $\{-2, -1.5, -1, -0.5, 0, 0.5, 1, 1.5, 2\}$. For each choice of λ one obtains a DIC, denoted DIC_{λ}. However, to compare the different DIC_{λ}s a

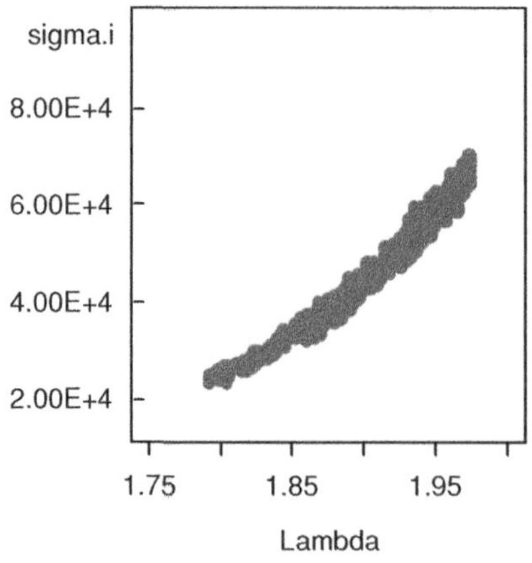

Figure 10.11 Dietary study: scatterplot of σ^k versus λ^k using WinBUGS.

correction term is needed to bring them back to the original scale of the response. Let the corrected DIC value be $\text{DIC}(\lambda)$ then

$$\text{DIC}(\lambda) = \text{DIC}_\lambda - 2\sum_{i=1}^{n} \log|J_i(\lambda)| = \text{DIC}_\lambda - 2(\lambda - 1)\sum_{i=1}^{n} \log(y_i), \tag{10.34}$$

with $J_i(\lambda)$ is the Jacobian when transforming y_i to $y_i^{(\lambda)}$. In the next example, we have assumed a Box–Cox distribution for the response in the dietary study with the aim to estimate the parameter λ from the data.

Example X.24: Dietary study: Estimating the Box–Cox transformation of the response
From Example X.10, we know that the logarithmic scale for cholesterol intake is preferred over the original scale since $6909.666 = \text{DIC}(0) < \text{DIC}(1) = 6991.300$.

We applied both the zeros and the ones trick, but we got no convergence with WinBUGS (and OpenBUGS). Neither did the SAS Markov chain converge. The problem is the posterior correlation of σ (SD of the measurement error) and λ. In Figure 10.11, the scatterplot of σ^k, λ^k from one chain shows that there is a strong relation between σ^k and λ^k. This can be explained by the fact that when λ^k increases, the variability of the measurement error must also increase. However, a solution with WinBUGS or SAS does not seem easy. □

10.3.5.3 Generalizing the link function

For BGLMs, the commonly used link functions can be embedded into more general classes. For instance, the log-link $g(\mu) = \log(\mu)$ in the Poisson regression model is a special case of $g_\lambda(\mu) = (\mu^{(\lambda)} - 1)/\lambda$ for $\lambda = 0$. For the binary case, say logistic regression, we can think of two kinds of generalizations. First, since the inverse of the logistic link is in fact the cumulative logistic distribution, we can generalize the link function by considering other distributions and/or embedding the current cdf into a larger class of cdfs. Secondly, we could embed the logistic link function into a family of link functions, say $g_\lambda(\pi) = \frac{1}{\lambda}\{[\pi/(1-\pi)]^\lambda - 1\}$

(Guerrero and Johnson 1982). Note that now there is no need to adjust the different DIC$_\lambda$-values.

10.3.5.4 Relaxing the linearity assumption

To allow for a nonlinear effect of the covariates polynomial and product terms can be introduced. One could also apply the Box–Cox transformation to some of the covariates. This is known in the literature as the Box–Tidwell transformation (Box and Tidwell 1962). Royston and Altman (1994) suggested *fractional polynomials* to discover the correct scale of a covariate x. A *fractional polynomial of degree m* in covariate x is a function $\phi_m(x, \boldsymbol{\alpha}, \lambda) = \alpha_0 + \alpha_1 x^\lambda + \sum_{j=2}^m \alpha_j x^\lambda [\log(x)]^{j-1}$, whereby the parameters $\alpha_0, \ldots, \alpha_m$ are estimated from the data. This is typically done for all candidate covariates. The model is gradually made more complex by subsequently replacing each original covariate x_j by its fractional polynomial and estimating its coefficients. An even more general approach to relax the linearity assumption in the systematic component of the model is *smoothing* or *nonparametric function estimation*. Smoothing is a well-established tool for exploratory data analysis and is treated comprehensively in Green and Silverman (1994), Ruppert *et al.* (2003) and Lee *et al.* (2006, pp. 267–291). For a quick introduction to smoothing and its relationship with mixed modeling (see expression (10.37) and paragraph below it; Gurrin *et al.* (2005)). We first look here at the classical approach.

To fix ideas, take the linear regression model introduced in Section 5.6.1 with one regressor x:

$$y_i = \beta_0 + \beta_1 x_i + \varepsilon_i,\ (i = 1, \ldots, n).$$

Smoothing the relationship implies replacing the linear relationship by

$$y_i = m(x_i) + \varepsilon_i,\ (i = 1, \ldots, n), \tag{10.35}$$

where $m(x)$ is an arbitrary smooth function. The smooth function is often modeled in practice using *splines*. There exists a variety of splines, we consider here two types: (a) splines based on truncated polynomials, and (b) B-splines. For the first type, the smooth function is a piecewise polynomial of degree d, namely,

$$m(x; \boldsymbol{\beta}, \boldsymbol{b}) = \beta_0 + \beta_1 x + \ldots + \beta_p x^d + \sum_{k=1}^{K} b_k (x - \kappa_k)_+^d,$$

where $c_+ = c$ if $c > 0$ and zero otherwise, $c_+^d = (c_+)^d$; $\boldsymbol{\beta} = (\beta_0, \ldots, \beta_d)^T$ and $\boldsymbol{b} = (b_1, \ldots, b_K)^T$ are vectors of regression coefficients. Expression (10.35) is called the *low-rank thin-plate spline representation* of $m(x)$. The function $m(x; \boldsymbol{\beta}, \boldsymbol{b})$ is constructed on an interval $[a, b]$ covering the range of x values and is split up into line segments at *(inner) knots* κ_k, i.e. $(a <)\kappa_1 < \kappa_2 < \ldots < \kappa_K (< b)$. The knots are often taken equidistant with $K \ll n$ or at the $k/(K+1)$ quantiles of the x-values. Note that $m(x; \boldsymbol{\beta}, \boldsymbol{b})$ has $(d-1)$ continuous derivatives. The functions $1, x, \ldots, x^d, (x - \kappa_1)_+^d, \ldots, (x - \kappa_K)_+^d$ are called the *basis functions*. Popular choices for d are 2 (quadratic splines) and 3 (cubic splines). One might also assume a different order for the polynomial and the truncated polynomial part. Simply estimating all coefficients $\boldsymbol{\beta}$ and $\boldsymbol{b}$, say by maximum likelihood, would yield a too wiggly estimated function $\widehat{m}(x; \boldsymbol{\beta}, \boldsymbol{b})$. A standard approach to control the smoothness of $m(x; \boldsymbol{\beta}, \boldsymbol{b})$ is to restrict the coefficients $b_1, \ldots, b_K$ since they represent changes in the gradient between consecutive line segments $[\kappa_{(k-1)}, \kappa_k]$. This can be done by minimizing the penalized least squares

$$\frac{1}{\sigma_\varepsilon^2}\sum_{i=1}^{n}[y_i - m(x_i; \boldsymbol{\beta}, \boldsymbol{b})]^2 + \frac{\lambda}{\sigma_\varepsilon^2}\boldsymbol{b}^T \mathrm{D}\boldsymbol{b} \tag{10.36}$$

with respect to all parameters. In expression (10.36), we assume that the term σ_ε^2 is fixed, its usefulness becomes clear below. The matrix D describes the penalty. A ridge penalty is obtained for $\mathrm{D} = \mathrm{diag}(1, \ldots, 1)$, but also other penalties are used. If $\lambda = 0$ then there is no smoothing, producing a possibly wiggly function while for $\lambda \to \infty$ the solution is a polynomial of degree $(d-1)$, which is the smoothest solution. The estimation procedure depends on λ. To find the optimal λ, one could choose different fixed values of λ and choose the one that gives the lowest AIC or the one that provides the best prediction of the responses evaluated by cross-validation. However, there is a more elegant procedure which uses the connection between smoothing and mixed models. Let $\boldsymbol{y} = (y_1, \ldots, y_n)^T$, $\boldsymbol{x}^s = (x_1^s, \ldots, x_n^s)^T$ for $(s = 1, \ldots, d)$, $\mathbf{1}$ the vector of 1's, $\boldsymbol{\varepsilon} = (\varepsilon_1, \ldots, \varepsilon_n)^T$, $\boldsymbol{X} = (\mathbf{1}, \boldsymbol{x}^1, \ldots, \boldsymbol{x}^p)$ (with p possibly different from d) and $\boldsymbol{Z} = ((\boldsymbol{x} - \kappa_1\mathbf{1})_+^d, \ldots, (\boldsymbol{x} - \kappa_K\mathbf{1})_+^d)$, then model $y_i = m(x_i; \boldsymbol{\beta}, \boldsymbol{b}) + \varepsilon_i$, $(i = 1, \ldots, n)$ can be rewritten as

$$\boldsymbol{y} = \boldsymbol{X}\boldsymbol{\beta} + \boldsymbol{Z}\boldsymbol{b} + \boldsymbol{\varepsilon}. \tag{10.37}$$

The formal equivalence between a mixed model and smoothing is obtained by interpreting (10.36) as the log-likelihood of a mixed model whereby $\boldsymbol{b} \sim \mathrm{N}(\mathbf{0}, \frac{\sigma_\varepsilon^2}{\lambda}\mathrm{D}^{-1})$. For a ridge penalty $b_k \sim \mathrm{N}(0, \sigma_b^2)$ $(k = 1, \ldots, K)$ with $\sigma_b^2 \equiv \sigma_\varepsilon^2/\lambda$, and hence we obtain a classical linear mixed model. For other choices of D a reparameterization delivers again a linear mixed model (see Example X.25). The advantage of reformulating smoothing is that mixed model software can be used and that the 'best' λ can be obtained from (RE)ML. Gurrin *et al.* (2005) provide an interesting alternative explanation why the b_k should be regarded as random rather than fixed to obtain a smooth curve. Namely, the estimated b_k are BLUPs which are known to shrink to zero and therefore show less variability.

In Section 5.7, we have established the analogy between ridge regression and a Bayesian normal linear regression analysis with a normal prior. In the same way, we may link the mixed model here to a Bayesian model whereby in model (10.37) $\boldsymbol{b}$ is given the normal prior $\mathrm{N}(\mathbf{0}, \frac{\sigma_\varepsilon^2}{\lambda}\mathrm{D}^{-1})$ and the other parameters have classical vague priors. We can then employ MCMC techniques (especially for complex smoothing exercises) to estimate all parameters. In the next example, we verify the linearity assumption in the osteoporosis data set.

Example X.25: Osteoporosis study: Smoothing the relationship of TBBMC with BMI using cubic splines

We wish to verify whether the linear regression model assumed in Example IV.7 is appropriate. In 'chapter 10 osteo study thin plate.R', we looked for the smooth relationship between BMI and TBBMC. For this, we adapted the WinBUGS program developed by Crainiceanu *et al.* (2005). Here we assume $m(x; \boldsymbol{\beta}, \boldsymbol{b}) = \beta_0 + \beta_1 x + \sum_{k=1}^K b_k(x - \kappa_k)_+^3$. The (r, s)th entry of the penalty matrix is $(\mathrm{D})_{r,s} = |\kappa_r - \kappa_s|^3$. With the reparameterization $\boldsymbol{b}^* = \mathrm{D}^{1/2}\boldsymbol{b}$ and $\boldsymbol{Z}^* = \boldsymbol{Z}\mathrm{D}^{-1/2}$ a classical linear mixed model is obtained. Twenty knots were chosen so that each segment contains roughly $100 \times (1/21)\%$ of the data. Further details on the program

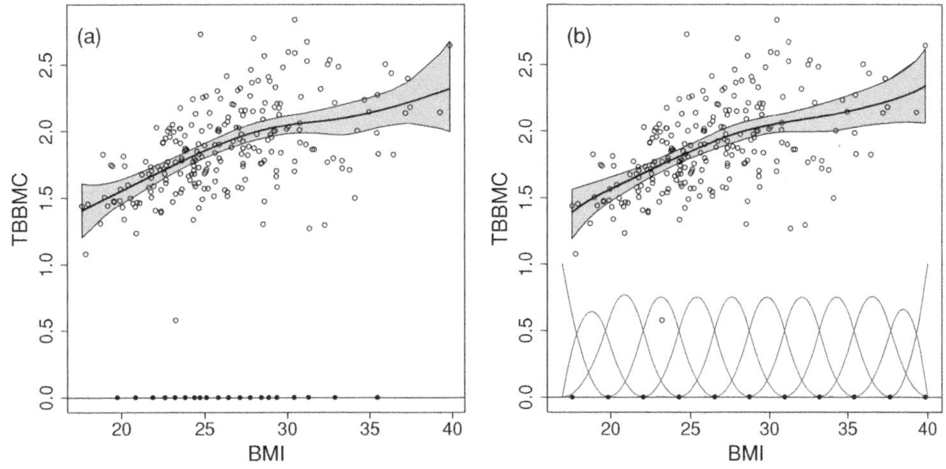

Figure 10.12 Osteoporosis study: smoothing the TBBMC–BMI relationship using (a) a Bayesian truncated cubic splines approach with 20 knots, (b) a Bayesian B-splines approach with ten inner knots and penalization. The thick line represents the posterior mean of $m(x)$ and the boundary lines represent the corresponding 95% pointwise equal-tail CIs. The circles at the bottom indicate the positions of the knots.

settings (number of iterations, burn-in part, number of chains, etc.) can be found in the R program. The large posterior median for the penalty parameter of $\lambda = 5799$ explains the minimal curvature of the smooth curve in Figure 10.12(a). We conclude that the relationship between BMI and TBBMC is approximately linear. The effective degrees of freedom of the smoothing model was estimated as $p_D = 5.96$ with DIC $= 78.3$. □

Another popular choice for spline smoothing makes use of *B-splines*. The B-spline representation of the smooth function $m(x)$ is

$$m(x; \boldsymbol{b}, r) = \sum_{q=1}^{Q} b_q B_q(x; r),$$

where the basis functions $B_q(x; r)$ are called *B-splines of degree r* which are piecewise polynomials of degree r on (most often) equidistant knots covering the range of the data. That is, a B-spline of degree 1 consists of linear functions that change at the knots, a B-spline of degree 2 consists of quadratic functions, a B-spline of degree 3 consists of cubic functions, etc. Note that the number of knots and the degree of the B-spline are related. The mathematical description of the B-spline is somewhat complicated, we therefore refer to de Boor (1978) for technical details. For a graphical depiction of cubic B-splines (degree $= 3$) (see Figure 10.12(b)). Smoothing with B-splines can be done by taking Q low without penalizing the regression coefficients b_q. Instead, Eilers and Marx (1996) suggested to take a large number of equidistant knots and to put a difference penalty on the b_q based on rth order differences. This is called the *P-splines approach*. For example, a first-order difference in the regression coefficients is $\Delta_q = b_q - b_{q-1}$; a second-order difference is given by $\Delta_q^2 \equiv \Delta_q - \Delta_{q-1} = b_q - 2b_{q-1} - b_{q-2}$. The idea is to penalize large values of these sth-order differences. That is, for the simple regression model, we minimize

$$\frac{1}{\sigma_\varepsilon^2}\sum_{i=1}^{n}[y_i - m(x_i; \boldsymbol{b}, r)]^2 + \frac{\lambda}{\sigma_\varepsilon^2}\boldsymbol{b}^T \mathrm{D}_s \boldsymbol{b}, \tag{10.38}$$

with now D_s a positive semidefinite matrix expressing the sth-order differences. Expression (10.38) is again recognized as the log-likelihood of a mixed model, i.e. $\boldsymbol{y} = \boldsymbol{Zb} + \boldsymbol{\varepsilon}$ (now there is no $\boldsymbol{X}$ part) and $\boldsymbol{b}$ having a normal distribution with mean zero and precision matrix $\sigma_b^{-2}\mathrm{D}_s$ and the smoothing parameter $\lambda = \sigma_\varepsilon^2/\sigma_b^2$. The optimal number λ is then determined from the estimates of the variance parameters.

The Bayesian version of B-splines and P-splines smoothing is obtained in analogy with cubic splines smoothing. In the next example, we applied both smoothing procedures on the osteoporosis data.

Example X.26: Osteoporosis study: Smoothing the relationship of TBBMC with BMI using B-splines
In 'chapter 10 osteo study B-splines.R' details can be found about the program settings for B-spline and P-spline smoothing both of degree 3. For B-spline smoothing with five inner knots, the relationship between TBBMC and BMI was linear up to BMI = 30 whereafter the curve bends. The effective degrees of freedom of the smoothing model was estimated as $p_D = 9.02$ with DIC = 80.7. P-spline smoothing with ten inner knots and second-order penalization produced Figure 10.12(b) which is quite similar as Figure 10.12(a). Now $\lambda = 35.1$ and the effective degrees of freedom were estimated as $p_D = 5.8$ with DIC = 77.6. Thus, the two penalization approaches produced basically the same smoothed models. □

The nonparametric regression model (10.35) has been extended in various ways. For the *semiparametric regression model* the response is related to several covariates, some in a linear manner and others in a smooth way. The extension of a generalized linear model (see Section 4.8) to include smooth functions of covariates was introduced by Hastie and Tibshirani (1986) and is called a *generalized linear additive model* (*GLAM*). More specifically, for a GLAM the linear predictor $g(\mu) = \eta = \beta_0 + \sum_{j=1}^{d}\beta_j x_j$ in model (4.33) is replaced by $g(\mu) = \eta = \beta_0 + \sum_{j=1}^{d}\beta_j m_j(x_j)$, with $m_j(x_j)$ smooth functions of x_j. Crainiceanu *et al.* (2004) further extended the GLAM by allowing the variance parameter to depend on covariates in a smooth manner. Smoothing can also be applied to hierarchical models. For instance, Crainiceanu *et al.* (2005) exemplified the use of a Bayesian longitudinal model whereby smoothing was applied to the overall curve as a function of time (fixed effect) and on the individual curves (random effects). Kooperberg *et al.* (1995) suggested to smooth the baseline hazard function in semiparametric survival models. Sharef *et al.* (2010) proposed to apply smoothing in mixed effects survival models, called frailty models. They smoothed the baseline hazard function as well as the frailty distribution in a frailty Cox proportional hazards model. Komárek and Lesaffre (2008) applied smoothing in a highly dimensional survival problem with interval-censored responses. Furthermore, the P-splines approach of Eilers and Marx (1996) was extended by Lang and Brezger (2004) to spatial models who also developed the Bayesian R package *BayesX* (`http://www.stat.uni-muenchen.de/~bayesx/bayesx.html`) for this purpose. This is not the end of the story. Indeed, smoothing has been and is still a very active area of research tackling increasingly complex problems.

In next example, we illustrate cubic-spline smoothing on a generalized linear mixed model.

Example X.27: Dietary study: Cubic-spline smoothing in a logistic random effects model There was interest in exploring the relationship of alcohol consumption with age, gender, length and weight. In addition, the subsidiary (eight subsidiaries) was given a normal random distribution. Preliminary data exploration hinted to a possible nonlinear relationship on the logit scale between the probability of alcohol consumption (p_A) and age. To verify this nonlinear relationship, the following model was fit with WinBUGS:

$$\text{logit}(p_{A_{ij}}) = \beta_0 + \beta_1 \text{age}_{ij} + \beta_2 \text{male}_{ij} + \beta_3 \text{length}_{ij} + \beta_4 \text{weight}_{ij} + \sum_{k=1}^{10} b_k(\text{age}_{ij} - \kappa_k)_+^3 + b_{\text{sub}_i},$$

with $j = 1, \ldots, n_i; i = 1, \ldots, 8$. The ten knots $\kappa_k (k = 1, \ldots, 10)$ were based on the quantiles of age. The random intercept $b_{\text{sub}_i} \sim \text{N}(0, \sigma^2_{\text{sub}})$ represents the subsidiary effect. As above, we assume $b_k \sim \text{N}(0, \sigma_b^2)$. The R2WinBUGS program that performs the Bayesian smoothing analysis can be found in 'chapter 10 dietary study cubic-splines.R'.

In the linear model ($p_D = 7.7$ and DIC $= 642.9$) significantly more males consumed alcohol, but none of the other covariates have a significant impact. In the next step, we smoothed the impact of age. In Figure 10.13(a), we plotted the smooth component of age versus age. There appears to be a slight quadratic effect in age, however, with wide confidence bands. Again gender was the only significant covariate and for this model: $p_D = 10.2$ and DIC $= 641.7$. Thus smoothing was no significantly improvement over the linear model. In Figure 10.13(b), we show the logit of the (posterior means of) predicted probabilities for alcohol consumption versus age. □

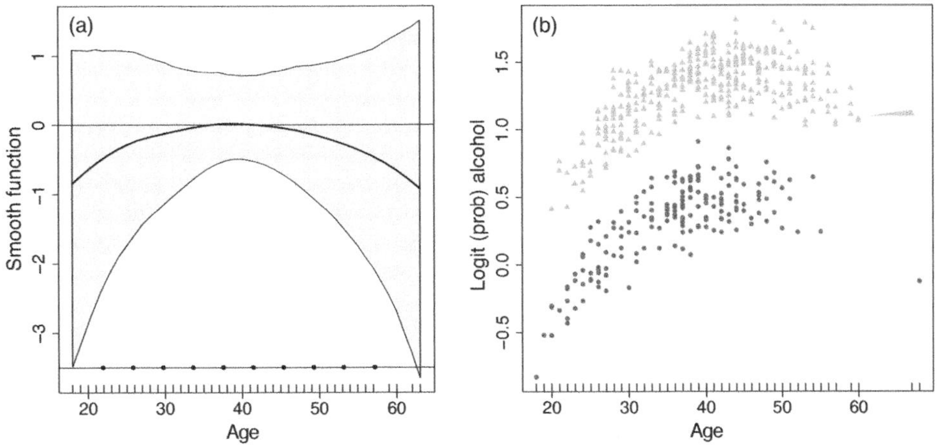

Figure 10.13 Dietary study: smoothing the relationship of logit(p_A) and age using cubic spline smoothing: (a) display of $\sum_{k=1}^{10} \widehat{b_k}(\text{age}_{ij} - \kappa_k)_+^3$ versus age and 95% pointwise equal-tail CIs, with $\widehat{b_k}$ the posterior mean of b_k. The circles at the bottom indicate the positions of the knots and (b) predicted probabilities of alcohol consumption, circles correspond to women and triangles to men.

In this section, we aimed to relax the assumptions in parametric Bayesian models. Note that models fit with WinBUGS are basically all parametric. Bayesian models with a nonparametric flavor, called *nonparametric Bayesian methods*, are beyond the scope of this book. In Chapter 17, some key references are given.

10.4 Closing remarks

In this chapter, we reviewed Bayesian exploratory techniques. In fact, we looked at the Bayesian toolbox for model building and model assessment. We do have to admit that some of these procedures are still too time consuming for reasonably sized problems. In addition, despite the existence of flexible Bayesian software such as WinBUGS, Bayesian software for diagnostic model tests is scattered around. A versatile software package with Bayesian routines for model checking would, therefore, be welcome.

Exercises

Exercise 10.1 Example X.8: Perform the longitudinal analyses using 'chapter 10 PotthoffRoy growthcurves.odc'. Run also the extra analyses in this program. Further, since normality of the random effects seems reasonable combine a bivariate normal distribution for $\boldsymbol{b}_i$ with various distributions for the measurement error. Evaluate the models with p_D and DIC. Report your final choice of the model.

Exercise 10.2 Example X.8: Assume in model M_1 three choices for the inverse Wishart prior IW(D, 2) for G the covariance matrix of the random effects, varying by the choice of D: (a) $\text{D} = \text{diag}(0.001, 0.001)$, (b) $\text{D} = \begin{pmatrix} 2 & -0.1 \\ -0.1 & 0.02 \end{pmatrix}$ and (c) $\text{D} = \text{diag}(100, 100)$. Evaluate the rate of convergence of the three Gibbs samplers and compare their posterior estimates with those obtained from a frequentist analysis using the SAS procedure MIXED. Use 'chapter 10 Pothoff-Roy growthcurves.odc'. What is your conclusion?

Exercise 10.3 Example X.8: Assume in model M_1 that (a) variances for random effects grow to infinity or (b) variances for random effects grow to zero. This can be done by fixing the respective variances in the WinBUGS to (a) large or (b) small values. Evaluate the models with p_D and DIC. How much evidence is there for the two extreme cases? How do you interpret these two extreme cases?

Exercise 10.4 Example X.8: Write a SAS program based on procedure MCMC to obtain parameter estimates for models M_1 to M_7. Procedure MIXED allows for a Bayesian mixed analysis. Check when this procedure can be used and compare the output with that of procedure MCMC.

Exercise 10.5 In 'chapter 10 dmft scores full data set.odc' a Poisson-gamma and a negative binomial distribution are fit to the dmft index of the 4352 seven-year-old children of the Signal-Tandmobiel study. In the negative binomial model the logical nodes 'alpha' and 'beta' are created to show the link with the Poisson-gamma model. Verify this correspondence by making use of formula (3.15) and the WinBUGS Manual. Verify that p_D and DIC differ considerably between the negative binomial and the Poisson-gamma model.

Exercise 10.6 Assume in Example X.10 alternative distributions for θ and choose the best model in combination with a normal distribution for *chol* or log(*chol*) using DIC.

Exercise 10.7 Evaluate which of the four models in 'chapter 10 Poisson models on dmft scores.odc': (1) Poisson model, (2) Poisson-gamma model, (3) zero-inflated Poisson model and (4) mixture of four Poisson models, fits best the dmft scores. Note that WinBUGS does not support p_D and DIC for models (3) and (4).

Exercise 10.8 Based on the data in Exercise 10.7 and using DIC, select the best fitting model from the following list: (1) Poisson model, (2) negative binomial model, (3) Poisson-gamma, (4) Poisson-lognormal, and (5) Poisson-log-logistic.

Exercise 10.9 Choosing a prior distribution in Exercise 10.7 for the Poisson model which is in conflict with the data and observe the change in p_D and DIC.

Exercise 10.10 Example X.11: Suppose that $\psi = 1/\theta^{\alpha}$ with $\alpha > 0$. Show that the prior of ψ is Pareto(α, 1) if the prior for θ is uniform on [0, 1]. Observe the change in p_D and DIC when α is increasing from 1 to 5.

Exercise 10.11 Example X.13: Verify that the posterior of the raw residuals is indeed a t_{n-d-1}-distribution. Produce also a similar (and additional) graph as Figure 10.3.

Exercise 10.12 In 'chapter 10 caries with residuals.odc' a logistic regression model is fitted to the CE data of the Signal-Tandmobiel study of Example VI.9 with some additional covariates, i.e. gender of the child (1 = girl), age of the child, whether or not the child takes sweets to the school and whether or not the children frequently brushed their teeth. Apply the program and use the option **Compare** to produce various plots based on ε_i. Are there outliers? Do the plots indicate a special pattern of the residuals?

Exercise 10.13 In 'chapter 10 caries with residuals.R' the dmft index is fitted with a Poisson regression model using R2WinBUGS. Use the approach of Exercise 10.12 to find outliers, if any.

Exercise 10.14 In 'chapter 10 osteo study-outliers.R' PPO_i and CPO_i are computed for the linear regression applied to the osteoporosis data. Apply this program. In addition, compare $\widehat{\text{PPO}}_{179}$ based on effectively removing subject 179 and $\widehat{\text{CPO}}_{179}$.

Exercise 10.15 Example X.13: Perform the various Bayesian residual analyses by making use of the SAS procedure GENMOD.

Exercise 10.16 Example X.15: Perform the various Bayesian residual analyses by making use of the SAS procedure GENMOD.

Exercise 10.17 Example X.16: Use 'chapter 10 lip cancer with residuals.R' and reproduce Figure 10.5. Verify whether the graphs change with a log-*t* regression model.

Exercise 10.18 Example IX.18: Assess the impact of varying the prior of the measurement error variance (σ^2) and the variance of the random intercept (σ_b^2) in ϕ_{2i} to (1) $\sigma^2 \sim \text{IG}(10^{-3}, 10^{-3})$, $\sigma_b^2 \sim \text{IG}(10^{-3}, 10^{-3})$, (2) $\sigma^2 \sim \text{IG}(10^{-3}, 10^{-3})$, $\sigma_b \sim \text{U}(0,10)$, (3) $\sigma^2 \sim \text{IG}(10^{-3}, 10^{-3})$, $1/\sigma_b \sim \text{U}(0,10)$.

Exercise 10.19 Example IX.18: Assess the impact of varying the distribution of the measurement error. Consider a t-distribution, a logistic distribution, etc. compare these models to the basic model of Example IX.18. Use R2WinBUGS.

Exercise 10.20 Show that the caterpillar option in WinBUGS can be used to construct a normal probability plot and apply it to the osteoporosis data set.

Exercise 10.21 Example X.8: Perform a sensitivity analysis on the seven models. More specifically, evaluate the effect of varying the distributions of the random effects and measurement error on the parameter estimates. Look also for influential observations and subjects.

Exercise 10.22 Example X.19: Test the normality assumption with the Shapiro–Francia test (Shapiro and Francia 1972), which consists of computing the Pearson correlation coefficients between the ordered values and the expected order statistics from a standard normal distribution. Produce also a Q–Q plot of the posterior means of the residuals versus the posterior means of the simulated residuals.

Exercise 10.23 Exercise 10.12: In 'chapter 10 caries with residuals.odc' also a Poisson model is fitted to the dmft indices. Apply a PPC with the χ^2-discrepancy measure to check the Poisson assumption.

Exercise 10.24 Example X.20: In 'chapter 10 lip cancer PGM PPC theta.odc' the gamma assumption of the θs is checked using a variety of measures. Use R2WinBUGS.

Exercise 10.25 Example X.18: Verify the normality assumption for the measurement error and the random effects in each of the two groups using a PPC.

Exercise 10.26 Example X.22: Check the choice of the logistic-link function in the toenail data set using WinBUGS.

Exercise 10.27 Example X.25: Check the linearity of the regression model of TBBMC as a function of age with or without assuming linearity in BMI. Apply both the B-splines as well as the cubic splines approach.

Exercise 10.28 Example X.27: Check the linearity of length, weight and age in predicting the probability of alcohol (consumption) using the B-splines as well as the cubic splines approach.

11

Variable selection

11.1 Introduction

This chapter reviews Bayesian variable selection techniques, also called (Bayesian) *subset selection techniques*, in observational studies. In explorative research, one looks for the explanation or prediction of a response using explanatory variables. When the aim is to 'explain' the response, we search for the real but unknown relationship between the response and the covariates. For a good understanding of the relationship, it is then important to select only those covariates that matter. When prediction is the aim, the actual choice of the covariates is of less interest as long as the fit to the data is good. But, also in this case selecting only the important covariates pays off in terms of prediction error (on future data). Variable selection is, indeed, in practice a standard first step especially when the number of candidate variables is large compared to the size of the study. When the sample size is much larger than the number of predictors, then it might sometimes be better not to select variables at all but to work with the full model (Draper 1999).

Formally, variable selection in a normal linear regression context is the exercise to prune the model

$$y_i = \alpha + \sum_{k=1}^{d} \beta_k x_{ki} + \varepsilon_i, \ \ (i = 1, \ldots, n), \tag{11.1}$$

by removing the regression coefficients β_k equal to zero. In matrix notation, the linear regression model is

$$\boldsymbol{y} = \mathbf{1}_n \alpha + \boldsymbol{X}\boldsymbol{\beta} + \boldsymbol{\varepsilon}, \tag{11.2}$$

with $\boldsymbol{y}$ the stacked response vector, $\mathbf{1}_n$ the $n \times 1$ vector of ones, $\boldsymbol{X}$ the $n \times d$ full rank design matrix and $\boldsymbol{\varepsilon} \sim \mathrm{N}(\mathbf{0}, \sigma^2\mathrm{I})$ the $n \times 1$ vector of error terms. In expression (11.2), the intercept α is separated from the other regressors. This reflects the classical approach to variable selection which is to fix the intercept in the model and to focus on the real regressors. Though, some

Bayesian Biostatistics, First Edition. Emmanuel Lesaffre and Andrew B. Lawson.

Bayesian variable selection algorithms are based on the entire vector of regression coefficients. In that case, we work with $\boldsymbol{\beta}^* = (\alpha, \boldsymbol{\beta}^T)^T$ and $\boldsymbol{X}^* = (\mathbf{1}_n, \boldsymbol{X})$. In addition, it is customary to standardize the covariates to have mean zero and norm one. In this way, the intercept is common to all models and $\boldsymbol{X}^T\boldsymbol{X}$ becomes the empirical correlation matrix.

Variable selection involves the exploration of submodels. Let $\boldsymbol{\gamma}$ be the $d \times 1$ indicator vector with kth element $\gamma_k = 0$ if $\beta_k = 0$ and $\gamma_k = 1$ if $\beta_k \neq 0$ and let $d_\gamma = \sum_{k=1}^{d} \gamma_k$. Further, let $\boldsymbol{\beta}_\gamma$ be the d_γ-dimensional subvector of $\boldsymbol{\beta}$ corresponding to $\gamma_k \neq 0$ $(k = 1, \ldots, d)$ and $\boldsymbol{X}_\gamma$ the corresponding design matrix. Let also $\boldsymbol{\beta}^*_\gamma = (\alpha, \boldsymbol{\beta}^T_\gamma)^T$ and $\boldsymbol{X}^*_\gamma = (\mathbf{1}_n, \boldsymbol{X}_\gamma)$. The normal linear regression model M_γ is then given by $\boldsymbol{y} = \mathbf{1}_n\alpha + \boldsymbol{X}_\gamma\boldsymbol{\beta}_\gamma + \boldsymbol{\varepsilon}$. For $\boldsymbol{\gamma} = \mathbf{0}$, the intercept model is obtained. Denote the number of different $\boldsymbol{\gamma}$s by K, then with d regressors $K = 2^d$. Clearly, K becomes quickly large, e.g. with $d = 15$ $K = 32\,768$ candidate models should be evaluated. In explorative research, it is not uncommon to have a few hundred regressors. In genome wide association (GWA) studies, even 2.5 million SNPs need to be explored for their relationship with phenotypes. Efficient search algorithms are, therefore, needed to explore all possible models or at least the most promising ones. This leads to automated variable selection techniques. For the final model, one might also need to consider interaction terms of the original regressors, look for transformations of the response and/or the covariates, check the distribution of the measurement error, etc. All of this adds to the complexity of the problem. In addition, a definition of 'promising' is needed, which means that we need an appropriate criterion that judges the quality of the visited models.

Automated variable selection procedures have received a lot of criticism and many statisticians prefer to build the statistical model that agrees with theory and data, thereby interacting intensively with the clinical researcher (Gelman and Rubin 1995). This is often possible with a limited number of covariates, but in clinical research, there are usually too many explanatory variables that can determine a response without a clear insight of which covariates should be excluded a priori. That is, in clinical research there is often an abundance of data but not often a clear theory behind the data. An initial selection is then still required.

In this chapter, we review not only the Bayesian approach to variable selection but also model selection will be considered. Selection will be based on the criteria introduced in Chapter 10. We start with a brief review of the classical approaches to variable selection since the issues encountered there are also relevant for the Bayesian case. Bayesian model selection, but especially subset selection techniques, have seen an explosion of developments over the last two decades with a significant impetus coming from genetic research. In the subsequent sections, various Bayesian strategies for subset selection are reviewed, focusing on the intuitive ideas behind the approaches rather than on mathematical derivations. Note that, throughout this chapter, we assume that there are no missing values in the covariate structure.

11.2 Classical variable selection

A sketch of the variable selection approaches developed in the classical/frequentist paradigm is given. Only normal linear regression will be treated in this review.

11.2.1 Variable selection techniques

'Variable selection' often means 'automated' variable selection. That is, a computational procedure searches through the K models for those models M_γ that exhibit a good performance, e.g. predictive ability. Well-known and still often used automated selection procedures are: forward, backward, stepwise and all subsets selection procedures. Besides F-values or P-values, other criteria can be used for subset selection such as the mean-squared error (MSE) for prediction which leads to Mallows statistic C_p and the PRESS residual. Alternatively, one could use the likelihood or likelihood-based criteria such as Akaike's Information Criterion (AIC) and Bayesian Information Criterion (BIC).

We illustrate the classical procedures on the well-known diabetes data set used in Efron *et al.* (2004), and make use of the SAS® software.

Example XI.1: Diabetes study: Classical automated selection techniques
Efron *et al.* (2004) analyzed a diabetes data set to illustrate the performance of shrunken regression estimators. This data set has been analyzed by many others afterward. In this study, 442 diabetes patients were measured on ten baseline variables: age, gender (0 = female, 1 = male), BMI, blood pressure (bp) and six serum measurements indicated as $s1$, $s2$, ..., $s6$. The question was how they relate with a measure of disease progression 1 year after baseline (response y). It was hoped that the selected model would produce accurate baseline predictions of the response for future patients and that the expression of the model would suggest which covariates are important for disease progression. Note that prior to variable selection the regressors but not the response were standardized.

In Table 11.1, we report the outcome of several regression analyses performed with the SAS procedure REG. The first analysis is based on all baseline variables, and hence no selection was applied. This model has an R^2 equal to 0.52 and an adjusted R^2 (R_a^2) equal to 0.51. Some fairly large variance inflation factors (VIFs) indicate moderate dependencies between some of the covariates producing correlation coefficients between 0.09 and 0.74.

Table 11.1 Diabetes study: estimates (SE) of regression coefficients.

Cov	LSE	(SE)	VIF	FW/BW/SW	RI	BRI	LA	BLA
int	152.13	(2.6)	0	152.13	152.13	152.13	152.13	152.13
age	−0.48	(2.9)	1.22		−0.17	−0.23		−0.11
gender	−11.42	(2.9)	1.28	−10.68	−10.79	−10.75	−9.42	−9.96
BMI	24.75	(3.2)	1.51	25.23	24.34	24.44	24.87	24.93
bp	15.44	(3.1)	1.46	15.58	14.93	15.00	14.15	14.44
$s1$	−37.72	(19.8)	59.20	−36.09	−7.69	−10.00	−4.95	−8.00
$s2$	22.70	(16.1)	39.19	25.65	−0.012	0.85		−0.14
$s3$	4.81	(10.1)	15.40		−7.94	−6.94	−10.66	−7.60
$s4$	8.43	(7.7)	8.89		5.43	5.68		4.46
$s5$	35.77	(8.2)	10.08	38.29	23.63	24.65	24.51	24.52
$s6$	3.22	(3.1)	1.48		3.69	3.58	2.69	3.11

FW, forward selection; BW, backward selection; SW, stepwise selection; RI, Ridge regression; BRI, Bayesian ridge regression; LA, LASSO regression; BLA, Bayesian LASSO regression. VIF, variance inflation factor.
Note: The classical LSE solution is based on all baseline covariates and is computed with the SAS procedure REG. Automated variable selection is done at significance level 0.15 with the procedure REG as also ridge regression. The SAS procedure GLMSELECT was used for classical LASSO estimation, but the Bayesian ridge and LASSO estimates are based on the R package 'monomvn'.

In addition, we performed automated variable selection techniques: forward, backward and stepwise (all at significance level 0.15, but the same selection was obtained with 0.05). While most often the three selection strategies yield different solutions, here all three methods delivered the same model (see Table 11.1). The all-subsets-variable selection procedure with R_a^2 as criterion selected in the best model the variables gender, BMI, bp, $s1$, $s2$, $s4$, $s5$ and $s6$ with $R_a^2 = 0.51$. But about 20 different models have an almost equal R_a^2. The program can be found in 'chapter 11 CVS diabetes study.sas'. □

Subset selection procedures seek a trade off between bias and variance in order to minimize the MSE for prediction. However, they select models with a too optimistic fit to the data (Miller 2002, p. 147). The failure to control the overall (familywise) error rate with automated selection procedures is well known. With a large study, we can protect ourselves against a too optimistic model choice by splitting the data set into a training, a validation and a test set. In the training part, the models can be estimated, the decision to end the variable selection can be based on the validation part and the performance of the chosen model on new data is quantified in the test data set. Unfortunately, in practice, the size of the data sets rarely allows for this ideal procedure.

11.2.2 Frequentist regularization

A different approach to find a compromise between bias and variance is to shrink the individual regression coefficients. A well-known example of such an approach is *ridge regression*, discussed in Section 5.7. According to expression (5.37), the ridge regression estimator $\widehat{\boldsymbol{\beta}}^R(\boldsymbol{\lambda})$ of $\boldsymbol{\beta}$ is obtained by minimizing

$$(\boldsymbol{y}^* - \boldsymbol{X}\boldsymbol{\beta})^T(\boldsymbol{y}^* - \boldsymbol{X}\boldsymbol{\beta}) + \lambda \sum_{k=1}^{d} |\beta_k|^r, \tag{11.3}$$

with $r = 2$ involving the L_2-norm, $\boldsymbol{y}^* = \boldsymbol{y} - \overline{y}\mathbf{1}_n$ and $\lambda \geq 0$ a penalty parameter to control the 'size' of the regression coefficients. It follows that $\widehat{\boldsymbol{\beta}}^R(\lambda) = (\boldsymbol{X}^T\boldsymbol{X} + \lambda\mathrm{I})^{-1}\boldsymbol{X}^T\boldsymbol{y}$ and $\widehat{\alpha} = \overline{y}$ (because covariates are standardized). For $\lambda = 0$ the least-squares estimate (LSE) is obtained. That the ridge regression estimator is constrained in size follows from the fact that minimizing (11.3) is equivalent to minimizing

$$(\boldsymbol{y}^* - \boldsymbol{X}\boldsymbol{\beta})^T(\boldsymbol{y}^* - \boldsymbol{X}\boldsymbol{\beta}), \quad \text{subject to } \sum_{k=1}^{d} |\beta_k|^r \leq t \tag{11.4}$$

with t inversely related to λ. For more background on ridge regression; see Section 3.4 in Hastie *et al.* (2009). In general, ridge regression decreases the MSE in estimating the regression coefficients and has good prediction properties.

Another shrinkage method was suggested by Tibshirani (1996) for simultaneous variable selection and estimation. The estimation method, called *LASSO (Least Absolute Shrinkage and Selection Operator) estimation*, is based on taking $r = 1$ in expressions (11.3) and (11.4) thereby replacing the L_2-norm by the L_1-norm. With increasing λ (decreasing t) the constraint in (11.4) becomes more restrictive and certain regression coefficients will be put effectively at zero. For λ large a 'sparse' model is obtained, which is the main motivation for using this approach. Note that for λ large enough, the LASSO technique also delivers estimators with a MSE for prediction smaller than the LSE estimators (Rosset and Zhu 2004).

The estimated regression coefficients depend on the choice of λ. A common strategy in ridge regression is to choose λ from the ridge trace (plot of λ versus $\widehat{\boldsymbol{\beta}}^R(\lambda)$) and the plot of VIF values. Then $\widehat{\lambda}$ can be taken as the smallest value of λ for which the regression coefficients become stable with a low value for the VIFs. This gives the ridge regression estimate $\widehat{\boldsymbol{\beta}}^R(\widehat{\lambda})$ for the regression coefficients. Alternatively, one could choose $\widehat{\lambda}$ that maximizes, say R^2 or BIC, while controlling the VIFs. In general, both regularization approaches produce a biased estimate of λ because of the double use of the data. Tibshirani (1996) suggested, therefore, to obtain the LASSO $\widehat{\lambda}$ from cross-validation (or generalized cross-validation). This renders the LASSO model selection *adaptive*.

Although both methods imply shrinkage of the regression coefficients, the L_2 penalty shrinks the regression coefficients uniformly, whereas the L_1 penalty implies a differential shrinkage and thereby puts some regression coefficients at zero especially for λ large. Computing standard errors of the parameter estimates might pose a problem in the classical approach. Because of computational difficulties, standard errors may not be available, but there is also no consensus on whether standard errors of biasedly estimated regression coefficients are useful (Kyung *et al.* 2010).

Both ridge and LASSO regression can be used to perform variable selection, but LASSO regression is definitely more popular for this job since it puts increasingly more regression coefficients at zero with increasing λ and thereby delivers a forward selection method.

Finally, we note that many variations of the basic LASSO approach have been proposed especially in the last decade. While these approaches can be applied beyond the linear model (e.g. generalized linear models (GLIMs) and survival models), most of these developments were theoretically investigated on the linear regression model. For a recent overview of frequentist and Bayesian LASSO approaches, we refer to Kyung *et al.* (2010). In Section 11.8.1, we treat the Bayesian LASSO approach. Now, we illustrate the two shrinkage methods with the diabetes example.

Example XI.2: Diabetes study: Shrunken regression estimates

With the SAS procedure REG, we performed ridge regression varying λ from 0 to 0.10 with steps of 0.002. Around $\lambda = 0.04$ the regression coefficients and VIFs stabilized (below 7 for all covariates) (see Figure 11.1). In Table 11.1, we see that the ridge regression coefficients are smaller in absolute value than the LSE estimates.

The recently released procedure GLMSELECT provides extensive variable selection facilities for linear models with a variety of selection strategies and selection criteria. The LASSO technique yields a forward selection technique with varying constraints t, but to select the best performing model, a criterion is needed. With BIC, the variables gender, BMI, bp, $s1$, $s3$, $s5$ and $s6$ were selected. As can be seen from Table 11.1, this model differs from the choice made by FW, BW and SW. In the same table it can be seen that often, but not always, the LASSO estimates are smaller in absolute value than the corresponding LSE estimates. In Figure 11.2, the LASSO variable selection procedure is summarized with curves that emanate at zero when the corresponding regressor is left out of the model. The vertical line indicates when BIC is maximal and indicates the selected model. □

GLMSELECT also offers cross-validation to evaluate the selection procedure, as well as estimating the selection procedure on a training set and evaluating it on a validation

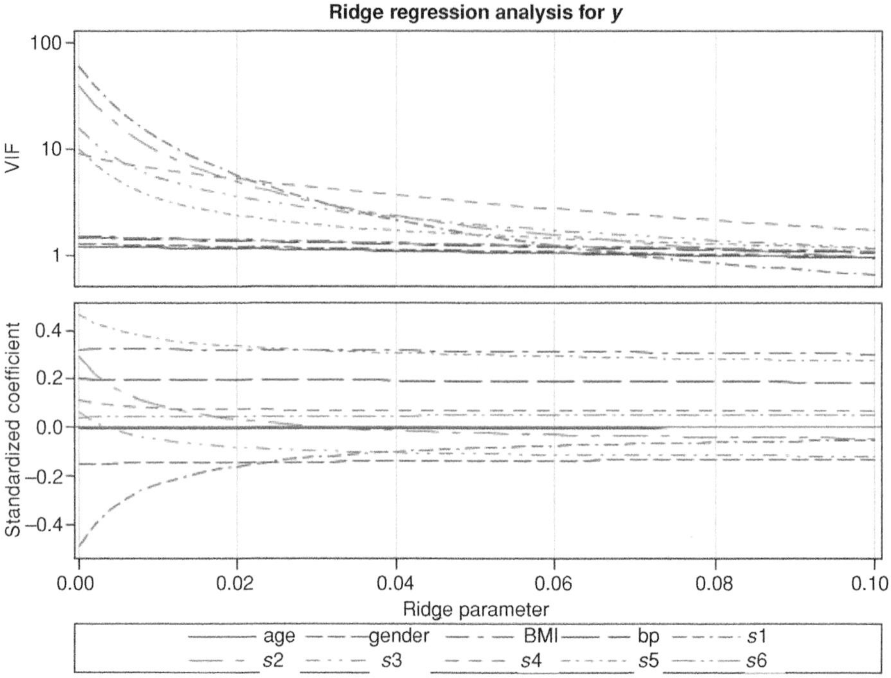

Figure 11.1 Diabetes study: ridge trace in VIF and standardized coefficients (output from SAS procedure REG) as a function of λ.

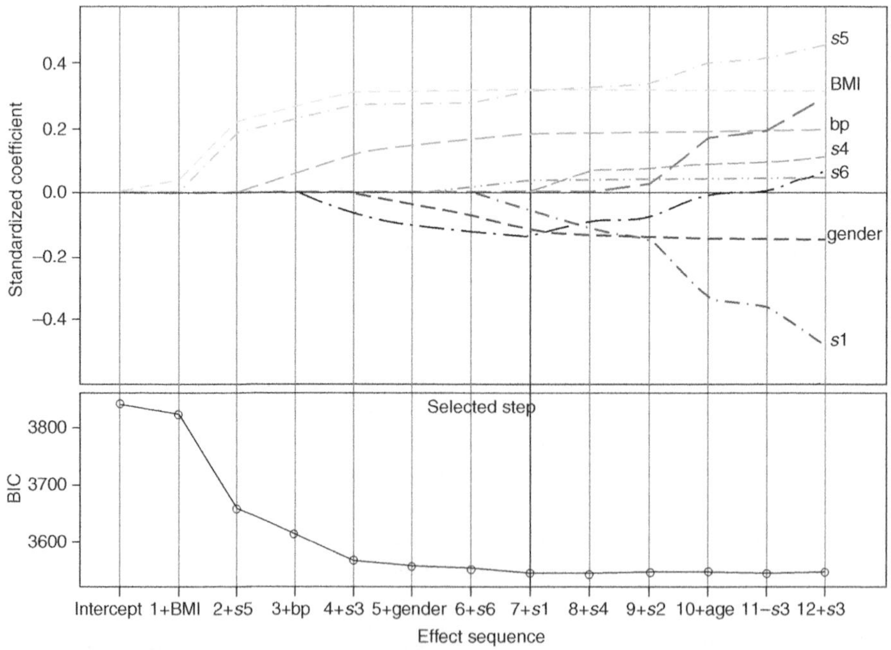

Figure 11.2 Diabetes study: coefficient plot and BIC determined by LASSO estimation as a function of t (output SAS procedure GLMSELECT).

and test set. On the other hand, the R software offers a rich scala of procedures to perform regularized estimation for various regression models (see the R packages `lars`, `penalized` and `monomvn`).

11.3 Bayesian variable selection: Concepts and questions

The last 20 years have seen an explosion of approaches for Bayesian variable selection (BVS). A review of the classical and BVS methods up to 2000 can be found in George (2000) and Miller (2002).

In this section, we focus on the principles of BVS techniques. Here, we are only interested in selecting variables, but we keep in mind that selecting the best model may also involve changing other aspects of the model. For sure, we apply selection techniques when we are uncertain about the statistical model itself.

Let the K models be indexed by $\boldsymbol{\gamma}_1, \ldots, \boldsymbol{\gamma}_K$. The vectors $\boldsymbol{\gamma}_k$ indicate which variables are included in the regression model with design matrix $\boldsymbol{X}_{\boldsymbol{\gamma}_k}$ and corresponding regression vector $\boldsymbol{\beta}_{\boldsymbol{\gamma}_k}$. The following alternative notation may and will also be employed whenever suitable. Namely, we will denote regression models also as $M_1, \ldots, M_K$, where $M_m \equiv M_{m(\boldsymbol{\gamma})} \equiv M_{\boldsymbol{\gamma}}$ with $m(\boldsymbol{\gamma})$ a sequential number that indexes the models. The k_m-dimensional vector of parameters of model M_m is denoted as $\boldsymbol{\theta}_m$, which for linear regression consists of σ^2, α and d_m regression coefficients $\boldsymbol{\beta}_m$ (hence $k_m = d_m + 2$) which correspond to the design matrix $\boldsymbol{X}_m$.

In principle, the Bayesian variable (and model) selection problem is relatively straightforward and only involves the computation of the posterior model probabilities. Let $p(M_m)$ be the prior probability for model M_m, then its posterior probability is

$$p(M_m \mid \boldsymbol{y}) = \frac{p(\boldsymbol{y} \mid M_m)p(M_m)}{\sum_{j=1}^{K} p(\boldsymbol{y} \mid M_j)p(M_j)}, \tag{11.5}$$

with

$$p(\boldsymbol{y} \mid M_m) = \int p(\boldsymbol{y} \mid \boldsymbol{\theta}_m, M_m)p(\boldsymbol{\theta}_m \mid M_m)\, \mathrm{d}\boldsymbol{\theta}_m, \tag{11.6}$$

which is the marginal distribution of the mth model averaged over the possible values of model parameters. The Bayesian principle dictates to choose the model with the highest posterior probability which is the *maximum a posteriori* (MAP) model. An alternative expression of the posterior probability is

$$p(M_m \mid \boldsymbol{y}) = \frac{\mathrm{BF}_{mk}\, p(M_m)}{\sum_{j=1}^{K} \mathrm{BF}_{jk}\, p(M_j)}, \tag{11.7}$$

where $\mathrm{BF}_{jk} = p(\boldsymbol{y} \mid M_j)/p(\boldsymbol{y} \mid M_k)$ is the Bayes factor of comparing model M_j to model M_k, say a reference model (e.g. saturated or null model). Besides the MAP model, it is also of interest to find all other promising models.

Although Bayes theorem tells us how to select the most promising model(s), we need to address some issues that are important for the practical implementation of variable (and model) selection. Namely:

- What do we take as prior probabilities for $p(M_m)$? Can we use expert knowledge or should we use automatic priors, such as equal probabilities $p(M_m) = 1/K$?

- Expression (11.7) shows that the posterior probability involves the Bayes factor which is known to depend critically on the prior distributions $p(\boldsymbol{\theta}_m \mid M_m)$. Therefore, it is important to reflect on the choice of these priors such that they do not greatly influence model selection.
- How can we compute the marginal likelihoods $p(\boldsymbol{y} \mid M_m)$ in an economical manner, as these integrals are typically high dimensional? We will see that it becomes again important to choose the priors $p(\boldsymbol{\theta}_m \mid M_m)$ such that $p(\boldsymbol{y} \mid M_m)$ can be determined analytically or well approximated (in a fast numerical sense). This will lead to automatic priors.
- When K is large, what search strategies can be implemented to quickly find the most promising models?

In addition, we need to address the problems that were mentioned in the section on classical variable selection. For instance, does it make sense to base statistical inference on one selected model? And, if other models should be taken into account, how should this be done?

The next two sections describe BVS techniques that employ the *model space* approach. This means that variable selection is directly based on the marginal likelihood. In Section 11.4, most of the developments are based on the BIC approximation to the marginal likelihood. That section serves also as an introduction to the various concepts in BVS. In Section 11.5, we focus on Zellner's g-prior which is an important conjugate prior to $p(\boldsymbol{y} \mid \boldsymbol{\theta}_m, M_m)$. Section 11.6 is devoted to the application of Reversible Jump MCMC to variable selection. In Section 11.7, various hierarchical model-based approaches for BVS are reviewed. Bayesian regularization approaches including, e.g. the Bayesian LASSO approach, are explored in Section 11.8. In Section 11.9, we briefly review the important case when d is large possibly exceeding n. In Section 11.10, it is shown that (Bayesian) variable selection techniques can do more than selecting variables. Finally, in Section 11.11, we review the Bayesian Model Averaging (BMA) approach.

While in the previous chapters, most of the computations were done with WinBUGS (or related software) or SAS; in this chapter, extensive use of dedicated R packages proved necessary. A lot of the illustrations are based on WinBUGS, but dedicated R programs are often considerably faster and benefit from the rich R programming environment.

11.4 Introduction to Bayesian variable selection

11.4.1 Variable selection for K small

We start the case when K is small, i.e. when a limited number of covariates are involved. In Section 10.2, the objective was to select 'the best model(s)', now the objective is to select models with a high model probability. To compute the posterior model probability (11.5) we need $p(\boldsymbol{y} \mid M_m)$, typically involving the evaluation of large dimensional integrals. Computations can be speeded up by using the BIC approximation (see paragraph below expression (10.10)), where BIC is defined in expression (10.9). Since $-2\log \text{BF}_{jk} \approx \text{BIC}_j - \text{BIC}_k$, we can rewrite expression (11.7) as

$$p(M_m \mid \boldsymbol{y}) \approx \frac{\exp(-\Delta\text{BIC}_m/2)p(M_m)}{\sum_{j=1}^{K} \exp(-\Delta\text{BIC}_j/2)p(M_j)}, \tag{11.8}$$

with $\Delta\text{BIC}_j = \text{BIC}_j - \text{BIC}_{\min}$ and $\text{BIC}_{\min}$ is the minimum BIC of the K models. To introduce the concepts in BVS, we first look at the normal linear regression model defined in expression (11.2). Note, however, that the BIC approximation works well only for large sample sizes compared to the number of parameters and for relatively simple models (Berger and Pericchi 2001).

In contrast to most variable selection procedures below, the intercept is not given a separate status here and thus now we work with the vector $\boldsymbol{\beta}_m^*$ and the corresponding design matrix $\boldsymbol{X}_m^*$. Recall that, according to a result in Section 10.2.2, the BIC for a normal linear regression model M_m is based on assuming $p(\boldsymbol{\beta}_m^* \mid M_m) = \text{N}\left(\widehat{\boldsymbol{\beta}}_m^*, n\widehat{\sigma}^2(\boldsymbol{X}_m^{*T}\boldsymbol{X}_m^*)^{-1}\right)$, with $\widehat{\boldsymbol{\beta}}_m^*$ the MLE (LSE) of $\boldsymbol{\beta}_m^*$ and $\widehat{\sigma}^2$ the MLE of σ^2. This prior represents the equivalent information of a sample of size one (with the same design matrix as the observed data) and hence the use of BIC for model/variable selection corresponds to a particular prior. To compute expression (11.8) the prior probabilities, $p(M_m)$ must be supplied. A first choice could be to assume that $p(M_m) = 1/2^d$.

Looking for only the most plausible model a posteriori may be not a good idea since often many models will do a good job. In the search for good models, it is of interest to have a unique ordering of the models. The following model indicator transforms the vector of binary indicators $\boldsymbol{\gamma}$ to a decimal number (Ntzoufras 2009):

$$m(\boldsymbol{\gamma}) = 1 + \sum_{k=1}^{d} \gamma_k 2^{k-1}. \tag{11.9}$$

For instance, the model containing only the intercept is put first, $m = 1$. In the diabetes study with $d = 10$, the indicator vector for the MAP model (see Example XI.3) is $\boldsymbol{\gamma} = (0, 1, 1, 1, 0, 0, 1, 0, 1, 0)^T$ which corresponds to $m = 1 + 2 + 4 + 8 + 64 + 256 = 335$. To find the vector $\boldsymbol{\gamma}(m)$ corresponding to m we used a self-written algorithm (included in the R software discussed in Example XI.3).

The assumption $p(M_m) = 1/2^d$ implies that all models are a priori (1) independent and (2) equally probable. Both assumptions may be unrealistic in practice. For instance, suppose that two covariates are highly collinear, like systolic and diastolic blood pressure in predicting heart failure. When two models contain the same covariates except for blood pressure, then inserting systolic blood pressure or diastolic blood pressure results in almost the same model. Another example is when interaction terms are involved. Good statistical practice suggests that the main effects should be included whenever the interaction terms have been selected, but this asks for a dependent selection of variables. Equal and independent prior probabilities may be fine for selecting different models, but for variable selection, we need to pay more attention. Note first that, if the prior probability assigned to each variable to be in the model is 1/2, i.e. $p(\gamma_k = 1) = 0.5$ $(k = 1, \ldots, d)$ and these probabilities are assumed independent, the prior probability for each $\boldsymbol{\gamma}$ is equal to $1/2^d$. But then the a priori expected size model size is $d/2$, because $d_{\boldsymbol{\gamma}} \sim \text{Bin}(d, 0.5)$. On its turn, this implies that the prior $p(M_m) = 1/2^d$ is informative on the size of the model and prefers a priori models of size $d/2$ which are possibly too complicated.

Two alternative suggestions have been proposed for choosing model priors. The first suggestion is to take the independent Bernoulli prior given by

$$p(M_{m(\boldsymbol{\gamma})}) \equiv p(\boldsymbol{\gamma} \mid \omega) = \omega^{d_{\boldsymbol{\gamma}}}(1-\omega)^{d-d_{\boldsymbol{\gamma}}}, \ \omega \in (0, 1) \tag{11.10}$$

and to impute a prior guess for the proportion of $\beta_k \neq 0$, i.e. for ω. By e.g. choosing ω close to zero prior preference is expressed for sparse models, useful for GWA studies. Note that the uniform distribution $p(\boldsymbol{\gamma} \mid \omega) = 1/2^d$ is again obtained by taking $\omega = 1/2$. Hence the parameter ω controls the number of covariates in the model. Another suggestion is to give ω a prior distribution and combine it with expression (11.10); see George and McCulloch (1993); Scott and Berger (2010). With $\omega \sim \text{Beta}(\alpha_\omega, \beta_\omega)$ the marginal prior for $\boldsymbol{\gamma}$ becomes

$$p(\boldsymbol{\gamma}) = \int_0^1 p(\boldsymbol{\gamma} \mid \omega)p(\omega)\mathrm{d}\omega = \frac{B(\alpha_\omega + d_\gamma, \beta_\omega + d - d_\gamma)}{B(\alpha_\omega, \beta_\omega)}. \quad (11.11)$$

A popular choice is to take $\alpha_\omega = \beta_\omega = 1$, then $p(\boldsymbol{\gamma}) = \frac{1}{d+1}\binom{d}{d_\gamma}^{-1}$. This prior is uniform on the size of the model. Scott and Berger (2010) called this special case of prior (11.11) the 'fully Bayesian' version of variable selection priors, but it is more referred to as the *dependent prior*. Scott and Berger (2010) demonstrated that this prior corrects for 'multiplicity'. Correction for multiplicity means classically that the statistical procedure corrects for false positives. Here, it means that the number of falsely selected variables (those with truly $\gamma_k = 0$) should be kept under control. For instance, Swartz and Shete (2007) reported an inflated false positive rate with prior (11.11) with $\omega = 0.5$ (which disappeared when $\omega = 0.25$) when searching for genetic markers of a disease in the absence of any association.

Finally, from the posterior model probabilities one can derive the marginal probability that a covariate x_k is included in the model. This is the *(marginal) posterior inclusion probability* for variable x_k given by

$$q_k = p(\gamma_k = 1 \mid \mathbf{y}) = \sum_{m:\gamma_k=1} p(M_m \mid \mathbf{y}). \quad (11.12)$$

The posterior inclusion probability is a useful summary as often all models will have small posterior probabilities. These probabilities are used to determine the *median probability (MP) model* which is the model consisting of those variables whose posterior inclusion probability is at least 1/2. Barbieri and Berger (2004) reported that the MP model is often better for prediction than the MAP model.

In Example XI.3, we illustrate the above concepts with the diabetes data.

Example XI.3: Diabetes study: BVS based on the BIC approximation

We have performed a BVS on the diabetes data and made use of the BIC approximation with the self-written R program 'chapter 11 BIC and Zellner diabetes.R'. With equal prior model probabilities, the MAP model contains gender, BMI, bp, $s3$ and $s5$. Note that the MAP model differs from the best model found with the classical variable selection procedures by the selection of $s3$ rather than $s1$ and $s2$. However, the models are competitive and differ in R_a^2 only in the third decimal.

In addition, our R program delivers all posterior model probabilities. In Figure 11.3(a), we show (part of the) the posterior model probabilities obtained by computing expression (11.8) with $p(M_m) = 1/2^{10}$. We highlighted the five models with posterior probability greater than 0.05. The MAP model corresponds to $m = 335$ with posterior probability equal to 0.28, while the model selected by the classical variable selection procedures corresponds to m=319 with posterior probability equal to 0.22. To find the median probability model, the marginal posterior inclusion probabilities are required. They were for age: 0.05, gender: 0.98, BMI:

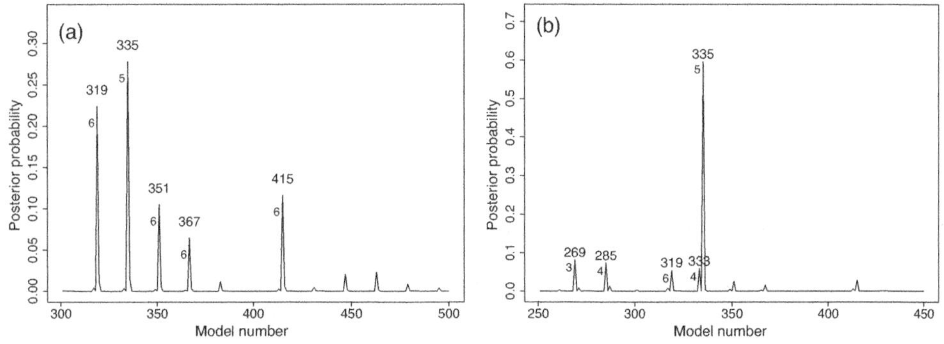

Figure 11.3 Diabetes study: index plot of model posterior probabilities obtained from a BVS combining the BIC approximation with (a) the independent model prior ($\omega = 0.5$) yielding equal prior model probabilities, and (b) with $\omega = 0.01$. The size of the model (number of variables) is indicated to the left of the vertical bar of the model.

1.0, bp: 1.0, $s1$: 0.57, $s2$: 0.38, $s3$: 0.57, $s4$: 0.20, $s5$: 1.0, and $s6$: 0.07. Thus, the MP model consists of gender, BMI, bp, $s1$, $s3$, $s5$ and is equal to the MAP model.

The first variable selection was based on the prior (11.10) with $\omega = 0.5$. In the next step, we varied ω to illustrate the effect of the hyperprior $p(\boldsymbol{\gamma} \mid \omega)$. For small values of ω, a greater prior weight is put on sparse models, while for large values of ω the reverse happens. For $\omega = 0.01$ the MAP model contains only three covariates (BMI, bp, $s5$) with posterior probability $= 0.61$ and the next most plausible model only two covariates (posterior probability $= 0.24$). For $\omega = 0.99$, the MAP model contained all covariates (posterior probability $= 0.50$). In Figure 11.3, the posterior probabilities for two values of ω are shown. With the dependent prior (11.11) the same MAP model as for $\omega = 0.5$ was obtained.

Further, in Figure 11.4, the effect of the model prior on the posterior probabilities of the model sizes is illustrated. Clearly, the dependent prior increases the posterior probability for smaller and larger models, which can be seen by comparing the independent and the dependent posteriors on the model size. □

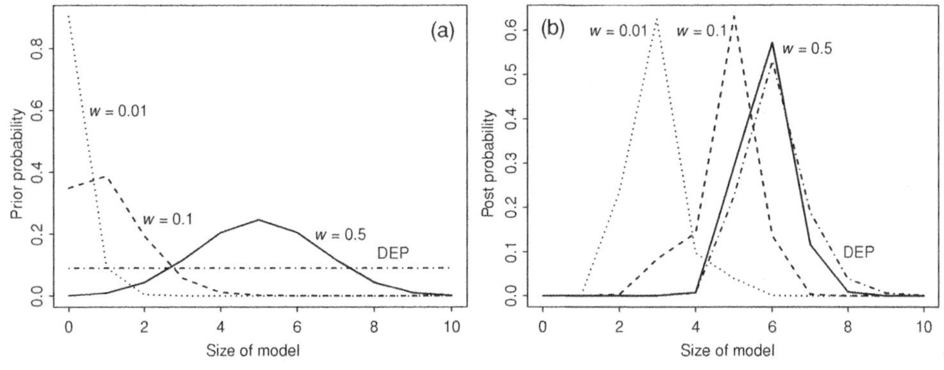

Figure 11.4 Diabetes study: (a) prior and (b) posterior probabilities of model size for various model priors (DEP = dependent prior).

The BVS principles can be immediately applied to all regression models. With the BIC approximation to the marginal likelihood the determination of the best models will again be relatively fast. This is illustrated later for a probit regression model. The choice of the probit was inspired by software availability and but also by computational difficulties with the logistic link in WinBUGS (see Chapter 8 and Example XI.7). Another reason for choosing the probit link is its latent representation of a discretized normal random variable. This was first suggested in Albert and Chib (1993) and was illustrated in Example VII.9. Sections 11.8 and 11.9 further highlight the usefulness of this representation.

Example XI.4: Rheumatoid arthritis study: BVS based on the BIC approximation
Rheumatoid arthritis (RA) is an autoimmune disease characterized by chronic synovial inflammation and destruction of cartilage and bone in the joints. The Rotterdam Early CoHort Study (REACH) was initiated in 2004 to investigate the development of RA in patients with early manifestations of joint impairment. Information regarding basic patient characteristics, serological measurements and patterns of disease involvement at baseline have been gathered in a total number of 681 recruited patients. For more information on the REACH study (see Geuskens *et al.* 2008; Alves *et al.* 2011).

It was of interest to know which of the following 12 factors are associated with the development of RA (binary outcome): *accp* (cyclic citrullinated peptide antibody), *age*, *esr* (erythrocyte sedimentation rate), *dc* (duration of complaints in days), *stiffness* (duration of morning stiffness in minutes), *rf* (rheumatoid factor), *gender*, *sym* (symmetrical pattern of joint inflammation yes/no), *sjc* (swollen joint count), *tjc* (tender joint count), *bcph* (bilateral compression pain in hands yes/no) and *bcpf* (bilateral compression pain in feet yes/no). The Spearman correlations between the covariates were all relatively low (below 0.25 in absolute value) except for cor(*accp*,*rf*) $= 0.67$ and cor(*sym*,*sjc*) $= 0.86$. Based on classical probit regression, the F-to-out backward selection significance level 0.05 yields a model with the following variables: *accp*, *esr*, *dc*, *sym*, *sjc and bcph*. The model with the most favorable value of the AIC criterion selected after an exhaustive model evaluation contains two extra variables: *rf* and *stiffness*.

The R program 'chapter 11 BIC and Zellner REACH.R' selects variables in a probit regression model using the BIC approximation. We used equal model probabilities for this exercise. The results are shown in Table 11.3 in the column *BF*. The MAP model contains only four variables: *accp*, *esr*, *sym* and *bcph*. Note that the best model obtained by a classical backward selection is among the five best models. □

To conclude this section, variable selection based on the BIC approximation is achieved through the evaluation of the following:

- *Posterior model probabilities* $p(M_m \mid \mathbf{y}) \equiv p(\boldsymbol{\gamma}(m) \mid \mathbf{y})$: This gives the MAP model and all other plausible models in the light of the observed data.
- *(Marginal) posterior inclusion probabilities (11.12)*: This gives the MP model by inspecting for which of the regressors the posterior inclusion probability exceeds 0.5.

11.4.2 Variable selection for K large

We now look at the case of large model spaces. Exploration of all 2^d models is not possible for d large, even when the marginal likelihood (and the Bayes factor) can be determined analytically. A search strategy needs to be installed to find the most promising models. We first review a deterministic strategy which is combined with restricting the set of models.

We again assume that we can efficiently compute $p(\boldsymbol{y} \mid M_m)$ for all M_m such that together with $p(M_m)$ we know $p(M_m \mid \boldsymbol{y})$ (up to a constant). Raftery and Madigan (1994) proposed a deterministic variable selection strategy in the context of Bayesian model averaging (see Section 11.11) based on two principles. The first principle narrows the selection to models with a high posterior probability which leads to the set of models satisfying

$$A' = \{M_m : \frac{p(M_m \mid \boldsymbol{y})}{\max_k p(M_k \mid \boldsymbol{y})} \geq C\}, \tag{11.13}$$

where C is a constant chosen by the user. The second principle, known as Occam's razor introduced in Section 10.2.2, excludes all models which are less supported by the data than their simpler versions. That is, models in

$$B = \{M_m : \exists M_k \in A', M_k \subset M_m, p(M_k \mid \boldsymbol{y}) > p(M_m \mid \boldsymbol{y})\} \tag{11.14}$$

are excluded from the set, where $M \subset N$ means that model N contains at least one extra covariate. The set of models to be considered is then reduced to $A = A' \setminus B$ and it is assumed that the omitted models are responsible for a small portion of the posterior probability. In that case, the posterior probabilities $p(M_m \mid \boldsymbol{y})$ computed with equation (11.5) and based on the set of models A are a good approximation to the true posterior probabilities based on all models.

A conceptual description of the algorithm goes as follows (Hoeting *et al.* 1999a). When for two nested models the simpler model is decisively rejected then the algorithm rejects also submodels of the simpler model. Second, when $p(M_0 \mid \boldsymbol{y})/p(M_1 \mid \boldsymbol{y}) > O_R$, with M_0 a submodel of M_1 and $O_R \geq 1$ then M_1 is rejected. When $p(M_0 \mid \boldsymbol{y})/p(M_1 \mid \boldsymbol{y}) < O_L$ with $O_L < 1$ and small, then M_1 is rejected. When $O_L < p(M_0 \mid \boldsymbol{y})/p(M_1 \mid \boldsymbol{y}) < O_R$, then neither model is rejected. The interval $[O_L, O_R]$ is called *Occam's window* which gives also the name to the method. Raftery *et al.* (1996) advised to take $O_R = 20$ and $O_L = 1/20$. More details are found in Raftery and Madigan (1994) who proposed backward and upward model search algorithms where models differ only by one variable. The actual search is then run as a combination of both.

Alternatives to purely deterministic methods such as Occam's window are those based on stochastic search. These methods introduce some randomness into the search and, therefore, are less vulnerable to getting trapped in the model space. The stochastic approach we consider here was suggested by Madigan *et al.* (1995) again in the context of Bayesian model averaging. The approach uses MCMC methods to sample from the posterior model distribution $p(M_m \mid \boldsymbol{y})$ assuming that $p(\boldsymbol{y} \mid M_m)$ can be determined efficiently for all models. The method has become known as MC^3, which means that it is a 'Model Composition using MCMC'.

Sampling is done via the classical MH-algorithm on the space of models. The Markov chain of models $\{M^k; k = 1, \ldots\}$ or equivalently the $\boldsymbol{\gamma}$s move locally in the neighborhood of the current model. Given the current position M_m, model M_{m^*} is sampled in the neighborhood of M_m by the proposal distribution $q(M_{m^*} \mid M_m) = 1/d$. Thus, all models in the neighborhood are accessible with the same probability and the corresponding $\boldsymbol{\gamma}$ and $\boldsymbol{\gamma}^*$ differ in one position. The sampled model M^* is then accepted with probability

$$\min\left(1, \frac{p(M_{m^*} \mid \boldsymbol{y})}{p(M_m \mid \boldsymbol{y})}\right), \tag{11.15}$$

otherwise the chain stays at model M_m. Although an improvement over Occam's window approach, sampling with the MC^3 approach still proceeds in small steps and therefore the mixing of the chain might not be ideal.

The MC^3 algorithm provides an empirical estimate of $p(M_m \mid \mathbf{y})$ by taking the proportion of times model M_m is selected over the total number of visited models, i.e.

$$\widehat{p}(M_m \mid \mathbf{y}) = \frac{1}{L}\sum_{l=1}^{L} I(M^l = M_m), \tag{11.16}$$

with M^l the model visited in iteration l of the Markov chain, $I(\cdot)$ the indicator function and L the total number of MCMC iterations. Further, the posterior inclusion probabilities (11.12) are computed by replacing $p(M_m \mid \mathbf{y})$ with (11.16).

The R package *BMA* provides functions for variable selection based on Occam's window and MC^3 in the context of Bayesian model averaging. For linear models, the conjugate NIG-prior for regression coefficients is taken with minimally informative priors (Raftery *et al.* 1997). For GLIMs, Raftery (1996) applies a Laplace approximation (3.19) on $h(\boldsymbol{\theta}_m) = \log\{p(\mathbf{y} \mid \boldsymbol{\theta}_m, M_m)\, p(\boldsymbol{\theta}_m \mid M_m)\}$ (see Section 10.2.2). Hereby an approximation to the marginal likelihood and the Bayes factor against the null model ($\boldsymbol{\beta}_m = \mathbf{0}$) is obtained for a user-defined but minimally informative prior. A further approximation is based on GLIM output. We now illustrate the use of the package BMA with the diabetes data.

Example XI.5: Diabetes study: BVS based on Occam's window and the MC^3 approach
The R package `BMA` hosts several BVS functions with, however, limited options for prior model probabilities. In this example we applied the functions `bic.glm` and `MC3.REG`. The first function is based on Occam's window in combination with the classical BIC approximation to the Bayes factor and provides variable selection in GLIMs. `MC3.REG` is based on MC^3 but can only be used with linear models and is based on the NIG conjugate prior for $p(\boldsymbol{\beta}_m^* \mid M_m)$. Both programs provide model averaging tools, but here we focus on the variable selection algorithms.

The program 'chapter 11 Occam diabetes.R' performs BVS on the diabetes data and is based on `bic.glm` and `MC3.REG`. The results of this exercise are given in Table 11.2 and

Table 11.2 Diabetes study: selection of the best models.

Covariates	BF	BO	B	MC^3	G
2,3,4,7,9	0.278	0.326	0.286	0.381	0.281
2,3,4,5,6,9	0.224	0.253	0.223	0.269	0.224
2,3,4,5,8,9	0.116	0.133	0.117	0.080	0.116
2,3,4,5,7,9	0.105	0.120	0.106	0.063	0.105
2,3,4,7,8,9	0.023	0.027	0.023	0.019	0.022

Note: Five best linear regression models according to their posterior model probability obtained from BIC-approximation with full exploration of all models (BF), BIC-approximation with Occam's window (OR = 20) (BO) and without Occam's window (B) (both using 'bic.glm'), MC3 based on 2000 iterations using MC3.REG, Zellner's g-prior (G). The variables are abbreviated with numbers as follows: age (1), sex (2), BMI (3), bp (4), *s*1 (5), *s*2 (6), *s*3 (7), *s*4 (8), *s*5 (9), *s*6 (10).

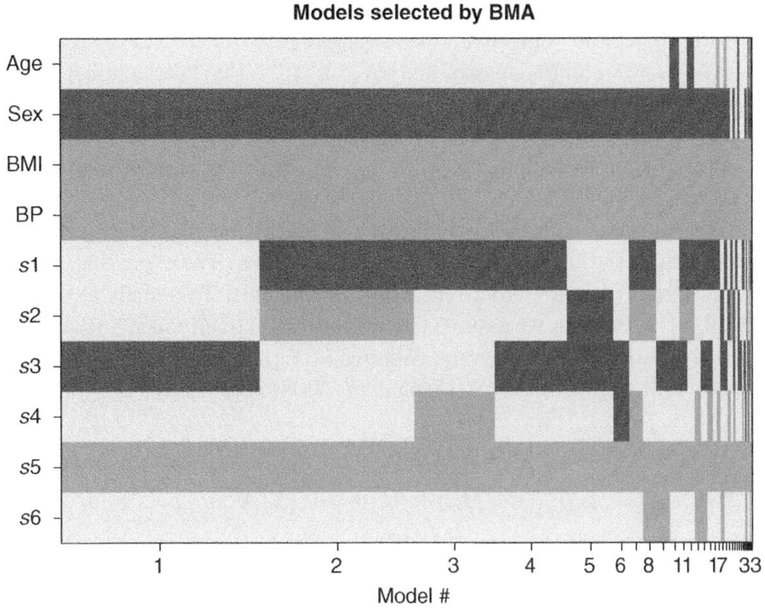

Figure 11.5 Diabetes study: included covariates in selected models obtained from 'bic.glm' (Occam's window option switched off). The models are sorted (on x-axis) in decreasing posterior probability. The horizontal strips indicate the variables that are included in the model with a positive/negative regression coefficient (grey/black).

tell us that (a) the posterior model probabilities for the five best models satisfy the inequality $BO \geq B \geq BF$ (for explanation of symbols, see Table 11.2), which is explained by the fact that the set of considered models increases from BO to BF and (b) the MC^3 estimates of $p(M_m \mid \mathbf{y})$ differentiate more the best fitting models. Despite some differences in the posterior model probabilities, the relative ranking of the five best models is the same. A graphical display of the selected variables for the respective models is given in Figure 11.5 (obtained from `bic.glm`). □

To conclude, variable selection based on Occam's window and MC^3 is achieved through the evaluation of $\widehat{p}(M_m \mid \mathbf{y})$ which delivers the MAP model. From the posterior inclusion probabilities computed with expression (11.16) the MP model is obtained.

11.5 Variable selection based on Zellner's g-prior

From Sections 3.8.3 and 10.2.1 it follows that for variable selection the prior $p(\boldsymbol{\theta}_m \mid M_m)$ needs to be chosen with care. In fact, while an improper prior leads to an indeterminate Bayes factor, with an informative prior there is the risk that prior considerations dictate the model choice. Thus, an appropriate prior needs to balance between a noninformative and an informative prior. Moreover, calculating the Bayes factor is often computationally demanding since it requires the marginal likelihood. A popular prior for the regression coefficients of a normal linear regression model in the context of BVS is the conjugate NIG-prior of Section 5.6.1, despite the problems mentioned there. This prior gives an analytical expression of the marginal likelihoods. More specifically, given σ^2, the conjugate prior for $\boldsymbol{\beta}^*$ is $\mathrm{N}(\boldsymbol{\beta}_0^*, g\sigma^2\Sigma_0^*)$. Popular choices for Σ_0^* are the identity matrix and $(\boldsymbol{X}_m^{*T}\boldsymbol{X}_m^*)^{-1}$. The latter choice corresponds to Zellner's g-prior when combined with $\sigma^2 \sim \mathrm{IG}(a_0, b_0)$. Zellner's g-prior enjoys an attractive property that it can be interpreted as the posterior from the analysis of an imaginary sample $\boldsymbol{y}_0$ (for $\boldsymbol{\beta}_0^* = \boldsymbol{0}$ it is $\boldsymbol{y}_0 = \boldsymbol{0}$) with the same design $\boldsymbol{X}_m^*$ as in the current sample and variance $g\sigma^2$, as shown in Section 5.6.1.

Working with the total vector $\boldsymbol{\beta}^*$ would shrink all regression coefficients, also the intercept α. Often, and certainly in GLIMs, we do not wish to shrink α. Therefore it is common to treat the intercept different from the other regression coefficients. This leads to using the model $\boldsymbol{y} = \boldsymbol{1}\alpha + \boldsymbol{X}_m\boldsymbol{\beta}_m + \boldsymbol{\varepsilon}$. Further, we assume that α is common to all models what happens when the covariates are centered since then the columns of $\boldsymbol{X}_m$ are orthogonal to the vector $\boldsymbol{1}$. The popular version of the g-prior in BVS (Liang *et al.* 2008) is given by

$$p(\alpha, \sigma^2) \propto \sigma^{-2}, \tag{11.17}$$

$$p(\boldsymbol{\beta}_m \mid \sigma^2, M_m) = \mathrm{N}\left(\boldsymbol{0}, g\sigma^2(\boldsymbol{X}_m^T\boldsymbol{X}_m)^{-1}\right). \tag{11.18}$$

Note that in expression (11.18) g controls the size of the $\boldsymbol{\beta}_m$ parameters. The prior for σ^2 can be taken the same for all models since the regression parameters are orthogonal to the variance in a linear model (Berger and Pericchi 2001). This version of the g-prior is not (conditionally) conjugate anymore but still leads to a closed expression of the marginal likelihood, namely,

$$p(\boldsymbol{y} \mid M_m, g) = \frac{\Gamma\left(\frac{n-1}{2}\right)}{(\pi n)^{(n-1)/2}} \frac{1}{\left(\sum_{i=1}^n (y_i - \bar{y})^2\right)^{(n-1)/2}} \frac{(1+g)^{(n-1-d_m)/2}}{(1+g(1-R_m^2))^{(n-1)/2}}, \tag{11.19}$$

where R_m^2 is the ordinary coefficient of determination of model M_m. When the null model M_k is the reference, $R_k^2 = 0$ and $d_k = 0$, the Bayes factor comparing model M_m to M_k is

$$\mathrm{BF}_{mk} = \frac{p(\boldsymbol{y} \mid M_m)}{p(\boldsymbol{y} \mid M_k)} = (1+g)^{(n-d_m-1)/2}\left[1 + g(1-R_m^2)\right]^{-(n-1)/2}; \tag{11.20}$$

see Liang *et al.* (2008) for more details on how to derive expressions (11.19) and (11.20). Zellner's g-prior needs a value for g. A popular choice is $g = n$ which leads to the unit information prior (Kass and Wasserman 1996), but other values have been proposed, see below. To arrive at the posterior model probabilities, Zellner's g-prior can be combined with the model prior (11.10) for a particular choice of ω or the dependent prior (11.11). When the number of variables is relatively small, BVS based on Zellner's g-prior can be combined with an exhaustive model search, otherwise a stochastic search algorithm should be used.

To define minimally informative Zellner's g-priors, many looked for the 'optimal' choice of g. In general, small values of g will result in a too strong prior, while very large values of g would favor the null model and thus induce the Lindley–Bartlett's paradox (Smith and Kohn (1996)). But, Smith and Kohn (1996) reported that the results were insensitive to values of g between 10 and 1000. George and Foster (2000) showed, that for σ^2 fixed, one can tune g and ω in (11.10) such that the MAP model obtained from Zellner's g-prior corresponds to the best model from a variable selection procedure based on popular model selection criteria such as AIC (e.g. $\omega = 0.5$ and $g \approx 3.92$) and BIC (e.g. $\omega = 0.5$ and $g = n$). Motivated by theoretical considerations and simulations, Fernandez *et al.* (2001) showed that $g = \max(n, d^2)$ leads to asymptotically selecting the correct model. This property is called *model selection consistency*. George and Foster (2000) argued that it is hard to make an a priori choice of ω and g and suggested to estimate these from the data using an empirical Bayes method. Instead, Liang *et al.* (2008) suggested a prior distribution for g and showed that for well-chosen priors, the BVS procedure achieves model selection consistency. These variable selection procedures appear to have better operational procedures. Finally, Krishna *et al.* (2009) suggested the prior $\mathrm{N}\left(\mathbf{0}, g\sigma^2(\boldsymbol{X}_m^T\boldsymbol{X}_m)^{\lambda}\right)$ as a replacement of expression (11.18). This extension yields again analytical results and allows to have control over correlated predictors, i.e. $\lambda > 0$ forces highly collinear predictors entering or exiting the model simultaneously, while $\lambda < 0$ has the reverse effect.

Extensions of Zellner's g-prior have been defined for other models such as GLIMs. Fouskakis *et al.* (2009) suggested $p(\boldsymbol{\beta}_m \mid M_m) = \mathrm{N}\left(\mathbf{0}_{d_m}, g\Im(\mathbf{0}_{d_m})^{-1}\right)$ with $g = n$, $\Im(\boldsymbol{\beta}_m)$ the Fisher (expected) information matrix evaluated in $\boldsymbol{\beta}_m$ and $\mathbf{0}_{d_m}$ the vector of zeros of dimension d_m. This leads to $p(\boldsymbol{\beta}_m \mid M_m) = \mathrm{N}\left(\mathbf{0}_{d_m}, 4n(\boldsymbol{X}_m^T\boldsymbol{X}_m)^{-1}\right)$ for logistic regression. Other proposals differ in the choice of the information matrix (observed versus expected) and in the vector wherein $\Im$ is evaluated; see Sabanés Bové and Held (2011b) for a review and additional references. These authors proposed a modification of the conjugate prior (5.35) of Chen and Ibrahim (2003) and suggested (in the notation of Section 5.6.2)

$$p(\boldsymbol{\beta}_m \mid \boldsymbol{y}_0, g, M_m) \propto \exp\left\{\frac{1}{g\phi}\sum_{i=1}^{n}[h(0)w_i\theta_i - w_i b(\theta_i)]\right\}, \tag{11.21}$$

with $h(0) = \mathrm{d}b/\mathrm{d}\theta(0)$ and w_i are weights. For $n \to \infty$ this prior converges to a generalized Zellner's g-prior

$$\boldsymbol{\beta}_m \mid g, M_m \sim \mathrm{N}\left(\mathbf{0}_{d_m}, g\phi c\left(\boldsymbol{X}_m^T\boldsymbol{W}\boldsymbol{X}_m\right)^{-1}\right), \tag{11.22}$$

with $c = \mathrm{d}^2b/\mathrm{d}\theta^2$(and $(\mathrm{d}b/\mathrm{d}\theta)^{-1}$) evaluated at zero and $\boldsymbol{W} = \mathrm{diag}(w)$. This boils down to the logistic regression g-prior of Fouskakis *et al.* (2009) when $g = n$ and $c = 4$, while for probit regression $c = \pi/2$. Fixing g to a particular value would imply that variable selection may not enjoy the model consistency property. Instead Sabanés Bové and Held (2011b) specified a hyperprior $p(g)$ for g and called therefore the resulting prior the *generalized hyper-g-prior*, which still needs to be completed with a prior for $\boldsymbol{\gamma}$. Their BVS algorithm, implemented in the R package `glmBfp`, is based on the following steps. First, the marginal likelihood $p(\boldsymbol{y} \mid M_m) \equiv p(\boldsymbol{y} \mid \boldsymbol{\gamma})$ is approximated with Laplace approximations combined with adaptive Gaussian quadrature. A MH-algorithm based on $p(\boldsymbol{y} \mid \boldsymbol{\gamma})$ then yields a sequence $\boldsymbol{\gamma}^1, \ldots, \boldsymbol{\gamma}^k, \ldots$. In addition (but not part of the BVS procedure), given $\boldsymbol{\gamma}$, an independent proposal density for $\log(g)$ is combined with a proposal density to sample α, $\boldsymbol{\beta}$.

Example XI.6: Rheumatoid arthritis study: BVS based on a generalized Zellner's g-prior
With the R package `glmBfp` variable selection can be done in a Bayesian generalized linear model (BGLIM). We used the package to select important covariates in a probit regression model for the REACH data. The package is based on prior (11.22) in combination with a variety of hyperpriors $p(g)$. Here, we have taken IG(0.1,0.1). In addition, different priors are allowed for $\boldsymbol{\gamma}$. We chose prior (11.10) with $\omega = 0.5$ and prior (11.11) with $\alpha_\omega = \beta_\omega = 1$.

Table 11.3 Rheumatoid arthritis study: selection of best models.

Covariates	BF	BO	B	L	G	RJ	SVSS2	SVSS4
1,3,8,11	0.250	0.316	0.255	0.273	0.027	0.170	0.310	0.058
1,3,8,9,11	0.133	0.168	0.136	0.115	0.046	0.139	0.168	0.061
1,3,4,8,11	0.105	0.133	0.107	0.109	0.033	0.074	0.077	0.029
1,3,6,8,11	0.059	0.075	0.060	0.076	0.019	0.043	0.069	0.043
1,3,5,8,11	0.051	0.065	0.053	0.055	0.016	0.036	0.048	0.022

Note: Five best probit regression models according to their posterior probability obtained from BIC approximation with full exploration of all models (BF); BIC approximation with Occam's window (OR = 20) (BO) and without (B) (both using 'bic.glm'); Raftery's Laplace approximation (L) using 'glib'; Generalized hyper-*g*-prior (G) using 'glmBfp'; RJMCMC (RJ) using the Jump Interface to WinBUGS; SSVS approach based on scenarios 2 (SVSS2) and 4 (SSVS4). The variables are abbreviated with numbers as follows: accp (1), age (2), esr (3), dc (4), stiffness (5), rf (6), gender (7), sym (8), sjc (9), tjc (10), bcph (11), bcpf (12).

Finally, we compared the solution based on an exhaustive search with the solution based on stochastic search. The commands can be found in the R program 'chapter 11 BIC and Zellner REACH.R' which incorporates the package `glmBfp`. The five best models with prior (11.10) are given in Table 11.3.

To compare the best models found by the hyper-*g*-prior, we applied the BMA routine `bic.glm` which is based on a BIC approximation with or without the use of Occam's window. The variable selection results are shown in the columns *BF*, *BO* and *B* of Table 11.3. Note that again $BO \geq B \geq BF$ with always the same MAP model (equal to that of Example XI.4). The BMA routine `glib` is based on a more accurate Laplace approximation to the marginal likelihood (Raftery 1996), applied to the REACH data produced column *L*. All programs can be found in 'chapter 11 BMA REACH.R'.

Compared with the other BVS algorithms, the posterior model probabilities are less outspoken with the hyper *g*-prior but nevertheless the algorithm gave the same five best models irrespective of whether a stochastic or an exhaustive search was done. Both search procedures gave also the same posterior model probabilities. Further, it is readily seen that, when switching from prior (11.10) to prior (11.11) with $\alpha_\omega = \beta_\omega = 1$ the posterior probabilities are proportional with a factor that depends on the model size. The posterior median of g was 28.3 (95% CI = [21.5, 39.7]) which is about 20 times lower than with the unit-information prior ($g = 681$). □

11.6 Variable selection based on Reversible Jump Markov chain Monte Carlo

The MC^3 method produces an MCMC chain which moves only within the model space, i.e. it moves from model M_m to model M_{m^*} bypassing the choice of regression coefficients since the MH-algorithm is based on $p(\boldsymbol{y} \mid M_m)$. Hence after selecting the model M_{m^*}, one needs to estimate the parameters $\boldsymbol{\theta}_{m^*}$. One could generalize the MC^3 approach by jointly sampling the parameters $\boldsymbol{\theta}_m$ and the model M_m using, say, a MH-approach. That is, given the current value $(\boldsymbol{\theta}_m, M_m)$ a proposal $(\boldsymbol{\theta}_{m^*}, M_{m^*})$ could be generated from the proposal distribution $q(\boldsymbol{\theta}_{m^*}, M_{m^*} \mid \boldsymbol{\theta}_m, M_m)$ which takes values in the combined space of parameter vectors and model identifiers. The proposal is then accepted with probability

$$\begin{aligned}\alpha_{MH} &= \min\left(1, \frac{p(\boldsymbol{\theta}_{m^*}, M_{m^*} \mid \mathbf{y})q(\boldsymbol{\theta}_m, M_m \mid \boldsymbol{\theta}_{m^*}, M_{m^*})}{p(\boldsymbol{\theta}_m, M_m \mid \mathbf{y})q(\boldsymbol{\theta}_{m^*}, M_{m^*} \mid \boldsymbol{\theta}_m, M_m)}\right),\\ &= \min\left(1, \frac{p(\mathbf{y} \mid \boldsymbol{\theta}_{m^*}, M_{m^*})p(\boldsymbol{\theta}_{m^*} \mid M_{m^*})p(M_{m^*})q(\boldsymbol{\theta}_m, M_m \mid \boldsymbol{\theta}_{m^*}, M_{m^*})}{p(\mathbf{y} \mid \boldsymbol{\theta}_m, M_m)p(\boldsymbol{\theta}_m \mid M_m)p(M_m)q(\boldsymbol{\theta}_{m^*}, M_{m^*} \mid \boldsymbol{\theta}_m, M_m)}\right),\end{aligned}$$

where the second line follows from Bayes theorem. The proposal is done in 2 steps with first a proposal for M_{m^*} and then a proposal for $\boldsymbol{\theta}_{m^*}$ which implies that $q(\boldsymbol{\theta}_{m^*}, M_{m^*} \mid \boldsymbol{\theta}_m, M_m) = q(M_{m^*} \mid \boldsymbol{\theta}_m, M_m)q(\boldsymbol{\theta}_{m^*} \mid \boldsymbol{\theta}_m, M_{m^*}, M_m)$. The challenge is to ensure that the detailed balance condition (see Section 6.4) holds which means that the move from model $(\boldsymbol{\theta}_m, M_m)$ to model $(\boldsymbol{\theta}_{m^*}, M_{m^*})$ should be as easy as the opposite move. It is, however, not immediately clear how to guarantee this condition when the dimensions of the models change which occurs with variable selection. Reversibility is guaranteed by the Reversible Jump MCMC approach (Green 1995) introduced in Section 6.6. Here, we describe the reversible jump strategy sketched in Lunn *et al.* (2009b) and implemented in the Reversible Jump to WinBUGS Interface (abbreviated as *RJWinBUGS*). The attractiveness of the procedure is its link with WinBUGS making it quite general. For specific applications, other RJMCMC algorithms for variable selection might be preferred. For instance, the R package `monomvn` is an efficient RJMCMC-based procedure for BVS in linear regression (Gramacy and Pantaleoy 2010). The RJWinBUGS strategy is to some extent also typical for many other RJMCMC algorithms (see Chen *et al.* 2011).

General strategy Let $\boldsymbol{\theta}_m$ be the k_m-dimensional vector of parameters of model M_m. The key element of the algorithm is the specification of a suitable proposal distribution to move from $(\boldsymbol{\theta}_m, M_m)$ to $(\boldsymbol{\theta}_{m^*}, M_{m^*})$. When the dimensions change ($k_m \neq k_{m*}$), the construction of the proposal distribution needs careful attention to assure reversibility. For the MC^3 method and the original RJMCMC approach, the moves were confined to only adding or deleting one variable, which correspond to the 'birth' and 'death' moves in the original paper of Green (1995). To allow for a quicker exploration of the spaces, Lunn *et al.* (2009b) generalized the RJMCMC algorithm and proposed three types of moves: (1) 'dimension moves' which represent the two transdimensional moves, i.e. 'birth' and 'death' but where the change in dimension is in general greater than one; (2) 'configuration moves' which randomly pick up several variables and replace them by the same number of other variables; and (3) 'coefficient moves' which update the model coefficients via standard sampling methods.

The moves Only the *dimension moves* are transdimensional. RJWinBUGS uses a MH-algorithm for this. First, it is proposed to update the dimension by adding a randomly chosen integer δ to (or subtracting from) k_m. Here, we concentrate on selecting variables and hence the relevant part to consider are the d_m regression coefficients such that k_m is in fact d_m. In a second step, a new regression vector is proposed by sampling from its full conditional distribution (only conjugate full conditionals are allowed). With the full conditional as proposal density the authors show that the acceptance probability becomes independent of the regression coefficients, but remains dependent on the prior covariance matrix. This latter dependence makes the sampling procedure dependent on the choice of the prior precision of the regression coefficients, and thus it is important to choose an appropriate value. In the *con guration moves* the dimensions remain the same but a new regression vector is sampled. Finally, in the *coef cient moves* only the regression coefficients are updated. In all of the moves, a bijective function h, as defined in Section 6.6, is explicitly or implicitly constructed.

The interface RJWinBUGS must first be installed to allow WinBUGS to perform a RJMCMC variable selection approach. The instructions for installing the interface can be found in `http://www.winbugs-development.org.uk/rjmcmc.html`. An option *Jump* is added to the menu to obtain summaries of the RJMCMC analysis. Note that RJWinBUGS uses new commands, beyond those available in WinBUGS.

Example XI.7: Rheumatoid arthritis study: BVS using RJMCMC

The WinBUGS program 'chapter 11 RJMCMC REACH.odc' contains the commands to select the important variables from the REACH study in a probit regression model using the RJMCMC approach. For an R program based on R2WinBUGS, see Exercise 11.4. Note that the software does not support the logistic regression model (no full conditionals are available), only the probit model can be used with the response expressed as a binarized latent normal random variable. We initiated five chains with initial values for the number of covariates: 0, 3, 6, 9 and 12. Each chain was run for 10 000 iterations with a burn-in of 5000 iterations. We monitored two aspects of the variable selection procedure (see WinBUGS program): the model indicator *id* and the estimated regression coefficients vector *e*. The posterior summary measures are obtained from the option **Jump**. The option 'table' in the box **Jump Summary Tool** shows the most promising models. The output of our analysis is shown in Figure 11.6. Note that the user can limit the display of the visited models by modifying the variable 'razor'.

It is important to take an appropriate value for the precision of the regression coefficients to provide a minimally informative prior. We have taken as prior precision for the regression coefficients, the common diagonal element of the precision matrix $\frac{2}{n\pi}\left(\boldsymbol{X}_m^T\boldsymbol{X}_m\right)$ in expression (11.22), here equal to $\tau_\beta^2 = 0.64$. Thus we assumed independent priors $\text{N}(0, 1/\tau_\beta^2)$ for the β_ks. The most often visited models are shown in Figure 11.6. In more than 17% of the times the chains visited model `101000010010` (variables 1, 3, 8 and 11) which makes it the MAP model. From the second part of the output we conclude that it is also the MP model. The posterior model probabilities were less outspoken than those of the other BVS techniques. In addition, we performed a sensitivity analysis by applying the BVS for $\tau_\beta^2 = 0.2, 0.4, 0.8$. We found that the best models were basically the same for the different values of τ_β^2, but that the posterior model probabilities were less pronounced with increasing τ_β^2 always yielding the same MAP and MP model.

The Jump facilities can be combined with the standard WinBUGS facilities. For instance, trace plots illustrate the mixing of the chains and the transdimensional moves. Density plots summarize the posterior information. Figure 11.7 shows the marginal (posterior) density of the regression coefficient of *sjc*. The bimodal density is generated by the jumps when including and excluding the regressor. This is an example of Bayesian model averaging (see Section 11.11). □

Finally, checking convergence of a chain created by a RJMCMC algorithm is more complicated than with a standard MCMC algorithm due to the changing dimensions. Algorithms that generalize the Brooks–Gelman diagnostic can be found in Brooks and Giudici (2000); Castelloe and Zimmerman (2002), but software does not seem to be available yet.

Model structure	Posterior prob.	Cumulative prob.
101000010010	0.16984	0.16984
101000011010	0.1388	0.30864
101100010010	0.07436	0.383
101100011010	0.07364	0.45664
101001011010	0.07044	0.52708
101001010010	0.04256	0.56964
101010010010	0.03616	0.6058

Variable no.	Marginal prob.
1	1.0
2	0.0446
3	0.99668
4	0.30388
5	0.17468
6	0.27052
7	0.04212
8	1.0
9	0.4708
10	0.06724
11	0.99796
12	0.10688

Figure 11.6 Rheumatoid arthritis study: output from RJWinBUGS when the prior precision of β_ks is equal to $\tau_\beta^2 = 0.64$, with 'razor = 0.60'. The output is based on (in total) 25 000 iterations (five chains with 5000 iterations).

With RJMCMC, BVS is based on purely exploring the MCMC output. Since sampling is done in the combined space of model and regression coefficients, posterior information of the regression coefficients is directly available.

11.7 Spike and slab priors

An increasingly popular approach to combine variable selection with estimation of the regression parameters makes use of *variable selection priors*, better known as *spike and slab*

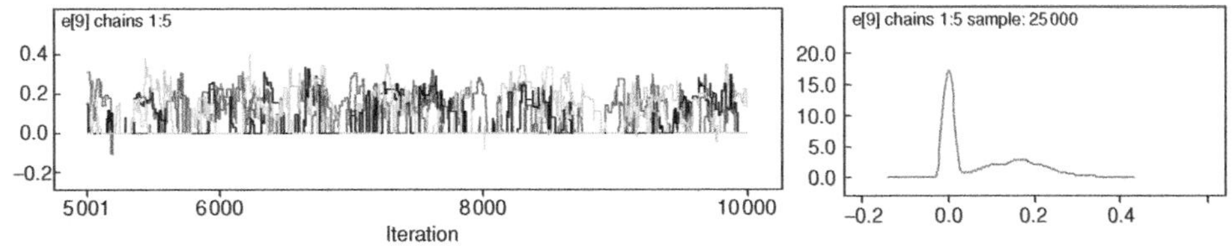

Figure 11.7 Rheumatoid arthritis study: trace plot and marginal posterior density of the regression coefficient of *sjc* using RJWinBUGS.

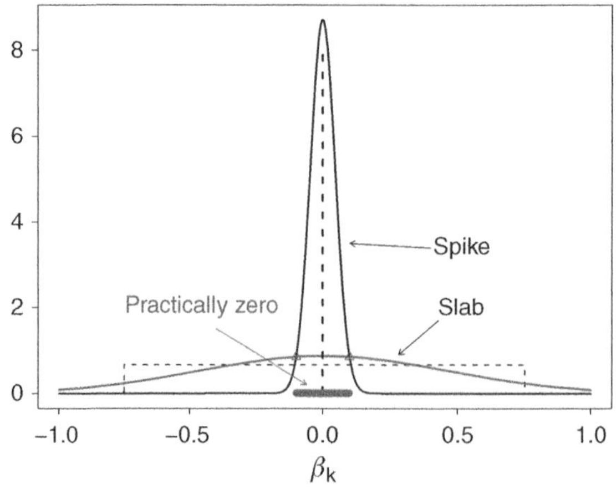

Figure 11.8 Spike and slab priors: the dashed lines correspond to the original approach of Mitchell and Beauchamp (1988), the solid lines correspond to the Gaussian mixture of George and McCulloch (1993).

priors. These priors were first suggested by Mitchell and Beauchamp (1988) for BVS with normal linear regression models. Spike and slab priors induce a positive prior probability on the hypotheses $H_0 : \beta_k = 0$ $(k = 1, \ldots, d)$. In the original formulation by Mitchell and Beauchamp (1988), the spike and slab distribution is defined as a mixture of a Dirac measure concentrated at zero and a uniform diffuse component. This mixture is shown in Figure 11.8 by the dashed lines. Here, we focus on an alternative spike and slab formulation due to George and McCulloch (1993). This choice of prior has computational advantages and can easily be implemented by the Gibbs sampler. Below, we elaborate on two BVS procedures based on spike and slab priors: *Stochastic Search Variable Selection* and *Gibbs Variable Selection*. For all approaches, we assumed that the intercept α has a flat prior or a vague normal prior $\mathrm{N}(0, \sigma_\alpha^2)$ with σ_α^2 large.

11.7.1 Stochastic Search Variable Selection

Stochastic Search Variable Selection (SSVS) was proposed by George and McCulloch (1993) for variable selection in the context of linear regression. Two versions of their variable selection procedure are circulating. In the first version, the linear predictor is given by

$$\alpha + \sum_{k=1}^{d} \beta_k x_k. \tag{11.23}$$

Further, the regression coefficients β_k are assumed to have a mixture prior of spike and slab Gaussian components. The spike element is concentrated closely around zero, reflecting the actual absence of the variable in the model (γ_k equals zero) and can be regarded as an approximation to the point mass prior in Mitchell and Beauchamp (1988). The slab component has a sufficiently large variance to allow for the 'nonzero' coefficients to be spread over larger values (γ_k equals one). The degree of separation between the two components is regulated by two tuning parameters τ_k and c_k, where $\tau_k^2 > 0$ is the variance in the spike component and $c_k^2\tau_k^2 > 0$ is the variance in the slab component (see Figure 11.8). In order to guide the choice of τ_k and c_k, it helps to note that the two Gaussian densities intersect at the points $\pm\varepsilon_k = \tau_k\delta_k$, where $\delta_k = \sqrt{2(\log c_k)c_k^2/(c_k^2 - 1)}$. The point ε_k can be regarded as a threshold for declaring 'practical significance' in that all coefficients falling into the interval $[-\varepsilon_k, \varepsilon_k]$ can be interpreted as zero. Given the parameter c_k, the variance τ_k^2 can be selected such that the intersection point reflects our perception of practical significance. The mathematical formulation of the SSVS hierarchical prior setup is then defined for $k = 1, \ldots, d$ by

$$\beta_k \mid \sigma_{\beta_k}^2 \sim \mathrm{N}(0, \sigma_{\beta_k}^2), \tag{11.24}$$

$$\sigma_{\beta_k}^2 \mid \tau_{0k}^2, \tau_{1k}^2, \gamma_k \sim (1 - \gamma_k)\delta_{\tau_{0k}^2}(\cdot) + \gamma_k\delta_{\tau_{1k}^2}(\cdot), \tag{11.25}$$

$$\sigma^2 \sim \mathrm{IG}(a_0, b_0), \tag{11.26}$$

$$\gamma_k \mid \omega_k \sim \mathrm{Bern}(\omega_k), \tag{11.27}$$

$$\omega_k \sim U(0,1), \tag{11.28}$$

with $a_0 = \nu_\gamma/2$ and $b_0 = \nu_\gamma\varsigma_\gamma/2$. Further, $\tau_{0k}^2 = \tau_k^2$ and $\tau_{1k}^2 = c_k^2\tau_k^2$; γ_k indicates the component of the mixture (for $\gamma_k = 0$ the kth regressor is 'practically zero'); $\delta_x(\cdot)$ is the Kronecker delta concentrated at point x; ν_γ and ς_γ are possibly depending on $\boldsymbol{\gamma}$ and ω_k is the prior probability that β_k is considered nonzero.

To construct the prior for the regression coefficients (combination of expressions (11.24) and (11.25)), George and McCulloch (1993) used a multivariate normal prior for $\boldsymbol{\beta}$:

$$\boldsymbol{\beta} \mid \boldsymbol{\gamma} \sim \mathrm{N}(\mathbf{0}, \mathrm{D}_\gamma \mathrm{R} \mathrm{D}_\gamma), \tag{11.29}$$

with $\boldsymbol{\gamma} = (\gamma_1, \ldots, \gamma_d)^T$, R the prior correlation matrix and $D_\gamma = \mathrm{diag}(a_1\tau_1, \ldots, a_d\tau_d)$, with $a_k = 1$ if $\gamma_k = 0$ and $a_k = c_k$ if $\gamma_k = 1$. The correlation matrix R can be taken as the identity matrix (what is used in the examples below) or $\mathrm{R} \propto (\boldsymbol{X}^T\boldsymbol{X})^{-1}$ which is a generalization of Zellner's g-prior.

Note that specifying priors (11.27) and (11.28) is equivalent to assuming the dependent prior (11.11). While prior (11.11) is preferred (see Section 11.4.1) George and McCulloch (1997) argued that model prior based on $\omega = 0.5$ (11.10) often yields sensible results and substantially reduces computational requirements. Most of our examples are, therefore, based on the latter prior, but some comparisons with the dependent prior were done.

It is important to notice that with SSVS the model is always maximal and hence there are no transdimensional jumps as with RJMCMC. Strictly speaking one could argue that SSVS is not a variable selection procedure as all variables remain in the model, but the γ_ks induce a differential shrinkage toward zero.

Due to the nonconjugacy of the priors, the analytical simplification of posterior distributions $p(\beta_k \mid \boldsymbol{y})$ and $p(\gamma_k \mid \boldsymbol{y})$ is not tractable. George and McCulloch (1993) suggested an MCMC approximation to the posteriors using the Gibbs sampler, which yields a Markov chain of regression coefficients and visited models $(\boldsymbol{\beta}^0, \sigma^0, \boldsymbol{\gamma}^0), \ldots, (\boldsymbol{\beta}^K, \sigma^K, \boldsymbol{\gamma}^K)$.

Ishwaran and Rao (2003) suggested to move the spike and slab element down in the hierarchy and place it on the variances rather than on the regression coefficients to diminish the sensitivity toward the tuning of hyperparameters. Their approach, referred to as *NMIG*

(Normal Mixture of Inverse Gammas), is equivalent to a spike and slab prior with scaled t-distributions (with $2a$ degrees of freedom and respective scales $s_1 = \sqrt{\frac{bv_0}{a}}$ and $s_2 = \sqrt{\frac{bv_1}{a}}$) as components; see Exercises 11.7 and 11.8 for practical examples.

SSVS can be extended to GLIMs without much difficulty (George *et al.* 1996). Indeed, the extension of the SSVS prior to a model $f(y \mid \boldsymbol{X\beta}, \varpi)$ with ϖ additional parameters involves replacing $p(\sigma^2)$ in the hierarchical prior by a suitable prior on ϖ. But all other priors remain the same. We now illustrate the application of the SSVS approach to a probit regression model on the REACH data set.

Example XI.8: Rheumatoid arthritis study: BVS using SSVS

In 'chapter 11 SVVS REACH.R', we applied the SSVS approach to a probit regression model to select variables from the REACH data. In addition to the original 12 covariates, 8 standardized noise variables were added for selection (see file for details). Four settings were implemented: (1) $\varepsilon = 0.01, \tau^2 = 1.1 \times 10^{-05}, c^2\tau^2 = 0.11$, (2) $\varepsilon = 0.05, \tau^2 = 0.00027$, $c^2\tau^2 = 2.7$, (3) $\varepsilon = 0.10$, $\tau^2 = 0.001$, $c^2\tau^2 = 10$, and (4) $\varepsilon = 0.10$, $\tau^2 = 0.0021$, $c^2\tau^2 = 0.21$. The first case represents a close approximation to a mass prior at zero. Mixing was good for all scenarios, 10 000 iterations were needed with 5000 burn-in iterations. The inclusion probabilities for the four scenarios are shown in Figure 11.9. It can be observed that in none of the scenarios the noise variables belonged to the MP model. Furthermore, only in scenario 1 the variables *rf* and *sjc* were selected in the MP model. In this scenario ε is the smallest, rendering it relatively easy for a variable enter the model. In Table 11.3 we show the model posterior probabilities based on scenarios 2 and 4 but based only on the 12 original variables. □

We conclude that the posterior model probabilities of a SSVS variable selection procedure show dependence on the choice of the spike and slab variances. This was also the conclusion of Rockova *et al.* (2012) in their simulation study. However, the marginal posterior inclusion probabilities, the marginal posterior summary measures of the regression coefficients and the MP model appear to be stable across the settings.

George and McCulloch (1997) introduced a variant of their SSVS procedure by setting the spike variance to zero ($\tau_{0k}^2 = 0$) and turning the spike prior into a point mass prior. For

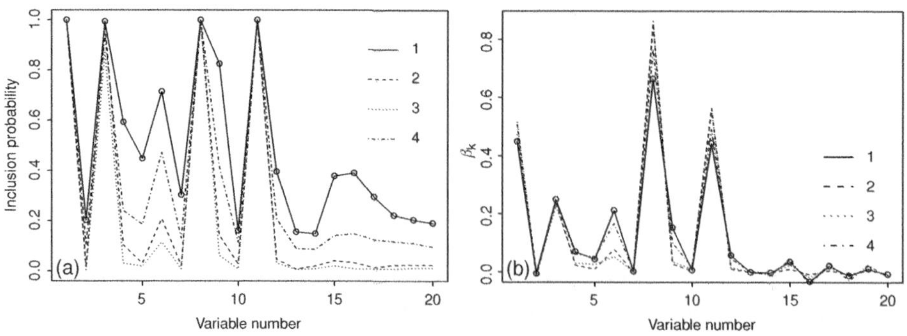

Figure 11.9 Rheumatoid arthritis study: comparison of (a) marginal posterior inclusion probabilities, and (b) posterior means of regression coefficients obtained from SSVS based on four scenarios (for details see Example XI.8).

such a prior the kth regressor is effectively removed from model (11.23) when $\gamma_k = 0$ such that in fact model (11.30) applies. Further, the authors suggested a conjugate version of the spike and slab algorithm by assuming $\beta_k \mid \sigma^2_{\beta_k}, \sigma^2 \sim \mathrm{N}(0, \sigma^2 \sigma^2_{\beta_k})$. With an inverse gamma prior for σ^2 the marginal prior $\beta_k \mid \sigma^2_{\beta_k}$ becomes a mixture of t-distributions. The advantage of this approach is that $\boldsymbol{\beta}$ and σ^2 can be integrated out from the joint posterior to yield $p(\boldsymbol{\gamma} \mid \mathbf{y})$ up to a constant. Based on this marginal posterior, a Gibbs-sampling algorithm can be constructed that yields a MCMC sequence $\boldsymbol{\gamma}^1, \ldots, \boldsymbol{\gamma}^K$. Alternatively, they suggested to use the MC^3 algorithm whereby regressors are randomly selected or deleted from the current model. The parameters $\boldsymbol{\beta}_{\boldsymbol{\gamma}}, \sigma^2$ can be sampled in an extra step given $\boldsymbol{\gamma}$. This SSVS version received recently quite some attention when many variables are involved (see Section 11.9)). In the nonconjugate case the authors suggested the sampling approaches of Carlin and Chib (1995) (see Section 11.7.2) or the RJMCMC algorithm.

In both SSVS implementations, BVS is achieved through the evaluation of the MCMC output as with RJMCMC but there are some differences especially with the first version. In the first version of SSVS no matter the value of $\boldsymbol{\gamma}$, all regressors remain in the model. Regressors corresponding to $\gamma_k = 0$ are considered to be practically zero implying thereby a change in definition of a MAP and a MP model. However, while a regressor is never removed from the model the marginal posterior of β_k might still be bimodal as with RJMCMC. When there is strong evidence against the inclusion of a variable, the spike will dominate the posterior and the posterior mean will be shrunk toward zero. Note that the decision on whether or not a variable enters the model (practical significance) can be done by *hard thresholding/selection shrinkage* where variables are only included if the absolute value of the estimated coefficient (e.g. posterior mean) exceeds some threshold value (say the intersection point ε). Finally, we have seen that the second implementation of SSVS has a similar flavor as RJMCMC.

11.7.2 Gibbs Variable Selection

Another approach for BVS based on a spike and slab prior was suggested by Dellaportas *et al.* (2002). In their approach, called *Gibbs Variable Selection (GVS)*, the variable indicator is introduced into the model. That is, the linear predictor of the model is equal to

$$\alpha + \sum_{k=1}^{d} \gamma_k \beta_k x_k. \tag{11.30}$$

Related variable selection techniques that allow for exclusion of regressors were proposed by George and McCulloch (1997) (second SSVS version), Carlin and Chib (1995), Kuo and Mallick (1998). It is now instructive to have a closer inspection of the full conditionals of the different spike and slab algorithms. First, we treat the regression parameters (neglecting additional parameters such as σ^2). For β_k we can write

$$\begin{aligned} p(\mathbf{y}, \boldsymbol{\beta}, \boldsymbol{\gamma}) &= p(\mathbf{y}, \beta_k, \boldsymbol{\beta}_{(k)}, \boldsymbol{\gamma}), \\ &= p(\mathbf{y} \mid \boldsymbol{\beta}, \boldsymbol{\gamma}) p(\beta_k \mid \boldsymbol{\beta}_{(k)}, \boldsymbol{\gamma}) p(\boldsymbol{\beta}_{(k)} \mid \boldsymbol{\gamma}) p(\boldsymbol{\gamma}), \end{aligned} \tag{11.31}$$

with $\boldsymbol{\beta}_{(k)}$ the vector of regression coefficients without β_k.

For the first version of SSVS, it is assumed that $p(\beta_k \mid \boldsymbol{\beta}_{(k)}, \boldsymbol{\gamma}) = p(\beta_k \mid \gamma_k)$ and, irrespective of $\gamma_k = 1$ or $\gamma_k = 0$, β_k is always contained in $p(\boldsymbol{y} \mid \boldsymbol{\beta}, \boldsymbol{\gamma})$. By removing the constant terms in expression (11.31) the full conditionals for the regression parameters are: $p(\beta_k \mid \boldsymbol{y}, \boldsymbol{\gamma}, \boldsymbol{\beta}_{(k)}) \propto p(\boldsymbol{y} \mid \boldsymbol{\beta}, \boldsymbol{\gamma}) p(\beta_k \mid \gamma_k)$.

Kuo and Mallick (1998) assumed that the prior of $\boldsymbol{\beta}$ is independent of $\boldsymbol{\gamma}$, i.e. $p(\boldsymbol{\beta})$ such that $p(\beta_k \mid \boldsymbol{\beta}_{(k)}, \boldsymbol{\gamma}) = p(\beta_k \mid \boldsymbol{\beta}_{(k)})$. Now, $p(\boldsymbol{y} \mid \boldsymbol{\beta}, \boldsymbol{\gamma})$ only contains β_k when $\gamma_k = 1$. Removing the constant terms then yields two expressions:

$$p(\beta_k \mid \boldsymbol{y}, \boldsymbol{\gamma}, \boldsymbol{\beta}_{(k)}) \propto \begin{cases} p(\boldsymbol{y} \mid \boldsymbol{\beta}, \boldsymbol{\gamma}) p(\beta_k \mid \boldsymbol{\beta}_{(k)}) & \text{if } \gamma_k = 1, \\ p(\beta_k \mid \boldsymbol{\beta}_{(k)}) & \text{if } \gamma_k = 0. \end{cases} \tag{11.32}$$

For GVS, it is again assumed that β_k depends only on γ_k, i.e. $p(\beta_k \mid \boldsymbol{\beta}_{(k)}, \boldsymbol{\gamma}) = p(\beta_k \mid \gamma_k)$. Further, Dellaportas *et al.* (2002) suggested to take

$$p(\beta_k \mid \gamma_k) = (1 - \gamma_k)\mathrm{N}(\mu_{0k}, \tau_{0k}^2) + \gamma_k \mathrm{N}(\mu_{1k}, \tau_{1k}^2), \tag{11.33}$$

for appropriate choices of $\tau_{0k}^2 \ll \tau_{1k}^2$ and μ_{0k}, μ_{1k}. When $\mu_{0k} = \mu_{1k} = 0$ expression (11.33) is equivalent to expressions (11.24, 11.25).

Note that $p(\boldsymbol{y} \mid \boldsymbol{\beta}, \boldsymbol{\gamma})$ contains β_k only when $\gamma_k = 1$ and combined with prior (11.33), the full conditional for β_k becomes

$$p(\beta_k \mid \boldsymbol{y}, \boldsymbol{\gamma}, \boldsymbol{\beta}_{(k)}) \propto \begin{cases} p(\boldsymbol{y} \mid \boldsymbol{\beta}, \boldsymbol{\gamma}) \mathrm{N}(\mu_{1k}, \tau_{1k}^2) & \text{if } \gamma_k = 1, \\ \mathrm{N}(\mu_{0k}, \tau_{0k}^2) & \text{if } \gamma_k = 0. \end{cases} \tag{11.34}$$

The distribution $\mathrm{N}(\mu_{0k}, \tau_{0k}^2)$ is the prior $p(\beta_k \mid \gamma_k = 0)$ and is called a *pseudo-prior*. This prior does not affect the posterior distribution but is regarded as a 'linking density' to increase the efficiency of the sampler (Carlin and Chib 1995). In principle, this linking density should be chosen such that sampling is optimized, e.g. here by choosing optimal values for μ_{1k} and τ_{1k}^2. But, in practice, such an exercise is considered impractical. In the WinBUGS program of Ntzoufras, $\mu_{1k} = 0$ while the spike and slab variances were taken as in the SSVS approach.

Finally, the full conditional for γ_k is Bernoulli with success probability $O_k/(1 + O_k)$ with the odds O_k equal to

$$\frac{p(\gamma_k = 1 \mid \boldsymbol{\gamma}_{(k)}, \boldsymbol{\beta}, \boldsymbol{y})}{p(\gamma_k = 0 \mid \boldsymbol{\gamma}_{(k)}, \boldsymbol{\beta}, \boldsymbol{y})} = \frac{p(\boldsymbol{y} \mid \boldsymbol{\beta}, \gamma_k = 1, \boldsymbol{\gamma}_{(k)})\, p(\boldsymbol{\beta} \mid \gamma_k = 1, \boldsymbol{\gamma}_{(k)})\, p(\gamma_k = 1, \boldsymbol{\gamma}_{(k)})}{p(\boldsymbol{y} \mid \boldsymbol{\beta}, \gamma_k = 0, \boldsymbol{\gamma}_{(k)})\, p(\boldsymbol{\beta} \mid \gamma_k = 0, \boldsymbol{\gamma}_{(k)})\, p(\gamma_k = 0, \boldsymbol{\gamma}_{(k)})}. \tag{11.35}$$

Expression (11.35) again illustrates the difference between the approaches. For instance for the SSVS approach, the first term on the RHS in expression (11.35) cancels out while for the approach of Kuo and Mallick (1998) the second term cancels out. Only for the GVS the whole expression is needed.

From the full conditionals we may conclude that, although regressors are effectively removed from the model by the γ_ks, the dimensionality of the model remains constant since all β_ks remain in the MCMC process. This is important for the computational procedure. In

Exercise 11.9, the REACH data are analyzed using the GVS approach. In Exercise 11.10, the approach of Kuo and Mallick (1998) is applied.

11.7.3 Dependent variable selection using SSVS

In Section 11.4, the dependent prior (11.11) was introduced to correct for multiplicity but this prior does not regulate the selection procedure when a particular ordering of the variables included in the model should be respected. Chipman (1996) suggested a mathematical way of expressing beliefs about the relationships between regressors. More specifically, he suggested priors that assign degrees of beliefs on including interactions and higher order polynomials, grouped regressors, competing regressors and restrictions on the number of regressors in the model. Prior (11.11) is an example of the last class where $p(\boldsymbol{\gamma})$ is in fact a function of $d_{\gamma} = \sum_{k=1}^{d} \gamma_k$, the size of the model.

Good statistical practice instructs to include interaction terms in a model only when main effects are included and that when rth order polynomial terms are in the model then also $(r-1)$th, $(r-2)$th, ... order polynomial terms should be included. None of the BVS algorithms forces variable selection to adhere to these principles. Chipman (1996) shows how to factorize the prior $p(\boldsymbol{\gamma})$ such that a particular selection ordering is respected. More specifically, when there are two regressors x_1 ($\gamma_1 = 1$), x_2 ($\gamma_2 = 1$) and their interaction $x_3 = x_1 \times x_2$ ($\gamma_3 = 1$), he suggested

$$p(\gamma_1, \gamma_2, \gamma_3) = p(\gamma_1, \gamma_2)\, p(\gamma_3 \mid \gamma_1, \gamma_2) = p(\gamma_1) p(\gamma_2)\, p(\gamma_3 \mid \gamma_1, \gamma_2), \tag{11.36}$$

assuming independence for the main effects but dependence of the interaction term on the main effects. For $p(\gamma_3 \mid \gamma_1, \gamma_2)$ there are four probabilities for including an interaction term: $p(\gamma_3 = 1 \mid \gamma_1 = 0, \gamma_2 = 0) = \pi_{00}$, $p(\gamma_3 = 1 \mid \gamma_1 = 1, \gamma_2 = 0) = \pi_{10}$, $p(\gamma_3 = 1 \mid \gamma_1 = 0, \gamma_2 = 1) = \pi_{01}$ and $p(\gamma_3 = 1 \mid \gamma_1 = 1, \gamma_2 = 1) = \pi_{11}$. Good statistical practice dictates: $\pi_{00} = \pi_{01} = \pi_{10} = 0$ and $\pi_{11} = \pi$, but Chipman (1996) also considers other cases. This prior can be implemented in WinBUGS by the inclusion of some extra commands. Namely, γ_1 and γ_2 could be given independent Bernoulli distributions with probability ω (say) $= 0.5$, while γ_3 could be given a Bernoulli distribution with probability $0.5\gamma_1\gamma_2$. Kuo and Mallick (1998) suggested another solution. That is, by choosing as regression coefficients $\beta_1\,[1-(1-\gamma_1)(1-\gamma_3)]$, $\beta_2\,[1-(1-\gamma_2)(1-\gamma_3)]$ and $\beta_3\gamma_3$, respectively, the regressors x_1 and x_2 are in the model once the product term is chosen; see Exercise 11.12 for testing interaction terms in the probit regression model on the REACH data. In addition, Chipman (1996) suggested prior distributions to select regressors in groups or competing regressors. This can be easily implemented in WinBUGS (see Exercise 11.13).

At the end of this chapter, we report on more recent approaches to perform dependent variable selection.

11.8 Bayesian regularization

The classical LASSO approach delivers L_1-penalized estimates of the regression coefficients and turns into a forward variable selection by gradually increasing the penalty term λ. BVS is computationally demanding primarily because the model space needs to be explored to find the most promising models. If this exploration could be replaced by an estimation technique, a considerable gain in computation time might be achieved.

11.8.1 Bayesian LASSO regression

The link between the classical ridge estimator and the MAP of a normal linear regression model with a Gaussian prior (Section 5.7) suggests that such a link also exists for the LASSO method. Indeed, Tibshirani (1996) noticed that, given σ^2 and λ, the LASSO estimate is the MAP of a normal linear regression model with independent and identical Laplace priors for the regression coefficients. Park and Casella (2008) built on this result but proposed a slightly different prior. They suggested to take the following conditional Laplace prior

$$p(\boldsymbol{\beta} \mid \sigma^2) = \prod_{k=1}^{d} \frac{\lambda}{2\sigma} \mathrm{e}^{-\lambda|\beta_k|/\sigma}. \tag{11.37}$$

This prior differs from the prior of Tibshirani by the inclusion of σ. Conditioning on σ guarantees the unimodality of the posterior of β_k $(k = 1, \ldots, d)$.

However, Gibbs sampling based on this prior yields unfamiliar full conditionals due to the absolute values $|\beta_k|$ in expression (11.37). Using a latent parameter τ^2 one can rewrite the prior (11.37) as a scale mixture of normals with an exponential distribution as mixing density (Andrews and Mallows 1974):

$$\frac{\lambda}{2}\mathrm{e}^{-\lambda|y|} = \int_0^\infty \frac{1}{\sqrt{2\pi\tau^2}} \mathrm{e}^{-y^2/(2\tau^2)} \frac{\lambda^2}{2} \mathrm{e}^{-\lambda^2\tau^2/2} \mathrm{d}\tau^2, \ \lambda > 0. \tag{11.38}$$

This leads to an hierarchical representation of the prior structure, namely,

$$\begin{aligned}
\beta_k \mid \sigma^2_{\beta_k} &\sim \mathrm{N}(0, \sigma^2_{\beta_k}), \ (k = 1, \ldots, d) \\
\sigma^2_{\beta_k} &= \sigma^2 \tau_k^2, \qquad\qquad (11.39) \\
\tau_k^2 &\sim \frac{\lambda^2}{2} \mathrm{e}^{-\lambda^2\tau_k^2/2}, \ (k = 1, \ldots, d) \\
\sigma^2 &\sim p(\sigma^2), \qquad\qquad (11.40)
\end{aligned}$$

which, together with the normal linear regression likelihood given by expression (11.2), is the basis for the *Bayesian LASSO*. Park and Casella (2008) suggested to use a Jeffreys prior or an inverse-gamma prior for σ^2. With these priors and for fixed λ, the Bayesian LASSO posterior mode is equal to the classical LASSO MLE. This follows from the derivations in Section 5.6.1.

Both the LASSO prior and the spike and slab prior are normal mixtures: the first prior is a continuous mixture of normal distributions while the second prior is a discrete mixture on the variances. Figure 11.10 shows that the LASSO prior provides an approximation to the spike and slab prior. One can, therefore, expect that the LASSO prior induces shrinkage of the regression coefficients toward zero. However, while the classical LASSO shrinks some of the coefficients to exactly zero, this happens with the Bayesian LASSO only with the posterior

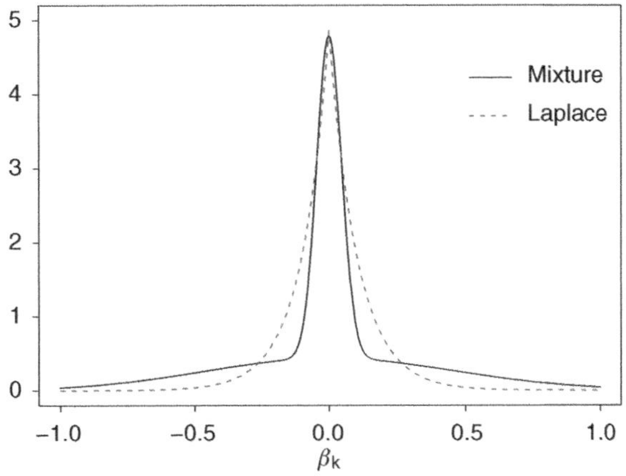

Figure 11.10 Comparison (Gaussian mixture) spike and slab prior with approximating Laplace prior.

mode (with σ fixed). Thus, Figure 11.2 can only show up with the Bayesian LASSO for the posterior mode and not for the posterior mean or median.

Which value of λ should be taken? For the classical LASSO the optimal λ is obtained from cross-validation, but for the Bayesian LASSO a more natural procedure is to give λ a hyperprior. Park and Casella (2008) suggested to give λ^2 the following vague gamma hyperprior

$$p(\lambda^2) = \frac{\delta^r}{\Gamma(r)}(\lambda^2)^{r-1}e^{-\delta\lambda^2}, \qquad r > 0, \delta > 0. \tag{11.41}$$

The choice of the gamma hyperprior for λ^2 ensures a conditional conjugate prior for λ^2 together with (11.40). The authors suggested small values for r and δ. For the posterior estimates of the regression coefficients one averages over the posterior distribution of λ, which produces more stable parameter estimates.

We have seen that for the classical LASSO approach there are computational problems (standard error is often estimated as zero) and statistical issues that prevent them to be reported, e.g. the R package `penalized` does not provide standard errors. However, Kyung *et al.* (2010) argued that standard errors are needed for prediction. From a numerical viewpoint, there is no reason why not to calculate standard errors with the Bayesian LASSO approach since the MCMC methods provide automatically posterior estimates of the standard errors with good behavior (Kyung *et al.* 2010).

We now illustrate Bayesian LASSO regression with the diabetes data. There are several R packages that offer classical LASSO regression, but only a few that do Bayesian LASSO regression. Here, we illustrate the use of the R package monomvn.

Example XI.9: Diabetes study: BVS using Bayesian LASSO

In 'chapter 11 Lasso and Blasso diabetes.R', penalized estimation approaches are applied with the R package monomvn. The `blasso` program is part of the R package and provides

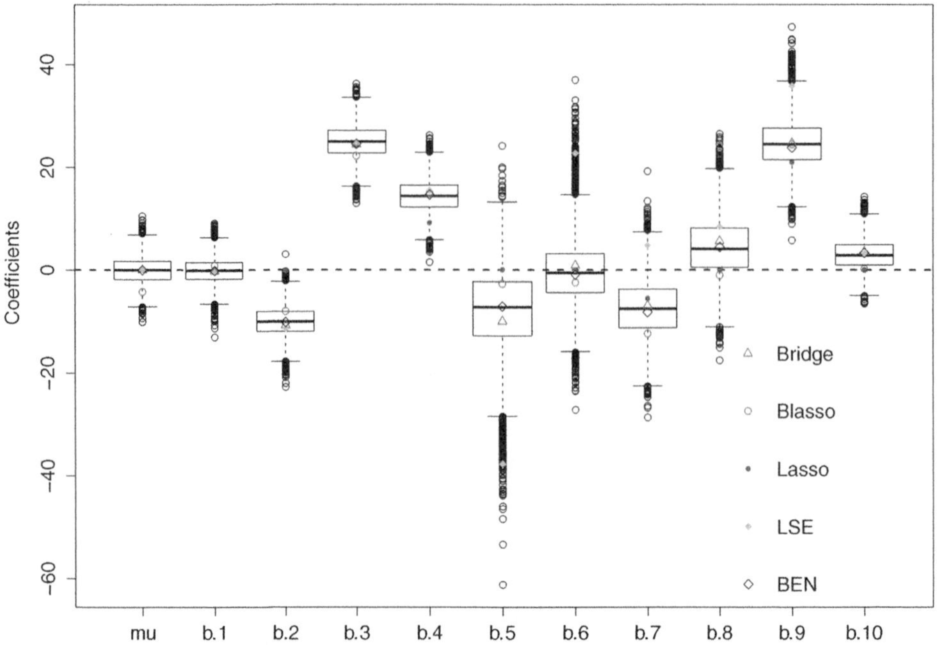

Figure 11.11 Diabetes study: Bayesian LASSO estimates (MAP) of regression coefficients compared to LSE, classical LASSO, Bayesian ridge (Bridge, posterior mean) and Bayesian Elastic Net (BEN, posterior mean) estimates.'mu' stands for intercept, 'b.x' represents the xth regression coefficient.

Bayesian LASSO regression using the approach of Park and Casella (2008). The package also provides classical and Bayesian ridge regression.

We performed here Bayesian ridge regression, classical and Bayesian LASSO regression on the diabetes data. The estimated regression coefficients are found in Table 11.1.

The classical LASSO solution was obtained by leave-one-out cross-validation based on the C_p-Mallows statistic; we obtained $\widehat{\lambda} = 224$. For the Bayesian LASSO, we applied `blasso` and a WinBUGS program with compatible settings for the prior distributions. In both cases a single chain was taken of length 10 000 with 2000 burn-in sample. In Figure 11.11, the ridge, LASSO and OLS estimates are contrasted with the Bayesian estimates. In this figure also the response is centered to enhance the legibility of the graph. The LASSO MAP is based on the marginal posterior mode of the regression coefficients (marginalized over the λ^2 posterior distribution). The following conclusions could be drawn: (1) the Bayesian LASSO estimates are often close to the classical LASSO estimates, (2) classical and Bayesian LASSO estimates may deviate considerably from the OLS estimate, and (3) more uniform shrinkage is seen with the ridge procedure. The MAP of the Bayesian LASSO (marginal mode) does not coincide with the classical LASSO estimate as it never shrinks to exactly zero. The posterior median of λ^2 is 0.081 with 95% CI = [0.052, 0.11]. A comparison of the classical and the Bayesian λ estimates is, however, not useful because of the different settings in the programs. In addition, we have implemented Bayesian LASSO in WinBUGS ('chapter 11 Blasso diabetes.odc'). The

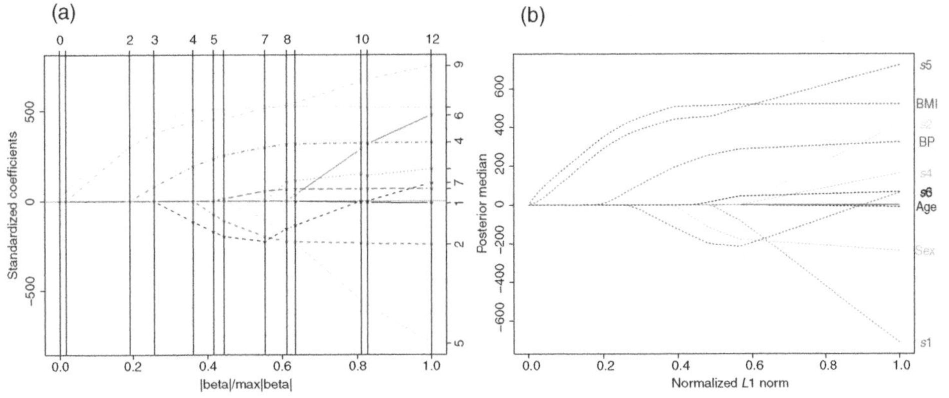

Figure 11.12 Diabetes study: paths of (a) classical LASSO estimates (MLE) and (b) Bayesian LASSO estimates (median) for varying values of λ.

posterior regression estimates were about the same as those from `blasso`, but the processing time for WinBUGS was 763 seconds compared to 5 seconds for `blasso`.

In Section 11.2.2, we have seen that the LASSO approach offers a variable selection procedure by varying λ (see Figure 11.2). A similar graph can be constructed with the Bayesian LASSO approach, but this option is not supported by `monomvn`. A self-written R program produced the graph in Figure 11.12(b) based on the posterior median value of the regression estimates. There is here a remarkable correspondence with the LASSO graph in Figure 11.12(a) produced by the R package `lars`. Note that, in general, the plot of the Bayesian LASSO path is more smooth when based on posterior medians or posterior means.

Finally, to evaluate the impact of the settings on the gamma hyperprior of λ^2 on the estimated λ, we varied the parameters of $p(\lambda^2)$ since their choice is not intuitively clear, besides that they should be small to ensure vagueness. We chose 16 combinations of r and δ from the set $\{0.01, 0.05, 0.5, 1\}$. The conclusion of our exercise was that the posterior median of λ showed more stability than the other posterior summary measures and hence appears preferable. □

We may be enthusiastic that the classical LASSO has been extended to the Bayesian LASSO. But, what is the advantage using the Bayesian version since it may take considerable more time to produce the solution? The advantage cannot be judged from our examples but should be deduced from simulation studies or analytical calculations. This was done by Kyung *et al.* (2010) who showed that the mean squared prediction errors evaluated on test data were often lower for the Bayesian LASSO (and variants).

The classical LASSO approach performs simultaneously variable selection and parameter estimation. Zou (2006) and Zhao and Yu (2006) showed that the classical LASSO procedure does not possess the *oracle property* which means it is not guaranteed that, when $n \to \infty$, the correct model is chosen with estimated regression coefficients that converge to the true values. The reason for this is that some regression coefficients need much more shrinkage (corresponding to unimportant regressors) than others. To resolve this problem, Zou (2006) suggested the *adaptive LASSO* approach which replaces $\lambda \sum_{k=1}^{d} |\beta_k|$ in expression (11.3) by

$\lambda \sum_{k=1}^{d} w_k|\beta_k|$ with $w_k = 1/|\widehat{\beta}_k^{\nu}|$ and $\widehat{\beta}_k$ the OLS estimate of β_k and $\nu > 0$ a user-chosen constant. He proved that (under some regularity conditions) the adaptive LASSO satisfies the oracle property. The *adaptive Bayesian LASSO* follows immediately by allowing τ_k^2 to have different priors, i.e. to replace expression (11.40) by

$$\tau_k^2 \sim \frac{\lambda_k^2}{2} e^{-\lambda_k^2 \tau_k^2/2} \ (k = 1, \ldots, d)$$

(Leng *et al.* 2009). A large posterior value of λ_k is then associated with a relatively larger shrinkage of β_k. Leng *et al.* (2009) noted important improvements in terms of variable selection in some of their examples.

There appears to be no R package that performs adaptive Bayesian LASSO, but it is quite easy to adapt a Bayesian LASSO WinBUGS program to the adaptive version; see Exercise 11.14 for an example. An extension of the Bayesian LASSO to probit regression can be found in Bae and Mallick (2004). They used the latent representation of the probit model whereby $Y = 1 \Leftrightarrow Z > 0$ and $Z \sim N(\boldsymbol{x}^T\boldsymbol{\beta}, 1)$ in combination with the settings of Park and Casella (2008) for $\sigma = 1$. In a similar manner the adaptive Bayesian LASSO can be extended to GLIMs. Again, no software appears to be available, though a WinBUGS program can easily be implemented.

11.8.2 Elastic Net and further extensions of the Bayesian LASSO

Recent efforts in generalizing the penalization methodology to more complex data structures crystalized in several innovations of the LASSO approach. Often these new approaches are first developed in classical statistics and then given a Bayesian analogue. In the linear regression setting, Tibshirani *et al.* (2005) proposed the *Fused LASSO* for predictors that have a natural ordering, where the penalty is a linear combination of a L_1 penalty on the coefficients and a L_1 penalty on their first order differences. Such a penalty induces similarity between neighboring regression coefficients. In case grouping among regression coefficients is suspected but unknown, Zou and Hastie (2005) suggested *Elastic Net*, which combines the LASSO and ridge penalties into one penalty and as such tends to keep the related variables in the model as a group with estimated coefficients nearly equal. This behavior is appreciated in modeling, for instance, with gene expression data where related genes should enter the model as a group.

When the groups of predictors are known (e.g. group of dummy variables or spline coefficients), Yuan and Lin (2006) proposed the *Grouped LASSO*, which penalizes elliptical norms of the coefficients for each group. The Bayesian counterparts of these LASSO alternatives emerge by adapting the prior (11.37) to the various penalties and reexpressing these priors as scale mixtures of normals (Kyung *et al.* 2010; Li and Lin 2010).

The *Bayesian elastic net (BEN)*, proposed by Zou and Hastie (2005) and Li and Lin (2010) in the context of linear regression, constitutes a compromise between LASSO and ridge regression enjoying the advantages of the two. The elastic net prior inherits the sparsity property from the LASSO, since it is also not differentiable at zero, and at the same time encourages grouping which is typical for the ridge prior.

The frequentist penalty term L_{net} for the 'naive' Elastic Net of Zou and Hastie (2005) is the linear combination of L_1 and L_2 penalties, i.e. $L_{net}(\boldsymbol{\beta}) = \lambda_1 \sum_{k=1}^{d} |\beta_k| + \lambda_2 \sum_{k=1}^{d} \beta_k^2$. For

BEN, the prior for $\boldsymbol{\beta}$ should depend on σ for the same reason as with the Bayesian LASSO:

$$p(\boldsymbol{\beta} \mid \sigma^2) \propto \exp\left\{-\frac{\lambda_1}{\sigma}\sum_{k=1}^{d}|\beta_k| - \frac{\lambda_2}{2\sigma^2}\sum_{k=1}^{d}\beta_k^2\right\}. \tag{11.42}$$

Using latent parameters $\tau_1^2, \ldots, \tau_d^2$ and identity (11.38), we obtain the hierarchical representation of the prior structure:

$$\begin{aligned} \beta_k \mid \sigma_{\beta_k}^2 &\sim \mathrm{N}\left(0, \sigma_{\beta_k}^2\right), \ (k = 1, \ldots, d) \\ \sigma_{\beta_k}^2 &= \sigma^2(\tau_k^{-2} + \lambda_2)^{-1}, \ (k = 1, \ldots, d) \\ \tau_k^2 &\sim \frac{\lambda_1^2}{2} \mathrm{e}^{-\lambda_1^2 \tau_k^2/2}, \ (k = 1, \ldots, d) \\ \sigma^2 &\sim p(\sigma^2). \end{aligned} \tag{11.43}$$

Diffuse hyperpriors for the two penalization parameters λ_1 and λ_2 are added in the formulation to circumvent the uncertainty in their selection. As λ_1 pertains to the LASSO part, λ_1^2 is given a gamma prior while λ_2 is given a gamma prior since it acts as a rate (σ^2/λ_2 plays the role of the prior variance of β_k). Ghosh (2007) raised concerns about the Elastic Net approach because it is based on the ordinary Bayesian LASSO on therefore cannot satisfy the oracle properties. He suggested, therefore, the *adaptive Elastic Net*. The *Bayesian adaptive Elastic Net* is constructed by replacing λ_1 in (11.43) with d different λs pertaining to the d regressors.

Finally, recently hybrid algorithms combining LASSO priors with MCMC procedures have been suggested. For instance, Hans (2009) complemented the LASSO prior with the point mass at zero and provided Gibbs sampling schemes (combined with RJMCMC) as an alternative to the approach of Park and Casella (2008). Also, the R package monomvn offers an hybrid sampling algorithm.

Example XI.10: Diabetes study: BVS using extensions of the Bayesian LASSO approach
The results from the Bayesian Elastic Net displayed in Figure 11.9 can be obtained from the WinBUGS program 'chapter 11 BEN diabetes.odc'. The posterior means of most regression coefficients are close to the ridge estimates, but for the important regressors the BEN estimates show more shrinkage. The two penalty parameters were estimated as $\widehat{\lambda}_1 = 3.94$ and $\widehat{\lambda}_2 = 8.94$ (posterior median).

We also applied the option in the R package monomvn which combines the Bayesian LASSO procedure with RJMCMC, but obtained basically the same posterior summary measures. Due to the RJMCMC option, variables are now effectively selected and dropped from the model. □

11.9 The many regressors case

Applications with many regressors (d large) pose computational and statistical challenges, especially when $d > n$. Examples of such applications are: (1) GWA studies where several thousands of genome variables are to be related with phenotypes (physical characteristics, the presence or absence of diseases in humans, animals, plants, etc); (2) functional Magnetic

Resonance Imaging (fMRI) data, where one aims to model brain effective connectivity from neuroimaging data and the number of nodes are small; (3) adverse event monitoring based on huge data bases, etc. For such applications the (classical and Bayesian) BVS techniques cannot be immediately applied, but a (slight) twist in the computational procedure could make them again suitable. That computational difficulties occur can be easily inferred for Gibbs-based sampling procedures from the full conditionals. With Bayesian LASSO the full conditionals of the regression coefficients involve the inversion of the covariance matrix pertaining to (a block of) regression coefficients (Kyung *et al.* 2010). When hundreds or more of variables are involved, either computational instability is implied ($d \approx n$) or sampling is impossible ($d \gg n$). Chen *et al.* (2011) suggested to combine the Bayesian LASSO approach with the RJMCMC procedure whereby the size of the model is given a truncated Poisson prior on the range $0 - d$. Nevertheless, variable selection is possible even when $d > n$ since in each step only part of the variable set is active. Another example of a combined LASSO-RJMCMC approach is provided by the R package `monomvn`.

Much of the recent developments in variable selection techniques have been inspired by studies involving DNA microarrays where the purpose is to classify and predict phenotypes from (a huge number of) gene expression profiles. Examples can be found in Lee *et al.* (2003), Sha *et al.* (2004), Yi *et al.* (2005), Tadesse *et al.* (2005), Swartz *et al.* (2006) and Pikkuhookana and Silanpää (2009).

Two recent contributions that are based on the probit regression model using the latent normal representation are from Yang and Song (2010) and Kwon *et al.* (2011). The approach of Yang and Song (2010) is an extension of the SSVS approach of George and McCulloch (1997) with a mass prior and it is based on a prior first proposed by West (2000). It can be verified (George and McCulloch 1993) that the full conditional of $\boldsymbol{\beta}_\gamma$ involves the inverse of $\boldsymbol{X}_\gamma^T\boldsymbol{X}_\gamma$. Hence, this computation collapses when $d_\gamma > n$, which also happens with Zellner's g-prior for $\boldsymbol{\beta}_\gamma$. The extension of Yang and Song (2010) consists of replacing the classical inverse $(\boldsymbol{X}_\gamma^T\boldsymbol{X}_\gamma)^{-1}$ by the Moore–Penrose generalized inverse $(\boldsymbol{X}_\gamma^T\boldsymbol{X}_\gamma)^{+}$. Another generalization is proposed by Kwon *et al.* (2011) who suggested a Correlation-Based Search algorithm, the *hybrid-CBS*, which extends SSVS to high-dimensional correlated regressors. Variable addition, deletion and swapping are done as in SSVS except that now correlation of the regressors is taken into account. That is, the added regressor is chosen such that it shows a low correlation with a (randomly chosen) regressor already in the model while the deleted regressor has a large correlation with a (randomly chosen) regressor already in the model. It is clear that these recent developments are algorithms that combine existing algorithms (in a clever manner) such as SSVS (or GVS), RJMCMC or Bayesian LASSO.

Example XI.11: Glioma study: BVS when $d > n$

Gliomas are the most common primary brain tumors with heterogeneous morphology and variable prognosis. Treatment decisions in patients rely mainly on histologic classification and clinical parameters. However, differences between histologic subclasses and grades are subtle, and classifying gliomas is subject to a large interobserver variability. To improve current classification standards, Gravendeel *et al.* (2009) have performed gene expression profiling on a cohort of glioma samples from 276 patients undergoing surgery at Erasmus University Medical Center (Rotterdam, the Netherlands) between 1989 and 2005 of all histologic subtypes and grades and related it to the patient's survival time (defined as time between death and surgery). We have selected for this exercise a subset of 100 patients which were analyzed for an expression of 115 selected genes which showed relatively high variability among the

100 samples. Note that each measurement quantifies the abundance of the corresponding messenger RNA transcript and thereby the intensity with which the gene is expressed.

Because censoring occurred in only 15% of the subjects it was ignored. In our sample for only 1 patient there was censoring. Further, we assumed that on the log-scale the survival time has a normal distribution in a regression model with the gene expression variables as covariates. The aim of this exercise is to determine the subset of genes associated with the survival time. To this end, we applied three variable selection techniques (see R program 'chapter 11 glioma data analysis.R'):

LASSO: Classical LASSO variable selection was performed with the R package `penalized`. The penalty parameter $\widehat{\lambda} = 1.09$ was found by locating the maximum of the cross-validated profile likelihood evaluated on a dense grid. Despite its appeal, LASSO variable selection possesses several deficiencies: in $d > n$ settings it is not possible to select more than n variables in the model (which is a problem, however, in extreme cases), the selection of the optimal penalty parameter is time consuming and the computation of the standard errors is not straightforward (if required). The variables selected by LASSO with $\widehat{\lambda} = 1.09$ were $X11075, X55800, X2861, X81031, X117154, X166752, X10643, X25834$ and $X158763$.

Bayesian LASSO: Bayesian LASSO variable selection was performed with the R package `monomvn` using the RJMCMC option. Based on 10 000 iterations with a burn-in period of length 1000, the posterior inclusion probabilities have been computed and plotted in Figure 11.13. Based on the MP model criterion, we selected 42 genes. The Bayesian LASSO model estimates (posterior means without the RJMCMC facility) are plotted in Figure 11.13.

Spike and slab: Spike and slab models were obtained from the `spikeslab` R package which provides BMA estimates. The BMA estimates are based on a rescaled spike and slab model, a variant of the spike and slab model that induces a nonvanishing penalization effect independent of the sample size (Ishwaran and Rao 2005). In the classical spike and slab models, the penalty effect becomes swamped by the likelihood as the sample size n increases, reducing the ability of the prior to impact model selection. Instead, in the rescaled spike and slab model the y responses are replaced with $\sqrt{n}$ rescaled values. This makes it possible for the prior to retain a nonvanishing effect with increasing sample size. First, the BMA estimates are computed using the rescaled spike and slab model. In the second step, d penalty parameters (unique to each coefficient) are determined such that the corresponding generalized ridge estimates are close to the BMA estimates. In the third step, the L_1 regularization path is determined using the R package `lars`. The optimal L_1 penalty parameter λ_1 is obtained as a value that minimizes the AIC criterion. This penalty leads to the inclusion of the genes $X11075$, $X55800$, $X81031$, $X166752$, $X10643$, $X25834$, $X158763$, $X9118$ and $X358$, and hence shows quite some overlap with the other two solutions.

Further testing is usually needed to find the real putative genes, but this was not the aim of this exercise (which was only based on part of the data). □

It must be clear from our exposition that the area of BVS is progressing fast. Over the last decade, there has been an explosion of new developments. That this is not going to stop quickly is illustrated below where we describe yet other original approaches to optimize BVS.

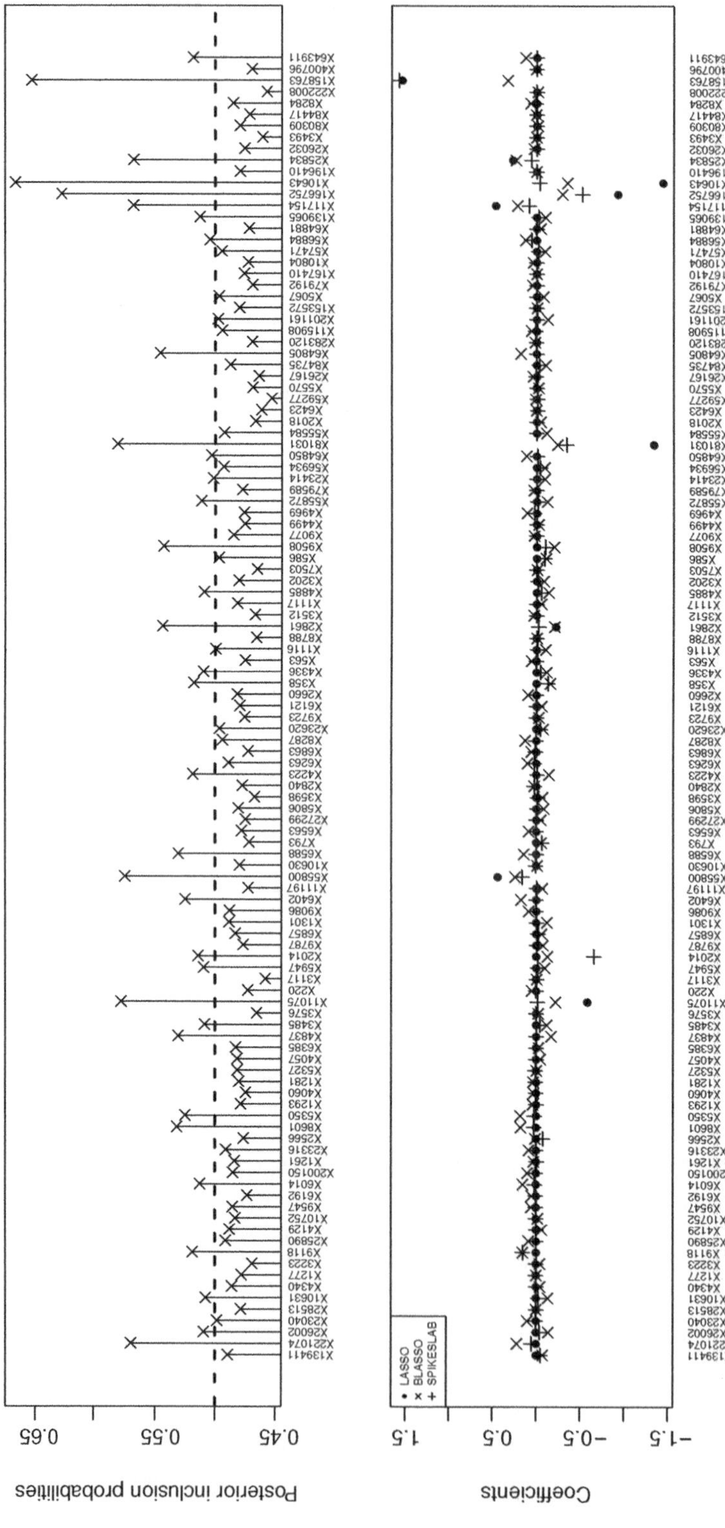

Figure 11.13 Glioma study: posterior inclusion probabilities (top) and estimated regression coefficients (bottom).

Population-based MCMC: The limitations of the classical Metropolis–Hastings- or Gibbs-based stochastic variable selection procedures are the inability to escape from steep local posterior peaks or to discover relevant but isolated parts of the model space. The difficulties with multimodal posterior landscapes can be overcome with the assistance of population-based MCMC algorithms (Jasra *et al.* 2007b). The idea is to run a population of chains in parallel, each chain being associated with one particular 'heated/tempered version' of the target distribution. In the model selection context, the target distribution is the posterior over the model space. Using the BIC approximation of Bayes factors, the posterior model probabilities $p(\boldsymbol{\gamma} \mid \mathbf{y})$ are approximately proportional to $\exp(-\frac{1}{2}\mathrm{BIC}_{\boldsymbol{\gamma}})$, where $\mathrm{BIC}_{\boldsymbol{\gamma}}$ stands for the BIC of a model $\boldsymbol{\gamma}$. The heated distribution $p_i(\boldsymbol{\gamma} \mid \mathbf{y})$ for a given temperature t_i is then defined to be proportional to

$$\exp\left(-\frac{1}{2t_i}\mathrm{BIC}_{\boldsymbol{\gamma}}\right).$$

The tempering has the effect of flattening the peaks of the true target distribution. The greater the temperature t_i of the tempered target density, the easier it is for the chain to escape from the abrupt peaks. Furthermore, the parallel chains interact and learn from each other making the exploration of the model space fluent and more efficient. The interaction is achieved by altering/swapping model configurations between/within the chains with different temperatures at each MCMC iteration. An extension of population-based MCMC to settings of varying dimension was considered by Jasra *et al.* (2007a) and Fouskakis *et al.* (2009). Liang and Wong (2000) suggested a hybrid procedure that combines the idea of parallel tempering together with genetic algorithms in the method called Evolutionary MCMC (EMC); see also Bottolo and Richardson (2010) for the application of EMC in Bayesian model selection.

Parallel tempering is closely related to simulated annealing (Kirkpatrick *et al.* 1983), where only a single chain is used to sample from a joint distribution of the temperatures and target distribution, where only values with 'zero' temperature are recorded.

Shotgun stochastic search: As an alternative to parallel tempering techniques Hans *et al.* (2007) suggested the *Shotgun Stochastic Search* (SSS) that is capable of sampling from vast discrete spaces of regression models. SSS can be regarded as a hybrid procedure that combines Occam's razor principle with Metropolis–Hastings MCMC ingredients. Similar to the Occam's window, SSS neither focuses on finding a point estimate nor it aims at closely approximating the posterior model distribution. The goal is rather to determine a bigger set of best models. As opposed to Occam's window the search is not entirely deterministic, since the explored models are subject to a randomized proposal mechanism (similarly as in the MH routines). In comparison to MC^3, in SSS all models from the neighborhood of the current state are evaluated and multiple models are stored at each iteration. In direct parallel to Occam's window, at each iteration the set of best models is deterministically updated by better models found in the neighborhood.

11.10 Bayesian model selection

Models may differ in more than just the set of included of covariates. For instance, GLIMs may differ in the choice of the link function and the distributional component. Ntzoufras *et al.* (2003) considered model selection in GLIMs whereby the link function and the included covariates are unknown. They suggested a RJMCMC algorithm for selecting the link function, the covariates and the regression coefficients in any order. The specification of the prior distribution needs some extra attention here since the meaning of the regression coefficients changes when the link function changes. The prior is specified hierarchically as $p(\boldsymbol{\beta}^*_{\gamma,L}, \boldsymbol{\gamma}, L) = p(\boldsymbol{\beta}^*_{\gamma,L} \mid \boldsymbol{\gamma}, L)p(\boldsymbol{\gamma} \mid L)p(L)$, where $\boldsymbol{\beta}^* = (\alpha, \boldsymbol{\beta}^T)^T$ and $p(L)$ is uniform on the considered link functions L. The prior $p(\boldsymbol{\gamma} \mid L)$ can be any of the previously described prior model functions (independent, dependent, etc). The problem lies in specifying $p(\boldsymbol{\beta}^*_{\gamma,L} \mid \boldsymbol{\gamma}, L)$. Indeed, suppose the prior is taken $\boldsymbol{\beta}^*_{\gamma,L} \mid \boldsymbol{\gamma}, L \sim \mathrm{N}(\boldsymbol{\beta}^*_{0\gamma,L}, \Sigma_{\gamma,L})$ then the question is how does this relate to a prior $\boldsymbol{\beta}^*_{\gamma,L'} \mid \boldsymbol{\gamma}, L' \sim \mathrm{N}(\boldsymbol{\beta}^*_{0\gamma,L'}, \Sigma_{\gamma,L'})$. Ntzoufras *et al.* (2003) developed transformation rules for the nonzero intercept α when changing the link function. Since $\boldsymbol{\beta}^*_{0\gamma,L}$ is usually taken zero, the transformation rule for the genuine regression coefficients is defined on the prior covariance structure of $\boldsymbol{\beta}_{\gamma,L}$. Software for doing the job does not seem to be available, though.

Sabanés Bové and Held (2011a) described an approach to combine variable selection with choosing appropriate scales for the covariates using fractional polynomials (Royston and Altman 1994) (see also Section 10.3.5). For each covariate x_k, at most two powers are chosen from the set $\{-2, -1, -1/2, 0, 1/2, 1, 2, 3\}$ (with $x_k^0 \equiv \log(x_k)$) and collected in $\boldsymbol{p}_k = (p_{k1}, p_{k2})^T$. The corresponding coefficients are collected in the vector $\boldsymbol{\alpha}_k$ and this yields a term $\boldsymbol{\alpha}_k^T \boldsymbol{x}_k^{\boldsymbol{p}_k}$. For instance, $\boldsymbol{x}_k^{\{2,0\}}$ represents two regressors x_k^2 and $\log(x_k)$ and $\boldsymbol{\alpha}_k^T \boldsymbol{x}_k^{(2,0)} = \alpha_{k1}x_k^2 + \alpha_{k2}\log(x_k)$. When $p_{k1} = p_{k2}$ then $\boldsymbol{\alpha}_k^T \boldsymbol{x}_k^{(2,2)} = \alpha_{k1}x_k^2 + \alpha_{k2}x_k^2\log(x_k)$. Variable selection is embedded in the framework because x_k is not included in the model when $\boldsymbol{p}_k = \boldsymbol{0}$. Then each model is defined by $\boldsymbol{\gamma} = (\boldsymbol{p}_1^T, \ldots, \boldsymbol{p}_d^T)^T$, the covariates are $\boldsymbol{x}_1^{\boldsymbol{p}_1}, \ldots, \boldsymbol{x}_d^{\boldsymbol{p}_d}$ and the vector of regression coefficients is given by $\boldsymbol{\beta}_\gamma = (\boldsymbol{\alpha}_1^T, \ldots, \boldsymbol{\alpha}_d^T)^T$. This combined procedure for selecting covariates and finding their appropriate scale is illustrated with the REACH data.

Example XI.12: Rheumatoid arthritis study: BVS and choosing the appropriate scale of the covariates

The R package `glmBfp` allows to check for nonlinear dependence of the covariates in the REACH data. In the variable selection step, the posterior model probabilities are determined allowing for fractional polynomials. However, of the first 50 most plausible models a posteriori only five models indicate some nonlinearity. Namely, there is some (minor) evidence for $DC^{-2}\log(dc)$ and esr^3. Note that first the variables need to undergo a linear transformation to make sure that logarithms can be computed. The program provides also graphical output to display the (non)linear relationship; see 'chapter 11 Zellner REACH FP.R' for the commands. □

Examples of other approaches that perform simultaneously variable selection and model verification can be found, e.g. Hoeting *et al.* (2002) who suggested to combine variable selection and transformation of both the response as well as the covariates in linear regression or in Gottardo and Raftery (2009). Hoeting *et al.* (1996) proposed a method for simultaneous variable selection and outlier detection (implemented in the `BMA` package with the function `MC3.REG`). The recently developed R package `spikeSlabGAM` is currently the most advanced and versatile model selection software, but restricted to the $d < n$ case. The package implements BVS and model selection with a spike and slab prior structure extending the approach of Ishwaran and Rao (2005) and allows to select single coefficients as well as blocks of coefficients for generalized additive mixed models. Gaussian, binomial and Poisson responses can be modeled as a function of smooth functions of covariates in the presence of random effects and their interactions, but the package also allows for fitting spatial models (Scheipl 2011).

11.11 Bayesian model averaging

It is a myth to assume that one can ultimately find the true model. Still in practice this is often hoped for. The different examples illustrate that searching for a true model is a useless exercise, at most one can find some good models. To base the final conclusions on one model may, therefore, not be a good strategy since hereby one neglects model uncertainty. An alternative strategy is to consider many models, estimate the measure of interest for each model, average this measure over the considered models and determine its statistical variability. This exercise is called *model averaging*. Specifically, suppose that the total set of possible models is $\{M_1, \ldots, M_K\}$ and that one is interested in estimating a measure Δ, e.g. the response of a future observation. Further, suppose that the model probabilities $p(M_m \mid \boldsymbol{y})$, $(k = 1, \ldots, K)$ are available, then the posterior distribution of Δ is

$$p(\Delta \mid \boldsymbol{y}) = \sum_{m=1}^{K} p(\Delta \mid \boldsymbol{y}, M_m) p(M_m \mid \boldsymbol{y}), \tag{11.44}$$

with $p(\Delta \mid \boldsymbol{y}, M_m)$ determined from the posterior of the model parameters $p(\boldsymbol{\theta}_m \mid \boldsymbol{y}, M_m)$ by marginalization. Often only the posterior mean and variance of Δ are needed:

$$E(\Delta \mid \boldsymbol{y}) = \sum_{m=1}^{K} \widehat{\Delta}_m p(M_m \mid \boldsymbol{y}), \tag{11.45}$$

$$\text{Var}(\Delta \mid \boldsymbol{y}) = \sum_{m=1}^{K} \left[\text{Var}(\Delta \mid \boldsymbol{y}, M_m) + \widehat{\Delta}_m^2\right] p(M_m \mid \boldsymbol{y}) - E(\Delta \mid \boldsymbol{y})^2, \tag{11.46}$$

with $\widehat{\Delta}_m = E(\Delta \mid \boldsymbol{y}, M_m) = \int \Delta(\boldsymbol{\theta}_m) p(\boldsymbol{\theta}_m \mid \boldsymbol{y}, M_m) d\boldsymbol{\theta}_m$ (Raftery *et al.* 1997). Expression (11.46) follows from the factorization $\text{var}(x) = E_y[\text{var}(x \mid y)] + \text{var}_y[E(x \mid y)]$ with y discrete (also seen in expression (5.13)).

Model averaging has been suggested both under the frequentist (Claeskens and Hjort 2008) as well as under the Bayesian paradigm. In the latter case, it is called *BMA*. In the frequentist world, the model probabilities $p(M_m \mid \boldsymbol{y})$ are typically taken as in (11.8) using either AIC, BIC or some other information criterion. This is only possible when the number of models is not too large. For large d, one needs to restrict to models with the highest model probabilities since they will have the most impact in the computation of the mean and variance of Δ. In the Bayesian context, a stochastic search algorithm will determine the most promising models. The mean and variance of Δ are then just a byproduct of the variable selection exercise, i.e. Δ is estimated in each visited model and the mean and variance are computed across the visited models. It must be said, however, that the average of regression coefficients across models is fraught with interpretation problems (see Draper 1999). Indeed, it is known from each classical regression textbook that the interpretation of a regression coefficient is conditional on the other regressors in the model. In a BMA exercise, we average β_k over models (a) with x_k, but where the other regressors vary in the model and (b) without x_k. In an MCMC context, the omission of x_k is seen in the density of the sampled $\widetilde{\beta}_k$ as a

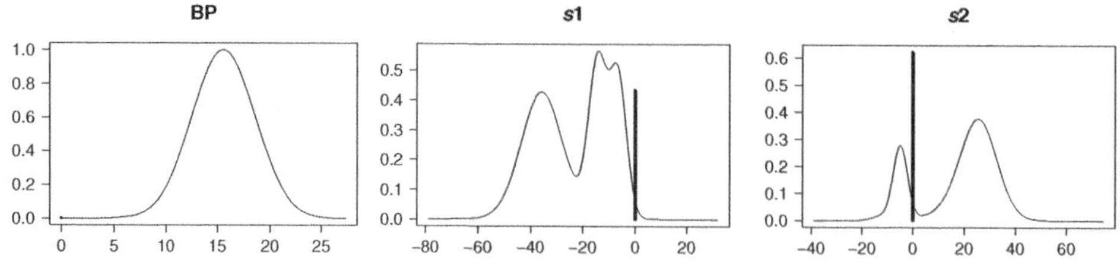

Figure 11.14 Diabetes study: marginal posterior densities of three regression coefficients obtained from bic.glm.

spike like in Figure 11.14. Hoeting *et al.* (1999b), though, gave arguments for taking BMA of regression coefficients and computed summary measures of individual regression coefficients in several publications (Gottardo and Raftery 2009; Hoeting *et al.* 1996, 2002). The posterior inclusion probability is easier to interpret and has been used above to determine the median probability model. It could even replace the classical P-value as it expresses how many times a regressor is considered necessary in the model.

There are no issues when Δ represents the predicted response of a new subject. In fact, much of the motivation for basing inference on BMA is that the technique provides better predictive ability as measured by the logarithmic scoring rule than for any single model M_l which implies:

$$-E\left\{\log\left[\sum_{m=1}^{K} p(\Delta \mid \mathbf{y}, M_m)p(M_m \mid \mathbf{y})\right]\right\} \leq -E\left[\log(p(\Delta \mid \mathbf{y}, M_l))\right],\ (l = 1, \ldots, K), \tag{11.47}$$

which follows from the Kullback–Leibler inequality (Raftery *et al.* 1997). An appealing feature of the Bayesian approach to model averaging is its complete generality. For instance, one can generalize the concept of the posterior predictive distribution to account for model uncertainty (Clyde and George 2004), i.e

$$p(\widetilde{y} \mid \mathbf{y}) = \sum_{m} p(\widetilde{y} \mid \mathbf{y}, M_m)p(M_m \mid \mathbf{y}).$$

Example XI.13: Diabetes study: Bayesian model averaging

We now return to the analysis of Example XI.5. The R function `bic.glm` in the package BMA allows for Bayesian model averaging for a linear regression problem. With an exhaustive search 36 models were visited. Figure 11.14 shows part of the graphical output obtained from `bic.glm`. The figure shows the marginal densities of three regression coefficients. For *bp* the density is unimodal since *bp* is in all models. For the two other regression coefficients, there is a vertical bar at zero with height equal to the proportion of models that does not contain the corresponding regressor in the model. Thus, the regressors $s1$ and $s2$ are not included in all models and when they are included in the model their regression coefficients change dramatically depending on which other regressors are in the model.

Posterior means and standard errors of the regression coefficients can also be obtained from `bic.glm`. Both unconditional (marginal over all selected models) as well as conditional (restricted to the models containing the regressor) posterior summary measures are available. In Table 11.4, we compared the marginal mean and SE of all regression coefficients based on two runs of the program: one with Occam's window switched on (nine models) and one

Table 11.4 Diabetes study: Bayesian model averaging using bic.glm based on Occam's window and exhaustive search.

	Occam's window on (OR = 20)			Occam's window off		
x_k	$E(\beta \mid \mathbf{y})$	$SD(\beta \mid \mathbf{y})$	$P(\beta \neq 0 \mid \mathbf{y})$	$E(\beta \mid \mathbf{y})$	$SD(\beta \mid \mathbf{y})$	$P(\beta \neq 0 \mid \mathbf{y})$
int	0.000	2.576	1.00	0.000	2.576	1.00
age	0.000	0.000	0.0	−0.012	0.584	0.04
gender	−10.958	2.877	1.00	−10.761	3.175	0.98
BMI	25.294	3.139	1.00	25.355	3.161	1.00
bp	15.599	3.002	1.00	15.546	3.024	1.00
$s1$	−13.317	15.962	0.55	−13.244	15.793	0.57
$s2$	7.065	12.464	0.37	6.748	12.477	0.38
$s3$	−7.633	7.119	0.57	−7.414	7.140	0.57
$s4$	1.787	5.004	0.18	1.950	5.202	0.20
$s5$	28.253	7.394	1.00	28.232	7.346	1.00
$s6$	0.132	0.898	0.04	0.216	1.141	0.07

where this feature is switched off. It is argued that these estimates are preferable above estimates based on a single 'best' model. However, most often researchers wish to discover a unique best model whereby the importance of the individual covariates are indicated by P-values. We further computed the mean-squared prediction error (MSPE) defined here as $\frac{1}{n}\sum_{i=1}^{n}(y_i - \widehat{y}_i)^2$, where the predicted value $\widehat{y}_i$ is obtained from either the MLE of the selected model (note that this definition of MSPE is different from that in Section 10.2.3) or is a BMA prediction. In Figure 11.15, we see that the BMA estimated model has a small MSPE but is not the smallest across the models. This does not contradict, however, result (11.47) since we are using a different metric here, and most importantly the MSPE is too optimistic for the individual models since the data are used twice. The R program can be found in 'chapter 11 BMA diabetes.R'. □

11.12 Closing remarks

Variable and model selection has always been one of the most complicated problems in statistics. This is also true in the Bayesian paradigm although the Bayesian approach has a lot to offer. Indeed, in the Bayesian world candidate models can be elegantly compared using posterior model probabilities if appropriate priors are specified.

In addition, the multitude of (new) developments offers a rich toolbox of BVS methods certainly when $d < n$. But with a variety of approaches practitioners will need guidance, otherwise they might fall back to the old standards such as forward, backward and stepwise selection techniques. It appears that a lot of empirical research is needed to find the trustworthy approaches. In Rockova *et al.* (2011), a simulation study was undertaken to compare Bayesian regularization approaches and the spike and slab approaches. Besides the observation that the performance of the considered approaches is vulnerable to prior settings, practical conclusions did not yet emerge.

Despite the wide overview of BVS procedure, this review is not comprehensive. For instance, we have omitted here the predictive approach to variable selection; see Gelfand and Ghosh (1998), and also variable model selection using the CART approach. A refinement of

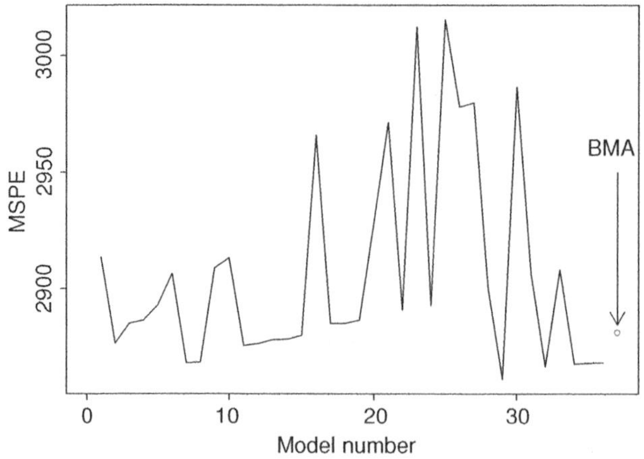

Figure 11.15 Diabetes study: MSPE for 36 models obtained from bic.glm with Occam's window switched off and MSPE based on the BMA estimate.

the CART approach (BART, see Chipman et al. 2010) does not assume any particular statistical model when selecting important covariates that relate to the response. The approach has been implemented in the R package `Bayes Tree` and appears to have excellent variable selection properties.

We did not discuss the many software developments, such as the approach of Kiiveri (2003). Some of these developments are described in some review papers such as (Chipman *et al.* 2001; Clyde and George 2004; Kadane and Lazar 2004; O'Hara and Sillanpää 2009). Finally, we refer to Ando (2010) for a somewhat more mathematical treatment of the Bayesian model selection techniques.

Exercises

Exercise 11.1 Dietary study: Predict body-mass index (kg/m^2) from age, gender, length (cm), weight (kg), and the food intake variables measuring the daily consumption of: alcohol (g/day), calcium (mg/day), cholesterol (mg/day), protein (g/day), iron (mg/day), potassium (mg/day), carbohydrates (g/day) containing mono and disachharides (g/day) and polysachharide (g/day), several parameters measuring fat intake (total fat intake (g/day), mono-unsaturated fat (g/day), poly-unsaturated fat (g/day), saturated fate intake (g/day), ratio poly-unsat/sat fat (PS), ratio mono+poly-unsat/sat fat (US)), sodium (mg/day), phosphorus (mg/day), fibres (mg/day) and energy intake (kcal/day); see excel file 'IBBENS.xls' for the data. In addition to a full linear regression analysis by making use of all variables, use as classical variable selection approaches: Forward, backward and stepwise selection techniques, ridge and LASSO shrinkage techniques. Determine the best fitting model(s) to the data. Search for appropriate R functions to do the job.

Exercise 11.2 Diabetes study: Find the MP models using the R functions `bic.glm` and `MC3.REG`.

Exercise 11.3 Rheumatoid arthritis study: Find the MP models using the R functions `bic.glm` and `glib`.

Exercise 11.4 Rheumatoid arthritis study: Use WinBUGS program 'chapter 11 RJMCMC REACH.odc' to check the dependence of the solution on the precision of the regression coefficients, i.e. MAP and MP model, marginal probabilities, posterior summary measures for the regression coefficients. Then call WinBUGS from within R to do the job.

Exercise 11.5 Diabetes study: Use R2WinBUGS to select the most important variables using a RJMCMC approach and compare it to the solution when applying the R program `monomvn`. Extend the set of covariates by adding all (45) double products and 9 quadratic terms and apply the R program `monomvn`.

Exercise 11.6 Diabetes study: Adapt WinBUGS program 'chapter 11 SSVS REACH.R' to select variables in a linear regression model and apply it to the diabetes data. Perform a sensitivity analysis by varying the spike and slab variances.

Exercise 11.7 Rheumatoid arthritis study: Use R2WinBUGS based on 'chapter 11 NMIG REACH.odc' to select variables in a logistic and a probit regression model using the approach of Ishwaran and Rao (2003). Perform a sensitivity analysis by varying the spike and slab variances.

Exercise 11.8 Diabetes study: Apply Exercise 11.7 to the diabetes data and compare the selected models from those selected with other BVS approaches.

Exercise 11.9 Rheumatoid arthritis study: Apply the WinBUGS program 'chapter 11 GVS REACH.odc' to select variables in a probit regression model using the GVS approach. Compare the selected models from those selected with other BVS approaches.

Exercise 11.10 Rheumatoid arthritis study: Adapt the WinBUGS program 'chapter 11 GVS REACH.odc' with the approach of Kuo and Mallick (1998).

Exercise 11.11 Diabetes study: Apply Exercise 11.9 to the diabetes data.

Exercise 11.12 Rheumatoid arthritis study: Adapt the WinBUGS program 'chapter 11 GVS REACH.odc' to check the importance of the product terms of all regressors with *dc* (duration of complaints in days). Use the approach of Chipman (1996).

Exercise 11.13 Rheumatoid arthritis study: Adapt the WinBUGS program 'chapter 11 GVS REACH.odc' to check whether *sjc* (swollen joint count) should be transformed with log, sqrt or inverse by making use of a variable selection technique suggested by Chipman (1996).

Exercise 11.14 Diabetes study: Apply the WinBUGS program 'chapter 11 blasso adaptive diabetes.odc' to perform Bayesian adaptive LASSO estimation on the diabetes data.

Exercise 11.15 Rheumatoid arthritis study: Apply the following Bayesian shrinkage regression approaches: ridge, LASSO, adaptive LASSO and Elastic Net to the REACH data. Use the latent representation of the probit model for this. Show that these approaches exhibit more shrinkage than SSVS and GVS. Further, show ridge regression induces more uniform shrinkage, while BL, ABL and BEN result in more differential shrinkage.

Exercise 11.16 Rheumatoid arthritis study: Apply Exercise 11.14 to the REACH data.

Exercise 11.17 Diabetes study: Apply the R program `glmBfp` to find nonlinear associations with the response y.

Exercise 11.18 Diabetes study: Apply any of the BVS techniques to produce the model averages of the regression coefficients and the predicted values of the responses. Compare your results to the results obtained from `bic.glm`.

Part III

BAYESIAN METHODS IN PRACTICAL APPLICATIONS

12

Bioassay

Bioassay, short for 'biological assay', is a type of scientific experiment where a substance of interest is introduced to a living organism to assess the effects of the substance. A classic example would be the introduction of a new drug or compound into a plated cell line to see if the product causes changes in the cells (e.g. mutation). Quantification of the effects of the substance leads to quantitative bioassay and its application lies mainly in the area of drug development and environmental pollution assessment. Environmental bioassays are generally a broad-range survey of toxicity, whereas in drug development, the focus may be on mutagenesis, carcinogenesis, teratogenesis as well as toxicity. In the latter field, early stage preclinical drug testing can require the use of assays that attempt to detect mutation in cell lines, cancer induction (carcinogenesis) or the detection of reproductive defects (teratology). In what follows, we focus on the aspects of bioassay that arise mainly in drug-development environments. Environmental bioassay is reviewed in Piegorsch and Bailer (2005).

12.1 Bioassay essentials

The basic idea of bioassay is very simple. A controlled experiment is set up where different dosages of a compound are administered to a biological agent. Over the progression of the experiment, changes to the biological agent are monitored.

12.1.1 Cell assays

The biological agent could be a cell line, and in that case, the monitored end point would be changes to cells. Such an assay is often called *in vitro* as it involves experiments within test tubes or plated cultures. A well-known example of such an assay is the Ames Salmonella assay (SAL) (Mortelmans and Zeiger 2000). The end point tested within the assay could be mutagenesis (mutation of the cell) which may be an indicator of carcinogenic potential, or the carcinogenesis (cancer causing) potential could be analyzed directly. There are many variants of these forms depending on the end point of interest. In what follows, we will consider two particular assays: the *Ames salmonella mutagenicity assay* and the *mouse lymphoma*

Bayesian Biostatistics, First Edition. Emmanuel Lesaffre and Andrew B. Lawson.

mutagenic assay. These assays have different foci in that the Ames assay focuses on short-term bacterial reversal mutagenesis whereas the mouse lymphoma focuses on mutation in mammalian cells.

12.1.2 Animal assays

Animal assays are termed *in vivo* as they are carried out in full life forms, such as mammals. These assays often follow *in vitro* assays and are scaled up to be relevant to larger life forms (such as humans). Once a compound passes a battery of *in vitro* assays, it may then be tested via animal assay. Animal assays are usually carried out on target drugs or compounds which may be of use in human or veterinary applications. Hence, they must be chosen with care toward matching the assay host to the target life form. For example, due to an inappropriate animal model to test the drug Thalidomide, the subsequent use of that drug in humans led to birth defects.

While it is not the purpose here to describe in detail the regulatory requirements for assays, we note that there are three broad classes of assays that are important in applications: lethal dose assays (such as LD50) used for toxicity testing, teratogenicity testing where the compounds are examined for their potential to yield birth defects and carcinogenicity testing where large scale long-term longitudinal animal studies are established to monitor the appearance of tumors. Here, we will focus solely on toxicity testing.

A particular assay arises from the need to establish toxicity of a compound prior to testing for other effects (such as mutagenic or carcinogenic potential). Toxicity is often established by setting up an experiment where different dose levels of a compound are administered to a biological entity (e.g. animal) and for each dose level the count of subjects that died is recorded after a fixed period of time. A survival curve is computed from these data which provides an estimate of the lethal dose that kills 50% of the subjects (LD50). A variant of this is the ED50, or the *effective dose* at which 50% of subjects reach an endpoint (ED 50%). The end point could be 'cured' or another state of improvement. The ED50 is used in dose finding in clinical trials whereas LD50 is used preclinically for toxicity testing.

Here, we examine a famous early example of LD50 testing: the beetle mortality data of Bliss (1935). In this, example sets of beetles (Tribolium confusum) were given different concentrations of carbon disulphide. Each of the dose groups consists of different numbers of beetles (ranging from 56 to 63), and out of these numbers, a proportion that died during the 5-hour exposure to the toxic agent was recorded. In this experiment, the number of beetles that died is assumed to be binomially distributed. There are $N = 8$ groups. Define r_i as the number of beetles killed out of n_i in each group, with subscript i denoting group ($i = 1, \ldots, N$). The dose level x_i is a covariate measured at group level. Notice that as the dose increases then more deaths occurred until at the highest dose all beetles have died. Table 12.1 displays these data. Figure 12.1 displays the proportion killed (r_i/n_i) for these data.

Assume the following model for the number of deaths:

$$r_i \sim \text{Bin}(n_i, p_i),$$

where p_i is the probability of death in the ith group. We want to relate this probability to the dose level and hence we employ a link function to relate p_i to x_i. The choice of the link function is quite important in this example and we will look at three different link functions: the logit, the probit and the complimentary-log-log (c-loglog). The link functions differ mainly in their tail behavior (at low or high doses) and can lead to quite different measures of GOF.

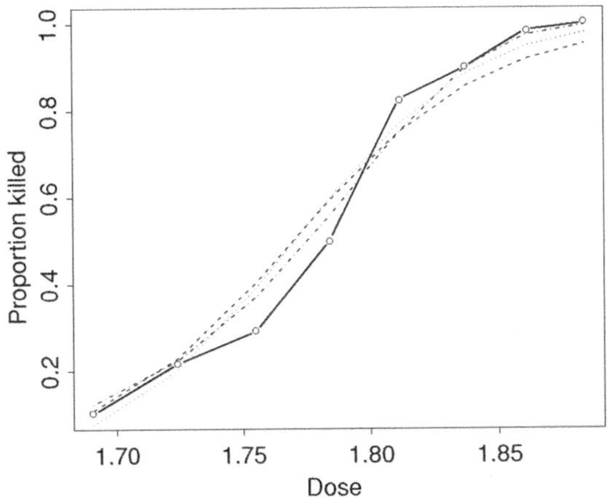

Figure 12.1 Bliss beetle mortality data: plot of proportion killed versus dose. Curve of predicted probabilities based on logit link (dashed line), probit link (dotted line) and c-loglog link (dot-dashed line).

The considered models are:

$$\text{logit}(p_i) = \beta_0 + \beta_1 x_i, \quad (12.1)$$

$$\text{probit}(p_i) = \beta_0 + \beta_1 x_i, \quad (12.2)$$

$$\text{cloglog}(p_i) = \beta_0 + \beta_1 x_i. \quad (12.3)$$

In model (12.1), we have $p_i = \exp(\beta_0 + \beta_1 x_i)/[1 + \exp(\beta_0 + \beta_1 x_i)]$, in model (12.2) we have $p_i = \Phi(\beta_0 + \beta_1 x_i)$, where $\Phi(.)$ is the standard normal cdf, and in (12.3) $p_i = 1 - \exp[-\exp(\beta_0 + \beta_1 x_i)]$. In Figure 12.2, we show the WinBUGS code for the logit bioassay model. The statement `logit(p[i]) <- alpha.star + beta * (x[i] -`

Table 12.1 Bliss beetle mortality data: dose concentration of carbon disulphide (x_i) and beetle mortality, with n_i is the number of beetles exposed and r_i is the number of beetles died.

x_i	n_i	r_i
1.6907	59	6
1.7242	60	13
1.7552	62	18
1.7842	56	28
1.8113	63	52
1.8369	59	52
1.8610	62	61
1.8839	60	60

```
model
        {
        for (i in 1:N ) {
        r[i] ~ dbin(p[i],n[i])
        logit(p[i]) <- alpha.star + beta*(x[i] - mean(x[]))
        rhat[i] <- n[i]*p[i]
        }
    alpha <- alpha.star - beta*mean(x[])
    beta ~ dnorm(0.0,tauB)
    alpha.star ~ dnorm(0.0,tauA)
    tauB <- pow(sdB,-2)
    sdB ~ dunif(0,5)
    tauA <- pow(sdA,-2)
    sdA ~ dunif(0,5)
        }
```

Figure 12.2 Bliss beetle mortality data: WinBUGS model code for the logit bioassay model.

`mean(x[]))` specifies the logit model. The code for the probit link is obtained by replacing `logit(p[i])` by `probit(p[i])`, and for the c-loglog link, we replace it by `cloglog(p[i])`. Further, in the WinBUGS code a derived variable `rhat[i]` is computed which represents the fitted value of r at different levels of dose.

Two chains were initiated with burn-in of 12 000 and sample size 5000. The convergence diagnostics suggested convergence and good chain mixing. The results of the fit are displayed in Table 12.2 along with the results of fitting the probit and c-loglog models. Clearly, the choice of the link function affects the GOF. We compared the models using Deviance Information Criterion (DIC) and obtained: (1) for the logit model: DIC $= 48.95$, $p_D = 1.809$ and (2) probit model: DIC $= 41.46$, $p_D = 1.957$ and for the c-loglog model: DIC $= 35.02$, $p_D = 1.727$. It is clear that the c-loglog model yields the best overall GOF. Table 12.2 demonstrates the ability of the c-loglog model to closely match the observed data. This is confirmed in the graphical representation of the three models in Figure 12.1, which also shows that the three fitted curves still deviate modestly from the observed data at moderate to low doses. For the c-loglog model

Table 12.2 Bliss beetle mortality data: comparison of estimated rhat with r for different link models.

r	Logit	Probit	c-loglog
6	6.45	4.50	7.28
13	13.73	12.14	13.39
18	24.99	24.28	22.95
28	33.24	33.50	31.22
52	47.26	48.49	47.26
52	50.47	52.18	52.98
61	56.9	58.78	60.34
60	57.19	58.73	59.76

the LD50 is solved in $\log(-\log(0.5)) = \beta_0 + \beta_1 x_i$, i.e. $\beta_0 + \beta_1 x_i = -0.3665$. In this case, the posterior mean of LD50 is 1.776 (95% CI: [1.768, 1.784]). Note that the plug-in value using the posterior mean estimates for β_0 (−35.28), β_1(19.66) is very close to this value: 1.7758.

Various Bayesian developments have been proposed in bioassay. Gelfand and Kuo (1991) proposed a general nonparametric Bayesian approach (see also final chapter) to the estimation of the tolerance distribution instead of assuming parametric forms. In that work, the ordered Dirichlet and product-beta prior distributions were explored for the mortal probability. Ramgopal *et al*. (1993) extended this work with constrained non-parametric prior distributions which address specific features of the tolerance distribution. For example, one might consider a threshold model for toxicity where a dose must reach a certain level before toxic effects are seen. Equally, there could be multiple levels of threshold that should be accounted for. Multivariate testing and multiple end points with competing risks are obvious extensions.

12.2 A generic *in vitro* example

A preclinical *in vitro* mutagenicity experiment is carried out to assess the mutagenic potential of a new drug (drug A). A dosage (L mg/L) of the drug is applied to a $N = 1,000$ cells *in vitro*. The cells are left for a defined time period (T) and then assessed for mutagenic transformation. The binary random variable y_i is defined as the cell state (0: untransformed; 1: transformed) of the ith cell after time T. The sum of these independent cell states is a binomial random variable ($r = \sum_{i=1}^{N} y_i$) with transformation probability p. The maximum likelihood estimate of p is simply $\widehat{p} = r/N$. In this case, it was found that, $r = 9$ and so $\widehat{p} = 0.009$. Hence, drug A appeared to have a very low mutagenic potential.

In a Bayesian analysis, p is given a prior distribution and often this is assumed to be a beta distribution, i.e. $p \sim \text{Beta}(\alpha, \beta)$. The posterior expectation of p is then $E(p \mid r) = (r + \alpha)/(N + \alpha + \beta)$. For the indifferent prior with $\alpha = \beta = 1$, we obtain $10/1002 = 0.00998$. An alternative might be to assume a more sophisticated model for p. If covariates are to be included then a link to a linear predictor may be required. The commonest of these would be a logit link to a simple intercept parameter (α_0), which in turn has a hyperprior distribution, so that

$$\begin{aligned} \text{logit}(p) &= \alpha_0 \\ \alpha_0 &\sim \text{N}\left(0, \sigma_{\alpha_0}^2\right), \end{aligned}$$

with precision $\tau_{\alpha_0} = \sigma_{\alpha_0}^{-2}$. This suggests the hierarchical model described by a directed acyclic graph as in Figure 12.3.

Note that a more general formulation can be suggested where the α_0 parameter is replaced by a linear predictor consisting of parameters (and possibly also covariates or random effects). Denote the dose response parameters for a single dose predictor as α_0 and α_1, and the associated variances (precisions) for the Gaussian prior distributions as $\sigma_{\beta_0}^2$ ($\tau_{\beta_0}^{-1}$) and $\sigma_{\beta_1}^2$ ($\tau_{\beta_1}^{-1}$), respectively. The linear predictor with single dose predictor (D_i) is $\text{logit}(p_i) = \beta_0 + \beta_1 D_i$. Further extensions of this example could be made in different settings. First, we could consider changes to the prior distributions for both regression parameters and precisions. Sensitivity to the prior specification is important and so we would be

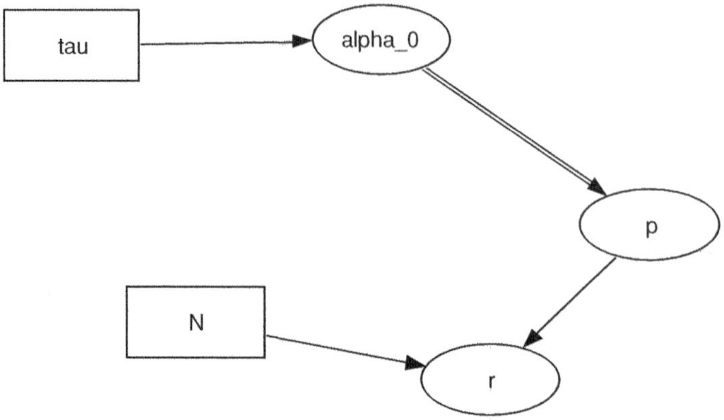

Figure 12.3 Generic *in vitro* study: directed acyclic graph of the generic binomial logit bioassay model.

concerned whether the Gaussian specification (for β_0 and β_1) or the fixed nature of σ_*^2 would be appropriate. Variants of the Gaussian could be the zero-mean t distribution or asymmetric alternatives such as the skewed Gaussian (see O'Hagan and Leonhard 1976) or the asymmetric Laplace. Hyperprior specification for the variance parameters (σ_*^2) would also be important to consider. Additionally, the link function chosen (in this case the logit) might be changed as it was found that the c-loglog link performed better in some examples (e.g. the beetle example above).

In other situations, the context may dictate further modifications to the procedures. For example, historical and active controls might need to be included in a study. Alternatively, multiple control groups are sometimes recommended (as in the Mouse Lymphoma assay (MLA)). The historical data may update the prior distributions and their parameters as in Section 5.6. Such dynamic updating is a fundamental feature of the Bayesian paradigm.

Finally, there is always the need to compare the effects of different drugs/substances in relation to dosage, either as new tests on the same drug (repeated testing) or simply making a comparison between aspects of the toxicity of one drug/substance to the other. Bivariate Bayesian generalized linear model (BGLM) and Bayesian generalized linear mixed model (BGLMM) models (see Sections 4.8 and 9.5.3) can be proposed whereby a count outcome for the ith subject with the jth drug is given by y_{ij} and then

$$E(y_{ij}) = \mu_{ij},$$

$$g(\mu_{ij}) = \beta_{0j} + \beta_{1j} D_{ij} \quad \text{(BGLM)},$$

or

$$g(\mu_{ij}) = \beta_{0j} + \beta_{1j} D_{ij} + \gamma_{ij} \quad \text{(BGLMM)},$$

with $\gamma_{ij} \sim \mathrm{N}(\gamma_j, \sigma_{\gamma_j}^2)$ a random effect of the combined effect of dose level and drug. Drug comparison could be made via the examination of the posterior functionals such as $d_i = \mu_{i1} - \mu_{i2}$, $\beta_{01} - \beta_{02}$ or $\beta_{11} - \beta_{12}$, for example. The comparison of multiple drugs/substances would lead naturally to the consideration of multivariate models.

In the following sections, we briefly discuss two specific assays and their analysis: the SAL and the MLA.

12.3 Ames/Salmonella mutagenic assay

In Chapter 5, we introduced the Ames/Salmonella assay in Example V.1 and discussed a simple analysis of replicate counts within that assay. The Ames/Salmonella microsome assay was developed to detect mutagenicity (Breslow 1984; Kim and Margolin 1999; Krewski *et al.* 1993; Margolin *et al.* 1989; Tarone 1982).

Various researchers have examined dose-response data for the Ames assay, where a dose level of a compound is given to a set of replicated plates and the resulting count of revertant colonies is the outcome. At the data level, we have

$$y_{ij} \mid \mu_{ij} \sim \text{Poisson}[\mu_{ij}(D_i)], \quad (i = 1, \ldots, N; \; j = 1, \ldots, n_i)$$

where y_{ij} is the revertant count in the ith plate/dose level, jth replication, with n_i replications. The model chosen for the expected count can be structured in a variety of ways and is assumed to be a function of dose D_i. Using biological considerations, Krewski *et al.* (1993) suggested using hit theory to propose two different models:

1. Short-term toxicity: $\mu_{ij}(D_i) = (\beta_{0i} + \beta_1 D_i)\exp(-\beta_2 D_i^{\theta})$
2. Long-term toxicity: $\mu_{ij}(D_i) = (\beta_{0i} + \beta_1 D_i)[2 - \exp(\beta_2 D_i^{\theta})]$

The parameter θ is a low-dose adjustment to allow for a threshold. It is assumed to be $\theta > 1$, but the value $\theta = 2$ is often assumed.

Krewski *et al.* (1993) used quasi-likelihood to allow for a mean-variance relationship but no more parametric assumptions. Here, we assume, at the data level, a conditional independent Poisson distribution for the ijth level. We assumed initially that $\beta_{0i} = \beta_0$ is fixed. Of course, to allow for overdispersion in the model, we allow prior distributions at higher levels of the hierarchy and hence are not limited by the Poisson data level assumption. To compare the Bayesian results to those of Krewski *et al.* (1993), we have examined the data for 1-Nitropyrene, TA 100-S9, Laboratory 10, Round 3 (dose in μ_g), reported from a collaborative trial by the International Programme on Chemical Safety (IPCS). Table 12.3 and Figure 12.4 display these data. In this case, $n_1 = n_2 = 2$ replications, and $N = 6$ dose levels.

The above two models were fitted for fixed values of θ and for a random θ. For the random model, we have assumed an Exp(1) prior distribution truncated at 1 for θ. Further, we have assumed zero mean Gaussian prior distributions for the $\boldsymbol{\beta}$ parameters with uniform hyperpriors for the standard deviations (see Section 5.7, Chapter 9).

Table 12.3 Ames assay IPCS data: dose and replication counts.

Dose	Rep 1	Rep 2
0.00	169	159
0.75	359	426
1.50	679	571
3.00	572	716
4.50	649	423
6.00	299	129

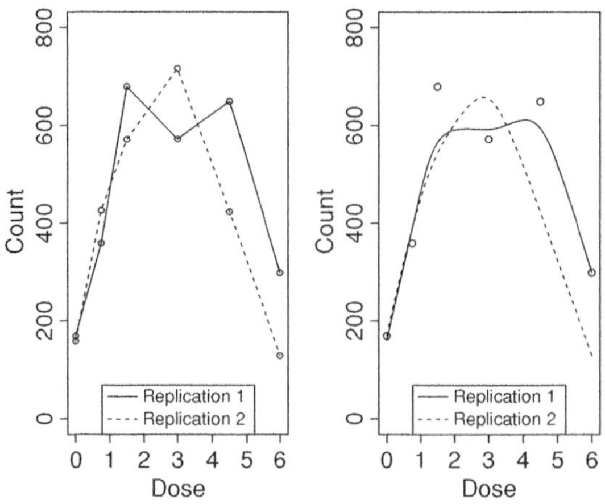

Figure 12.4 Ames assay IPCS data: scatter plot of replications 1 and 2. Left panel displays both replications with no smoothing, right panel displays a kernel regression smoothing of each replication superimposed on replication 1 data only.

Table 12.4 and Figure 12.5 display the results of fitting a range of models to the IPCS data. It is clear that the short-term toxicity model provides the lowest DIC and mean-square predictive error (MSPE) with the fixed $\theta = 2$. This model yields a considerably lower DIC than the other models. Note that this corresponds to a Gaussian-like decline with dose. On the other hand, for the long-term toxicity model and based on MSPE, $\theta = 1$ or a random θ seem most appropriate for these data.

The posterior median regression parameter estimates (and standard errors) for the short-term toxicity model with $\theta = 2$ are $\widehat{\beta_0} = 120.1$ (3.534), $\widehat{\beta_1} = 144.6$ (3.498), $\widehat{\beta_2} = 0.02883$ (0.00115). The posterior mean and median estimates are identical for this model fit. The estimated dose-response curve using the posterior median values from a sample of K iterations, $\widehat{\mu}_{ij}(D_i) = \text{med}_K[(\beta_{0i}^k + \beta_1^k D_i)\exp(-\beta_2^k D_i^2)]$ are displayed in Figure 12.6.

Table 12.4 Ames assay IPCS data: comparison of overall goodness-of-fit via DIC, p_D, and MSPE for short-term and long-term models for the IPCS data.

Model: short term	p_D	DIC	MSPE
$\theta = 1$	1.77	1984.6	59990.0
$\theta = 2$	1.98	1309.9	38960.0
θ random	1.57	6613.8	141300.0
Model: long term	p_D	DIC	MSPE
$\theta = 1$	1.50	13300.5	170500.0
$\theta = 2$	1.41	13355.5	170600.0
θ random	1.62	13306.7	170500.0

Node	Mean	sd	MC error	2.5%	Median	97.5%	start	sample
b0	120.1	3.534	0.06278	112.9	120.1	127.2	10001	20000
b1	144.6	3.498	0.07987	137.8	144.6	151.4	10001	20000
b2	0.02883	0.001148	1.89E-05	0.02657	0.02883	0.03109	10001	20000
Deviance	1308	41.42	0.7515	1228	1308	1391	10001	20000

Figure 12.5 Ames assay IPCS data: posterior estimates of regression parameters based on the short-term toxicity model with $\theta = 2$, obtained from WinBUGS.

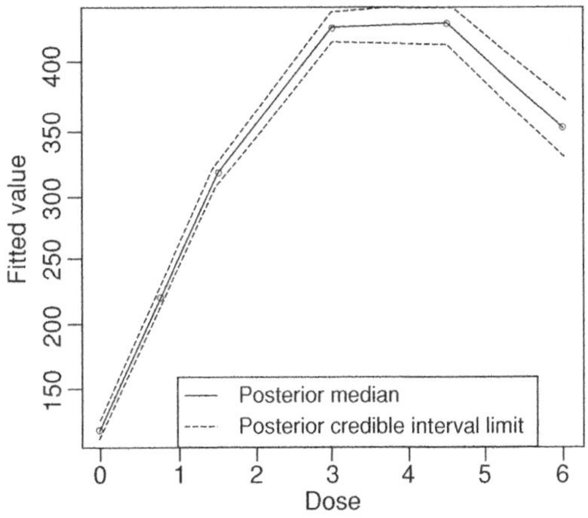

Figure 12.6 Ames assay IPCS data: posterior average estimate of the mean revertant level with associated 95% CI based on the short-term toxicity model with $\theta = 2$.

In conclusion, for the IPCS data the short-term model seems to describe the variation reasonably well and certainly leads to a much improved DIC. The resulting estimated average revertant-dose relation has a relatively narrow 95% credible interval.

12.4 Mouse lymphoma assay (L5178Y TK+/−)

A different assay arises when the focus is on changes in DNA cell structure. The MLA focuses on thymidine kinase locus mutation caused by base pair changes, frameshift and small deletions (Clements 2000; Moore *et al.* 2003). Thymidine kinase is part of a system that recycles free thymidine that is eventually incorporated into DNA. Trifluorothymidine (TFT) is a toxic analog of thymidine and interferes with DNA metabolism, killing the cell. However, if the functional copy of the *TK* gene is lost through mutation, the TFT is not metabolized and is no longer toxic.

L5178Y cell cultures are treated with various concentrations of a test compound in both the presence and the absence of a metabolite production enhancer. Duplicate cultures are used at each experimental point. Usually, at least four dose levels of the compound are assessed with the highest dose level being either that expected to reduced survival by 80–90% based on a scaled down preliminary test or, for nontoxic compounds, the standard limit of 5 mg/mL or to the limit of solubility. The treated cells are grown for an expression period to allow fixation of mutations.

Many of the statistical modeling principles already discussed above apply to this assay (and indeed many variants). Usually, we observe counts of cells at fixed dosage and we wish to estimate the underlying dose-response behavior of the test substance. For the MLA, the outcomes are often expressed as mutation frequency (MF) (per 10^4 survivors) and this can be considered as a count. MF can be modeled with concentration of test substance as predictor, as in other assays. Often both positive and negative controls are employed and these can be modeled via factor effects.

Finally it is worth noting that many of these mutational assays are considered to provide evidence of carcinogenicity also and can be used in combination as preliminary tests for cancer agents. Comparisons of these tests in this regard is given in Tennant *et al.* (1987) and an account of general statistical methods for a range of cell assays is provided in Kirkland (2008).

12.5 Closing remarks

In this short review, we have attempted to provide an introduction to the issues found in the analysis of biological assay data. We have not attempted to cover all aspects of the subject and indeed we did not consider more complex problems, for example, as found in litter-based teratology studies. However, from a practical viewpoint, the important topics of LD50 estimation was approached in the beetle assay as was evaluation of goodness of link, repeated dosage updating for the Ames assay, and long- and short-term toxicity via hit theory was examined for the Ames assay also. We believe that this should motivate those who work in preclinical testing (both *in vitro* and *in vivo*) to consider the benefits of Bayesian approaches.

All analyses were done with WinBUGS but could have been done also using SAS® procedures. More specifically, the procedure GENMOD can be used to analyze the beetle data while the procedure MCMC is needed for the Ames assay.

13

Measurement error

In a wide range of biostatistical applications, the modeling approach adopted can depend on the specification of the degree of error observed in variables of interest. In the simplest case, for example, a random sample of a normally distributed random variable (y) with mean μ and precision τ, can be assumed to be described by a first-level model hierarchy such as

$$y_i \sim \mathrm{N}(\mu, \sigma^2),$$

where the precision is given by $\tau = \sigma^{-2}$. Hence, the error in the random variable can be plainly seen from the relation

$$y_i = \mu + v_i,$$

where $v_i \sim \mathrm{N}(0, \sigma^2)$. In this simple case, the true value of y_i, μ, is contaminated by the zero-mean error term which is assumed to be additive. This illustrates a basic concept of measurement error: any variable deemed to be observed with error can be expressed as a combination of a true value and an error term. The importance of this idea will become clearer with more advanced examples in the following sections. In Section 13.1, the continuous measurement error case is considered. In the subsequent section, discrete measurement error models are treated. For reviews of this area see Gustafson (2004), Carroll *et al.* (2006) and Buonaccorsi (2010).

13.1 Continuous measurement error

In Chapter 4, we considered a simple hierarchical regression model. Here, we initially examine the extension of this model to the situation where the predictor x is measured with error.

13.1.1 Measurement error in a variable

Assume that a variable is measured with error, i.e. $x_i^* = x_i + u_i$, with x_i the true value for the variable measured at the ith subject and u_i the error made when recording the variable.

Bayesian Biostatistics, First Edition. Emmanuel Lesaffre and Andrew B. Lawson.

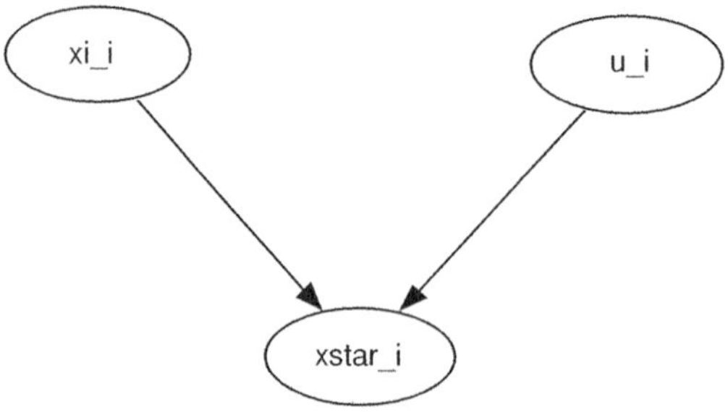

Figure 13.1 A graphical model (DAG) representation of the classical measurement error problem with continuous data. Here, the model is $x_i^* = x_i + u_i$.

Classically one assumes that $u_i \sim \mathrm{N}(0, \sigma_u^2)$. This assumption can be rewritten as the following model:

$$x_i^* \sim \mathrm{N}(x_i, \sigma_u^2). \tag{13.1}$$

Hence, $E(x_i^*) = x_i$. Thus, the observed value is assumed to be a contaminated version of the true value. The observed variable is, therefore, also called a *surrogate measurement*. The contamination is assumed to be symmetric with variance σ_u^2. This is known as *classical* measurement error. Figure 13.1 displays a DAG for the classical measurement error problem.

Note that we could extend this model by assuming different forms of error besides u_i. For example, when subjects are examined repeatedly two kinds of error may appear: a subject specific and a pure measurement error. Such a dual decomposition of error has been proposed by Kipnis and coworkers in the analysis of food frequency questionnaires (FFQ) in nutritional studies (Kipnis *et al.* 1999, 2001, 2003). Their model for the variable obtained from the ith subject at the jth repeated administration of an FFQ is given by

$$x_{ij}^* = \alpha_0 + \alpha_1 x_i + v_{ij},$$
$$v_{ij} = u_i + u_{ij}$$

with u_i representing the subject-specific measurement error and u_{ij} the pure measurement error both having a normal distribution. Alternative proposals involving non-normal and asymmetric errors have been made for FFQ data (Song *et al.* 2010).

13.1.2 Two types of measurement error on the predictor in linear and nonlinear models

If we now assume that x_i^* is a variate that is included in a regression model as an explanatory predictor then we must consider how to include the measurement error on x_i within the model formulation. We first consider the classical measurement error model and then the Berkson error model.

Let us first assume that there is no measurement error and that a dependent variable y_i is thought to relate to x_i via a simple linear regression model:

$$y_i = \beta_0 + \beta_1 x_i + \varepsilon_i, \tag{13.2}$$

with $\varepsilon_i \sim \mathrm{N}(0, \sigma_y^2)$ representing the variability of the y_i around the regression line. Suppose now that there is measurement error in y_i and x_i and we replace y_i by $y_i^* = y_i + v_i$ and x_i by $x_i^* = x_i + u_i$. Further, suppose that we again assume a linear regression model relating the response and the predictor yielding the model

$$y_i^* = \beta_0^* + \beta_1^* x_i^* + \varepsilon_i^*, \tag{13.3}$$

with $\varepsilon_i^* \sim \mathrm{N}(0, \sigma_y^{*2})$. Then the slope, β_1^*, in the above model does not represent the true relationship between the response and the predictor, which we would like to know.

To fix ideas, let us take the following example taken from the IRAS multicenter study, introduced below. Blood is taken from a patient and high-density cholesterol *hdl*) and blood low-density cholesterol (*ldl*) are measured. Most likely, both *hdl* and *ldl* are measured with error. A natural assumption is that the true underlying relation between *hdl* and *ldl* will be based on the true value of *ldl* (x_i) and *hdl*(y_i) and not on their observed values. In Figure 13.2, a scatterplot of these data together with the least-squares estimate (LSE) solution is shown.

From model (13.2), we can see that if there was only measurement error on y_i, then the induced extra variability can be incorporated into the variance of ε_i. The question is, therefore, what effect the error on the predictor has on the estimated slope. In other words, what does β_1^* in model (13.3) estimate? To see the effect of measurement error on the estimated regression coefficients, one can compute the MLE of a bivariate normal model with responses y_i^* and x_i^* (Carroll *et al.* 2006). This computation shows that the estimated slope in model (13.3) is attenuated compared to the estimated slope in model (13.2). Namely, not β_1 is estimated but $\beta_1^* = \lambda\beta_1$, where

$$\lambda = \frac{\sigma_x^2}{\sigma_x^2 + \sigma_u^2}, \tag{13.4}$$

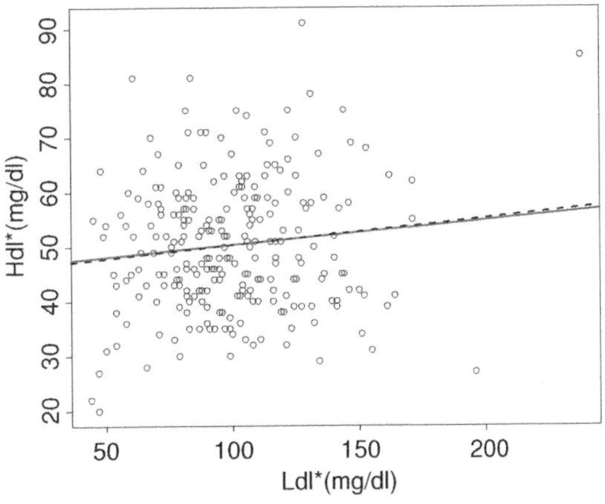

Figure 13.2 Hdl–ldl example: scatterplot of blood cholesterol measurements (*hdl*, *ldl*) for 254 study participants. The LSE (solid line) and the corrected (for measurement error) regression line (dashed line) are added.

with σ_x^2 the inter-subject variability of the predictor. Thus, error in the prediction variable creates a bias in the estimated regression coefficient. This bias is known as the *attenuation bias*. Further, one can show that the residual variance has increased from σ_y^2 to $\sigma_y^2 + \beta_1^2\sigma_u^2\left(\frac{\sigma_x^2}{\sigma_u^2+\sigma_x^2}\right)$. Thus, measurement error in the predictor will also cause a decrease in power, due to an increased residual variance.

Measurement error can appear also in another way. Namely, *Berkson error* occurs when $x_i = x_i^* + u_{Bi}$ where $u_{Bi} \sim \mathrm{N}(0, \sigma_{Bu}^2)$. In other words, in the case of Berkson error, $E(x_i) = x_i^*$, which is just the reversed situation of the classical measurement error model. This occurs for instance when, in an industrial process, one wishes to control the temperature or pressure at a particular level (x_i^*) but the actual level (x_i) fluctuates around it (Carroll *et al.* 2006). Notice that model (13.3) can then be written as (error in response is integrated in ε^*):

$$y_i = \beta_0 + \beta_1 x_i^* + \beta_1 u_{Bi} + \varepsilon_i^*.$$

Since $E(u_{Bi}) = 0$, there is no *attenuation bias* in the Berkson error model, but the residual variance will increase to $\sigma_y^2 + \beta_1^2\sigma_{Bu}^2$.

If more than one predictor with measurement error is included in the model, then things become more complex. Namely, if there are two predictors in the model with x measured with error and z perfectly measured, then there is again attenuation in the regression coefficient of x, but also the regression coefficient of z may be distorted.

The effects of classical measurement error in nonlinear models are roughly the same as in the normal linear model, i.e. reduced power for testing associations and bias in the estimation of the regression coefficients. However, while Berkson error does lead to unbiased estimation of the regression coefficients in the linear case, in general, this will not be true anymore in the nonlinear case. In addition, the impact of measurement error on other parameters in the regression model (such as shape parameters) will not be straightforward.

13.1.3 Accommodation of predictor measurement error

There are two basic ways to accommodate for the error in a single predictor x_i:

1. *Structural modeling*: Given that we have two sources of observed data y_i and x_i^*, we can consider two models that are linked: (1) a structural model (13.3), which links y_i to x_i and (2) a measurement error model (13.1), which links the observed value x_i^* to x_i. These two models would now be fitted simultaneously and x_i would be estimated as a *latent* variable. This is an example of a structural equation model with two components:

   Structural model: $y_i \sim \mathrm{N}(\beta_0 + \beta_1 x_i, \sigma_y^2)$,
   Measurement error model: $x_i^* \sim \mathrm{N}(x_i, \sigma_u^2)$.

   In order to make the parameters estimable, several strategies could be adopted depending on the available data and/or prior information. For instance, substantive considerations could lead to strong prior information on σ_u^2 or to fix this variance as done in, e.g. Gössl and Küchenhoff (2001). If validation data relating x_i^* to x_i are available as in Section 13.2.3, then a joint modeling exercise is involved. If no extra information is available, the model can still be identifiable for particular choices of the prior distribution $p(x_i \mid \gamma)$. It is usually not advisable to assume a Gaussian prior distribution for x_i unless highly constrained, as this may allow for nonpositive values. But

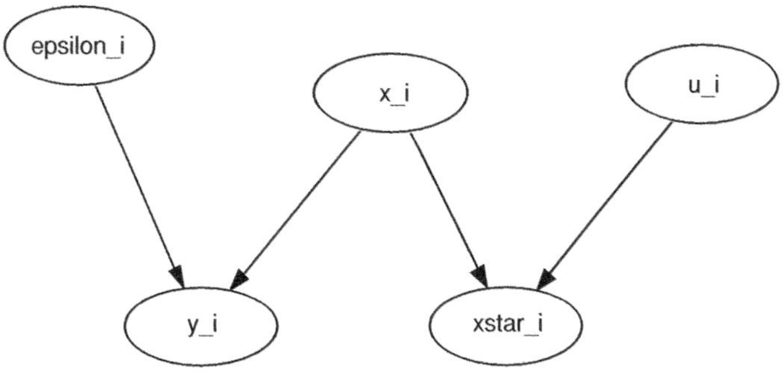

Figure 13.3 Graphical model for the structural equation model with latent variable x_i.

this choice may also lead to an unidentifiable model when combined with the Gaussian error model. Instead, if a gamma prior distribution is realistic for the true covariate values, such as $x_i \sim \text{Gamma}(\gamma^2, c\gamma)$ with mean equal to γ/c and variance equal to $1/c^2$, then the parameters of the measurement error model as well as the parameters of the structural model are estimable. Hyperparameters can also be specified. Figure 13.3 displays the graphical model for the structural equation.

2. *Random effects modeling*: Another approach is to simply add a random effect to the linear relation $y_i = \beta_0^* + \beta_1^* x_i^* + \varepsilon_i^*$ so that the model becomes:

$$y_i = \beta_0 + \beta_1 x_i^* + u_i + \varepsilon_i,$$

where $u_i \sim \text{N}(0, \sigma_u^2)$ and $\varepsilon_i \sim \text{N}(0, \sigma_y^2)$.

In this model, there are now two components of variation that need to be estimated. In addition, the identification of these two components may be of concern at the individual level as the total noise variation for any unit could be swapped between the two errors. Note that the Kipnis model is essentially the same but has a repeated measure error term (u_{ij}) and this may help identification.

13.1.3.1 Analysis of the hdl–ldl example

We have analyzed the *hdl–ldl* data for the 254 study participants of the cholesterol study, which were collected in the context of the IRAS multicenter study. Figure 13.4 displays the WinBUGS code for analyzing the *hdl–ldl* data with the structural modeling approach. In this case, relatively diffuse prior distributions were assumed for the hyperparameters of the variance components as well as for the gamma parameter `gamma2`. A single chain was run for 70 000 iterations with 30 000 burn-in iterations. Figure 13.6 displays the posterior expected sample results for several main parameters for the model in Figure 13.4. From Figure 13.6, we learn that the posterior mean of λ is 0.9834 with SD $= 0.03488$, hence the attenuation bias is minimal. In fact, the uncorrected posterior mean of β_1 was 0.0478 while the corrected posterior mean increased to only 0.0451. Figure 13.5 displays the posterior marginal density estimate of the attenuation bias and confirms that the attenuation bias is quite close to 1. This suggests that the error in the overall model is quite large (`sdldl`) compared to the error in the *ldl* predictor (`sdldlu`). In Figure 13.2, we observe that the corrected regression line is close to the LSE. The estimated true *ldl* appears to be well estimated with low standard deviations

```
model
     {
        for (i in 1:N) {
        hdl[i] ~ dnorm(mu[i], tau.e)
        mu[i] <- beta0 + beta1*ldl[i]
        ldlstar[i] ~ dnorm(ldl[i],tau.u)
        ldl[i] ~ dgamma(gamma2,cgamma)
        }
     gamma2 <-gamma*gamma
     cgamma <- c*gamma
     c2 <- tau.ldl
     c <- pow(c2,0.5)
     gamma ~ dgamma(0.05,0.005)
     tau.e ~ dgamma( 0.05,0.005)
     tau.u ~ dgamma(0.05,0.005)
     tau.ldl ~ dgamma(0.05,0.005)
     sige <- 1/tau.e
     sigldlu <- 1/tau.u
     sigldl <- 1/tau.ldl
     sde <-  pow(sige,0.5)
     sdldlu <- pow(sigldlu,0.5)
     sdldl <- pow(sigldl,0.5)
     lambda <- sigldl/(sigldl+sigldlu)
     beta0 ~ dnorm(0,0.00001)
     beta1 ~ dnorm(0,0.001)
     }
```

Figure 13.4 Hdl–ldl example: WinBUGS code for structural modeling.

for each observation in the posterior sample. Figure 13.7 displays the density estimate of the posterior expected value of *ldl*.

The WinBUGS code for the random effects approach is given in Figure 13.8. The results of this analysis (not shown) suggest that the general random variation is much larger than the overall model error. However, there is an additional issue that should be considered in this case, i.e. the *nonidenti ability* of the two different additive errors at the same level within the hierarchy (unit level). Hence, while the posterior expected value of `Rat` is very small (0.00119), suggesting a very large random effect variance, it should be borne in mind that the

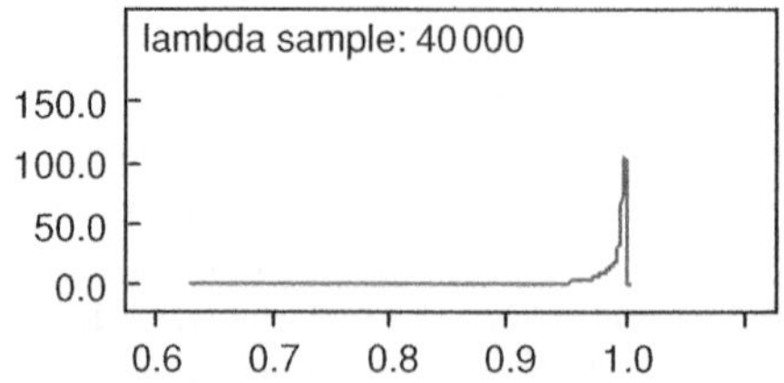

Figure 13.5 Hdl–ldl example: attenuation bias for structural modeling.

Node	Mean	sd	MC error	2.5%	Median	97.5%	Start	Sample
beta0	45.79	2.801	0.017	40.26	45.81	51.23	30001	40000
beta1	0.04511	0.02709	1.637E-4	-0.007479	0.045	0.0986	30001	40000
lambda	0.9834	0.03488	0.002154	0.8814	0.996	1.0	30001	40000
sde	11.96	0.5319	0.002729	10.97	11.94	13.06	30001	40000
sdldl	27.99	1.472	0.04518	25.13	27.97	30.94	30001	40000
sdldlu	2.566	2.545	0.1678	0.09351	1.789	9.61	30001	40000

Figure 13.6 Hdl–ldl example: WinBUGS posterior summary measures for the main parameters of the model in Figure 13.4.

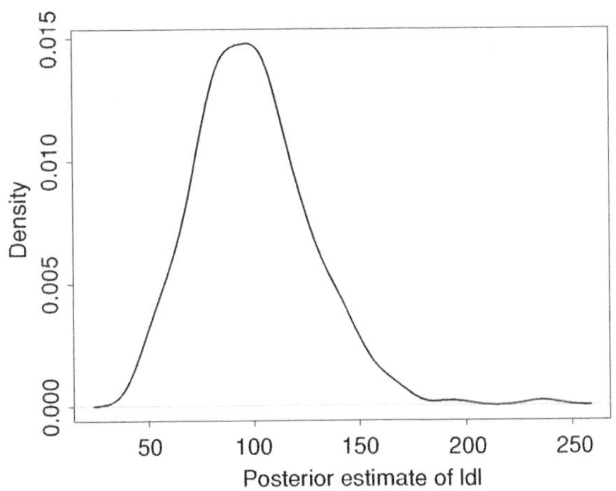

Figure 13.7 Hdl–ldl example: density estimate of the posterior expected value of the latent (true) variable *ldl* over the 254 participants.

```
model
    {
    for (i in 1:N) {
    hdl[i] ~ dnorm(mu1[i],tau.e)
    mu1[i] <- beta0 + beta1*ldl[i]+eps[i]
    eps[i] ~ dnorm(0,tau.eps)
    }
tau.e ~ dgamma( 0.05,0.005)
tau.eps ~ dgamma(0.05,0.005)
sige <- 1/tau.e
sigeps <- 1/tau.eps
Rat <- sige/(sige+sigeps)
beta0 ~ dnorm(0,0.00001)
beta1 ~ dnorm(0,0.001)
}
```

Figure 13.8 Hdl–ldl example: unit level random effect model for the cholesterol data.

nonidentification of the effects may influence this result. Identification is discussed further in Chapter 9.

13.1.4 Nonadditive errors and other extensions

In the previous discussion, attention has been placed solely on additive error. In many situations, this a natural assumption. However, it is quite possible that errors are not additive. For example, it could easily be that the error depends on the level of the measured variable and so an error such as

$$x_i^* = x_i \times u_i$$

or even

$$x_i^* = x_i^{u_i}$$

is quite possible. Indeed, a model could be formulated to allow different forms such as

$$x_i^* = l(x_i), \quad \text{where} \quad l(z) = \beta_0 + \beta_1 z^{\gamma}.$$

Nonlinearity in the error can cause problems in the analysis, especially if additive error is assumed but was misspecified.

Finally, in many studies, ME is not independent between responses within sampling units and so the assumption of independent prior distributions for error may not be appropriate. For example, in a questionnaire survey there may be correlation between responses to different questions and so joint prior distributions may need to be assumed. Further, ME may also be correlated between sampling units. For example, underlying but unobserved stratification could cause correlated response errors within strata. Further discussion of these problems, however, is beyond the scope of this book.

13.2 Discrete measurement error

13.2.1 Sources of misclassification

Discrete measurement error arises when outcomes or predictors are measured with error on discrete scales. In that case, measurement error is sometimes also called *misclassi cation*. Perhaps the commonest example of this would be found in questionnaire responses where a finite set of possible responses yields integer values. These response outcomes may be ordered (ordinal) or not (nominal). When a response is not correct then some form of error is found. A simple example of this would be a question which has a yes/no answer. In this case, an error is introduced if the correct (true) answer were *yes* (1) but the respondent answered *no* (0). More generally, for a multilevel response with k levels, if the true response were l then any response $l^* \neq l$ has error. Note that when the binary response is possibly misclassified, then correction for misclassification is explicitly needed and cannot be ignored as in the continuous case where the y-measurement error is assumed to be part of the model.

Errors in discrete variates could be ascribable to a number of causes. There may simply be a recording error that leads to the wrong response. In the case of questionnaire surveys, this could be due to interviewer bias, or in the case of switching systems, operator error. In many cases this could be a relatively random error as it may be assumed that the error is not intentional. However, there could also be systematic bias in these errors. For example, recording of a particular respondent could be affected by their speech patterns and so multiple errors could arise across surveys. Equally systematic errors could occur in switching systems if they were operated differently at different times. For example, weather conditions might affect the operation of some systems and might produce a systematic bias.

Another error source arises when self-reported information is sought, but the responses may be biased due to perceptual errors or even intentional errors. For example, a respondent in a survey may perceive that they eat low amounts of high fat food, when in fact they eat large amounts. Alternatively, due to their wish to be seen as eating nutritiously they may underestimate high-fat foods. This underestimation of 'bad' food and overestimation of 'good' food relates to theories of social desirability (Crowne and Marlowe 1960; Fisher 1993). Social desirability is the need to appear socially acceptable in the eyes of others and so this produces distortions in responses to certain questions.

Ultimately various sources of bias could lead to misspecification bias in the variables and they might be combined in one study. For example, self-report of dietary intake may have error due to social desirability concerns, and then recorded by an interviewee who then induces further bias. In the context of regression models, the effect of such misclassification errors is a distorted picture of the relationship between the response and the predictor (see Neuhaus 1999; Mwalili *et al.* 2005).

13.2.2 Misclassification in the binary predictor

Here, we examine a simple case where a discrete binary covariate is included in a linear model with continuous outcome. More complex scenarios can be found in Gustafson (2004).

Define the independent binary variable as x_i, and assume model (13.2). This implies that $E(y \mid x) = \beta_0 + \beta_1 x_i$. Assume now that the observed predictor is x_i^*. We also assume that the distribution of x_i^* only depends on x_i, and not on y_i. In that case we speak of a *nondifferential* measurement error. Based on this assumption, we can summarize the misclassification by $S_n = p(x^* = 1 \mid x = 1)$ and $S_p = p(x^* = 0 \mid x = 0)$, which are the sensitivity and specificity of the classification, respectively. Note that under the above linear model it can be shown that $E(y \mid x^*) = \beta_0^* + \beta_1^* x_i^*$ where $\beta_0^* = \beta_0 + \beta_1 p(x = 1 \mid x^* = 0)$ and the attenuation bias (expressed as a proportion) is

$$\frac{\beta_1^*}{\beta_1} = 1 - p(x = 0 \mid x^* = 1) - p(x = 1 \mid x^* = 0). \tag{13.5}$$

Expression (13.5) demonstrates that the degree of bias depends on the degree of misclassification given the apparent classification. In terms of sensitivity and specificity, expression (13.5) can be written as

$$\frac{\beta_1^*}{\beta_1} = (S_n + S_p - 1)\frac{\psi(1 - \psi)}{\psi^*(1 - \psi^*)},$$

where $\psi = p(x = 1)$ and $\psi^* = p(x^* = 1) = (1 - S_p) + (S_n + S_p - 1)\psi$. The interpretation of these results follows immediately in that when $S_n = S_p = 1$ then the attenuation proportion is 0, and increases when S_n or S_p increases.

Bayesian approaches to accommodating discrete measurement error usually involve the assumption of certain distributional forms for model components. We now look at an example of such an approach with an outcome variable y and a vector of continuous predictor variables (z) and a binary exposure variable x. A simple example could be a logistic regression for a binary outcome y so that for a single observation

$$\text{logit}\, p(y = 1 \mid x, z) = \beta_0 + \beta_1 x + \boldsymbol{\beta}_2^T z \tag{13.6}$$

and

$$\text{logit}\, p(x = 1 \mid z) = \rho_0 + \boldsymbol{\rho}_1^T z, \tag{13.7}$$

with $\boldsymbol{\beta}_2$ and $\boldsymbol{\rho}_1$ regression vectors pertaining to the continuous covariates. These two relations define the joint distribution of $y, x \mid z$ and the conditional distribution of x given y, z. It is also straightforward to show that

$$\text{logit}\, p(x = 1 \mid y, z) = \rho_0 + \beta_1 y + \boldsymbol{\rho}_1^T z + h(z, \boldsymbol{\beta}), \tag{13.8}$$

which frames the problem in terms of an '*exposure given outcome*' model. One simplification then is to ignore the final nonlinear term $h(z, \beta)$, and so we have a linear model in y and z. We could use either expression (13.6) with expression (13.7) or use the simpler exposure given outcome model based on expression (13.8).

13.2.2.1 Example: The IRAS multicenter study

In the IRAS multicenter study (Insulin Resistance and Atherosclerosis Study) (Liese *et al.* 2004), the relationship between insulin resistance and cardiovascular disease (CVD) and its risk factors in a tri-ethnic (African–American, Hispanic, and non-Hispanic white) population aged 40–69 years at baseline was examined. In addition, it was the aim to identify the genetic determinants of insulin resistance and visceral adiposity.

Here we look at the relationship between blood pressure (*CurrBPMd*) and nutrition and exercise. Participants were asked to respond to two binary questions of current activity: the first of these was the current healthy diet (*CurrD*: yes(2)/no(1)) and the second was the current physical activity level (*CurrE*: low(1)/high(2)). These questions were self-assessed and so may be prone to misclassification. The outcome of interest for subjects was current blood pressure state (*CurrBPMd*: high (2)/low(1)) and a continuous blood chemistry covariate (*FG*: fasting glucose $\times 10^{-1}$) was also measured.

There were 152 participants. Table 13.1 displays a partial listing of the data. We regard *CurrD* and *CurrE* as surrogate measures for 'healthy lifestyle' behavior. Hence, they both represent an aspect of 'healthy' lifestyle behavior and could be regarded as reasonable surrogates. In this example we have 53/152 exposed to exercise and 63/152 have healthy diet. We also have high blood pressure registered for 29/152 participants. The first ratios are estimates of proportion 'exposed' in the study. Figure 13.9 displays various marginal and conditional

Table 13.1 IRAS study: blood pressure (*CurrBPMd*) measured with a covariate *Glychem* (*FG* = Fasting Glucose $\times 10^{-1}$) and discrete possibly misclassified covariates consisting of self-reported dietary intake (*CurrD*) and exercise (*CurrE*).

CurrD	CurrE	FG	CurrBPMd
1	1	10.90	1
1	1	7.56	1
1	1	9.18	1
2	1	7.72	1
2	1	12.92	2
1	1	6.02	1

plots of the variables in the data set. Fasting glucose seems to show a slight relation with level of *CurrBPMd* whereas the conditioning plots also show some relationship.

We have fitted two models to this data example using WinBUGS. For simplicity we have only examined a single exposure surrogate (current diet). However, the analysis can be extended to incorporate more surrogates (as in this case). The first model is the joint surrogate model with

$$\text{logit}\, p(y = 1 \mid x, z) = \beta_0 + \beta_1 x + \beta_2 z,$$

$$\text{logit}\, p(x^* = 1 \mid x, z) = \alpha_0 + \alpha_1 x + \alpha_2 z,$$

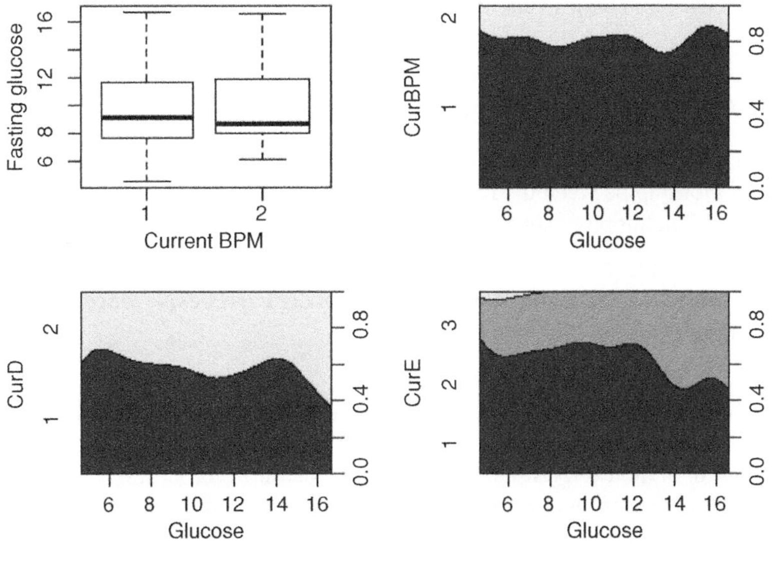

Figure 13.9 IRAS study: (1) top left: box plots of *glucose* against *CurrBPMd* and (2) three conditional plots of the discrete predictors and outcome against *glucose*.

Table 13.2 IRAS study: posterior estimates of model parameters from a converged MCMC sampler for models 1 and 2: median and 95% credible interval.

Model 1	Estimate (95% CI)	Model 2	Estimate (95% CI)
β_0	−0.5394 (−1.796, 0.3486)	β_0	−0.10230 (−0.7467, 0.2606)
β_1	−0.2069 (−1.775, 0.8136)	β_1	−0.04419 (−0.7472, 0.4456)
β_2	−0.0759 (−0.179, 0.0440)	β_2	−0.06642 (−0.6505, 0.2793)
		β_3	−0.00496 (−0.0560, 0.0561)
α_0	−0.3898 (−1.447, 0.4475)	α_0	5.27E-4 (−0.6365, 0.6475)
α_1	0.1590 (−1.712, 0.9114)	α_1	0.00105 (−0.6194, 0.6359)
α_2	0.0185 (−0.071, 0.1231)	α_2	0.00259 (−0.6208, 0.6138)

with x as the true current diet (acting as a latent variable), x^* is the observed current diet, y is the current blood pressure level, and z is the continuous fasting glucose $\times 10^{-1}$. The second model is the exposure given outcome model. In particular, we considered

$$\text{logit } p(x^* = 1 \mid x, y, z) = \beta_0 + \beta_1 x + \beta_2 y + \beta_3 z,$$

$$\text{logit } p(x = 1 \mid y, z) = \alpha_0 + \alpha_1 y + \alpha_2 z,$$

as a joint exposure given outcome model variant. The results of fitting these two models to the data are displayed in Table 13.2. For both models, not only convergence of the deviance was attained by 20 000 iterations but also for the individual parameters convergence was found. The posterior median parameter estimates for the converged samples from both models are displayed in Table 13.2. In either model there is little evidence of significant relations between the outcome and the continuous covariate, although in model 1 there is stronger evidence of association between *blood pressure* and *glucose* and *diet* and *glucose*, given the values of β_2 and α_2.

13.2.3 Misclassification in a binary response

When a categorical response is suspected to have misclassification error then this will also affect the relationship between the response and the covariate(s). We will now illustrate this with the Signal-Tandmobiel® study.

13.2.3.1 Example: Misclassification error in scoring caries experience in the Signal-Tandmobiel® study

The Signal-Tandmobiel® study was introduced in Example II.3. Here, we consider data collected in the last year (2001) on 100 children, randomly selected from the total sample. One of the purposes of this study was to search for predictors of caries experience (CE). CE can be analyzed on mouth level, i.e. whether there is caries (yes = 1, 0 = no) in the mouth somewhere. However, of more interest to the dentists is to look for predictors of CE on the surface level, i.e. whether there is CE on the surface. The data have a three-level structure: (1) surfaces, (2) within teeth, and (3) within mouths. Therefore, a multilevel logistic regression model was considered to explore the effect of predictors at subject level, tooth level and surface level. The covariates at subject level were *age* at examination (note there was still considerable age variation despite that the children were examined around the age of 11 years) and *gender*. We considered one covariate at tooth level, i.e. whether the tooth is *deciduous* or *permanent*. At surface level, we have included four binary covariates: (1) *lingual* surface (surface where the tongue would be), (2) *mesial* surface (surface visible from the side closest to where the middle line of the face would be), *distal* surface (surface visible from the side furthest from where the middle line of the face would be), and (3) *occlusal* surface (surface of a tooth that occludes with or contacts an opposing surface of a tooth in the opposing jaw). The buccal (frontal) surface was chosen as baseline surface. Note that only premolars and molars have five surfaces, the other teeth have four surfaces.

In oral health surveys, the detection of CE is prone to misclassification for several reasons, thereby affecting the quality of the obtained data. For this reason, calibration exercises, which aim to assess and improve the scoring behavior of dental raters, were organized. During a calibration exercise, a sample of children is examined by the benchmark scorer and the dental examiners allowing the estimation of misclassification probabilities. This misclassification information can be used for correction purposes in the main data.

In this sample, there were 53 boys with a mean (SD) age of 11.6 (0.36) years. There were 311 surfaces with CE from a total of 10 800 surfaces. Most caries were found on the occlusal surface (162/311). To simplify matters, we assumed here that there was only one dental examiner (hence lumping together all 16 dental examiners into one). The misclassification Table 13.3 obtained from the calibration exercises, allows us to estimate the S_n (=428/(428+146)=0.75) and the S_p (=4684/(4684+146)=0.98). We assumed nondifferential misclassification, which means that the probability of misclassification only depends on the true status of the surface.

The multilevel logistic regression model at surface level is defined as follows. Let y_{mts} denote the true binary CE outcome obtained from the benchmark scorer for surface $s = 1, \ldots, S$ in tooth $t = 1, \ldots, T$ of subject $m = 1, \ldots, M$. This model involves two random effects: $b_m \sim \mathrm{N}(0, \sigma_m^2)$ for the mouth level and $b_t \sim \mathrm{N}(0, \sigma_t^2)$ for the tooth level. Without misclassification, the multilevel logistic regression model is given by

$$\text{logit}\,[p(y_{mts} = 1 \mid \boldsymbol{x}_{mts}, \boldsymbol{b})] = \boldsymbol{x}_{mts}^T \boldsymbol{\beta} + b_m + b_t,$$

where $\boldsymbol{\beta}$ represents the fixed effects. Denote the possibly corrupted binary score obtained from the dental examiner as y_{mts}^*. From the above misclassification table S_n and S_p are available. The corrected multilevel logistic regression model (corrected for misclassification) is given by

$$p(y_{mts}^* = 1 \mid \boldsymbol{x}_{mts}, \boldsymbol{b}) = (1 - S_p) + [S_n + S_p - 1][\text{expit}(\boldsymbol{x}_{mts}^T \boldsymbol{\beta} + b_m + b_t)],$$

Table 13.3 Signal-Tandmobiel study: misclassification table.

		Benchmark	
		0	1
Examiner	0	4684	146
	1	87	428

Table 13.4 Signal-Tandmobiel study: parameter estimates of corrected and uncorrected multilevel logistic models.

Parameter	Uncorrected estimate (SD)	95% CI	Corrected estimate (SD)	95% CI
Fixed effects				
Intercept	−5.973 (0.558)	[−7.250, −5.112]	−9.378 (1.205)	[−11.592, −6.894]
Gender				
Girls	−0.043 (0.476)	[−1.024, 0.851]	−0.266 (0.885)	[−1.951, 1.374]
Boys	...	...	...	...
Age	0.370 (0.273)	[−0.161, 0.879]	0.600 (0.571)	[−0.536, 1.790]
Dentition type				
Permanent	−2.550 (0.308)	[−3.151, −1.969]	−4.273 (0.610)	[−5.588, −3.169]
Deciduous	...	...	...	...
Surface type				
Distal	0.407 (0.299)	[−0.162, 0.997]	1.107 (0.626)	[−0.027, 2.440]
Mesial	0.847 (0.291)	[0.299, 1.435]	2.153 (0.618)	[1.062, 3.517]
Lingual	0.294 (0.297)	[−0.265, 0.868]	1.093 (0.617)	[−0.041, 2.429]
Occlusal	3.755 (0.286)	[3.224, 4.322]	6.806 (0.837)	[5.313, 8.505]
Buccal	...	...	...	...
Random effects				
σ_m^2	4.946 (1.530)	[2.810, 8.747]	16.836 (5.632)	[8.275, 30.907]
σ_t^2	4.450 (0.730)	[3.226, 6.114]	11.540 (2.646)	[7.194, 16.879]

where *expit* represents the inverse of the logit function. Plugging in the obtained values for S_n and S_p allows us to estimate the regression coefficients, $\boldsymbol{\beta}$, expressing the relationship between the true CE outcome and the covariates.

For the regression coefficients $\boldsymbol{\beta}$, we assumed vague normal priors, i.e. with mean 0 and variance 10^6. The prior distribution for the standard deviations of the random effects was taken as uniform, i.e. $\sigma_m \sim U(0, 100)$ and $\sigma_t \sim U(0, 100)$. The analysis was performed using JAGS 3.1.0. Three MCMC chains each of 2000 iterations were run with 200 burn-in iterations for both models. Convergence was assessed using Brooks, Gelman and Rubin's (BGR) diagnostic ($\hat{R}$) which was close to 1 for all the parameters. In Table 13.4, we show the posterior estimates of the parameters.

We found that *age* and *gender* do not contribute significantly to CE. Permanent teeth show less CE than deciduous teeth, which can be explained from the fact that deciduous teeth have been exposed for a longer period to acid-producing bacteria. Further, compared to the buccal surface there is more CE on the mesial and occlusal surfaces. Further, there appears to be an important mouth and tooth variability. Finally, one can observe that all corrected regression coefficients are greater in absolute value than the corresponding uncorrected ones, which again illustrate the attenuation effect due to measurement error.

Note that we have assumed in our analysis that the misclassification probabilities S_n and S_p are known. However, a proper analysis should take into account the uncertainty with which these correction terms are estimated. This can be easily done by an appropriate change in the (WinBUGS, JAGS, etc.) program. For details on how this could be done and for correction for misclassification in other categorical models we refer to Mwalili *et al.* (2005), Lesaffre *et al.* (2004), Mwalili *et al.* (2008), Lesaffre *et al.* (2009), Mutsvari *et al.* (2010), and Garcia-Zattera *et al.* (2010).

13.3 Closing remarks

In this brief overview of measurement error, we have deliberately demonstrated simple examples with simple models for outcomes. Measurement error, and in particular Bayesian approaches to measurement error, is a broad topic with a relatively large literature associated with it. The reader is directed to Gustafson (2004), Carroll *et al.* (2006) and Buonaccorsi (2010) for more detailed coverage of this important topic area. Finally, it should be stated that, for many problems involving measurement error, the Bayesian paradigm in combination with powerful software such as WinBUGS provides an ideal approach or set of methods, not only for handling unobserved or latent effects, but also for allowing the use of prior distributions and the ability to control the estimation of effects appropriately. Many measurement error problems cannot be approached easily via the use of conventional frequentist methods. Finally, note that all examples can also be analyzed with the SAS procedure MCMC.

14

Survival analysis

Survival analysis is a fundamental part of modern biostatistics. It is focused on the analysis of 'time to event' type of data where the variable or outcome of interest is *time* itself. Examples abound of this kind of data come from reliability testing (where the time to failure of a device is of interest), finance (time to maturity), clinical trials (time to cure or adverse outcome), etc. In biostatistical practice, time to an event is common in a clinical trial setting where groups of subjects are given treatments and then the subjects are followed up in time. In the clinical setting, it is often a concern to monitor patient survival under different treatment regimes and relate this to other treatment outcomes.

At the population level, survival data can be found in cancer registries, where each case is logged with date of diagnosis and also (possibly) vital outcome. Many countries now have registries for diseases such as cancer. Cancer occurrence is commonly found in national registries. Cancer-registry data usually consist of unique individual records where date of diagnosis, cancer type and severity and basic individual demographic data are lodged. In addition, the individual record can often be linked to vital outcome so that duration of illness may also be recorded. In this type of data, date of diagnosis can be regarded as an endpoint, as well as date of vital outcome.

14.1 Basic terminology

Define the random variable t as the time to an end point (death, cure, changed state etc.). We will focus on the *failure* or *endpoint* density denoted by $f(t)$ and related quantities. The function $f(t)$ is a probability density on the times to endpoint. There are various special functions related to this density that are useful in survival analysis.

We can define the cumulative distribution function of failure times as $F(t) = \int_0^t f(u)\mathrm{d}u$ and the survivor function as $S(t) = 1 - F(t)$, which is the probability of failure/endpoint given no failure endpoint prior to t. Other important relations follow: $f(t) = -\mathrm{d}S(t)/\mathrm{d}t$ and the hazard function defining the instantaneous failure rate conditional on surviving to t is defined by the ratio

$$h(t) = f(t)/S(t).$$

Bayesian Biostatistics, First Edition. Emmanuel Lesaffre and Andrew B. Lawson.

The hazard function can be derived directly from the survivor function as $h(t) = -d\log(S(t))/dt$. A cumulative hazard can also be defined by $H(t) = \int_0^t h(u)du = -\log(S(t))$. These relations lead to further important identities:

$$S(t) = \exp[-H(t)] = \exp\left[-\int_0^t h(u)\,du\right],$$

$$f(t) = h(t).S(t) = h(t).\exp\left[-\int_0^t h(u)\,du\right].$$

Assume that a sample of individuals have associated endpoint times $\{t_i\}$, $(i = 1, \ldots, n)$. For now assume that these times are all observed exactly. In addition to these ingredients, each observation unit can have covariates associated and, for the ith unit/person these are denoted by the vector $\boldsymbol{x}_i$. These covariates could be individual or contextual/ecological. Reviews of Bayesian survival methods can be found in Gustafson (1998a) and Ibrahim *et al.* (2000). For Bayesian proportional hazard modeling see Carlin and Hodges (1999).

14.1.1 Endpoint distributions

Often a failure time or endpoint distribution is specified for the time to endpoint and this is often chosen from distributions on the R^+ line. Common choices are among the Weibull or extreme value, lognormal or gamma families. Hence, for a parametric survival model, at the first level of the hierarchy, the data model consists of an endpoint distribution. For flexibility, we will initially assume a Weibull distribution in the following. The probability of an endpoint at time t_i under a Weibull distribution is specified by

$$f(t_i) = \rho\mu t_i^{\rho-1}\exp(-\mu t_i^{\rho}), \tag{14.1}$$

where $\rho > 0$ and $\mu > 0$. The survival and hazard functions derived from this specification are

$$S(t_i) = 1 - \int_0^{t_i} f(u)\,du = \exp(-\mu t_i^{\rho}),$$

$$h(t_i) = f(t_i)/S(t_i) = \rho\mu t_i^{\rho-1}.$$

The parameterization emphasizes the modeling of a function of the mean of the distribution via μ. Note that this allows a straightforward interpretation of the model component for this distribution: covariates (and contextual effects, see Section 14.1.3) can be included within μ and the parameter ρ provides the shape of the distribution. Often modeling proceeds via the hazard function, rather than the density, and for the Weibull this decomposes into two components:

$$h(t_i) = h_0(t_i) \times h_1(t_i) = \rho t_i^{\rho-1} \times \mu_i.$$

Here $h_0(t_i)$ is regarded as a baseline hazard, while $h_1(t_i)$ is a nonbaseline component which is most often the focus of modeling. Usually, it is assumed that a predictor term is linked to the parameter μ_i and each unit will have a different μ_i depending on covariates. A log-linear specification is often assumed, for example,

$$\log(\mu_i) = \boldsymbol{x}_i^T \boldsymbol{\beta}, \tag{14.2}$$

where $\boldsymbol{x}_i$ is the vector of individual unit-level covariates and $\boldsymbol{\beta}$ the corresponding parameter vector. This leads to a hazard, modulated by covariates, where the baseline risk is decreasing for $\rho < 1$, constant for $\rho = 1$ and increasing for $\rho > 1$:

$$h(t_i) = \rho t_i^{\rho-1}.\exp(\boldsymbol{x}_i^T \boldsymbol{\beta}).$$

Note that the Weibull model displays a feature termed *proportionality of hazard*, whereby the baseline hazard is modulated by the covariates in a multiplicative (log-linear) relation. This is an example of a proportional hazards (PH) model, and these models are discussed more fully in Section 14.1.5.

While the Weibull is a flexible distribution, there are many alternatives, some of which do not impose the constraints of proportionality of hazard. A wider class of models is the accelerated failure time (AFT) models. These models replace the t_i within the survival and hazard functions with a modulated function of covariates: $t_i \exp(\boldsymbol{x}_i^T \boldsymbol{\beta})$. This leads to a covariate acceleration/deceleration of risk. The Weibull is a special case of this general class. Note that the AFT model is in fact a linear model in the log of time:

$$\log(t_i) = \alpha + \boldsymbol{x}_i^T \boldsymbol{\beta} + \varepsilon_i,$$

where ε_i is an error term independent of $\boldsymbol{x}_i$ (not necessarily zero centered) and α is an intercept.

14.1.2 Censoring

Censoring occurs when the time of event endpoint is not observed exactly. Censoring is always an important issue in survival analysis as it is often the case that times are not observed exactly. For example, the most common form of censoring is right censoring where a study ends but individual observation units have not experienced the endpoint. This leads to two forms of data: observations with exact uncensored times $\{t_u\}$ and observations with censored times $\{t_c\}$. Under right censoring the censored times will be a time beyond which no observation was made. This could be a time of drop out or study end. For parametric models, this can be treated via a survivor function term product in the likelihood. For example, for right censoring we can assume

$$L = \prod_u f(t_u) \prod_c S(t_c),$$

where u denotes uncensored and c denotes right censored, and $S(\cdot)$ is the probability of surviving beyond a censoring time t_c. Note that this likelihood simplifies if you assume a censoring indicator γ which takes 0 for censored and 1 for uncensored, as

$$L = \prod_{all\ t} h(t)^\gamma S(t).$$

Other likelihood forms can similarly be derived for alternative censoring mechanisms.

14.1.3 Random effect specification

As most survival data are observed at the individual unit level, there could be either individual covariates or random or contextual effects relating to the individual. For example, the age of an individual could be a personal covariate and the location coordinates of the individual's address could be regarded as personal covariates also. In addition, there could be an individual level random effect which allows for frailty among individuals. This could be correlated or uncorrelated. The correlation could be induced by a grouping in the data, e.g. a common region or stratum. Survival models that involve individual frailties are called *frailty models*.

An example of a frailty model is obtained by adding a random intercept to expression (14.2), i.e.

$$\log(\mu_i) = \boldsymbol{x}_i^T \boldsymbol{\beta} + v_i, \tag{14.3}$$

with v_i an uncorrelated random effect given a prior distribution, i.e. $v_i \sim \text{N}(0, \sigma_v^2)$ where $\sigma_v^2 = \tau_v^{-1}$. This model was suggested by Carlin and Hodges (1999). We can extend this formulation by consideration of additional effects within the log-linear predictor. For example, we could specify

$$\begin{aligned} \log(\mu_i) &= \boldsymbol{x}_i^T \boldsymbol{\beta} + \Omega_i \\ \Omega_i &= v_i + u_i + \dots, \end{aligned} \tag{14.4}$$

where Ω_i contains the unit specific random effect terms. These effects could be individual unit level or they could be contextual in that they could relate to population groups, regions or other strata within the hierarchy. Note that, in this case, the PH assumption is not satisfied anymore.

The AFT model can also be extended to a frailty version by the addition of random effects which are individual or contextual in the form of

$$\log(t_i) = \alpha + \boldsymbol{x}_i^T \boldsymbol{\beta} + \Omega_i + \varepsilon_i,$$

where Ω_i is a random effect term (as in expression (14.4) above).

14.1.4 A general hazard model

In the context of cancer registry data, Banerjee and Carlin (2003) proposed a relaxation of the Weibull model to allow a semiparametric formulation whereby, with subject i ($i = 1, \dots, n_j$) in the jth (county) group:

$$h(t_{ij}|\boldsymbol{x}_{ij}) = h_{0j}(t_{ij}) \exp(\boldsymbol{x}_{ij}^T \boldsymbol{\beta} + v_j),$$

where h_{0j} denotes the county-specific baseline hazard. For an individual with censoring indicator γ_{ij} (0 if alive, and 1 if dead), the likelihood contribution is then

$$h(t_{ij}; \boldsymbol{x}_{ij})^{\gamma_{ij}} \exp[-H_{0j}(t_{ij}) \exp(\boldsymbol{x}_{ij}^T \boldsymbol{\beta} + v_j)],$$

where $H_{0j}(t_{ij}) = \int_0^{t_{ij}} h_{0j}(u)du$ is a county-specific cumulative baseline hazard and the covariates are assumed to be time independent. The baseline hazard appears in this likelihood and so must be estimated. Different approaches have been proposed for the estimation of the baseline hazard. One approach assumes a gamma process which is a function of a parametric cumulative hazard (see Ibrahim *et al.* 2000; Lawson and Song 2010). Another approach involves the use of beta mixtures (Banerjee and Carlin 2003). A related spatial model was developed by Bastos and Gamerman (2006) whereby they assumed time-dependent covariates which are fixed within small time periods and a correlated spatial frailty. They assumed no separate baseline risk, however.

14.1.5 Proportional hazards

Proportionality of the hazard is a common assumption in basic survival applications. For ordered times $\{t_{(1)}, \ldots, t_{(m)}\}$ with no censoring, Cox (1972) derived a partial likelihood which is free of the baseline hazard. It is given by

$$\prod_i \exp(\boldsymbol{x}_{(i)}^T \boldsymbol{\beta}) / \sum_{j \in R_i} \exp(\boldsymbol{x}_j^T \boldsymbol{\beta}),$$

where R_i is the set of those individuals at risk just before the ith event time. This approach allows the estimation of regression parameters without estimating the baseline hazard function because the baseline hazard is factored out of the likelihood. This semiparametric approach is often referred to as the *Cox model*. If, in addition, also the baseline hazard needs to be estimated then a nonparametric estimator can be used. For the PH model, we can further estimate the survivor function for a given covariate pattern via the identity

$$S(t|\boldsymbol{x}_i) = S_0(t)^{\exp(\boldsymbol{x}_i^T \boldsymbol{\beta})},$$

where $S_0(t)$ must be estimated separately.

14.1.6 The Cox model with random effects

The Cox proportional hazards model has been applied in a spatially correlated context by Henderson *et al.* (2002). Note that contextual effects can be included by extending the specification of the intensity term $\exp(\boldsymbol{x}_i^T \boldsymbol{\beta})$ to include random effects

$$\exp(\boldsymbol{x}_i^T \boldsymbol{\beta} + v_i), \tag{14.5}$$

where v_i are random contextual effects which could be at an aggregate level such as strata, geographic region or other grouping unit. In addition, these effects could also be purely individual (in the sense of frailty rather than context).

14.2 The Bayesian model formulation

For a Bayesian model formulation, it is common to assume a full likelihood (rather than a partial likelihood) as $h_0(t)$ and hence $S_0(t)$ can be modeled via flexible prior distributional specifications. For example, gamma processes can be assumed or a mixture of beta distributions for the hazard (Banerjee and Carlin 2003; Dunson and Herring 2005; Ibrahim *et al.* 2000). Two examples of Bayesian models with such a form are a Weibull model with random effects at the individual level and a nonproportional competitor: the AFT model with random effects.

14.2.1 A Weibull survival model

Let us take the general formulation of the Weibull model introduced above. The hazard is of the form

$$h(t_{ij}|\boldsymbol{x}_{ij}) = \rho t_{ij}^{\rho-1} \exp(\boldsymbol{x}_{ij}^T\boldsymbol{\beta} + \Omega_i),$$

where Ω_i can have a range of effects included depending on the application. For example, in the situation where individual and treatment group effects are important then a form such as $\Omega_i = v_i + \lambda_{i(i\in j)}$ might be considered where v_i is an individual effect and $\lambda_{i(i\in j)}$ is a group effect shared by all individuals within the jth group.

There is a facility in WinBUGS for the specification of a censoring mechanism within the definition of a distribution. This facility allows the use of a censoring variable to denote censoring times and can be used for different types of censoring (e.g. right, left and interval). The format is defined, in general, for a time variable `t[i]` and distribution `dist()` as

```
t[i]~dist()I(,)
```

The indicator notation is used to define limits for the censoring mechanism. I (lower, upper) specifies the lower and upper limits for the observed quantity. For example, right censored data with a censoring vector `Tlow` would have `I(Tlow,)` specified. An example of the type of specification for a Weibull distribution with right censoring would be

```
t[i]~dweib(rho,lambda[i])I(tcen[i],).
```

Here, `rho` is the shape parameter of the distribution, `lambda[i]` is the nonbaseline parameterized hazard, and `tcen` is a vector of censored observation times. An example of some code for a simple Weibull model is

```
for(i in 1: n)
t[i] ~ dweib(rho,lambda[i])I(tcen[i],)
lambda[i] <- exp(beta0+v[i])
v[i] ~ dnorm(0,tauv)
median[i] <- pow((log(2) /lambda[i]), 1/rho)
log(surv[i]) <- -lambda[i]*pow(t[i],rho)
```

Here, the `n` subjects have noncensored times (`t[i]`) or censored times (`tcen[i]`). The nonbaseline hazard is log linear and defined to have a constant term (`beta0`) and an individual level random effect (`v[i]`), which is assumed to have a zero mean Gaussian prior distribution: `v[i] ~ dnorm(0,tauv)`. For the Weibull distribution, the median survival time and the survivor function have closed forms and can be computed within a MCMC sampler. The median survival time is given by $\text{med}(S_i) = [\log(2)/\exp(\boldsymbol{x}_{ij}^T\boldsymbol{\beta} + \Omega_i)]^{1/\rho}$ for linear predictor $\boldsymbol{x}_{ij}^T\boldsymbol{\beta} + \Omega_i$ and this is given by code

```
median[i] <- pow((log(2) /lambda[i]), 1/rho).
```

The survivor function or log survivor function can also be specified for a linear predictor and is given simply by $\log(S_{ij}) = -[\exp(x_{ij}^T\beta + \Omega_i)]t_{ij}^{\rho}$, and in terms of code, is specified as `log(surv[i])<- -lambda[i]*pow(t[i],rho)`. The censoring mechanism requires that two different vectors are specified for the censoring. We demonstrate this with a simple example of ten individuals with two censored observations (items 3 and 4) and eight uncensored observations. In WinBUGS, any censored or missing observation must be specified as NA, and then in the censored vector, the time of censoring is specified for all the data. In the case of uncensored data, the censoring time would be 0 for right censoring. The censoring time for the censored data is 6.0 in this example. Hence, in list format, we could read data in as

```
list(t=c(2.3,2.3,NA,NA,3.5,4.1,4.5,4.5,5.4,5.6),
tcen=c(0,0,6.0,6.0,0,0,0,0,0,0),...)
```

In the initialization, however, missing values of the vector `t` must be given 'credible' initial values. If the censoring time is 6.0 then the initial values must be $\geq$ 6.0. Hence in the inits statement in WinBUGS we could have

```
list(...,t=c(NA,NA,7.0,7.0,NA,NA,NA,NA,NA,NA),...),
```

where the observed data are denoted NA and the censored data are given an initial value.

A full WinBUGS program for this arbitrary example is given in Figure 14.1. In this program, the prior distributions for the parameters are taken relatively noninformative: $\rho \sim$ Gamma(1.0, 1.0×10^{-4}), $\beta_0 \sim N(0, 1.0 \times 10^{-4})$, $v_i \sim \mathrm{N}(0, \sigma_v^2)$, $\tau_v = \sigma_v^{-2}$, $\sigma_v \sim$ U(0, 10).

```
model{
    for (i in 1:10){
    t[i] ~ dweib(rho,lambda[i])I(tcen[i],)
    lambda[i] <- exp(beta0+v[i])
    v[i] ~ dnorm(0,tauv)
    median[i] <- pow((log(2) /lambda[i]), 1/rho)
    log(surv[i]) <- -lambda[i]*pow(t[i],rho)
    }
beta0 ~ dnorm(0,0.0001)
rho ~ dgamma(1.0,0.0001)
tauv <- pow(sdv,-2)
sdv ~ dunif(0,10)
}
# data
list(t=c(2.3,2.3,NA,NA,3.5,4.1,4.5,4.5,5.4,5.6),
tcen=c(0,0,6.0,6.0,0,0,0,0,0,0))
# inits
list(v=c(0,0,0,0,0,0,0,0,0,0),
t=c(NA,NA,7.0,7.0,NA,NA,NA,NA,NA,NA),
sdv=0.1,rho=0.1,beta0=0.1)
```

Figure 14.1 A WinBUGS program for the arbitrary survival example with log linear predictor with intercept and zero mean Gaussian random effect.

14.2.2 A Bayesian AFT model

Alternative specifications which do not require proportionality of hazard assumptions are sometimes favored. One such is the AFT model. This model provides a simple option for this and is specified as

$$\log(t_{ij}) = \alpha + \boldsymbol{x}_{ij}^T\boldsymbol{\beta} + \Omega_{ij} + \sigma\varepsilon_i,$$

where $\alpha + \boldsymbol{x}_{ij}^T\boldsymbol{\beta}$ is a linear predictor subset with intercept and linear combination of regression predictors and parameters, Ω_{ij} is a set of random effects, and finally ε_i is the error term. Let $f(\cdot)$ denote the density function of t and $f_0(\cdot)$ denote the density function of ε. $S(\cdot)$ and $S_0(\cdot)$ denote the survival functions and $h_0(\cdot)$ and $h(\cdot)$ represent the hazard functions corresponding to $f_0(\cdot)$ and $f(\cdot)$, respectively. Then, we have

$$f(t_{ij}|\lambda_{ij}) = \frac{1}{\sigma t_{ij}} f_0\left(\frac{\log(t_{ij}) - \lambda_{ij}}{\sigma}\right),$$

$$S(t_{ij}|\lambda_{ij}) = S_0\left(\frac{\log(t_{ij}) - \lambda_{ij}}{\sigma}\right),$$

$$h(t_{ij}|\lambda_{ij}) = \frac{1}{\sigma t_{ij}} h_0\left(\frac{\log(t_{ij}) - \lambda_{ij}}{\sigma}\right).$$

This leads to the following likelihood

$$L = \prod_{i=1}^{n}\prod_{j=1}^{n_i}\left[\frac{1}{\sigma t_{ij}} f_0\left(\frac{\log(t_{ij}) - \lambda_{ij}}{\sigma}\right)\right]^{\delta_{ij}} S_0\left(\frac{\log(t_{ij}) - \lambda_{ij}}{\sigma}\right)^{1-\delta_{ij}}, \tag{14.6}$$

where $\lambda_{ij} = \alpha + \boldsymbol{x}_{ij}^T\boldsymbol{\beta} + \Omega_{ij}$, $f_0(\cdot)$ and $S_0(\cdot)$ are the base failure distribution and corresponding survival distribution. The choice of $f_0(\cdot)$ is varied and target distributions include the Gaussian distribution, the logistic distribution and the extreme value distribution. For the logistic model, we have that $S_0(\varepsilon) = \frac{1}{1+\exp(\varepsilon)}$ and so $S(t_{ij}|\lambda_{ij}) = S_0\left(\frac{\log(t_{ij})-\lambda_{ij}}{\sigma}\right) = \frac{1}{1+[t_{ij}\exp(-\lambda_{ij})]^{1/\sigma}}$ and $f(t_{ij}|\lambda_{ij}) = S_0\left(\frac{\log(t_{ij})-\lambda_{ij}}{\sigma}\right)^2 \exp\left(\frac{\log(t_{ij})-\lambda_{ij}}{\sigma}\right)$. The logistic AFT model will be applied to a gastric cancer data set in Section 14.3.1.

14.3 Examples

14.3.1 The gastric cancer study

In this example, we examine a data set analyzed originally by Moreau *et al.* (1985) and provided at `http://cancercenter.mayo.edu/mayo/research/biostat/therneau-book.cfm` by T. Therneau. This consists of survival times of 90 patients suffering from gastric cancer. In addition to a covariate for two treatment modalities (treatment: chemotherapy, OR chemotherapy and radiation), the data are censored individually (outcome: death = 1, censored = 0). Figure 14.2 displays box plots for treatment group and an overall histogram of the survival times. There is a clear median difference between the groups although the overall variability is similar. Figure 14.3 displays the empirical Kaplan-Meier survival curves for the two treatments.

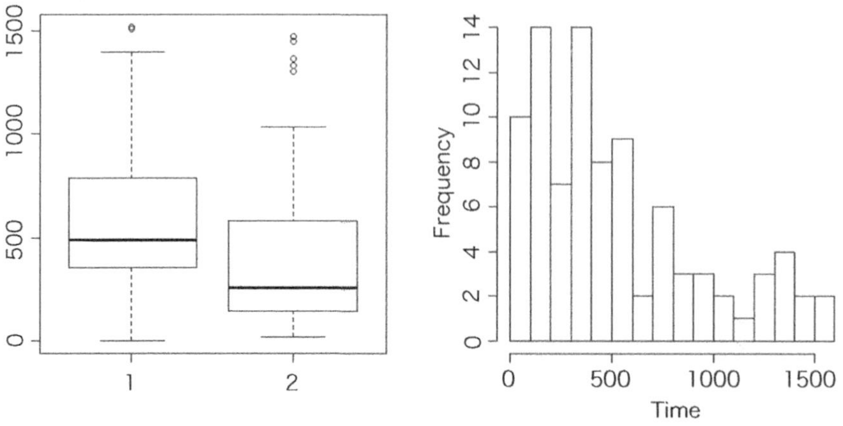

Figure 14.2 Gastric cancer study: comparison of treatment groups in terms of survival times.

There appears to be an effect of treatment, particularly in the early stages. To model this effect we have examined both Weibull and AFT models with relevant treatment effects and also variants with different specifications for random effects and survival rates. Table 14.1 displays the results in terms of DIC, $\overline{D}$, effective number of parameters (p_D) and MSPE for different Weibull model fits to the gastric cancer data. The first model (model 1) is a simple specification with $t_i \sim \text{Weibull}(\rho, \lambda_i)$ where the rate parameter is defined as $\log(\lambda_i) = \beta_0 + \mu_{j(i\in j)}$, $(j = 1, 2)$ which is an overall rate with a treatment effect for the jth group (in which the ith person lies). The remainder of the hierarchical model is specified as follows:

$$\beta_0 \sim \text{N}(0, \sigma_\beta^2),$$
$$\mu_j \sim \text{N}(0, \sigma_\mu^2),\ \forall j$$
$$\log(\rho) \sim \text{N}(0, \sigma_\rho^2),$$

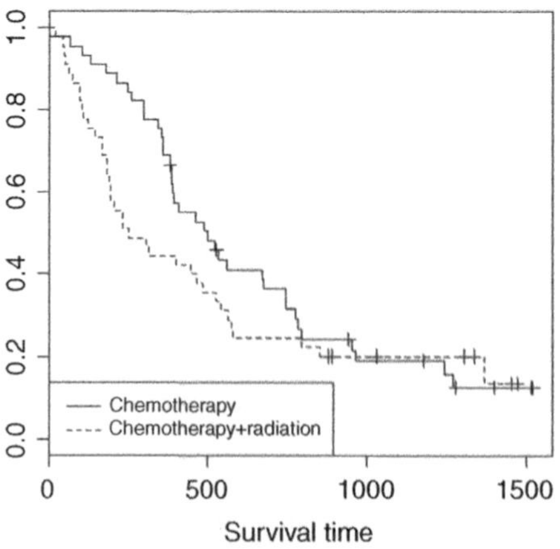

Figure 14.3 Gastric cancer study: Kaplan–Meier nonparametric survival curve estimates for the treatment groups plotted as separate curves.

Table 14.1 Gastric cancer study: Weibull model goodness of fit, with model 1: intercept + treatment effect, model 2: as model 1 + random effect and model 3: as model 2 but with individual scale parameters.

Model	p_D	$\overline{D}$	DIC	MSPE
1	3.00	1043.60	1046.54	213900.0
2	12.03	1035.40	1047.04	204200.0
3	4.50	1053.70	1058.30	453800.0
4	3.55	1043.00	1046.55	230800.0

with all precisions specified with the σ-uniform prior distributions (Gelman 2006), i.e. $\sigma_* \sim \text{U}(0, c)$, with $c = 5$. The second model (model 2) extends model 1 by adding an individual frailty (random) effect. Here, $\log(\lambda_i) = \beta_0 + \mu_{j(i \in j)} + v_i$ and $v_i \sim \text{N}(0, \sigma_v^2)$ and $\tau_v = \sigma_v^{-2}$, $\sigma_v \sim \text{U}(0, c)$, with $c = 5$. It is clear from Table 14.1 that this addition lowers the average deviance ($\overline{D}$) but due to the increased parameterization leads to a slightly higher DIC than model 1. It does have a lower MSPE. The next model considered allows the shape parameter ρ to vary with the individual so that $t_i \sim \text{Weibull}(\rho_i, \lambda_i)$. In this model, we assumed that the prior distribution for ρ_i is lognormal so that $\log(\rho_i) \sim \text{N}(0, \sigma_\rho^2)$ and excluded the individual level random effect. This model allows for a variation in shape. Applied to our data leads to a higher $\overline{D}$, and DIC and also MSPE, hence would not be favored as a parsimonious description of the data. Finally, we considered a model (model 4) where the shape parameter is a function of the treatment group: $t_i \sim \text{Weibull}(\rho_{j(i \in j)}, \lambda_i)$. In this case, DIC is close to that of the model 1 with a slightly lower $\overline{D}$ but a slightly higher p_D. The MSPE is higher than for model 1 or 2. Hence, based on DIC, models 1, 2 and 4 are to be favored. Model 1 is favored based on parsimony, although model 3 has a lower $\overline{D}$. From a predictive view point, model 2 would be favored due to its relatively low MSPE.

Figure 14.4 displays for Weibull model 1 (lowest DIC) the posterior mean of the estimated uncensored survival times. It should be noted that the posterior mean estimates of the μ_j are not well estimated under this model. However, under the competing model (model 4) where the shape parameter is modeled by group, the separate group shape parameters are well estimated: $\widehat{\rho_1}$:1.525 (SD = 0.2073) and $\widehat{\rho_2}$:1.19 (SD = 0.137).

There is a possibility that the hazards are nonproportional in this example and so we also considered an AFT model. We assumed here a logistic base distribution for $f_0(\cdot)$ and so the survival probability will be $\frac{1}{1+[t_{ij}\exp(-\lambda_{ij})]^{1/\sigma}}$. Further, we assumed that the likelihood (14.6) is relevant. To fit this model within the WinBUGS framework, we can use a a programming trick that is available for arbitrary likelihoods (the zeros or ones trick). This trick was explained in Section 10.3.5. The zeros trick for this example is shown in Figure 14.5. The arbitrary likelihood is defined in `L[i]`, the survival probability is `s[i]` and `indic[i]` is the binary censoring indicator. A log-linear model is taken for the rate (`lam[i]`) with $\beta_0 + \mu_{j(i \in j)}$ and with $\sigma \sim \text{U}(0, 5)$.

The next model considered is one with a frailty term included for individuals ($v_i \sim N(0, \sigma_v^2)$). We already noted that this was not a competitive model when a Weibull distribution was used, and in this case, we have found little change in the overall DIC. In addition we examined the pseudo-marginal likelihood which is a cross-validated measure of goodness of fit and can be estimated via $\text{M}_{pl} = \sum_i \log(CPO_i)$, where CPO_i is the conditional predictive ordinate for the ith observation (see Section 10.2.1 and Ibrahim *et al.* 2000, Chapter 6.3). In

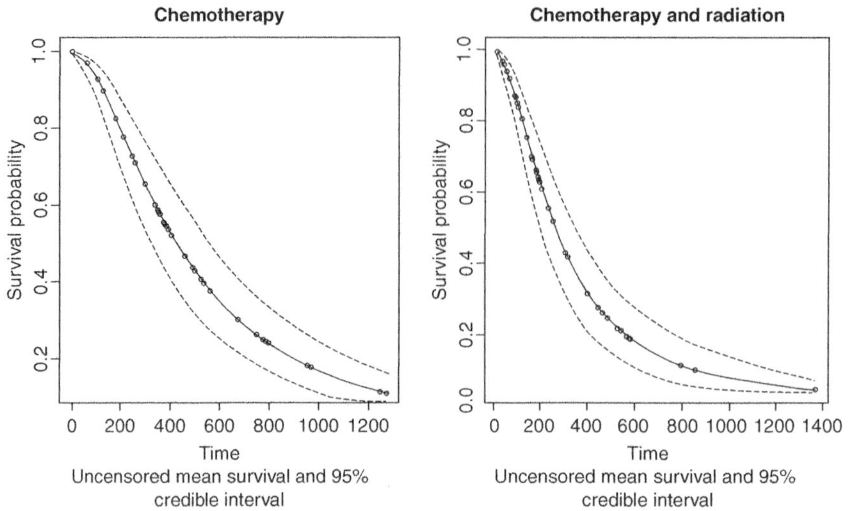

Figure 14.4 Gastric cancer study: Weibull model fit (model 1): posterior mean estimated survival with 95% credible interval (dashed line) (uncensored data only shown).

general, the larger the value of M_{pl} the more favored is the model. For different data sets, an averaged value can be used (M_{pl}/n). For the AFT models of the gastric cancer data set, we have the following results for M_{pl}/n: model 1: −466.1, model 2: −527.1, model 3: −527.1. Based on these results, it appears that model 1 remains the best model in terms of cross-validatory prediction. Assuming this model, we derived the posterior mean survival probability and 95% credible intervals from the posterior sampler.

Figure 14.6 displays the results for model 1 for a posterior sampler based on MH updating. The estimated mean rate parameters for the treatment groups ($\mu_{j(i\in j)}$) are 2.132 (SD = 1.151)

```
    C <- 10000
    for (i in 1:90) {
    temp[i] <-  (log(timeF[i]+0.01)-log(lam[i]))/sigma
    log(lam[i]) <- beta0+mu[treat[i]]
#logistic
    s[i]<-1/(1+exp(temp[i]))
    f[i]<-exp(temp[i])*pow(s[i],2)
# log likelihood
    L[i]<-indic[i]*log(f[i]/(sigma*(timeF[i]+0.01)))+(1-indic[i])*
log(s[i])
# Poisson  zeroes trick
    zeros[i] <- 0
    new[i] <- -L[i]+C
    zeros[i] ~ dpois(new[i])
     }
```

Figure 14.5 Gastric cancer study: WinBUGS code which uses a zeros trick to allow sampling of a arbitrary AFT survival density with censoring.

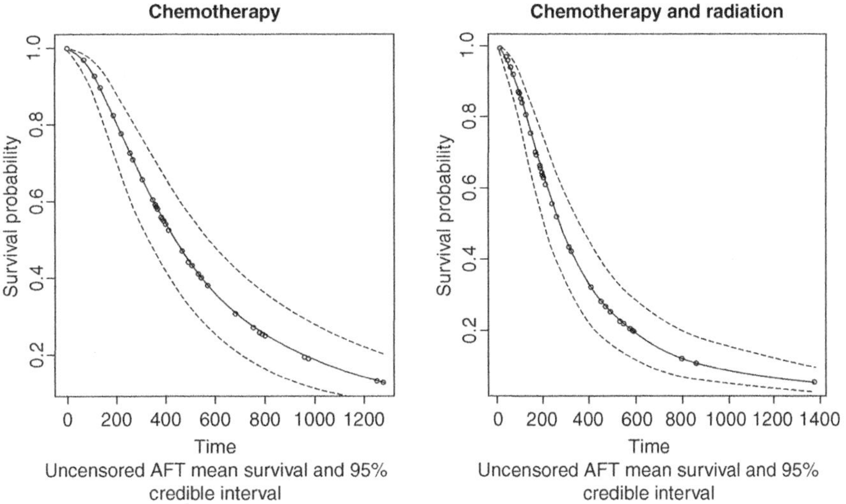

Figure 14.6 Gastric cancer study: posterior sample estimates for the mean survival probability $1/[1+(t_{ij}\exp(-\lambda_{ij}))^{1/\sigma}]$ and sample-based pointwise 2.5% and 97.5% credible limits using an AFT model.

and 1.652 (SD = 1.129) and so it seems that the overall posterior mean treatment difference $(\mu_1 - \mu_2)$ is 0.4969 (SD = 0.1964) and this demonstrates that we have an average treatment effect.

In both the Weibull and AFT model versions, we can see that the treatment regimes do affect the survival probability with chemotherapy alone seeming to lengthen survival in this comparison.

14.3.2 Prostate cancer in Louisiana: A spatial AFT model

In the US, a number of states have designated Surveillance, Epidemiology and End Results (SEER) cancer registries which are federally standardized registries for all reported cancers. In these state-based registries any new diagnosis of cancer is logged with relevant basic patient information such as *date of diagnosis*, *age*, *gender*, *marital status*, *cancer severity* (grade, stage) and *residential address*. The registries can sometimes be linked to vital outcomes also and so in some cases there is also data on whether and when a patient died.

A SEER registry has existed from 2001 for the state of Louisiana and is continuously operational up to the present. In this example, we demonstrate the possibility of contextual modeling of survival outcomes. In particular, we demonstrate that geographical context (county of residence) can be incorporated in a survival setting to explain spatial variations in survival risk. Some of the model components presented here were introduced in Chapter 16. A fuller description of this example is given in Zhang and Lawson (2011).

Let t_{ij} denote the survival time after diagnosis for patient i in county j, and $\boldsymbol{x}_{ij}$ denotes possible risk effects corresponding to t_{ij}, where $i = 1, \cdots, n_j$, $j = 1, \cdots, n$. The AFT model can be expressed as:

$$\log(t_{ij}) = \mu + \boldsymbol{x}_{ij}^T\boldsymbol{\beta} + \sigma\varepsilon_{ij} \,,$$

where $\boldsymbol{\beta}$ is the unknown coefficient vector, μ and σ are the shape parameter and the scale parameter, respectively, and the ε_{ij}'s are independent random errors.

The spatial structure and models are discussed in detail in Chapter 16. In this application, a spatial structure can be considered by adding a random effect reflecting the location or county of residence to the AFT model. The AFT spatial model is specified as

$$\log(t_{ij}) = \mu + \boldsymbol{x}_{ij}^T \boldsymbol{\beta} + W_j + \sigma \varepsilon_{ij}, \tag{14.7}$$

where the W_js are spatial random effects $W_j \equiv W_{j(i \in j)}$. The advantage of the AFT spatial model is that interpretation of risk/spatial effects on the failure time are easy since the AFT spatial model simply regresses the logarithm of the survival time over covariates and random spatial effects.

Then, we have

$$f(t_{ij}|W_j) = \frac{1}{\sigma t_{ij}} f_0 \left(\frac{\log(t_{ij}) - \mu - \boldsymbol{x}_{ij}^T \boldsymbol{\beta} - W_j}{\sigma} \right),$$

$$S(t_{ij}|W_j) = S_0 \left(\frac{\log(t_{ij}) - \mu - \boldsymbol{x}_{ij}^T \boldsymbol{\beta} - W_j}{\sigma} \right).$$

From the relationship between the survival functions, we can see that the spatial random effects have a direct effect on the survival probability. Note that the hazard rate keeps changing over time even when the spatial random effect is fixed, while it keeps changing at the same rate given the specific region in the proportional hazard model. It is more reasonable to assume the hazard rate changes over time even in the same location.

It is common to assume that $S_0(\cdot)$ comes from the standard normal distribution, the standard extreme value distribution or the logistic distribution. More general distributions are suggested by Komárek *et al.* (2005). The $S_0(\cdot)$ expressions and their corresponding $S(\cdot)$s are summarized in Table 14.2, where $\lambda = \mu + \boldsymbol{x}_{ij}^T \boldsymbol{\beta} + W_j$, and $\Phi(\cdot)$ denotes the cumulative density function from the standard normal distribution.

Corresponding to the distribution of ε, the survival distribution of t follows the lognormal distribution, Weibull distribution or the log-logistic distribution with parameters λ and σ.

We consider survival data $(t_{ij}, \delta_{ij}, \boldsymbol{x}_{ij})$, where δ_{ij} is the censoring indicator. We assume that censoring is independent and noninformative. Let $\mathbf{W} = (W_1, \ldots, W_n)$, and $\boldsymbol{\phi} = \{\mu, \sigma, \boldsymbol{\beta}\}$

Table 14.2 Common distributions in the AFT spatial model, where $\lambda = \mu + \boldsymbol{x}_{ij}^T \boldsymbol{\beta} + W_j$.

Distribution	$S_0(\cdot)$	$S(\cdot)$
Normal	$1 - \Phi(\varepsilon)$	$1 - \Phi\left(\frac{\log(t)-\lambda}{\sigma}\right)$
Extreme value	$\exp(-\exp(\varepsilon))$	$\exp\left[-\exp(-\lambda)t\right]^{\frac{1}{\sigma}}$
Logistic	$\frac{1}{1+\exp(\varepsilon)}$	$\frac{1}{1+\left[\exp(-\lambda)t\right]^{1/\sigma}}$

denote the parameters to be estimated. Given the spatial random effect, the likelihood function can be written as

$$L(t|\boldsymbol{\phi}, \mathbf{W}) = \prod_{j=1}^{n} \prod_{i=1}^{n_j} f(t_{ij})^{\delta_{ij}} S(t_{ij})^{1-\delta_{ij}}.$$

The spatial random errors can be correlated among counties. We refer to mutually uncorrelated county-specific effects as spatially uncorrelated heterogeneity and model this situation with independent Gaussian distributions defined as $W_{1j} \sim \mathrm{N}(0, \sigma_v^2)$. It is worthwhile pointing out that the AFT spatial model under independence is similar to the AFT frailty model with normal random effects, albeit with frailty effects at the county level rather than individual level. In the correlated situation, we can consider the conditional autoregressive (CAR) model, which is discussed more fully in Chapter 16 and is widely used for smoothing in disease mapping. This formulation permits correlation among the random effects according to a neighborhood structure:

$$W_{2j}|(\{W_{2k}\}, \sigma_s^2) \sim N(\overline{W}_{2\delta_j}, \sigma_s^2/n_{\delta_j}),$$

where $\overline{W}_{2\delta_j}$ is the mean over the neighborhood (δ_j) of the jth area. The number of neighbors is n_{δ_j}. With this CAR model prior specification, we call W_{2j} spatially correlated heterogeneous. We also include both spatially correlated and uncorrelated random effects in a single model ($W_j = W_{1j} + W_{2j}$) to permit a trade-off between independence and a purely local spatially structured dependence of the random effects (Besag *et al.* 1991). This combined spatially correlated and uncorrelated heterogeneity yields a convolution prior with spatially varying variance: σ_s^2/n_{δ_j}.

In the AFT spatial model, we considered three different cases according to different spatial correlation, which are summarized as follows:

- Case 1: W_j is spatial uncorrelated. That is, W_j follows a zero mean Gaussian distribution.
- Case 2: W_j is spatially correlated. That is, W_j follows the CAR model.
- Case 3: $W_j = W_{1j} + W_{2j}$, where W_{1j} is the spatial uncorrelated random effect and W_{2j} denotes the spatial correlated random effect. This case considers both spatial correlated and uncorrelated effects.

Multiple chains were run and the first 10 000 iterations used as preconvergence burn-in, retaining 10 000 iterations as the posterior sample. The DIC and p_D for the models are listed in Table 14.3.

Table 14.3 displays results for the normal error AFT model only. From this table, we can see that the model with spatially correlated random effects under the normal baseline is the best among these cases, which has the smallest DIC value and p_D value. The estimated parameters for case 2 is summarized in Table 14.4.

From Table 14.4, we can see that age, race and stage have significant influence on the survival probability of the *PrCA* (as indicated by * in the table). *Marital status* does not display significance. More than 75% of patients in this study are married, so there may not be enough evidence to show the effect of *marital status*.

Table 14.3 Prostate cancer example: a comparison of goodness of fit (DIC, p_D) for the AFT model and the three cases of the AFT spatial model.

Distribution of $S_0(\cdot)$	DIC	p_D
Normal AFT	11950.0	6.133
Normal+case 1	11960.0	65.42
Normal+case 2	11930.0	17.59
Normal+case 3	12000.0	85.01

Table 14.4 Prostate cancer study: the best fitting AFT spatial model (case 2): posterior means and SDs, and quantiles.

	Mean	SD	MC error	2.5%	50%	97.5%
Age	−0.0336*	0.00184	0.0001	−0.0374	−0.0335	−0.0301
Marital	−0.0096	0.0299	0.0016	−0.0688	−0.0100	0.0494
Race	0.1843*	0.0360	0.0019	0.1171	0.1835	0.2553
Stage	−0.9643*	0.0569	0.0025	−1.080	−0.9617	−0.8578

In order to show the spatial effect, we present the median of the posterior spatial random effect in Figure 14.7, which displays considerable spatial structure in the middle eastern area of the state.

For illustration purposes, we compare the estimated survival curves for the five regions indicated in Figure 14.7 since the survival curve on each region will be affected by the spatial random effects. The estimated survival curves for the different race based on the AFT spatial model and the Kaplan–Meier approach according to the different regions are displayed for regions 1 and 5. In the Kaplan–Meier approach, we only considered the race effect. In the

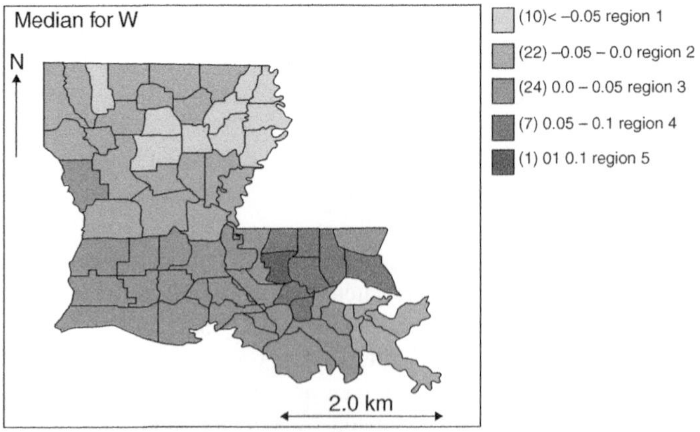

Figure 14.7 Prostate cancer study: median value of spatial random effects from fitted AFT spatial model (case 2), Louisiana counties.

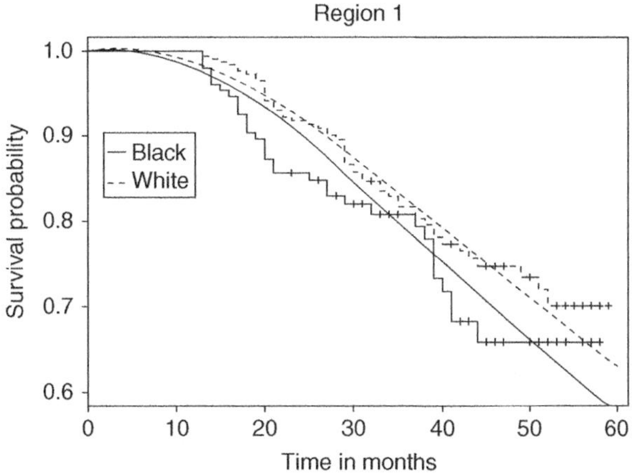

Figure 14.8 Prostate cancer study: fitted survival curve from the KM approach and AFT spatial model, region 1.

AFT spatial model, we considered the median value of age, marital status and the stage for each race and median of the estimated spatial random effects in each region. The survival curves for regions 1 and 5 are illustrated in Figures 14.8 and 14.9.

We conclude first that the survival curves from the AFT spatial model are similar to those from the KM approach, which indicates that the AFT spatial model fits the data set well. Second, we can see that the survival probability for white men is higher than that for the blacks in all regions, which is consistent with PrCA being more aggressive in the black than the white racial group. Finally, we find that the survival probability is affected by the geographical region. For example, the survival rate for black men at 60 months is around 0.6 in region 1 from the AFT spatial model, 0.67 from the KM approach, while in region 5 it is

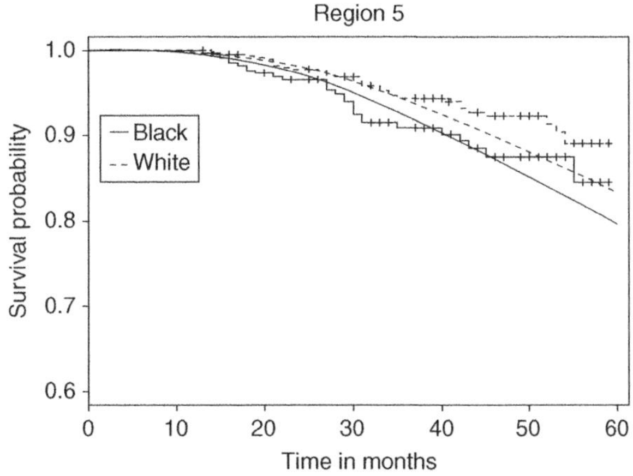

Figure 14.9 Prostate cancer study: fitted survival curve from the KM approach and AFT spatial model, region 5.

around 0.8 from the AFT spatial model and 0.83 from the KM approach. Similar effects can be found in other regions.

14.4 Closing remarks

In this chapter, we have examined a range of survival models applied in different contexts both clinical and observational. These modeling scenarios could be extended in a number of ways. First, more complex censoring structures could be encountered. Second, we could have considered hierarchies of contextual effects in different strata or groupings. We only considered individual and county level effects here. Finally, some smoothing terms rather than linear terms could be allowed for covariate modeling and hence semiparametric forms could be employed.

Finally, note that for some of the above Bayesian analyses also the SAS® procedures LIFEREG, PHGLM and MCMC could be used.

15

Longitudinal analysis

Longitudinal data arise in many biostatistical applications, both in clinical settings and at the population level. Here, we define 'longitudinal' as meaning any data that is repeatedly measured over time on individual study units (e.g. patients, regions and images). Usually the focus of the study is to determine whether changes over time have occurred, perhaps between groups, as in the clinical trial setting, or to simply model the system behavior over time. At the simplest level, the comparison of a marker in a group of patients between two time periods is an example of an analysis of a longitudinal problem. More complexity arises both when multiple time points are envisaged or when the observation time is a random variable itself. In this chapter, we focus on Bayesian methods for longitudinal data analysis. We examine both Gaussian and non-Gaussian response models. In addition, we address point referenced event data. We also treat missing data in generality. A practical example is given for the complex case of a not-at-random missingness process. This will be done by joint modeling longitudinal and a dropout process.

With respect to general references in this area, we refer the reader to Gelfand *et al.* (1990), Gelfand *et al.* (1992), Lange *et al.* (1992), Chib and Carlin (1999), Daniels and Hogan (2008), Clayton (1994), Ishawaran and James (2004), and Cook and Lawless (2007). In what follows, we give exemplars of analyses that represent typical applications of longitudinal methods.

In Chapter 9, we examined some examples of longitudinal studies. In this chapter, we examine additional examples some of a more advanced nature.

15.1 Fixed time periods

15.1.1 Introduction

Assume that individual (observational) units have been repeatedly measured. Denote these measurements as y_{ij} where i refers to the individual label and j to the time label. Define $i = 1, \ldots, n$ units and $j = 1, \ldots, m_i$ time periods. In this section, we assume that the evaluations were done at preplanned time periods t_{ij}. Here, we assume that all subjects in the study

Bayesian Biostatistics, First Edition. Emmanuel Lesaffre and Andrew B. Lawson.

are evaluated at the same time periods, i.e. $t_{ij} \equiv t_j$. If there are no missing responses then $m_1 = m_2 = \ldots = m_n$. In this case, we call the data set *balanced*. Imbalance in the repeated data can occur because some subjects were no measured at some occasions, or dropped out after some time. Another reason is that subjects come at different time periods. The latter case will be considered in Section 15.2.

The sequence of $\{y_{ij}\}_{j=1,\ldots,m_i}$ forms a time series of repeated measurements for each individual unit. Let the mean parameter associated with each observation be denoted as μ_{ij}. In the longitudinal setting, the focus is on modeling the mean structure μ_{ij} as a function of time-independent and time-dependent covariates. Examples of time-independent covariates are age (at entry of the study), gender, treatment, etc., while a straightforward example of a time-dependent covariate is time, but all covariates that vary during the study also belong to this class. Models for μ_{ij} will vary depending on the application. For example, in a two-period study ($j = 1, 2$) estimation of μ_{i1}, μ_{i2} will usually be of interest and a simple linear relation between the time points may be assumed: $\mu_{ij} = \alpha\mu_{i,j-1}$. Alternatively, the focus might be on the difference between period 1 and period 2, i.e. on $\delta_{\mu_i} = \mu_{i2} - \mu_{i1}$. When averaged over the sample, this difference mimics the paired two-group comparison often found in a clinical setting. A further subdivision of the individual units within a study is often of interest. For example, in clinical trials we would usually have dose groups. With grouping included within the analysis, there are then two possible foci: between-group effects and temporal effects. These effects could be averaged or be group specific. When additional covariates are put into the model the treatment effect is estimated conditional on the values of the covariates. While the main interest lies in the mean structure, modeling the covariance matrix of the responses, V_i, is also of importance in a longitudinal setting. For instance, an appropriate covariance structure may increase the power of the study. Moreover, establishing the appropriate covariance increases in importance when missing data are involved (see Section 15.3).

We will mainly consider mixed models introduced in Chapter 9. Recall that this involves the following model:

$$\begin{aligned} y_{ij} \mid \mu_{ij} &\sim \mathrm{N}(\mu_{ij}, \sigma^2), \\ \mu_{ij} &= \boldsymbol{x}_{ij}^T\boldsymbol{\beta} + \boldsymbol{z}_{ij}^T\boldsymbol{b}_i, \end{aligned}$$

with $\boldsymbol{x}_{ij}^T\boldsymbol{\beta}$ a linear predictor, $\boldsymbol{z}_{ij}^T\boldsymbol{b}_i$ a set of random effects for the ith individual at the jth time. While the random effects act on the linear structure they also imply a particular shape of the covariance matrix V_i. Apart from the variability due to inter-subject variability governed by the random effects, also the intrasubject variability contributes to the covariance matrix and is expressed by the covariance matrix of the residual term. We will explore in this section how the modeling of longitudinal studies is typically done via the well-known growth curve data first analyzed in Gelfand *et al.* (1990).

15.1.2 A classical growth-curve example

Previous examples of a growth-curve analysis appeared in Example IX.18 and X.8. Gelfand *et al.* (1990) looked at a weight gain experiment where 30 rats in each of two groups (control and treatment) were weighted repeatedly over a period of 36 days. There were five observation points in time (8, 15, 22, 29 and 36 days), and thus, $t_{ij} \equiv t_j$ ($j = 1, \ldots, 5$). Since $m_1 = \ldots, m_5 = 30$, the data set is balanced. We will only partly exploit the balanced nature

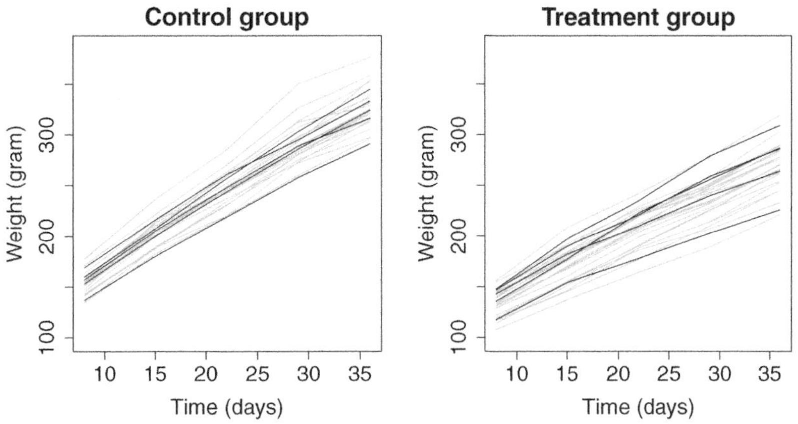

Figure 15.1 Rats study: weight profiles of the 30 rats (five rats randomly highlighted) from control and treatment groups (Gelfand *et al.* 1990).

of the data here. Indeed, most of the techniques we consider in this analysis can also be applied to unbalanced repeated measurements data sets.

In this example, the outcome of interest is the temporal weight progression. Figure 15.1 displays the temporal weight profiles for the rats in the experimental control group and the treatment group.

Assume that the outcome has a Gaussian distribution centered on the mean weight μ_{ij}, so that

$$y_{ij} \mid \mu_{ij} \sim \mathrm{N}(\mu_{ij}, \sigma^2).$$

Below, we look for the appropriate mean and variance structure of the repeated measurements.

15.1.2.1 The linear structure

At first, we assume that the gain in weight is approximately linear in time. Figure 15.2 shows that the variance increases with time. According to Section 9.5.2, this may hint to a linear mixed model with a random intercept and a random slope. Therefore, as a first model we could take

$$y_{ij} = \mu_{ij} + \varepsilon_{ij} = \beta_0 + \beta_1 t_j + b_{0i} + b_{1i} t_j + \varepsilon_{ij},$$

where b_{0i} is the deviation of the intercept of the ith rat to the population intercept, and b_{1i} is the deviation of the slope of the ith rat to the population slope. Note that we subtracted 8 from the time variable to give β_0 the meaning of the population intercept at day 8. Hence, each rat has a different intercept at day 8 equal to $\beta_{0i} = \beta_0 + b_{0i}$ and a different slope equal to $\beta_{1i} = \beta_1 + b_{1i}$. However, this model assumes that the two groups (control, treatment) have

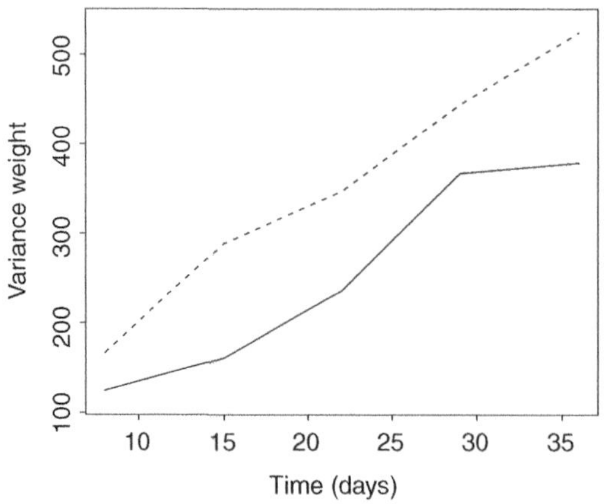

Figure 15.2 Rats study: variance weight of the measurements at each examination in the control (solid line) and the treatment group (dashed line).

the same population intercept and slope, which does not appear to be the case here according to Figure 15.1. Therefore, we prefer to take for the mean structure:

$$\mu_{ij} = \beta_{01} + \Delta_0 treat_i + \beta_{11} t_j + \Delta_1 treat_i \times t_j + b_{0i} + b_{1i} t_j, \quad (15.1)$$

where $treat_i = 1$ for the treatment group, and 0 elsewhere. Let $\beta_{02} = \beta_{01} + \Delta_0$ and $\beta_{12} = \beta_{11} + \Delta_1$, then the mean of β_{0i} is β_{01} for rats from the control group and β_{02} for rats from the treatment group, and similarly for the slopes.

The linear dependence on time in model (15.1) can be relaxed. For instance, in the fixed effects part of the model polynomial terms could be introduced. This could also be done in the random effects part, or in both parts. We have considered here a cubic polynomial relationship in each group, but only in the fixed part. Graphical explorations showed that linearity in the random effects structure can be assumed for the Rats data.

Model (15.1) could be expanded even further, as shown in Section 10.3.5. For instance, one could fit a fractional polynomial model in each group in the fixed and/or the random effects part. Alternatively, one could model the mean structure using splines. However, the Rats data set is balanced and only five time points are involved and thus not enough degrees of freedom are available to apply a smoothing approach.

15.1.2.2 The covariance structure

The above linear structure does not specify any distributional assumptions of the random effects nor of the residual error term. In Section 9.5.2, we have seen that the classical distributional assumptions for a linear mixed model is

$$\boldsymbol{b}_i \equiv \begin{pmatrix} b_{0i} \\ b_{1i} \end{pmatrix} \sim \mathrm{N}(\mathbf{0}, \mathrm{G}) \; (i = 1, \ldots, n),$$

where G is the covariance matrix of the random intercept and slope, with elements $G_{11} = \sigma^2_{\beta_0}$, $G_{22} = \sigma^2_{\beta_1}$ and $G_{12} = \sigma_{\beta_0, \beta_1}$. In addition, it is assumed that the residual error is independent of the random effects and has a normal distribution, i.e. $\varepsilon_{ij} \sim \mathrm{N}(0, \sigma^2)$. As seen in Section 9.5.2, these assumptions imply that the variance of the response increases quadratically over time. However, in Figure 15.2, we rather observe a linear trend for the Rats data. Therefore, one might look for further extensions of the classical BLMM.

The first extension is to assume that $\boldsymbol{b}$ has a different covariance matrix in the two groups, i.e. G_1 for the control group and G_2 for the treatment group. Another extension could be to assume that there are two residual variances: σ_1^2 for the control group and σ_2^2 for the treatment group. Further extensions could be assumed, such as letting the residual variance also change over time and different in the two groups. However, we did not pursue this generalization.

In all of the above models, it has been assumed that the error terms are uncorrelated. This assumption may not be appropriate for all forms of longitudinal data. That is why we may wish to allow for correlated errors. The simplest correlation model corresponds to independence of the residuals, which was assumed in the above models. Let the covariance matrix for the error term be R, then for the independence model a simple diagonal form is obtained, shown here for four time points:

$$\mathrm{R} = \sigma^2\,\mathrm{C} = \begin{pmatrix} \sigma^2 & 0 & 0 & 0 \\ 0 & \sigma^2 & 0 & 0 \\ 0 & 0 & \sigma^2 & 0 \\ 0 & 0 & 0 & \sigma^2 \end{pmatrix},$$

where C is the (independence) correlation matrix of the residuals. In general, the off-diagonal elements of the correlation model are nonzero. There are two popular correlation models in longitudinal analyses. The first assumes an autoregressive dependence on previous errors:

$$\begin{aligned} y_{ij} &= \mu_{ij} + \varepsilon_{ij}, \\ \varepsilon_{ij} &\sim \mathrm{N}(\psi\varepsilon_{i,j-1}, \sigma_\psi^2), \end{aligned}$$

with $0 \leq \psi < 1$. Note that if $\psi = 1$, a Gaussian random walk prior distribution arises. This autoregressive lag 1 assumption gives the *AR(1) correlation model* with correlation matrix

$$\mathrm{C} = \begin{pmatrix} 1 & \psi & \psi^2 & \psi^3 \\ \psi & 1 & \psi & \psi^2 \\ \psi^2 & \psi & 1 & \psi \\ \psi^3 & \psi^2 & \psi & 1 \end{pmatrix}.$$

Thus, for the AR(1) model the correlation of the residuals decreases with lag time in a geometrical manner. In the *compound symmetry (CS) correlation model*, it is assumed that the correlation remains the same irrespective of the lag time. In that case, the correlation matrix for four time points is

$$\mathrm{C} = \begin{pmatrix} 1 & \psi & \psi & \psi \\ \psi & 1 & \psi & \psi \\ \psi & \psi & 1 & \psi \\ \psi & \psi & \psi & 1 \end{pmatrix},$$

with $0 \leq \psi < 1$. Note that the combination of a general covariance matrix G with a correlated error structure is often challenging to fit, both in the frequentist as well as in the Bayesian way.

We could go even further in modeling the covariance matrix. For instance, we could let the correlation matrix and the residual variance(s) depend on continuous covariates. However, this extension is beyond the scope of this chapter and we refer to Pourahmadi and Daniels (2002), and Daniels and Pourahmadi (2002) for such models.

Finally, in Chapter 10, it is seen that the normality assumption of random effects and/or the residual term can be easily relaxed with Bayesian software. However, we did not pursue this further relaxation of the model.

15.1.2.3 Prior distributions

The distribution of the random effects, in a Bayesian context, is often referred to as a prior distribution. However, this prior belongs in fact to the likelihood part of the model and was, therefore, treated above. In the models that we consider for the Rats data, we need prior distributions for: the regression coefficients, the covariance matrix of the random effects, the variance(s) of the residuals and, if applicable, the correlation structure of the residuals.

Vague priors were assigned to the regression coefficients, i.e. $N(0, 10^6)$. For the residual standard deviations, we have taken uniform priors on [0, 20]. For correlated errors, we assumed for the AR(1) and the CS model that $\psi \sim U(0, 1)$. For the covariance matrix of the random effects, we looked at two ways to specify the prior for G. First, one could assume a noninformative Wishart prior distribution for the precision matrix (G^{-1}), i.e. $G^{-1} \sim \text{Wishart}(D, \nu_0)$. According to Section 5.3.3, ν_0 must be small for a NI prior. We have taken for the Rats data $\nu_0 = 2$, equal to the rank of the matrix. In addition, the matrix D was taken as ε times the identity matrix, with ε small. We have taken here $\varepsilon = 10^{-6}$. A second possibility is to give separate priors for the diagonal elements of D and for the correlation matrix C. For the Rats data, G is a 2×2 matrix. We have chosen as priors for the variance part: $\sigma_{\beta_0} \sim U(0, 20)$ and $\sigma_{\beta_1} \sim U(0, 20)$, which are the standard deviations of the random intercept and slope, respectively. For the correlation of the random terms we assumed $\rho \sim U(-1, 1)$

15.1.2.4 Application to the Rats data

We explored a variety of models and tested their appropriateness to fit the data. For all models, we ran a single chain for 30 000 iterations leaving out 10 000 burn-in iterations and determined DIC and p_D on the last 10 000 iterations. In addition, we computed MSPE defined here as ave $\sum_{ij}(y_{ij} - \widetilde{y}_{ij})^2$.

First we considered model (15.1), which we call *model 1*. We obtained for this model: DIC = 1950.75, $p_D = 104.2$ and MSPE = 16 580. In *model 2*, we allow the covariance matrix of the random effects to be group dependent, i.e. G_1 for the control rats and G_2 for the treated rats. This resulted in DIC = 1952.18, $p_D = 105.0$ and MSPE = 16 670. Clearly, model 2 is not an improvement over model 1 and hence we assumed that $G_1 = G_2$. In *model 3*, we allowed the residual variances to differ between the two groups and obtained DIC = 1952.18, $p_D = 105.0$ and MSPE = 16 750. According to DIC, model 3 is an improvement over model 1, but its MSPE is higher than that of model 1. This apparent contradiction can be explained by the different way the outlyingness of an observation is taken into account in the two prediction measures. In *model 4*, we added an AR(1) correlation model to model 3. However, immediately a trap error occurred. The same was true for *model 5* where we combined model 3 with a CS correlation model. The reason for this bad behavior is that the off-diagonal elements of the random effects part in the covariance matrix of the *i*th response, $V_i = \mathbf{Z}_i G \mathbf{Z}_i^T + R$, are competing with the residual correlation part. To illustrate this, we have fitted a model whereby the random intercept and slope were assumed to be independent and combined it with an AR(1) correlation model. No computational problems occurred now. But this model is worse than the previous one, with DIC = 2108.6 with $p_D = 39.6$. The same is true for the model with a CS correlation part. So, neither of these two models were considered any further.

It is generally advised to make at the start the mean structure as complex as possible. Here, we chose to start with a simple linear structure, which was inspired by the profiles shown in Figure 15.1. Nevertheless, we decided to check the linear structure of model 3 by expanded the mean model with quadratic and cubic terms. In *model 6*, we assumed these extra terms to have a different impact in the two groups. With DIC = 1775.5 and $p_D = 115.7$, MSPE = 9231, this model has the best fit up to now. The regression estimates of model 6 suggest to keep only the quadratic and cubic term for the treatment group, which results in *model 7*. This model gave a worse fit (DIC = 1870.5 with $p_D = 109.5$ and MSPE = 14 600) than model 6 and was therefore not kept. The correlation of the random intercept and random slope was low in model 6, with posterior mean (SD) equal to −0.13 (0.14). Therefore, we assumed in model 8 independence of the random effects and obtained: DIC = 1775.4 with $p_D = 114.2$ and MSPE = 9290.0. Consequently, model 8 is our choice.

The parameter estimates (SD) for this model are shown in Table 15.1. Apart from the model parameters we also estimated the difference in means of the weight response at the five time points (Δ_x with $x = 8, 15, 22, 29, 36$).

Table 15.1 Rats study: posterior mean estimates and SDs of the final model.

Parameter	Estimate	SD
	Control group	
β_{01} (intercept)	95.65	5.207
β_{11} (linear)	7.106	0.819
β_{21} (quadratic)	0.0037	0.0407
β_{31} (cubic)	−6.62E−4	6.13E−4
σ_1	4.373	0.332
	Treatment group	
β_{02} (intercept)	81.97	4.317
β_{12} (linear)	7.235	0.645
β_{22} (quadratic)	−0.0915	0.0320
β_{32} (cubic)	0.0010	4.81E−4
σ_2	3.453	0.262
	Random effects	
σ_{b_0} (intercept)	0.5455	0.0568
σ_{b_1} (slope)	12.78	1.319
	Comparison means	
Δ_8	−13.68	6.731
Δ_{15}	−27.47	3.906
Δ_{22}	−38.97	4.495
Δ_{29}	−48.91	5.268
Δ_{36}	−53.82	6.099

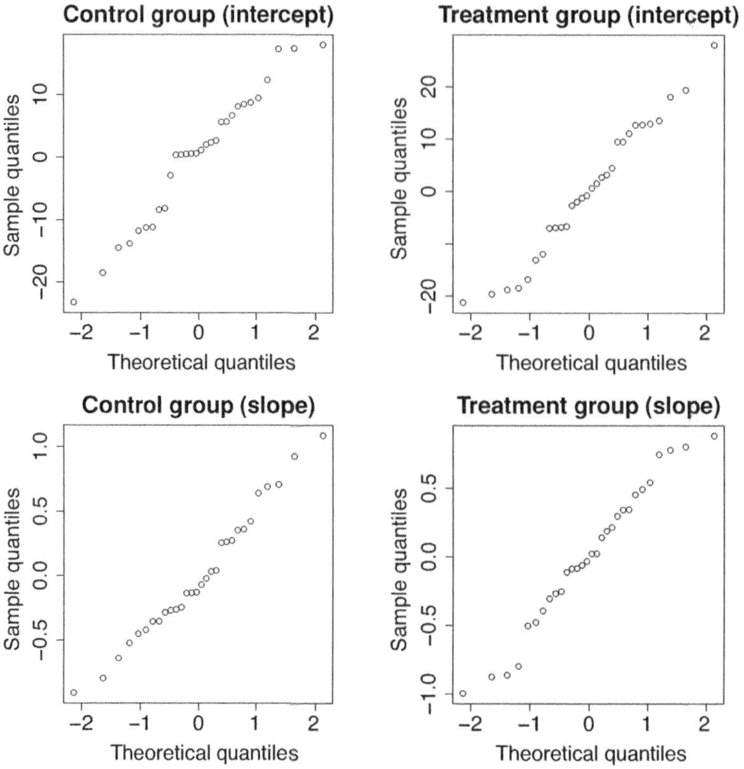

Figure 15.3 Rats study: normal probability plots of (the posterior mean of) the intercept and slope estimates for the control and the treatment group.

Finally, we checked for the final model the distributional assumptions of the random effects and of the residual term. In Figure 15.3, we show the normal probability plots based on the posterior means of the random intercept and slope in each group. We conclude that the random effects appear to have a normal distribution in each group. The same could be concluded for the residual errors, ε_{ij} (plot not shown)

15.1.3 Alternate data models

So far, we have assumed that the response has a Gaussian distribution. With Bayesian software such as WinBUGS and the Bayesian SAS® procedures, alternate response distributions are readily available. For instance, for a positive response, we might consider a gamma distributed error such as

$$y_{ij} \sim \text{Gamma}(\alpha, \beta).$$

Thus, $E(y_{ij}) = \alpha/\beta$ and the variance is equal to $\alpha/\beta^2 = E(y_{ij})/\beta$. Hence, specifying the mean also involves the variance. Other possible data models could be considered instead, such as an asymmetric or skew Gaussian distribution (Song *et al.* 2010). As seen in Chapter 9, a variety of data models and hence likelihoods can be specified within a Bayesian framework, not limited to continuous data.

For discrete outcomes, typically Poisson or binomial data models are assumed and these fall within the Bayesian generalized linear model (BGLM) framework. Note that overdispersion or extra variation within these models does not necessarily require alteration of the data model (to negative binomial or beta-binomial) as such overdispersion can be accommodated within higher levels of the model hierarchy. In addition, nonlinear models can be considered for longitudinal data (Bennett *et al.* 1996).

15.1.3.1 Epilepsy example

An example of discrete longitudinal data is the epilepsy trial first examined by Thall and Vail (1990). In this clinical trial, 59 patients suffering from epilepsy were given two different treatments: 28 patients were given placebo and 31 patients were given an anticonvulsant therapy. The seizure count for each patient was monitored at four visits: y_{ij}, $(i = 1, \ldots, 59, j = 1, \ldots, 4)$. Hence, y_{ij} is a discrete outcome. Also measured was the *baseline seizure count* (x_{1i}: included as $z_i = \log(x_{1i}/4)$), *treatment* (x_{2i}) and *age* (x_{3i}). The individual profiles of seizure counts are given per treatment group in Figure 15.4.

In this case, we could assume that the seizure count at any time is Poisson distributed and so $y_{ij} \sim \text{Poisson}(\mu_{ij})$ with

$$\log(\mu_{ij}) = \beta_0 + \beta_1 z_i + \beta_2 x_{2i} + \beta_3 x_{3i} + \beta_4 z_i x_{2i} + b_{ij}.$$

We included an interaction between baseline count and group ($z_i x_{2i}$). Here, the random effect term, b_{ij}, consists of an individual frailty term κ_i and an individual-visit interaction term ψ_{ij}. The prior distributions assumed for the parameters are as follows: $\beta_* \sim \text{N}(0, \sigma_*^2)$, $\sigma_* \sim \text{U}(0, c)$ and zero mean Gaussian random effect prior specifications as follows:

$$\kappa_i \sim \text{N}(0, \sigma_\kappa^2),$$
$$\psi_{ij} \sim \text{N}(0, \sigma_\psi^2).$$

This model can be extended by allowing the individual random intercept to have a temporal correlation. For example,

$$\gamma_j \sim \text{N}(\lambda \gamma_{j-1}, \sigma_\gamma^2), \tag{15.2}$$

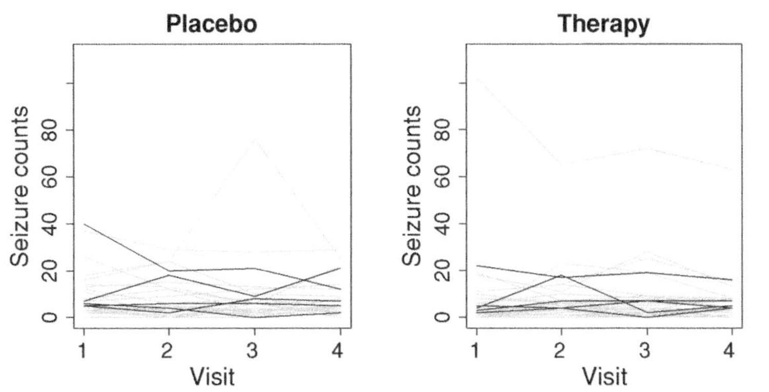

Figure 15.4 Epilepsy study: individual profiles of seizure counts per treatment group.

Table 15.2 Epilepsy study: posterior average parameter estimates and SDs for the model with individual and interaction random effects (RE) only.

Parameter	Estimate	SD
β_0 (intercept)	−1.403	1.262
β_1 (log baseline seizure)	0.884	0.138
β_2 (treatment)	−0.939	0.413
β_3 (log age)	0.342	0.210
β_4 (base-treat interaction)	0.476	0.371
σ_κ (SD individual RE)	0.372	0.0434
σ_ψ (SD interaction RE)	0.507	0.0727

with an additive effect. Hence: $b_{ij} = \kappa_i + \gamma_j + \psi_{ij}$, which is an AR(1) random effect. We considered the above model with and without such an effect and compared the goodness of fit using the DIC criterion.

We initiated for each model three chains of each 40 000 iterations and left out $3 \times 20\,000$ iterations. DIC was based on the last $3 \times 10\,000$ iterations. The model without the AR(1) effect has a marginally lower DIC equal to 1156.0 with $p_D = 121.3$ than the AR(1) effect model with DIC equal to 1156.5 and $p_D = 122.0$. Therefore, we have opted for the model without the AR(1) correlation part; see Table 15.2 for the parameter estimates.

It is noticeable that the baseline seizure and the base line seizure-treatment interaction are significant. Furthermore, the effect of treatment is significant and negative suggesting that over the study period the therapy has significantly reduced the number of seizures compared to the placebo treatment while allowing for the baseline level of seizure counts.

We then checked the distributional assumption of the individual random effects (κ_i) and the individual-visit interaction random effects (ψ_{ij}). In Figure 15.5, we show the NPPs of κ_i. There appears no deviation from the normality assumption. The same was done for ψ_{ij} (plot not shown). Now there was a bit more deviation from normality, but not alarming. To examine the itemwise fit of the model, we also examined the posterior average standardized residuals from

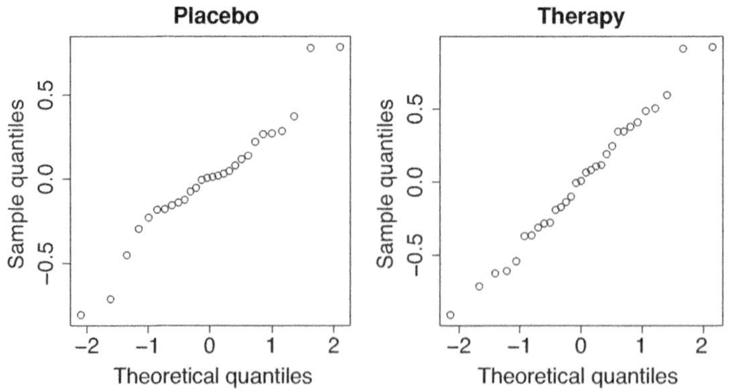

Figure 15.5 Epilepsy study: normal probability plots of the individual random effects (κ_i) in the two treatment groups.

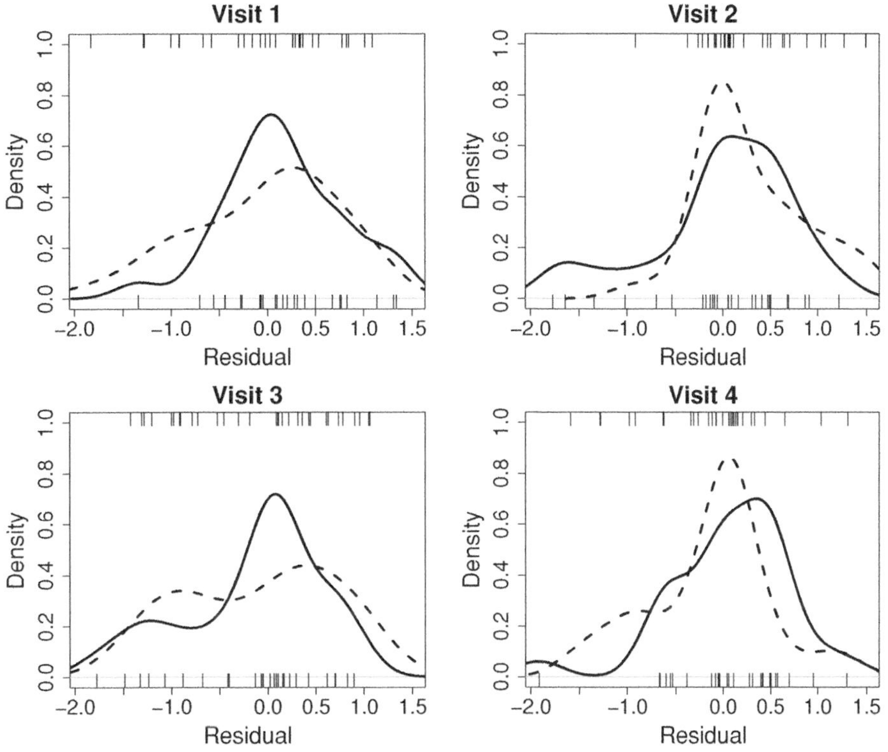

Figure 15.6 Epilepsy study: density plots of the standardized residuals based on the model with individual and interaction random effects only. The solid line represents the placebo group, the dashed line corresponds to the therapy group. The bottom ticks correspond to the placebo group and the top ticks to the therapy group.

this model for each visit. Figure 15.6 displays these residuals ($r_{ij} = \text{ave}_k[(y_{ij} - \mu_{ij}^k)/\sqrt{\mu_{ij}^k}]$). Overall, the fit seems reasonable across groups. At each visit, there is always a deviating patient, but there seems to be no systematic behavior.

15.2 Random event times

In the previous section, the examination times were considered taken at fixed and regular time points. In many applications, these examination times are irregular and should be treated also as such. An example is the *Jimma Infant study*. This is an Ethiopian study conducted between 11-9-1992 and 10-9-1993, set up to establish risk factors affecting infant survival and to investigate socioeconomic, maternal and infant-rearing factors that contribute most to the child's early survival. There was also interest in documenting the growth of the child in the first year measured by its length, weight and other anthropometric measurements such as arm circumference.

The 1501 singleton live births from the town Jimma were examined each 2 months during the first year of their life. In Lesaffre *et al.* (1999) a subgroup of 495 children was examined

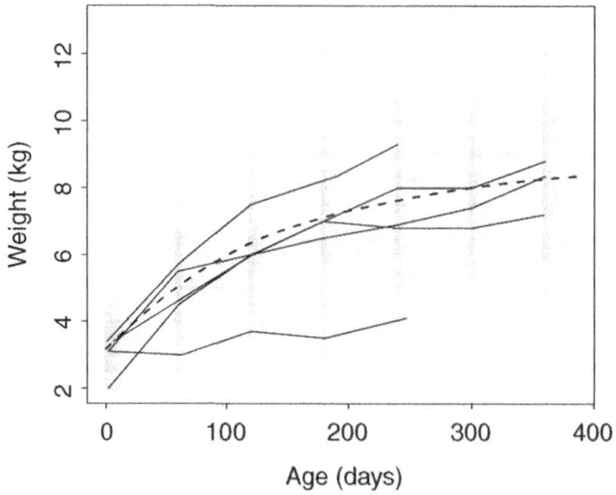

Figure 15.7 Jimma Infant study: weight measurements versus age and the profiles of some randomly selected children together with a LOESS smoother (dashed line) to express the average relationship.

for their first year's weight gain. However, there was quite some variation in the actual times of examination. Ignoring this variation by assuming fixed time points at 0, 2, ..., 12 months would produce a too rough analysis since children in this age period evolve rapidly. The weight profiles in the first year of the babies are plotted in Figure 15.7. One can observe the variability of actual times of examinations. However, the irregularity of the measurement times had no relationship with the physical condition of the children. Mixed effects models involving a random intercept and slope are, therefore, the first choice for the analysis of these weight profiles in combination with the smoothing techniques of Section 10.3.5.

In the above growth study, the timing of the visits was regulated by the examiners, and not by the children nor by the parents of the children. It is a different situation when the subjects themselves regulate their visits. In this case, the pattern of examination times could bear itself information on the response, and the timing of events could then become the focus of interest. An example is the pattern of visits to a general practitioner. The timing and amount of visits are indicative for the subject's health status. In general, a point process of events will then occur for each individual observation unit and hence for an individual unit a time series of events is available. Note that these data are just the finest level of resolution and, in fact, when observation units are aggregated into fixed time periods then data in the form of counts would arise. Hence, with aggregation the resulting data could be analyzed via standard discrete data BGLMMs, such as a random effects Poisson or binomial model. The means of these distributions could then also be made dependent on covariates, such as treatment, to verify whether with one treatment there on average more examination times than with another treatment.

With random times, there are no fixed observation points or intervals and hence binary time series do not arise (like when there is intermittent missingness, see Section 15.3). Instead, the data are the event times themselves: $\{t_{ij}\}$ $(i = 1, \ldots, n;\ j = 1, \ldots, m_i)$, and most often the m_i are different.

A basic model for such data, is a *Poisson process (PP) model* where the intensity of events is governed by an intensity function $\lambda(t)$, which is allowed to vary with time. This intensity represents the local rate of the process and is the focus of most modeling. Assuming a PP model, the event times are independently distributed. Conditional on m_i events in T (= fixed total time), the probability of an event at a given time t is just $\lambda(t)/\int_T \lambda(u)\,du$. If we are not willing to condition on m_i but wish to model the event counts as well as the times, then an unconditional probability is also available. Define the normalized conditional density as $p_i(t \mid m_i) = \lambda_i(t)/\int_T \lambda_i(u)\,du$ for the ith observation unit. We can define a joint likelihood for this model as

$$L(\mathbf{t} \mid \mathbf{m}) = \prod_{i=1}^{n} \prod_{j=1}^{m_i} p_i(t_{ij} \mid m_i),$$

with log-likelihood

$$\ell(\mathbf{t} \mid \mathbf{m}) = \sum_{i=1}^{n} \left[\sum_{j=1}^{m_i} \log \lambda_i(t_{ij}) - m_i \log(\Lambda_i) \right],$$

with $\Lambda_i = \int_T \lambda_i(u)du$. This likelihood depends on the definition of $\lambda_i(t_{ij})$ and on the evaluation of the integral Λ_i. While this form is not a standard distribution, it is reasonably simple to evaluate. First the integral can be approximated either by a numerical scheme whereby a fixed weighted sum is assumed (i.e. $\Lambda_i \approx \sum w_{ik}\lambda_{ik}$ where λ_{ik} is the value of $\lambda_i(t)$ at the kth evaluation point and w_{ik} is the corresponding integration weight), or by Monte Carlo integration whereby values of $\lambda_i(u)$ are simulated and averaged. Note that a simple quadrature rule could be used for the evaluation of Λ_i and with the arbitrary likelihood model facility on WinBUGS (zeroes or ones trick) this likelihood could be easily evaluated.

The specification of $\lambda_i(t_{ij})$ remains. It is common to consider a log link for this specification to a linear or nonlinear predictor. Hence, for example, we might assume

$$\lambda_i(t_{ij}) = \exp\left[\boldsymbol{x}_{ij}^T\boldsymbol{\beta} + f_i(t_{ij}) + b_{ij}\right],$$

where $\boldsymbol{x}_{ij}$ are individual level predictors (possibly time varying), $\boldsymbol{\beta}$ a parameter vector, $f_i(t_{ij})$ a function of time, and b_{ij} a set of random effects. Note that a common group effect can be incorporated via nested indexing across individuals. It should also be clear in this situation that we are modeling the internal structure of the event times and do not have any baseline behavior to contrast with in this specification. Instead, we might wish to include an overall baseline intensity within the specification so that

$$\lambda_i(t_{ij}) = \lambda_0(t_{ij}) \exp\left[\boldsymbol{x}_{ij}^T\boldsymbol{\beta} + f_i(t_{ij}) + b_{ij}\right]. \tag{15.3}$$

Without additional information or data concerning the baseline effect, we must assume a prior distribution which allows for temporal variation. The gamma process is a convenient tool for this specification (Ibrahim *et al.* 2000), whereby the increments of the baseline effect are gamma distributed with the scaling dependent on the time gap:

$$\lambda_0(s+t) - \lambda_0(s) \sim \text{Gamma}(\alpha, \beta).$$

Note that the parameters α, β can have hyperprior distributions and hence can be estimated. An alternative would be to assume that $\log(\lambda_0(t_{ij}))$ followed a Gaussian random walk so that $\log[\lambda_0(s+t)] \sim \text{N}\left[\log[\lambda_0(s)], \sigma_\lambda^2 t\right]$ which would also allow the variance to increase with time. Other considerations besides, the functional form of expression (15.3) could follow as defined for ordinary BGLMMs, with the caveat that any time dependent effects must be scaled per unit time as the times are not fixed intervals. We do not pursue these models here, but for further discussion of these and more advanced model variants, we refer to Clayton (1994), Ishawaran and James (2004), and Cook and Lawless (2007).

15.3 Dealing with missing data

15.3.1 Introduction

In this section, we discuss in more detail the issue of missing observations and their impact on the analysis of longitudinal data. Missing data occur in almost every longitudinal study. For example, patients enrolled in a clinical trial may fail to return for assessment. Hence, over (say) a five period trial, we may have some patients who attend all assessments called *completers*, some who *dropout* from the study which means that they stopped attending the assessments and some who miss an assessment but then return to the study (*intermittent missingness*). In some cases, one can even have subjects that drop-in the study. In the previous chapters, we have managed to analyze many studies that involved missing data, such as the toenail randomized controlled clinical trial (RCT) study, the Signal-Tandmobiel® study and the Jimma Infant study. Each time there was an appreciable number of subjects that missed a visit or that dropped out from the study and for a variety of reasons.

Most often, if not always, it is important to utilize as much of the data that is available. In fact, the principle of *Intent to Treat* (ITT) (Fisher *et al.* 1990) as employed in RCTs requires that all valid data available from the trial should be used, even when dropout happens. When a patient missed an examination, then all data are missing but data may be missing also for other reasons. For instance, when subjects are asked to fill in a questionnaire they might refuse to answer some sensitive questions. In that case part of the data are missing.

In the literature, missing data is dealt with in a variety of ways. The default in almost all statistical packages is to leave out in an analysis those subjects with somewhere a missing value. This is clearly an inefficient procedure, but may create also bias in the estimation process. This is called a *complete-case analysis*. Other approaches try to get rid of the missing data by imputing values for the missing data. An ad hoc and still often used technique in longitudinal studies, and especially in clinical trials, is the *Last Observation Carried Forward (LOCF)* approach. In this approach the missing response is replaced by the last observed value for that response. This can be regarded as a simple form of imputation. However, the method assumes a constant profile for the outcome, an assumption which is usually too strong within a clinical trial setting and underestimates the variability of the response. There are more intelligent imputation methods on the market. In the frequentist world a well accepted procedure is *multiple imputation* (Little and Rubin 2002). In the multiple imputation approach, a rich statistical model (not necessarily related to the longitudinal model) is used to impute M multiple values for the missing data. In practice, often $M = 3$ to $M = 5$ times a value is imputed for each missing value, hereby one emulates the variability of the observed data. Afterward one has to perform M times the statistical analysis on the (M) completed data sets and use expression (5.13) to compute the standard errors of the parameter estimates. The above imputation approaches perform *explicit imputation*. Here, we will look at *implicit imputation* approaches. Depending on whether the response is missing or the predictor is missing, the missingness process is called *response/outcome missingness* or *covariate/predictor missingness*.

15.3.2 Response missingness

Let the response for the ith unit and jth time be y_{ij}. We also need a missingness indicator r_{ij} with

$$r_{ij} = \begin{cases} 1 & \text{if } y_{ij} \text{ is observed,} \\ 0 & \text{otherwise.} \end{cases}$$

In vector notation we have for the ith individual, the vector of responses: $\boldsymbol{y}_i$ and the indicator vector of missingness: $\boldsymbol{r}_i$. The full data consists of all responses (missing and observed) and the information on the missingness. Therefore, the full data density is given by

$$p(\boldsymbol{y}_i, \boldsymbol{r}_i \mid \boldsymbol{x}_i, z_i, \boldsymbol{w}_i, \boldsymbol{\theta}, \boldsymbol{\psi}), \tag{15.4}$$

where $\boldsymbol{x}_i, z_i, \boldsymbol{w}_i$ are the covariates for the fixed effects part, the random effects part and the missingness mechanism, respectively, of the ith subject. Furthermore, $\boldsymbol{\theta}$ contains the fixed and random parameters and $\boldsymbol{\psi}$ is the set of missingness parameters.

Depending on how the full data density is split up, we distinguish between a *selection model* and a *pattern-mixture model*:

- Selection model:

  $$p(\boldsymbol{y}_i, \boldsymbol{r}_i \mid \boldsymbol{x}_i, z_i, \boldsymbol{w}_i, \boldsymbol{\theta}, \boldsymbol{\psi}) = p(\boldsymbol{y}_i \mid \boldsymbol{x}_i, z_i, \boldsymbol{\theta})\ p(\boldsymbol{r}_i \mid \boldsymbol{y}_i, \boldsymbol{w}_i, \boldsymbol{\psi}),$$

  where $p(\boldsymbol{y}_i \mid \boldsymbol{x}_i, z_i, \boldsymbol{\theta})$ describes the longitudinal model. Hence, this is the model we have used in the above examples to fit the longitudinal data. The function $p(\boldsymbol{r}_i \mid \boldsymbol{y}_i, \boldsymbol{w}_i, \boldsymbol{\psi})$ describes the mechanism for missingness. Note that this is a function of $\boldsymbol{y}_i$.

- Pattern mixture model:

  $$p(\boldsymbol{y}_i, \boldsymbol{r}_i \mid \boldsymbol{x}_i, z_i, \boldsymbol{w}_i, \boldsymbol{\theta}, \boldsymbol{\psi}) = p(\boldsymbol{y}_i \mid \boldsymbol{r}_i, \boldsymbol{x}_i, z_i, \boldsymbol{\theta})\ p(\boldsymbol{r}_i \mid \boldsymbol{w}_i, \boldsymbol{\psi}).$$

  Note that now the missingness is modelled directly without involving the responses, and that the response is modeled conditional on the missingness pattern. Hence, the modeling is quite different from before.

Finally, there is also a *shared parameter model*. In this case, it is assumed that the joint model (15.4) can be written as

$$p(\boldsymbol{y}_i, \boldsymbol{r}_i \mid \boldsymbol{x}_i, z_i, \boldsymbol{w}_i, \boldsymbol{\theta}, \boldsymbol{\psi}) = \int p(\boldsymbol{y}_i \mid \boldsymbol{x}_i, z_i, \boldsymbol{\theta}, \boldsymbol{b}_i) p(\boldsymbol{r}_i \mid \boldsymbol{w}_i, \boldsymbol{\psi}, \boldsymbol{b}_i)\, d\boldsymbol{b}_i. \tag{15.5}$$

In other words, in this model it is assumed that the measurement process is independent from the missingness process given some latent random structure defined by $\boldsymbol{b}_i$. Despite the attractiveness of the latter two approaches, we will not pursue them any further but refer to Daniels and Hogan (2008).

It is important to distinguish between the observed part of $\boldsymbol{y}_i$, namely $\boldsymbol{y}_i^o$ and the missing part, namely $\boldsymbol{y}_i^m$. Then, for the selection model,

$$p(\boldsymbol{r}_i \mid \boldsymbol{y}_i, \boldsymbol{w}_i, \boldsymbol{\psi}) = p(\boldsymbol{r}_i \mid \boldsymbol{y}_i^o, \boldsymbol{y}_i^m, \boldsymbol{w}_i, \boldsymbol{\psi}).$$

Further, we assume that the parameters in the measurement model and the missingness model have nothing in common. In Bayesian terms, it is reformulated as that $\boldsymbol{\theta}$ and $\boldsymbol{\psi}$ are a priori independent, i.e. $p(\boldsymbol{\theta}, \boldsymbol{\psi}) = p(\boldsymbol{\theta})p(\boldsymbol{\psi})$.

15.3.3 Missingness mechanisms

15.3.3.1 Missing completely at random

We speak of a missing completely at random (MCAR) mechanism when the response is not related to the missingness mechanism, so that

$$p(\boldsymbol{r}_i \mid \boldsymbol{y}_i, \boldsymbol{w}_i, \boldsymbol{\psi}) = p(\boldsymbol{r}_i \mid \boldsymbol{w}_i, \boldsymbol{\psi}).$$

In this case, the outcomes are not related to the missingness process and so

$$p(\boldsymbol{y}_i, \boldsymbol{r}_i \mid \boldsymbol{x}_i, \boldsymbol{z}_i, \boldsymbol{w}_i, \boldsymbol{\theta}, \boldsymbol{\psi}) = p(\boldsymbol{y}_i \mid \boldsymbol{x}_i, \boldsymbol{z}_i, \boldsymbol{\theta})\, p(\boldsymbol{r}_i \mid \boldsymbol{w}_i, \boldsymbol{\psi}).$$

Hence, the observed data are independent of the missingness process and thus

$$p(\boldsymbol{y}_i^o, \boldsymbol{r}_i \mid \boldsymbol{x}_i, \boldsymbol{z}_i, \boldsymbol{w}_i, \boldsymbol{\theta}, \boldsymbol{\psi}) = p(\boldsymbol{y}_i^o \mid \boldsymbol{x}_i, \boldsymbol{z}_i, \boldsymbol{\theta})\, p(\boldsymbol{r}_i \mid \boldsymbol{w}_i, \boldsymbol{\psi}). \tag{15.6}$$

This implies that the missingness mechanism can be ignored in the analysis of the observed outcomes, given the predictors in the model. In fact, one can show that the only effect of the missing data generated by a MCAR mechanism is a loss of efficiency. Descriptive statistics and basing the statistical analysis on $p(\boldsymbol{y}_i^o \mid \boldsymbol{x}_i, \boldsymbol{z}_i, \boldsymbol{\theta})$ are appropriate. For a practical example of a MCAR missingness process, take an RCT to compare (say) the effect of two lipid-lowering medications on serum cholesterol then examples of a MCAR mechanism are: (a) the patient's blood tube has been dropped and consequently no value was recorded at that visit, (b) a patient missed a visit because he stayed at home with a broken leg, etc. These examples are straightforward illustrations. However, another less obvious example is when there is an unequal dropout rate in the two arms of the study, but in each arm the reason for dropping out has nothing to do with the response.

Although one can never be sure about the missingness mechanism, it appears reasonable to assume that missing data in the Signal-Tandmobiel study have been generated by a MCAR process. Indeed, the reasons for the children to miss an examination time were: they moved to another geographical location, left the school or were ill at the day of the examination, but it is unlikely that they were absent because of a tooth problem.

15.3.3.2 Missing at random

In this case, the probability of missingness is conditionally independent of the unobserved data, given the observed data

$$p(\boldsymbol{r}_i \mid \boldsymbol{y}_i, \boldsymbol{w}_i, \boldsymbol{\psi}) = p(\boldsymbol{r}_i \mid \boldsymbol{y}_i^o, \boldsymbol{w}_i, \boldsymbol{\psi}),$$

so that

$$p(\boldsymbol{y}_i^o, \boldsymbol{r}_i \mid \boldsymbol{x}_i, \boldsymbol{z}_i, \boldsymbol{w}_i, \boldsymbol{\theta}, \boldsymbol{\psi}) = p(\boldsymbol{y}_i^o \mid \boldsymbol{x}_i, \boldsymbol{z}_i, \boldsymbol{\theta})\, p(\boldsymbol{r}_i \mid \boldsymbol{y}_i^o, \boldsymbol{w}_i, \boldsymbol{\psi}). \tag{15.7}$$

Since the two parameter vectors $\boldsymbol{\theta}$ and $\boldsymbol{\psi}$ have nothing in common, the missingness process is called *ignorable* and then a likelihood or a Bayesian analysis on only the observed data gives a valid answer. Note that now the descriptive statistics give a distorted picture of the parameters. For an example of a missing at random (MAR) process take again the randomized controlled clinical trial (RCT) on lipid lowering medications. Suppose that the study physician removes the patient from the study because his past profile does not show any decline in serum cholesterol. In that case, the missingness mechanism is MAR.

Notice that if the missingness process is MCAR but the longitudinal model is misspecified, say a covariate has been omitted, then the missingness mechanism can look more like an MAR process. The same is true for a process that is MAR under the correct model. If an incorrect model is fitted to the data then the missingness process can resemble more the MNAR process below. For this reason, it is important to model carefully the longitudinal process, i.e. the mean and the variance structure. The longitudinal models that we have fitted in Chapter 9 were based on the MAR assumption.

Most often one cannot be sure that the missingness mechanism is only MAR and not the more complicated MNAR as described in the following text. However, all classical mixed effects analyses are based on the MAR assumption and this was assumed, e.g. in the toenail RCT analyses. A motivation for assuming MAR in the toenail study is that the disease slowly evolves and the failure or success of the treatment, and hence also the probability of dropout, may be easily predicted from the patient's profile in the past.

15.3.3.3 Missing not at random

In this case the probability of a missing outcome is dependent on the *unobserved* response y^m. In general, the observed data and missingness process are convolved as

$$p(\boldsymbol{y}_i^o, \boldsymbol{r}_i \mid \boldsymbol{x}_i, \boldsymbol{z}_i, \boldsymbol{w}_i, \boldsymbol{\theta}, \boldsymbol{\psi}) = \int p(\boldsymbol{y}_i \mid \boldsymbol{x}_i, \boldsymbol{z}_i, \boldsymbol{\theta})\, p(\boldsymbol{r}_i \mid \boldsymbol{y}_i, \boldsymbol{w}_i, \boldsymbol{\psi})\, d\boldsymbol{y}_i^m. \tag{15.8}$$

In this case, the missingness must be modeled. Again in the context of the lipid lowering study, an example of a missing not at random (MNAR) mechanism is when the general practitioner of the patient, not involved in the conduct of the trial, suggests the patient to leave the study. When this is done without notifying the study physician (and the last patient's serum cholesterol was not recorded) then the patient dropped out because of a nonobserved response.

Most likely in practice the reasons for missing data and for dropping out are various, some have nothing to do with the response (MCAR), some can be predicted from the past (MAR) and some not (MNAR). In the Jimma Infant study children missed a visit or dropped out from the study for a variety of reasons: their parents were simply not present at the time the examiner arrived at their home, the parents moved to a different area or, more dramatically, the child died. From the 1501 live births involved at the start of the study, only 1152 children were still in the study at 12 months of which 141 died during the first year. Looking at the weight profiles of the children, some of the deaths are predictable but not all, rendering the dropout process MNAR. In addition, death is an absorbing state and in the classical statistical models that are used for the analysis of incomplete data, such as mixed models, the missing data are implicitly imputed. In the case of death, such imputation is not natural. We will not handle this problem here, however, but refer to Daniels and Hogan (2008).

The statistical analysis under MNAR is far more complex than under MAR. In Section 15.4, we treat a possible approach for analyzing longitudinal data involving a MNAR dropout mechanism. The approach is based on jointly analyzing the longitudinal data and assuming a survival model for the dropout times. However, it is important to stress that this is only one possible approach. In general, one recommends to perform a sensitivity analysis varying various aspects of the missingness model and evaluate their effect.

15.3.4 Bayesian considerations

The classification of the missing data mechanisms was described above in a largely classical context. However, the Bayesian approach to missing data problems is quite similar and differs only in the addition of prior distributions for the parameters. A full discussion of Bayesian issues in missing data problems can be found in Daniels and Hogan (2008).

Finally, in the Bayesian approach, it is straightforward to generate the missing values under the assumed model via the posterior predictive distribution. As seen before, this is also quickly done with WinBUGS and SAS.

15.3.5 Predictor missingness

Predictor missingness is common to many kinds of analyses besides longitudinal studies. As most analytical models assume conditioning on predictors, we usually do not consider predictors as having random variation. However, when missingness appears in predictors a mechanism is needed to allow for the estimation of the missing data. This can be achieved within the Bayesian paradigm by assuming a prior distribution for the predictor variable, which is justified in the same way that any parameter that is unobserved within a Bayesian model must be assigned a prior distribution. Consequently, this allows the missing predictor values to be imputed as parameters within a posterior sampling algorithm. For further details (see Daniels and Hogan 2008).

15.4 Joint modeling of longitudinal and survival responses

15.4.1 Introduction

Joint modeling is a statistical technique to estimate common parameters of two or more models jointly. The first approaches on joint modeling were primarily developed in AIDS clinical trials in the 1990's and combined longitudinal data with survival data (see Tsiatis *et al.* 1995; Wulfsohn and Tsiatis 1997). The method was proposed in the context of survival analysis in the presence of time-dependent covariates which were measured only periodically and with measurement error. However, it can also be seen as an approach to model informative dropouts where the survival time is taken to be the time to dropout (Guo and Carlin 2004; Ibrahim *et al.* 2001). Joint modeling offers less biased and more efficient estimates of treatment effects in the survival part of the model but equally so in the longitudinal part when the survival endpoint is the time for dropping out (see also Ibrahim *et al.* 2001).

We apply here a joint modeling approach to longitudinal data of which we suspect that the missing data process, in fact here the dropout process, is MNAR. We assume that the joint model of observed longitudinal and survival data is given by

$$p(\boldsymbol{y}_i^o, d_i \mid \boldsymbol{x}_i, z_i, \boldsymbol{w}_i, \boldsymbol{\theta}, \boldsymbol{\psi}) = \int\int p(\boldsymbol{y}_i \mid \boldsymbol{x}_i, z_i, \boldsymbol{\theta}, \boldsymbol{b}_i)\, p(d_i \mid \boldsymbol{w}_i, \boldsymbol{\psi}, \boldsymbol{b}_i)\, \mathrm{d}\boldsymbol{y}_i^m\, \mathrm{d}\boldsymbol{b}_i,$$

$$= \int p(\boldsymbol{y}_i^o \mid \boldsymbol{x}_i, z_i, \boldsymbol{\theta}, \boldsymbol{b}_i)\, p(d_i \mid \boldsymbol{w}_i, \boldsymbol{\psi}, \boldsymbol{b}_i)\, \mathrm{d}\boldsymbol{b}_i, \quad (15.9)$$

where d_i indicates the time of dropout, e.g. $d_i = 3$ when $\boldsymbol{r}_i = (1, 1, 0, 0, \ldots)$. In expression (15.9), we assumed that, conditional on a latent vector $\boldsymbol{b}_i$ the measurement and dropout process are independent.

15.4.2 An example

The example considered here was first analyzed by Guo and Carlin (2004). They combined a longitudinal model for treatment with a model for the survival experience of the patient during treatment. In a clinical trial to compare the efficacy and safety of two antiretroviral drugs in treating patients who had failed or were intolerant of zidovudine (AZT) therapy. In this example, 467 HIV-infected patients were enrolled (who met the inclusion and exclusion criteria), and randomly assigned to two treatment groups: *didanosine* (ddI) or *zalcitabine* (ddC). CD4 counts were recorded at five time points: baseline, 2, 6, 12 and 18 months. Figure 15.8 shows the individual longitudinal profiles of the response over time. Figure 15.9 displays the Kaplan–Meier survival curves for the two treatments groups (ddI and ddC).

We denote the $\sqrt{CD4}$ count for the ith individual at time j as y_{ij} ($i = 1, \ldots, n = 467$; $j = 1, \ldots, m_i$). There are four explanatory variables which were included in the analysis: *drug* (ddI = 1, ddC = 0), gender (male = 1, female = −1), previous infection at study entry (*prev* = 1 when AIDS was diagnosed and −1 otherwise), and *stratum* (AZT failure = 1, AZT intolerance = −1).

We now separately discuss the used longitudinal and survival model.

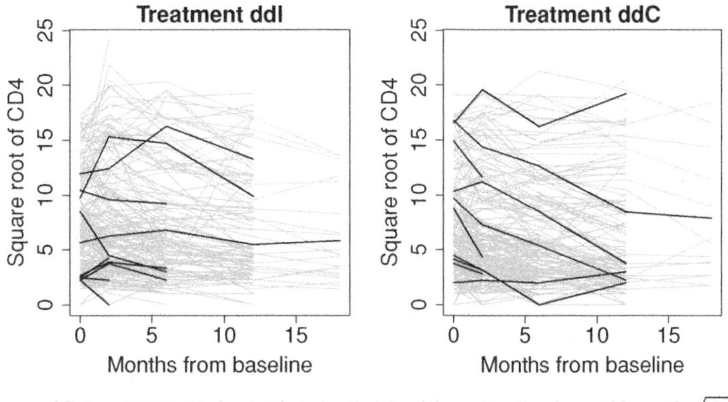

Figure 15.8 AZT clinical trial: individual longitudinal profiles of $\sqrt{CD4}$.

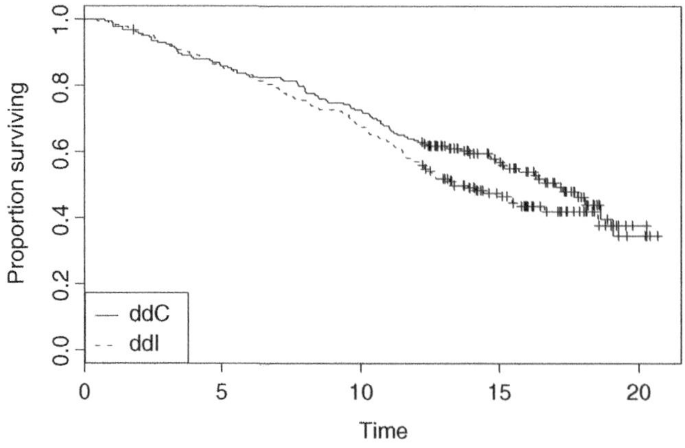

Figure 15.9 AZT clinical trial: Kaplan–Meier survival curves for the two treatment groups (ddI and ddC).

15.4.2.1 The longitudinal model

Assume that the longitudinal model is given by

$$y_{ij} \mid \mu_{ij} \sim \mathrm{N}(\mu_{ij}, \sigma^2),$$

with $\mu_{ij} = \boldsymbol{x}_{ij}^T\boldsymbol{\beta} + z_{ij}^T\boldsymbol{b}_i$, which corresponds to a linear mixed model described in Chapter 9. Denote the times of observation for the ith individual as s_{ij}. Then we have here

$$\boldsymbol{x}_{ij}^T\boldsymbol{\beta} = \beta_{10} + \beta_{11}s_{ij} + \beta_{12}s_{ij} \times \text{drug}_i + \beta_{13}\text{gender}_i + \beta_{14}\text{prev}_i + \beta_{15}\text{stratum}_i,$$

$$z_{ij}^T\boldsymbol{b}_i = W_{1i}(s_{ij}),$$

with $W_{1i}(s_{ij}) = b_{0i} + b_{1i}s_{ij}$. The two random effects represent a random intercept and a random slope for time. They are classically assumed to have a bivariate normal prior distribution with covariance G, i.e. $\boldsymbol{b}_i \sim \mathrm{N}(\boldsymbol{0}, \mathrm{G})$.

The regression parameters were assumed to have a noninformative zero mean multivariate normal prior distribution, whereas an inverse gamma distribution was assumed for $\sigma^2 \sim \mathrm{IG}(0.1, 0.1)$. With respect to the prior of G, we have evaluated three choices: (a) IW(D,2), with D = diag(0.001, 0.001); (b) IW(D,2), with D = diag(100, 100), which is the choice in Guo and Carlin (2004); and (c) uniform priors for the standard deviations of random intercept and slope, and their correlation: $\sigma_{b_0} \sim \mathrm{U}(0, 20)$, $\sigma_{b_1} \sim \mathrm{U}(0, 20)$ and $\rho \sim \mathrm{U}(-1, 1)$. In all analyses that we performed the uniform priors resulted in a lower DIC value followed by choice (b). Hence, we report here only the results based on the uniform priors.

15.4.2.2 The survival model

For the survival model, we considered a general Weibull model for the baseline distribution of the time of death, denoted for the ith individual as t_i, in combination with a Cox proportional hazards model to analyze the time-to-event data. This model was discussed in Chapter 14. A Weibull distribution has two parameters: ϕ the scale and a mean level ψ_i,

$$t_i \sim \text{Weibull}(\phi, \psi_i).$$

Note that when $\phi = 1$ an exponential model results which implies a constant hazard model over time. We also consider a log intensity specification so that

$$\log(\psi_i) = \boldsymbol{x}_{2i}^T \boldsymbol{\beta}_2 + W_{2i},$$

where the linear predictor is $\boldsymbol{x}_{2i}^T \boldsymbol{\beta}_2 = \beta_{20} + \beta_{21}\,\text{drug}_i + \beta_{22}\,\text{gender}_i + \beta_{23}\text{prev}_i + \beta_{24}\,\text{stratum}_i$, and the random effect term is defined as $W_{2i} = \gamma_0 b_{0i} + \gamma_1 b_{1i}$.

Similar to the longitudinal part, the regression parameters are assumed to have a noninformative zero mean multivariate normal prior distribution. The Weibull parameter ϕ was given a Gamma(1, 1) prior. We also fitted an exponential distribution to the survival data.

15.4.2.3 The joint model

Linkage between the two models is accommodated from two separate sources. First we have included common covariates in each model. Hence, both survival and CD4 count is thought to be related to drug, gender, prev and stratum. The second source of linkage is the use of common random effect terms. In this case, we have assumed that b_{0i} and b_{1i} appear in both models but in the survival model they are scaled by parameters γ_0 and γ_1. This does imply that these effects are jointly estimated within the two models.

For each joint model, we initiated one chain of total length 200 000 with thinning's factor = 10 and removed the first 100 000 iterations.

15.4.2.4 Modeling results

The models reported here consist of a linear mixed model for the longitudinal data fitted jointly with a survival model, first the Weibull model (ϕ estimated) and then the exponential model ($\phi = 1$). WinBUGS was used for the analysis. We only considered *model XI* of Guo and Carlin.

Table 15.3 displays the overall goodness-of-fit results in terms of DIC. In the original paper, Guo and Carlin only reported the exponential model results as they found a negative correlation between the ϕ parameter and a regression parameter in the full Weibull model. Hence, a constant hazard was assumed. In this analysis, we have found that the full Weibull

Table 15.3 AZT clinical trial: comparison of goodness of fit of joint models based on Weibull and exponential survival model. The subindex 'L' refers to the GOF measures of the longitudinal part of the model, 'S' refers to the survival part of the model and 'T' represents the total.

Model	DIC_L	$p_{D,L}$	DIC_S	$p_{D,S}$	DIC_T	$p_{D,T}$
Weibull	6128	517.6	931	204.4	7059	722.1
Exponential	6115	545.8	1665	82.5	7780	628.3

Table 15.4 AZT clinical trial: posterior means estimates and 95% credible intervals for the joint model with Weibull part.

Parameter	Estimate	95% CI
	Longitudinal analysis	
Intercept	7.979	(7.264, 8.692)
Time	−0.2426	(−0.2855, −0.2011)
Time × drug	−0.00153	(−0.0591, 0.0557)
Gender	−0.05209	(−0.6975, 0.6072)
Prev	−2.367	(−2.835, −1.889)
Stratum	−0.1331	(−0.6087, 0.3453)
G_{11}	16.07	(13.9, 18.56)
G_{22}	0.04304	(0.02989, 0.05757)
$\rho = G_{12}/\sqrt{G_{11}G_{22}}$	−0.01534	(−0.1626, 0.1348)
σ^2	3.152	(2.846, 3.486)
	Survival analysis	
Intercept	−21.64	(−26.39, −16.06)
Drug	1.106	(−0.3265, 2.695)
Gender	−1.013	(−2.479, 0.3493)
Prev	3.556	(2.275, 4.991)
Stratum	0.1696	(−0.7694, 1.005)
γ_0	−1.035	(−1.417, −0.6713)
γ_1	−33.67	(−43.77, −23.44)
ϕ	6.238	(4.552, 7.672)

yields a lower DIC than the exponential. In Table 15.4, we present the posterior average parameter estimates for the full Weibull model.

For the longitudinal part of this model, we found that time and prev have a significant negative effect on CD4 cell count, whereby 'significance' should be interpreted in a Bayesian sense (95% CI excludes zero). This implies that the CD4 cell count is lower for patients diagnosed at baseline with AIDS and it further decreases with time. No significant effects were established for the drug by time interaction. The posterior correlation estimate of the random effects was basically zero. For the survival part of the model, only prev is positive and significant indicating that patients who enter the study with AIDS diagnosis have a lower life expectancy. Both linking parameters γ_0 and γ_1 are negative and significant, providing strong evidence of an association between the two submodels and indicating that both the initial level and slope of CD4 count is negatively associated with the hazard of death. Finally, the scale parameter of the Weibull distribution is large and excludes the exponential model. In contrast to the original analysis, our model converged although at the expense of many more iterations than in Guo and Carlin (2004).

We further explored the distributional assumptions of the model. For instance, we checked the distribution of the random intercept and slope, by plotting their posterior means in a normal probability plot. For each of the treatment groups, we found that normality was achieved.

15.5 Closing remarks

This final longitudinal example served to highlight the great flexibility of joint modeling and the ability of WinBUGS to accommodate complex data structures within its programming capability. It is also a great feature of this package that sensitivity to model specification (in particular, prior specification) can be easily tested. For these more complex models it is always important to consider such sensitivity when assumptions cannot be directly tested in analysis. It must also be stated that similar sensitivity analyses are as easily possible with the SAS procedure MCMC. It will depend on the programming skills of the user which package will be used for the task.

Finally, we note that the area of longitudinal analyses is quite rich. Further complexity can be introduced without great difficulties. For instance, the following models have been analyzed in the literature: longitudinal models with a multivariate response (say not exceeding three to four dimensions), longitudinal models embedded in an extra multilevel structure, longitudinal models with censored responses, amongst others.

16

Spatial applications: Disease mapping and image analysis

16.1 Introduction

In this chapter, we outline approaches to two areas of study that feature spatial models and that have received considerable attention within the fields of Bayesian analysis: *Disease Mapping* and *Image Analysis*. These two areas have both featured in the early development of both modeling in Bayesian analysis and also in the development of algorithms for posterior sampling of Bayesian models. In fact, the earliest statistical applications of the Gibbs sampler were in image segmentation problems (see Geman and Geman 1984; Besag *et al.* 1991).

16.2 Disease mapping

Bayesian disease mapping is a wide subject and encompasses a range of topics where the geographical or spatial distribution of a disease is of importance. In what follows there is an emphasis on disease analysis as opposed to other aspects of public health sciences (such as health services research, health promotion or education). There is a need to employ particular *spatial* statistical methods which are designed for such data. The basic characteristic of data encountered in this application area is its discrete nature, whether in the form of spatial locations of cases of a disease, or counts of a disease within defined geographical regions. Hence, methods developed for continuous spatial processes, such as *Kriging* (Schabenberger and Gotway 2004, Chapter 5), are not directly applicable or only approximately valid. Often geographical hypotheses of interest focus on whether the residential address of cases of disease yields insight into etiology of the disease, or, whether adverse environmental health hazards exist locally within a region (as exemplified by local increases in disease risk). For example, in a study of the relationship between malaria endemicity and diabetes in Sardinia, a strong negative relationship was found (Bernardinelli *et al.* 1995; Lawson 2006, Chapter 9). This relation had a spatial expression and the geographical distribution of malaria was important in

Bayesian Biostatistics, First Edition. Emmanuel Lesaffre and Andrew B. Lawson.

generating explanatory models for the relation. In public health practice, it is of considerable importance to be able to assess whether localized areas, which have larger than expected numbers of cases of disease are related to any underlying environmental cause. Here, spatial evidence of a link between cases and a source is fundamental in the analysis. Evidence of such as a decline in risk with distance from the *putative* source of hazard or elevation of risk in a preferred direction is important in this regard.

16.2.1 Some general spatial epidemiological issues

Before considering the study of the spatial distribution of disease, there are some fundamental epidemiological ideas that should be considered.

16.2.1.1 Relative risk

Within any geographical area, the local density of cases of disease can be studied. We often want to examine this as it gives information about local variations in disease. If we have census tracts, then the counts of cases of a particular disease could be the data of interest. These crude counts of disease cannot be used on their own as the density of cases will be affected by the variation in the population of the area. This is true whether we observe case addresses (the residential address of a disease case) or the aggregated count of cases within small areas.

Hence, underlying the disease incidence is the variation in the population 'at-risk' of the disease. This background population will vary in its composition (age, gender, susceptibility groups) and in its density with spatial location. Hence, this variation should be accounted for in any analysis of the disease occurrence. Clearly, if areas of high susceptibility (with frail population groups) coincide with areas of high disease occurrence then there is likely to be less interest in these areas (in terms of adverse disease presence), than areas where there is high disease occurrence and a low number of susceptibles. Local occurrence of disease (counting of cases within areas) within short time spans (e.g. individual months or years) is termed *incidence*. Longer term accumulation of disease cases is often termed *prevalence*. Here, the term incidence is used throughout. In general, prevalence can be analyzed as for incidence.

To simplify discussion, initially, we will assume that we have a small administrative area (such as a census tract, postcode, zip code, county, etc.) within which we observe the disease incidence. Often we want to compare the observed counts of disease with what would have arisen from the underlying population. This will tell us if there is any excess disease risk in the local area. Let us assume that there are $i = 1, \ldots, n$ tracts or small areas in a study area. Often a ratio of the observed count y_i, in the ith tract to the expected count e_i derived from the background population is used to examine excess risk: the *relative risk* of a disease within the ith area can be estimated by y_i/e_i. This ratio represents the relative risk compared to that the local population suggests should be seen in the area. Often, we consider this to be given by a parameter θ_i and so the crude estimate of relative risk in an area is $\widehat{\theta_i} = y_i/e_i$. Usually, the count y_i will be available from government public health data sources and the expected count (or rate) is usually computed from known rates for the disease in population subgroups (broken by age and gender). This is known as *standardization*. The calculation of expected rates can be very important and different methods of calculation could lead to different conclusions about disease risk. Note that this relative risk definition implies a multiplicative model for risk. This is a common assumption in epidemiology.

16.2.1.2 Standardization

Expected rates in the small areas or tracts $\{e_i\}$ are calculated (estimated) from the local population structure. We do not consider different methods of standardization of expected rates here, but we assume that they are fixed in the further discussion. The reader is referred to Elliott *et al.* (2000) for more details. Expected rates are commonly used to allow for population effects when count data are observed. Count data are often available readily from government sources. However, for some purposes, there is a need to examine the spatial distribution of cases at finer spatial resolution. Commonly the residential address of cases is the finest level of resolution that can be found. Usually, this is only relevant if a small geographic study region is examined. In this case, the data form a spatial point process. As for count data, there is a need take the population variation into account when examining the risk at this spatial resolution level.

Expected rates are usually only available at aggregated geographic scales (census tracts or such like areas) and cannot be used effectively at fine resolutions to control for population variations. An alternative is to use the incidence of a *control disease* within the study region. A control disease is matched closely to the risk structure of the disease of interest, but must not display the incidence effect under investigation. For example, we could use live births as a control for childhood leukemia in clustering studies. In that case the address locations of all births would be used as a population surrogate. This leads to two point processes: (1) the leukemia case distribution, and (2) the live birth distribution. Of course, live birth is not a disease, but in this case, is a population indicator. Note that this control disease is a *geographical* control and is not matched to specific cases. The common feature of each control disease is that it should not be related to the effect of interest. There is some debate about use of these controls as opposed to expected rates from external sources.

16.2.1.3 Confounders and deprivation indices

All disease maps contain the influence of variables affecting the local population which are not accounted for in standardized rates or control diseases. We can try to allow for these effects in two ways:

1. Include as many known explanatory variables in the expected rate or regression model to allow for these effects. These variables are called *known confounders*.
2. Include the effect of unmeasured confounders via the use of *random effects*.

In the first case, the solution is to include in the study as many known variables that affect the outcome so that extra variation is explained. Of course, it may not be feasible to include all know confounders simply due to (realistic) study limitations. To make allowance for unmeasured confounders (whether known or unknown), it is possible to admit random effects into any regression model. These are additional unobserved variates that will soak up extra variation of various kinds.

Often adverse disease incidence is known to be related to a range of poverty-related explanatory variables, e.g. unemployment, housing type, welfare status and car ownership. That is, we expect that there is measurable adverse risk in areas where these variates indicate low income and poverty. These variables are often available from a national census. There has been some effort to combine such variables in composite measures known as *deprivation indices* (Carstairs 1981). In North America, these are often termed urbanicity indices. Deprivation indices are now routinely available from government census data organizations and can be incorporated directly into a disease map as a covariate or as an offset term.

16.2.2 Some spatial statistical issues

A fundamental feature of geo-referenced data available for analysis is that it is usually discrete (either in the form of a point process or counting process), and the cases of concern arise from within a local human population which varies in spatial density and in susceptibility to the disease of interest. Hence, any model or test procedure must make allowance for this background (nuisance) population effect. The background population effect can be allowed for in a variety of ways. For count data, it is commonplace to obtain *expected* rates for the disease of interest based on the age–sex structure of the local population (see Elliott *et al.* 2000, Chapter 3), and some crude estimates of local relative risk are often computed from the ratio of observed to expected counts (e.g. standardized mortality/incidence ratios: *SMR*s). For case event data, expected rates are not available at the resolution of the case locations and the use of the spatial distribution of a control disease has been advocated. In that case, the spatial variation in the case disease is compared to the spatial variation in the control disease. A major issue in this approach is the correct choice of the control disease. It is important to choose a control which is matched to the age–sex structure of the case disease but is unaffected by the feature of interest. For example, in the analysis of cases around a putative health hazard, a control disease should not be affected by the health hazard. Counts of control disease cases could also be used instead of expected rates when analyzing count data. In the following, we focus on count data models and their Bayesian implementation. Case event data are considered in more detail in Lawson (2009) and Lawson and Banerjee (2010).

16.2.3 Count data models

Figure 16.1 displays a typical count data example: male lip cancer mortality in the Landkreise of the former East Germany. Displayed is the SMR map for the 195 Landkreise (administrative regions). This example first appeared in Chapter 9.

A considerable literature has developed concerning the analysis of count data in spatial epidemiology (see reviews in Banerjee *et al.* 2004; Lawson 2006; Lawson and Banerjee 2010).

The usual model adopted for the analysis of region counts $\{y_i,\ i = 1, \ldots, n\}$ assumes that they are independent Poisson random variables with parameters $\{\lambda_i,\ i = 1, \ldots, n\}$. Often the $\lambda_i s$ are assumed to be constant within areas. Usually, the expected count is modeled as

$$E(y_i) = \lambda_i = e_i\theta_i,\ (i = 1, \ldots, n),$$

and so the data level model is

$$y_i \sim \text{Poisson}(e_i\theta_i).$$

Note that the parameter of interest in this model is the relative risk (θ_i). This model may be extended to include unobserved heterogeneity between regions by introducing a prior distribution for the log relative risks ($\log(\theta_i),\ i = 1, \ldots, n$). Incorporation of such heterogeneity has become a common approach and the Besag, York and Mollié (*BYM*) convolution model is now a standard model (Mollié 1999). A full Bayesian analysis using this model is available in WinBUGS.

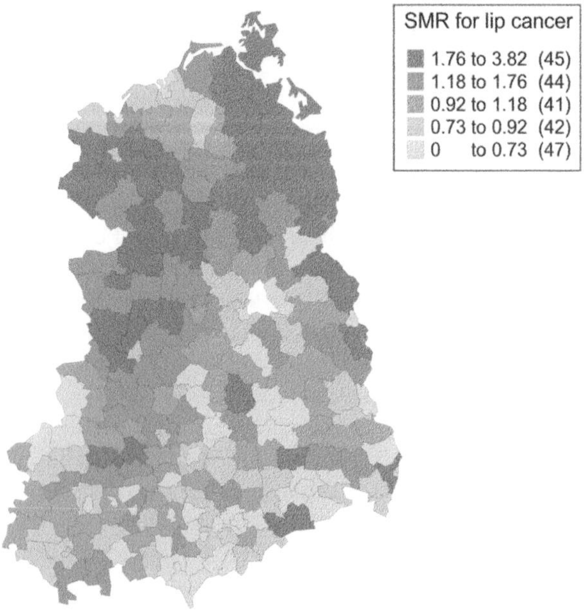

Figure 16.1 Lip cancer study: graphical display of standardized mortality ratios for male lip cancer in 1989 within the Landkriese of Eastern Germany.

16.2.4 A special application area: Disease mapping/risk estimation

In this area, focus is on the processing of the disease map to take out the random noise. Often applications in health services research require the production of an 'accurate' map of relative risks. Models for relative risk range from simple SMRs to posterior expected estimates from Bayesian models. In the count data situation, define the model for the observed counts as

$$y_i \sim \text{Poisson}(e_i\theta_i)$$
$$\log(\theta_i) = \boldsymbol{x}_i^T \boldsymbol{\beta} + \text{random terms},$$

where $\boldsymbol{x}_i^T$ is the ith row of a covariate design matrix and $\boldsymbol{\beta}$ is a regression parameter vector.

The simplest model assumes no linkages to covariates or random terms and the ML estimator of θ_i is the SMR: i.e. $\widehat{\theta_i} = y_i/e_i$. More often, and more generally, $\log(\theta_i)$ is assumed to be equal to a linear predictor involving covariates and regression parameters ($\boldsymbol{x}_i^T \boldsymbol{\beta}$). The final extension includes random effect terms to allow for overdispersion (uncorrelated heterogeneity UH: v_i) and spatially correlated heterogeneity (CH: u_i). The model would then take the form

$$\log(\theta_i) = \boldsymbol{x}_i^T \boldsymbol{\beta} + v_i + u_i.$$

In applications without covariates, when simple smoothing of rates is required, a simpler intercept random effect model would be used:

$$\log(\theta_i) = \alpha_0 + v_i + u_i.$$

This model assigns noise to two components: UH and CH, while identifying the overall rate via α_0. Both random components are usually fitted to capture all the noise components thought to be present. This is often termed the BYM convolution model. To be able to estimate these components, prior distributions are assumed for each component. Usually, these consist of an uncorrelated zero mean normal distribution for the overdispersion:

$$v_i \sim \mathrm{N}(0, \sigma_v^2), \tag{16.1}$$

where $\tau_v = \sigma_v^{-2}$ is the precision, and a spatial correlation prior distribution for the CH component. This could be chosen in a variety of ways. Commonly a Markov random field (MRF) is assumed. The intrinsic singular Gaussian distribution (Besag *et al.* 1991; Kunsch 1987; Rue and Held 2005) is used where the conditional mean of the region effect is based only on a neighborhood of the region:

$$u_i | \ldots \sim \mathrm{N}(\overline{u}_{\delta_i}, \sigma_u^2/n_{\delta_i}) \tag{16.2}$$

where δ_i is a neighborhood of the ith area, n_{δ_i} is the number of regions in the ith neighborhood, and $\sigma_u^2 = \tau_u^{-1}$ is a variance parameter that controls the degree of smoothing. This distribution can be relatively simply sampled using a posterior distribution sampling algorithm. An alternative to this specification is to assume a fully parameterized covariance and a multivariate normal distribution for CH:

$$\mathbf{u} \sim \mathrm{N}_n(\mathbf{0}, \Sigma)$$

where the elements of Σ are $\sigma_{ij} = \mathrm{cov}(u_i, u_j)$. This is a joint model for the $\mathbf{u}$, more heavily parameterized than the MRF model above and the model also requires the inversion of a $n \times n$ covariance matrix. This, of course, allows for more detailed covariance modeling.

In a Bayesian analysis, all parameters $(\boldsymbol{\beta}, \mathbf{u}, \mathbf{v}, \sigma_*, \ldots)$ would be assigned prior distributions and posterior sampling of these parameters, usually via MCMC algorithms, would be required.

For the lip cancer example above, we have fitted a range of basic models to exemplify these approaches. Table 16.1 displays the results of fitting a range of models to these data that are typical of models assumed for such small area health data. The models were run for an initial burn-in period of 10 000 iterations and convergence was checked on the deviance as an overall measure as well as on individual parameters, using Brooks–Gelman–Rubin (BGR) statistics. A sample of 5000 was then taken to compute Deviance Information Criterion (DIC). An mean-square predictive error (MSPE) could also be computed in this example but we did

Table 16.1 Lip cancer study: goodness of fit of a variety of models.

Model for $\log(\theta_i)$	DIC	p_D
(1) $\alpha_0 + v_i$	1122.19	125.6
(2) $\alpha_0 + u_i$	1090.08	103.6
(3) $\alpha_0 + v_i + u_i$	1092.96	107.5
(4) $\alpha_0 + v_i + \alpha_1(x_i - \overline{x})$	1109.90	114.8
(5) $\alpha_0 + v_i + u_i + \alpha_1(x_i - \overline{x})$	1091.25	100.3

not pursue this here as we are simply interested in overall goodness of fit and adjustment for parameterization.

Our philosophy in defining these models is that we would want to provide a parsimonious description of the relative risk variation on the map. To this end, we included different random effect terms and also considered the inclusion of a covariate *AFF* (% population employed in agriculture, Fisheries, and Forestry). This covariate would be thought a priori to be associated with sunlight exposure and hence enhancing lip cancer risk. The first model (UH only) has relative risk defined by $\log(\theta_i) = \alpha_0 + v_i$, with prior distributions defined as $\alpha_0 \sim \mathrm{N}(0, c)$, with $c = 10^6$, and $v_i \sim \mathrm{N}(0, \sigma^2)$ where $\sigma \sim \mathrm{U}(0, 10)$. In this model, an overall rate is assumed (e^{α_0}) and an exchangeable random effect is defined. Both the intercept and random effect have zero mean Gaussian distributions. The intercept has a fixed but large variance, whereas the variance of the random effect is parameterized and the standard deviation is assumed to have a uniform distribution on a large range. Other models consist of different combinations of random effects and the covariate. In model 2, a spatially correlated random effect is assumed where an intrinsic Gaussian prior distribution is introduced (as defined in 16.2). This prior distribution is zero centered but allows for correlation and smoothing via neighborhood effects. The variance is σ_u^2 and $\sigma_u \sim \mathrm{U}(0, 10)$. Model 3 is an example of a *convolution* model where an uncorrelated and correlated random effect are additively included. Finally, models 4 and 5 both include the covariate (*AFF*: x_i) as a mean-centered effect. This centering often allows for faster convergence within the sampler, as seen in Section 7.3. The prior distribution for α_1 is also assumed to be zero mean Gaussian where $\alpha_1 \sim \mathrm{N}(0, c)$. Overall, it is apparent from Table 16.1 that the models with the lowest DIC are models 2, 3 and 5. They are all within three DIC units, with the lowest being the 'CAR only model', followed closely by the 'convolution with covariate model'. It is notable that the covariate itself does not provide a good model and the model with *AFF* only included and no random effects yielded a DIC of 1424.49 with p_D of 2.03. Hence, from the point of view of DIC this is not a competitive model for describing the relative risk variation and *AFF* does not add to the degree of explanation of true risk in this case. For the lowest DIC model (model 2), the box plots for a posterior sample of size 5000 of the standardized residuals ($r_i = (y_i - \widehat{\lambda})/\sqrt{\widehat{\lambda}}$) are shown in Figure 16.2. A map of

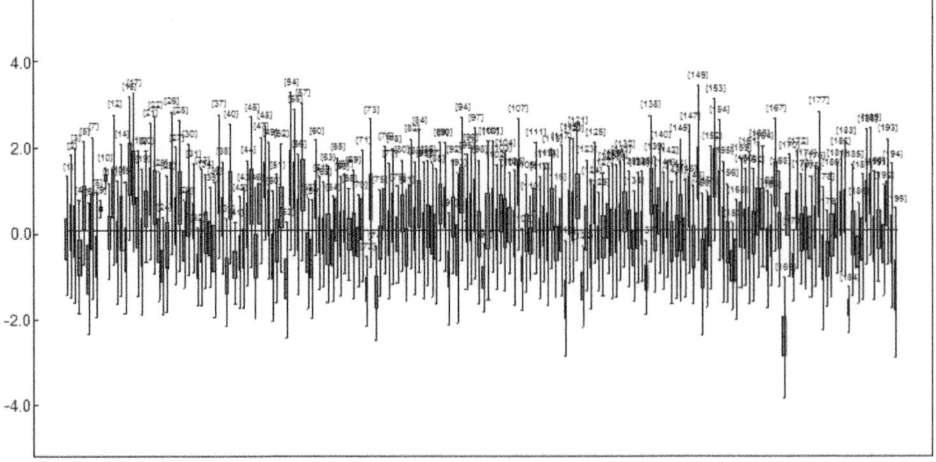

Figure 16.2 Lip cancer study: box plots of the standardized residuals from a posterior sample of size 5000 for the conditional autoregressive (CAR) only model.

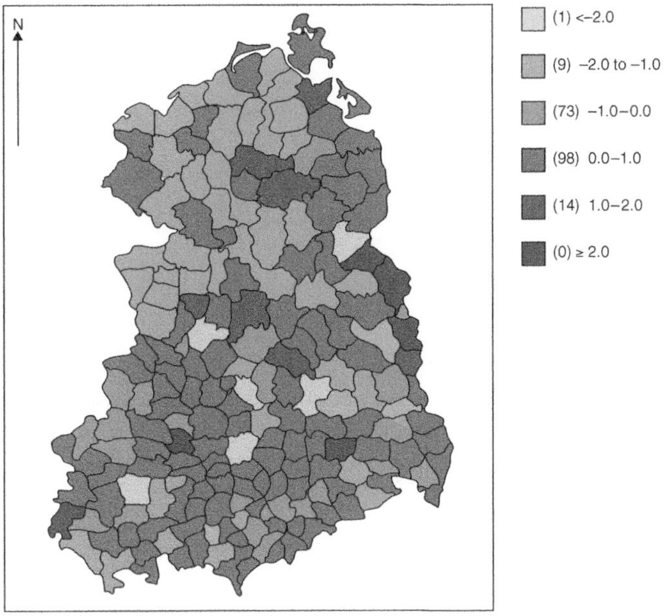

Figure 16.3 Lip cancer study: map of posterior averaged standardized residuals.

the posterior averaged standardized residuals is displayed in Figure 16.3. The spatial pattern of residuals seems to show a reasonable random pattern although there is some suggestion that northern areas have higher positive residuals.

The WinBUGS code for this model is displayed in Figure 16.4. Note that the improper CAR model is defined for an multivariate node within a single statement:

```
b1[1:n] ~ car.normal(adj[],weights[],num[],tau.u).
```

This statement defines the CAR prior distribution with neighborhood adjacencies defined in the vector `adj` with the number of neighbors specified in `num`. A weight matrix (`weights`) is also included and in this case set to 1 for all neighbor pairs. Further examples of the use of this model can be found in the GeoBUGS user manual in WinBUGS.

Another approach that could be taken to this analysis is to focus on whether a covariate is related to the health outcome at the aggregate level. In that case, the emphasis is not on the model that yields the best goodness of fit or describes best the 'true' relative risk, but on whether the parameter α_1 is well estimated, while allowing for confounding via random effects. Often evidence for this is taken from the 95% credible interval. An interval straddling a zero value suggesting that parameter values have been sampled at negative and positive levels and hence little evidence of a predictor effect, whereas an interval completely positive or completely negative suggesting stronger evidence for a predictor effect. In the model (5) above, the best fitting model including the AFF predictor, the posterior mean estimate was 0.831 with 95% credible interval limits: (0.0982, 1.536). This suggests that there is consistent evidence for a positive relation between the AFF predictor and lip cancer at the Landkreise level even allowing for a spatially correlated random effect. Of course, this model is not the best fitting model in terms of DIC.

```
model
    {
    for (i in 1:n ) {
    # Poisson likelihood for observed counts
    observe[i] ~ dpois(lambda[i])
    lambda[i] <- theta[i]*expect[i]
    # SMR
    smr[i] <- observe[i]/expect[i]
    aff1[i] <- aff[i]
    # Relative risk without hierarchical centering
    log(theta[i]) <- ab[i]
    ab[i] <- beta0+b1[i]
    pex[i] <- step(theta[i]-1)
    r[i] <- (observe[i]-lambda[i])/sqrt(lambda[i])
    }
b1[1:n] ~ car.normal(adj[],weights[],num[],tau.u)
    for(k in 1:sumNumNeigh)
    {weights[k] <- 1}
tau.u <- pow(sdu,-2)
sdu ~ dunif(0,10)
# Prior distributions for "population" parameters
beta0 ~  dnorm(0,1.0E-6)
}
```

Figure 16.4 Lip cancer study: WinBUGS code for the CAR only model (model 2).

16.2.5 A special application area: Disease clustering

In this area, the focus is not on reduction of noise, per se, but rather the assessment of the clustering tendency of the map and in particular the assessment of which areas of a map display clustering. Here, clustering could be around a known putative source of hazard (*focused* clustering) or have no known locations of clustering (*nonfocussed* clustering).

It is possible to consider Bayesian models for clusters. In general, the model formulation may not differ greatly from that of relative risk estimation, depending largely on the definition of clusters and clustering.

16.2.5.1 Focused clustering

Focused clustering is the simplest case and usually assumes that some form of distance decrease in risk happens around a (known) fixed point or points(putative source(s) of hazard). For example, the count data model can be defined as

$$\begin{aligned} y_i &\sim \text{Poisson}(e_i\theta_i) \\ \log(\theta_i) &= \log[1+\exp(-\alpha d_i)] + \boldsymbol{x}_i^T\boldsymbol{\beta} + z_i^T\boldsymbol{\gamma}, \end{aligned}$$

where d_i is a distance measured to the small area from the focus point(such as a chimney, mobile phone mast, or waste dump site). Here, the extra covariates appear in $\boldsymbol{x}_i$ while z_i represents the random effects and $\boldsymbol{\gamma}$ is a unit vector. In this case, focus is on inference concerning α, as this defines the distance relation. Within $\boldsymbol{x}_i$, there could also be directional terms such as $\cos(\phi)$ and $\sin(\phi)$, where ϕ is the angle between the area (centroid) and the focus point. This can be used to detect any directional concentration of risk (which could be important particularly if an air pollution risk is possible). Details of this type of approach appear in Wakefield and Morris (2001), and Lawson (2009), Chapter 7.

All parameters (α, $\boldsymbol{\beta}$, etc.) have prior distributions and the resulting posterior distribution would usually be sampled. Some examples of prior distributions used would typically be zero mean Gaussian for the regression parameters and uniform for the standard deviations:

$$
\begin{aligned}
\alpha &\sim \mathrm{N}(0, \sigma_\alpha^2), \\
\sigma_\alpha &\sim \mathrm{U}(0, 10), \\
\beta_* &\sim \mathrm{N}(0, \sigma_{\beta_*}^2), \\
\sigma_{\beta_*} &\sim \mathrm{U}(0, 10).
\end{aligned}
$$

16.2.5.2 Nonfocused clustering

When locations of clusters are unknown then the statistical task becomes more difficult. Not only are the locations of putative clusters unknown but their number and size are also not predefined. This area can be further divided into *general* clustering, where the overall tendency of an area to cluster is assessed, and *specific* clustering where the locations of clusters are to be assessed. Here, we examine only specific clustering.

Non-Bayesian approaches to this problem often focus on testing procedures (such as SatScan: Kulldorff and Nagarwalla 1995). Bayesian modeling of specific clustering can be approached in a variety of ways. First, if clustering of excess risk is simply and liberally regarded as *significant excess risk found anywhere on a map* then pointwise determination of excess can be pursued. This is known as hotspot clustering. For example, for count data we could assume

$$y_i \sim \mathrm{Poisson}(e_i\theta_i)$$

as before, and examine either (i) estimates of θ_i for unusual features (usually significantly elevated values) or (ii) the residuals from a fitted model:

$$\widehat{r_i} = y_i - e_i\widehat{\theta_i}$$

to find out if, after model fitting, whether there are areas of excess unexplained by the model.

The first approach assumes a model for risk and under that model some form of cluster identification may take place. Alternatively a model which simply cleans noise out may be considered i.e. a model for $\log(\theta_i)$ is assumed such as $\log(\theta_i) = \boldsymbol{x}_i^T\boldsymbol{\beta} + v_i$. This model allows for covariate adjustment and some extra variation but does not model CH (smoothing) as this may reduce its ability to detect aberrations in risk at the single-region level. Following the model fit, an assessment of the significance of $\widehat{\theta_i}$ could be made. Often, counting exceedences ($\theta_i > 1$) from posterior converged samples will provide an estimate of $P(\theta_i > 1)$. Figure 16.5 displays an example of this approach where the posterior averaged value of $I(\theta_i > 1)$, computed from the sample as $\sum_{g=1}^{G} I(\theta^g > 1)/G$, can be used as an estimate of

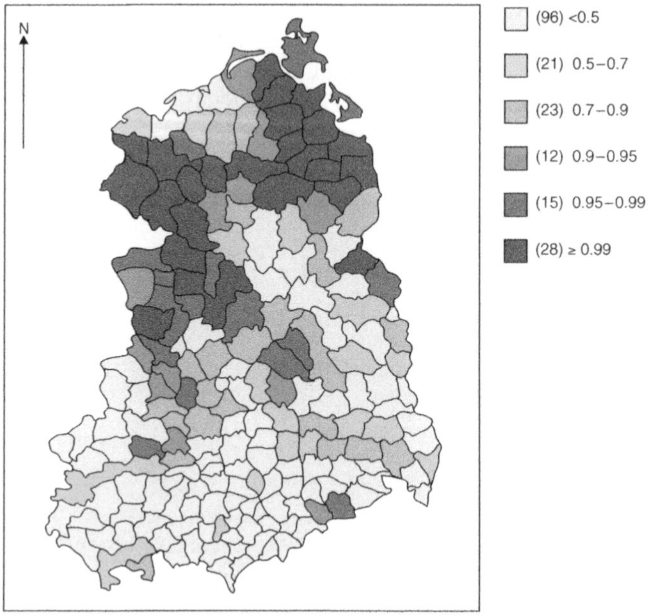

Figure 16.5 Lip cancer study: posterior average exceedence probability map for the CAR only model (model 2).

exceedence probability. It is notable that a number of northern areas (28) have a probability >0.99 suggesting very high risk in northern areas.

This approach to hotspot detection has been advocated by Richardson *et al.* (2004) and Abellan *et al.* (2008). There are concerns about the use of these exceedence probabilities, however. As they are estimated from the upper tail areas of the relative risk distribution they are very sensitive to model assumptions (see Ugarte *et al.* 2009). In fact, in some cases different models can yield markedly different spatial distributions of exceedence. As an example of this problem, we present below another data example. In this case, we examine county level congenital abnormality mortality within the 46 counties of South Carolina, USA. Figure 16.6 displays the standardized mortality ratio for 1990 for this example with expected counts computed from the 1990 statewide abnormality rate. Figure 16.7 displays the marginal histogram and box plot for these data. The pattern suggests that there is one area with particularly elevated risk (>4.0) and two other areas with relative risk in excess of 2.0 in the upper area of the state.

Figure 16.8 displays the spatial distribution of exceedence probabilities from a converged sampler for the model with a simple spatial trend in the (x, y) coordinates of the centroids of the counties: $\log(\theta_i) = \alpha_0 + \alpha_1 x_i + \alpha_2 y_i$ where $\alpha_0 \sim \text{N}(0.0, 1000)$, $\alpha_1 \sim \text{N}(0.0, 1000)$, $\alpha_2 \sim \text{N}(0.0, 1000)$. The areas with highest exceedence are areas in the north west where the highest values of relative risk are found. Figure 16.9 displays the exceedence map for a model with only an uncorrelated random effect ($\log(\theta_i) = \alpha_0 + v_i$; $\alpha_0 \sim \text{N}(0.0, 1000)$, $v_i \sim \text{N}(0, \sigma^2)$, $\sigma \sim \text{U}(0, 10)$). Now the relative risk is assumed to be randomly varying across the study area with no trend assumed. In this case, the exceedence map shows markedly different spatial

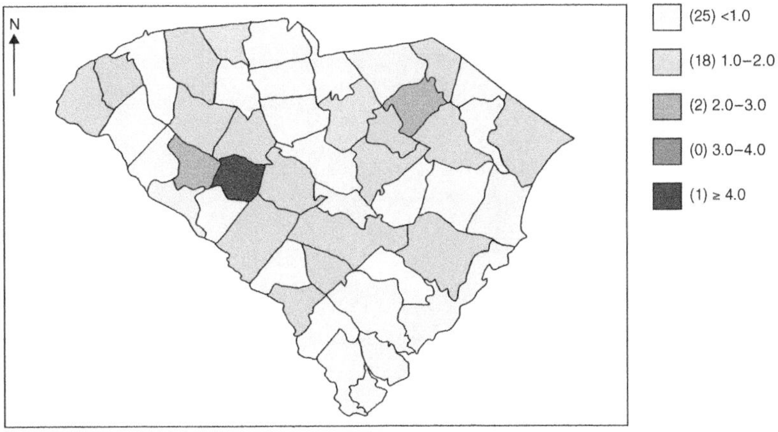

Figure 16.6 South Carolina study: county level congenital abnormality mortality in 1990, standardized Mortality Ratio (SMR) map using the total statewide rate with no age × gender stratification.

patterning than under the trend model. Figure 16.10 displays the resulting exceedence map for a convolution model with additive uncorrelated and correlated effects ($\log(\theta_i) = \alpha_0 + v_i + u_i$; $\alpha_0 \sim \text{N}(0.0, 1000)$, $v_i \sim \text{N}(0, \sigma_v^2), \sigma_v \sim \text{U}(0, 10), u_i \sim \text{CAR}(\tau_u), \tau_u = \sigma_u^{-2}$and $\sigma_u \sim \text{U}(0, 10)$). This map display is similar to the uncorrelated map in that a more random distribution of higher exceedences is found. Note that, as shown in Table 16.2, these different models were all within three DIC values of each other and the trend only model (model 1) has lowest DIC and p_D overall (170.9, 2.42). The concern about this effect is clear: exceedences are highly model dependent and the choice of a convolution model may not lead to stable estimates of clustering behavior. If a simple trend model were included in the possible models considered here then it would fit best and yield a different exceedence map.

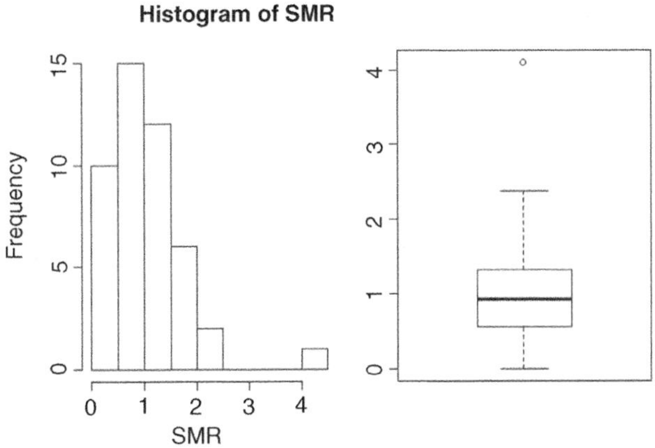

Figure 16.7 South Carolina study: histogram and box plot of the standardized mortality ratio.

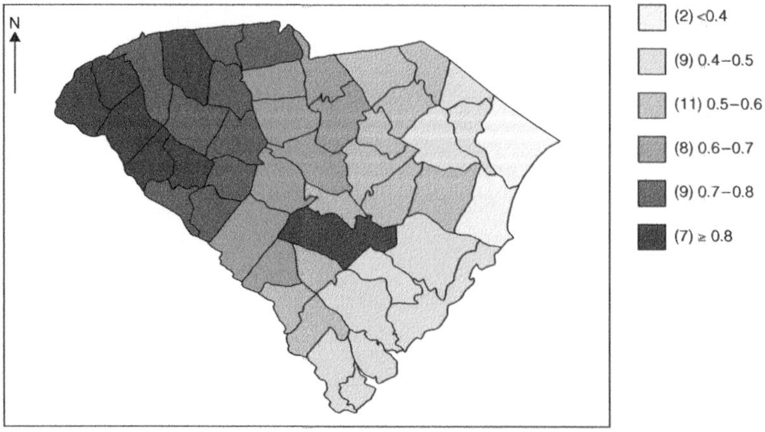

Figure 16.8 South Carolina study: map of $p(\theta_i > 1)$ for model with trend only components.

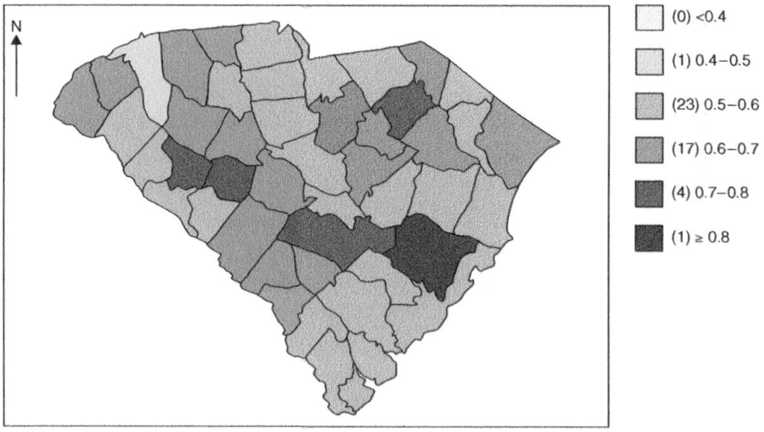

Figure 16.9 South Carolina study: map of $p(\theta_i > 1)$ for an uncorrelated heterogeneity model with no trend.

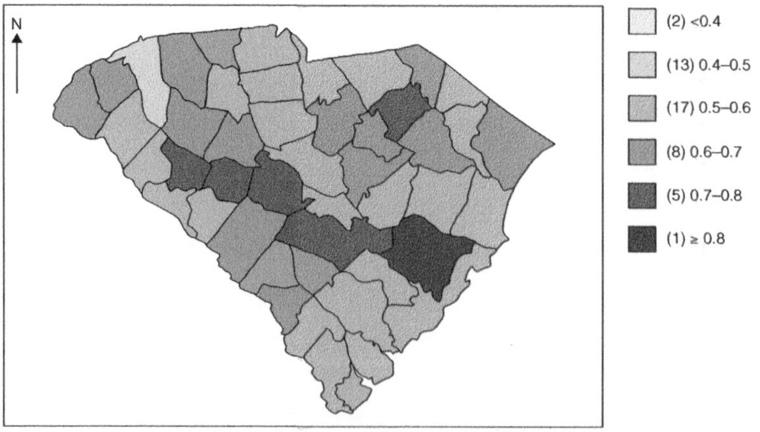

Figure 16.10 South Carolina study: map of $p(\theta_i > 1)$ under a convolution model.

Table 16.2 South Carolina study: model DIC results.

Model	DIC	p_D
(1) $x + y$	170.9	2.42
(2) $x + y + v_i$	173.3	7.60
(3) v_i	170.9	4.98
(4) $v_i + u_i$	172.6	7.90

16.2.5.3 Formal models

If, on the other hand, a specific structure for clusters is assumed then a formal clustering model may be assumed. There is a gray area between relative risk estimation (which focuses on the estimation of θ_i) and examining estimates of θ_i for significant excess. If some form of cluster identification is included into the model then that can be checked for location and size of clusters. This can be useful when data are sparse and other global CH models can not describe the cluster form. One proposal is for risk to be related to a set of hidden (unobserved) cluster locations:

$$\log(\theta_i) = \mathbf{x}_i^T \boldsymbol{\beta} + v_i + \log\left[1 + \sum_{k=1}^{K} h(\mathbf{s}_i; \xi_k)\right],$$

where there are K unknown clusters with locations $\{\xi_k\}$, $\mathbf{s}_i$ is the centroid of the ith small area and $h(\mathbf{s}_i; \xi_k)$ is a cluster distribution function that describes the relation of any point to a cluster location. Usually, $h(\mathbf{s}_i; \xi_k)$ is designed to have a decline in risk with distance from ξ_k, but a range of forms are available. Unfortunately, given that K is unknown, a number of assumptions must be imposed on the analysis to allow for estimation of parameters. Often, reversible jump MCMC is employed here (see Gangnon 2006; Lawson and Clark 1999; Lawson and Denison 2002).

The second approach, that of examining residuals such as $\widehat{r_i} = y_i - e_i\widehat{\theta_i}$, may be useful if a noise reduction model is used in the estimation of $\widehat{\theta_i}$. However, the residual will always include some form of noise unrelated to clustering. Even a perfect model will always have Poisson noise around the true risk: $e_i\theta_i$. Hence, it would be important to specify the risk model carefully to allow for only clustering effects to appear in the residual as far as possible. 'Unusual' residuals can be examined via Monte Carlo procedures using the predictive distribution.

Finally, alternative approaches that assume that clusters are defined within areas or neighborhoods (as opposed to single regions) can be considered and diagnostics for these have been proposed (Hossain and Lawson 2006).

16.2.6 A special application area: Ecological analysis

In this area, the relation between disease incidence and explanatory variables is the focus, and this is usually carried out at an aggregate level, such as with counts in small areas. Many issues of bias and misclassification error can arise with ecological data and the interested reader is referred to Wakefield (2004), Wakefield and Shaddick (2006) and Gustafson (2004) for further insights.

Two important areas of concern are related to scale aggregation issues: MAUP and MIDP. The Modifiable Areal Unit Problem (MAUP) concerns the scalability of models and whether, at different spatial scales, a model is valid. In general, this is unlikely to be the case as far as covariance structure is concerned as this would lead to fractal covariances which are not found commonly. However, the labeling of scales of relevance of models is important and the extent to which a model can be scaled is relevant in many applications. A related but different issue is how to use different scales of data within one analysis, i.e. should individual level data be used in preference to aggregated data or can they be combined. This is a focus of current research.

The MIDP is related to the last issue, but specifically addresses the issue of combining data from different spatial scales to provide analysis at one level. For example, health outcomes (disease incidence, etc.) may be observed within census tracts and we may have available pollution measurements at monitoring sites around the study area. To make inferences about the health outcomes, we want to use the pollution data relevant to the census tracts. One simple solution would be to block Krige the pollution data to provide block estimates for each of the tracts (see Banerjee *et al.* 2004, Chapter 6). This would ignore the error in the interpolation of the pollution data of course and a better approach is to consider a model where the true exposure is modeled within the health model but the pollution model is jointly estimated (see Kim *et al.* 2010).

16.3 Image analysis

Bayesian models for images have a relatively long history. In recent decades, methods have been developed linked to technological innovations in image technology. In the 1980s, much attention was focused on Bayesian modeling of Positron emission tomography (PET) and Single photon emission computerized tomography (SPECT) (see Green 1990). More recently, functional magnetic resonance imaging (fMRI) has been developed and achieves good spatial resolution. fMRI is used to measure hemodynamic response (blood flow) related to neural activity in the brain and spinal cord. It is a cornerstone of modern neuroimaging. It has become popular in part because it is less invasive and does not require radiation exposure of patients unlike tomography procedures (CAT, PET and SPECT).

Images provide a regular array of data which can be analyzed as a lattice. Various features could be of interest on an image. For example, we might simply want to clean up noise to yield the 'true' underlying scene. Much early Bayesian modeling was focused on this aspect of imaging (Besag 1974, Besag 1977, Besag 1986, Ripley 1988, Molina and Ripley 1989, Besag and Green 1993). In addition, it might be important to identify objects in images. This might require some form of boundary or edge detection or special prior distributions relating to the objects of interest, such as template priors (Hansen *et al.* 2002), Markov inhibition priors (Baddeley and M. van Lieshout 1993) or landmark models (Dryden and Mardia 1997).

One of the major challenges of image data is the fact that correlation between array elements or sites (pixels or voxels) naturally arises and so models usually must allow for such correlation. At the likelihood level, this is a complication as the joint density of observations cannot be formulated as a simple product of sample point densities. Usually awkward normalizing constants arise when correlated models are assumed at this level of the hierarchy. A common solution to this problem is to assume that features of interest in the image can be specified completely via prior distributions at higher levels and thereby allowing the assumption of conditional independence at the data level. In this way a conventional likelihood model can be assumed with component correlation confined to higher levels, and conditional independence assumed at the data level.

Often the correlation model is described by special spatially defined prior distributions. One general model is to assume that the hidden structure ($\boldsymbol{x}$ say) has its values governed by a multivariate normal distribution such as $\boldsymbol{x} \sim \mathrm{N}(\mu_x, \Sigma)$ where the correlation between sites depends on distance between them. Hence, an element of Σ, the covariance σ_{ij} say, is defined as $\sigma_{ij} = f(d_{ij})$ where d_{ij} is the intersite distance. A common example of such a spatial covariance would be the exponential where $\sigma_{ij} = \tau \exp(-\rho d_{ij})$. Here, τ describes the variability of the field and ρ the distance dependence or correlation. This type of model is often assumed for continuous fields especially in environmental and agricultural applications (see the spBayes and geoRglm packages in R). In these applications there is usually a relatively small number of measurement sites, which is an important consideration as this full multivariate normal model requires the inversion of the covariance matrix during estimation. In fact, this would be required at each iteration of an MCMC sampler if a Bayesian model were assumed. To reduce the computational burden for these models, various alternative formulations have been proposed: predictive process models (Banerjee *et al.* 2008), process convolutions (Higdon 2002), reduced rank Kriging or splines (Kim *et al.* 2010). For images, resort is usually made to Markov random field (MRF) models which assume only local dependence on neighborhoods. Figure 16.11 displays a 25 site mesh where site 13 has 8 (immediately) adjacent neighbors and 4 main neighbors and 24 second-order neighbors. In MRF models, dependence is purely defined conditionally via neighborhood values.

For example, a Gaussian first-order MRF could be defined for a component $\{u_i\}$ as

$$u_i|\{u_j\}_{j\neq i} \sim \mathrm{N}\big(\gamma \overline{u}_{\delta_i}, \sigma_\tau^2/n_{\delta_i}\big),$$

where $\sigma_\tau^2 = \tau^{-1}$, δ_i, the neighborhood of the ith site, n_{δ_i} the number of neighbors of the ith site, and $\overline{u}_{\delta_i}$ the mean of values for the neighborhood of the ith site. For regular arrays of pixels/voxels, $n_{\delta_i} = 8$ for first order except at edges where $n_{\delta_i} = 5$ and censoring occurs. Hence, the edge area sites would have greater variability. The parameter γ is a measure

1	2	3	3	5
6	7	8	9	10
11	12	13	14	15
16	17	18	19	20
21	22	23	24	25

Figure 16.11 Grid mesh of 25 sites: site 13 has 8 adjacent neighbors (first order): {7, 8, 9, 12, 14, 17, 18, 19}, and 24 second-order neighbors (including all other sites).

of neighborhood correlation. Notice that the component is defined conditionally and only depends on the average of neighboring values. If $\gamma = 1$, an improper CAR model arises which has a major advantage over other models in that it does not require the inversion of a covariance matrix during estimation. This model is commonly assumed in disease mapping applications also (see Section 16.2). We denote this model as $\text{CAR}(\gamma, \tau)$. A general review of these models is available in Rue and Held (2005). A review of MRF models for images is available in Winkler (2006).

There is a range of applications for Bayesian modeling of images which have their own special requirements. For example, PET is used to detect brain glucose dynamics (early detection of Alzheimer's disease) and also for tumor form detection in oncology. PET data yields counts of photons emitted from a light source activated by a radio-labeled tracer. Early Bayesian work in this area focused on EM algorithm solutions (see Green 1990). More recently MRI has become more prominent particularly in neuroscience applications and next we discuss modeling issues related to fMRI.

16.3.1 fMRI modeling

Here, we examine a few issues related to the analysis of fMRI images from a Bayesian modeling perspective. There is a wide and growing literature in the analysis of fMRI data and for a recent review of statistical issues the reader is referred to Lazar (2008). Functional MRI has become an important tool in diagnostic medicine and, in particular, in neuroscience. In the discussion here, we assume that postprocessing of the fMRI image has taken place and the resulting BOLD voxel image or sequences of BOLD images or time series are to be analyzed. We do not discuss the details and issues of image postprocessing here although in any substantive analysis these would have to be considered in relation to the models assumed. BOLD stands for *blood oxygenation level dependent* and there is a direct link between magnetic susceptibility of blood and oxygenation. BOLD response as measured in fMRI reflects pooled local neuronal activity (which reflects behavioral or cognitive activity). Hence, sites of elevated BOLD values reflect higher neuronal activity. A general comprehensive source for analysis in functional brain imaging is found in Friston *et al.* (2007) and Part 5 of that work focuses on Bayesian approaches.

We assume that the BOLD image consists of a $t \times p \times m \times n$ set of voxels where p represents slices through the brain area, t represents time, and the spatial voxel array has dimension $m \times n$ for an individual subject. Further, it is assumed that time is fixed at the $t = 1$ period in the next section. Later, we will also consider temporal models.

Figure 16.12 displays a single slice BOLD image from a finger tapping experiment. Areas of activation (signal) are shown as darker areas, while lighter areas show less or no activation. This image consists of an array of 69×79 voxels.

16.3.1.1 Spatial models

BOLD values are continuous measures and bounded away from zero and so the assumption of a Gaussian model for BOLD data is a reasonable first assumption. A simple spatial model for a slice (e.g. $p = 1$) and time ($t = 1$) could take the form, for j-kth site/voxel,

$$y_{jk} = \beta_0 + w_{jk} + e_{jk}.$$

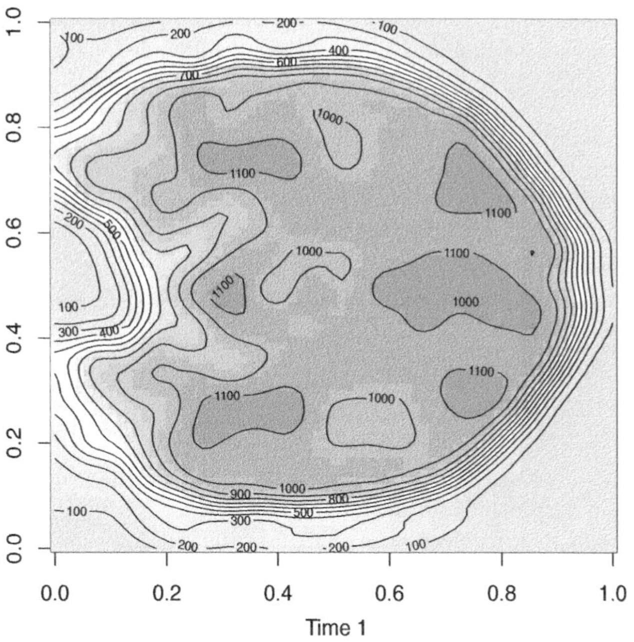

Figure 16.12 Finger-tapping experiment.

Here we assume a Gaussian error with $e_{jk} \sim \mathrm{N}(0, \sigma_y^2)$, with an intercept and a random effect term (w_{jk}) which can consist both of uncorrelated (unstructured salt and pepper) noise and correlated (spatially structured) noise. A convolution assumption is often made for the random effects so that $w_{jk} = v_{jk} + u_{jk}$ where $v_{jk} \sim \mathrm{N}(0, \sigma_v^2)$ and $u_{jk}|\{u_{lm}\}_{l.m \neq j,k} \sim \mathrm{CAR}(\gamma, \tau_u)$ so that we have

$$y_{jk} = \beta_0 + v_{jk} + u_{jk} + e_{jk} \tag{16.3}$$

as the basic model for a single-slice image. Such models have been assumed by Gossl *et al.* (2001), albeit in a spatio-temporal (ST) context. Note that so far we have only considered smoothing models and have not included either individual effects or stimulus effects.

More general models will include individual level data and also grouped data (Lange 2003). We assume, first, that the ith subject scanned has a single slice with a voxel array of $m \times n$ elements. Define the BOLD response at the j-kth voxel as y_{ijk}, $(i = 1, \ldots, N;$ $j = 1, \ldots, m; k = 1, \ldots, n)$. Hence,

$$y_{ijk} = \mu_{ijk} + e_{ijk}.$$

We assume that the error term at this level is uncorrelated random noise and so we assume

$$\boldsymbol{e}_i \sim \mathrm{N}(\mathbf{0}, \sigma^2 \mathrm{I}).$$

In addition, we assume that the underlying mean level μ_{ijk} is a smoothed representation of the data y_{ijk}. In that case, we could have a model for the ith individual and lth group:

$$y_{ijkl} = \boldsymbol{x}_{ijkl}^T \boldsymbol{\beta} + z_{ijk}^T \boldsymbol{b}_{il} + e_{ijkl}, \tag{16.4}$$

where $\boldsymbol{x}_{ijkl}$ is a predictor vector indexed by individual, voxel and group, with associated parameter vector $\boldsymbol{\beta}$, and $z_{ijk}^T \boldsymbol{b}_{il}$, an individual and group level random effect term, and an overall error term $e_{ijkl} \sim \mathrm{N}(0, \sigma_y^2)$.

We now assume a model for the mean BOLD level for the ith subject. We assume a general form of a mixed model where

$$\mu_{ijk} = \boldsymbol{x}_{ijk}^T \boldsymbol{\beta} + z_{ijk}^T \boldsymbol{b}_i.$$

When covariates are present, they may be spatially varying or they may be simply baseline measures (such as demographic information for individuals). Specifically, when a stimulus is present which is spatially referenced, then a link function is usually employed that can match the stimulus to the BOLD signal. Often a hemodynamic response function is used for this purpose ($h(s, \theta)$). Assume that the stimulus value obtained at a lagged time is z_{ijks}, then the link is often $x_{ijk}^* = \sum_s h(s, \theta) z_{ijks}$ where the lag is s. Then x_{ijk}^* could be added linearly or nonlinearly into the model for μ_{ijk}.

In what follows, we assume that there are no covariates and so our linear predictor $\boldsymbol{x}_{ijk}^T \boldsymbol{\beta} = \boldsymbol{\beta}_0$, is a constant intercept term representing the overall average level. The second term includes random effects and can include spatial correlation. A range of models of varying complexity are now possible:

1. Uncorrelated voxel noise model: $\mu_{ijk} = \beta_0 + v_{jk}$; $v_{jk} \sim \mathrm{N}(0, \sigma_v^2)$
2. Uncorrelated individual voxel-level model: $\mu_{ijk} = \beta_0 + b_i + v_{jk}$; $b_i \sim \mathrm{N}(0, \sigma_b^2)$, $v_{jk} \sim \mathrm{N}(0, \sigma_v^2)$
3. Uncorrelated and correlated voxel noise model: $\mu_{ijk} = \beta_0 + v_{jk} + u_{jk}$; $v_{jk} \sim \mathrm{N}(0, \sigma_\psi^2)$; $u_{jk} \sim \mathrm{CAR}(\gamma, \tau_u)$
4. Weighted mixture model: $\mu_{ijk} = \beta_0 + p_{jk} v_{jk} + (1 - p_{jk}) u_{jk}$; $p_{jk} \sim \mathrm{Beta}(1, 1)$
5. Extended weighted mixture with jump honoring: $\mu_{ijk} = \beta_0 + p_{jk} v_{jk} + (1 - p_{jk})\{q_{jk}[u_{jk}] + (1 - q_{jk})[u_{jk}^*]\}$; $q_{jk} \sim \mathrm{Beta}(1, 1)$ and $u_{jk}^* | \{u_{lm}^*\}_{l,m \neq jk} \sim \mathrm{CAR}.L1(u_{jk}^*)$

Model 1 is the least important as it does not include any structural assumptions. Model 2 contains both individual level effects and voxel-based effects. Model 3 is commonly termed a convolution model and provides a parsimonious description of the spatial variation. Figure 16.13 displays the posterior average of μ_{ijk} for a single subject for the finger data for model 3. For model 3, we also obtain the posterior average of the spatial heterogeneity component (u_{jk}).

Figures 16.14 and 16.15 display these random effects. Model 4 shows the mixing parameter field p_{jk} (between uncorrelated and correlated effects) which reflects the edge areas mainly where random noise is highest perhaps as edge effects (Figure 16.16).

For the extended mixture model (model 5) we display both p and q fields and the overall μ_{ijk} estimate (Figures 16.17, 16.18 and 16.19). Note that we use a posterior functional

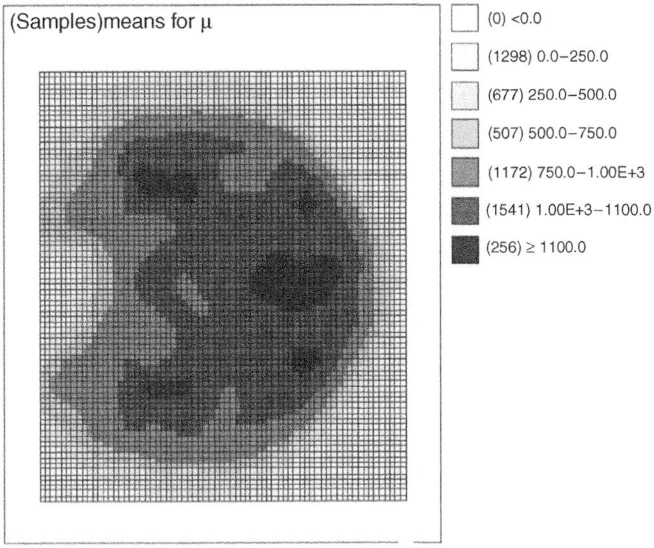

Figure 16.13 Finger tapping experiment: posterior mean estimate of μ_{ijk} under a convolution model for a single slice and single time.

(exceedence probability) to display the probability fields (see also Section 16.2.5). From the posterior sample $\{p^g_{1,1}, \ldots, p^g_{m,n}\}$, $g = 1, \ldots, G$ we have for each voxel $P_{jk} = \widehat{\Pr}(p_{jk} > 0.5) = \sum_{g=1}^{G} I(p^g_{jk} > 0.5)/G$. Suitable threshold values of P_{jk},such as 0.95 or 0.99 could be employed. This idea can be used more generally to isolate areas of highest BOLD activity or to detect clusters of high activation.

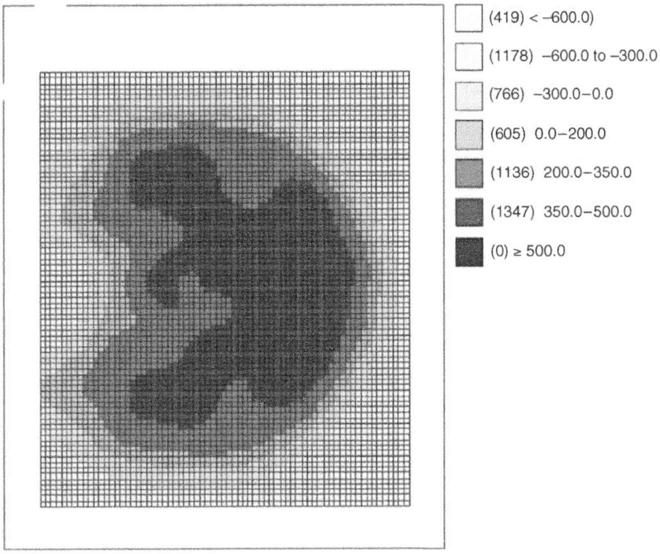

Figure 16.14 Finger-tapping experiment: posterior mean estimate of u_{jk} under a convolution model for a single slice and single time.

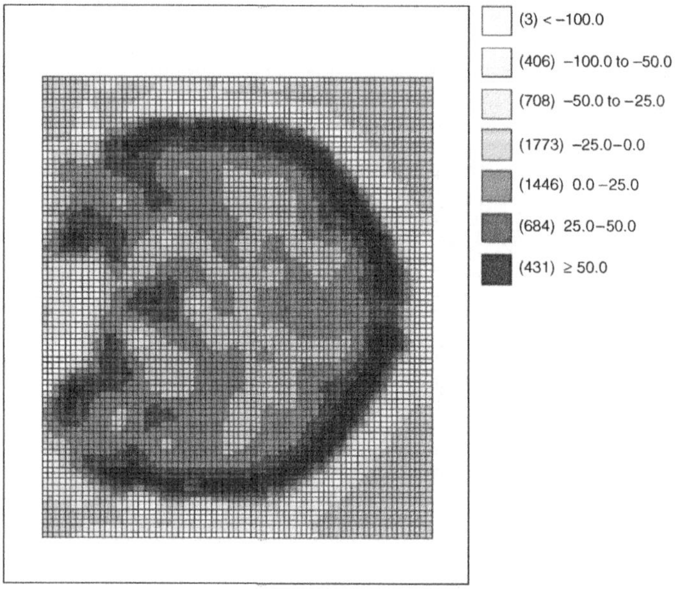

Figure 16.15 Finger-tapping experiment: posterior mean estimate of v_{jk} under a convolution model for a single slice and single time.

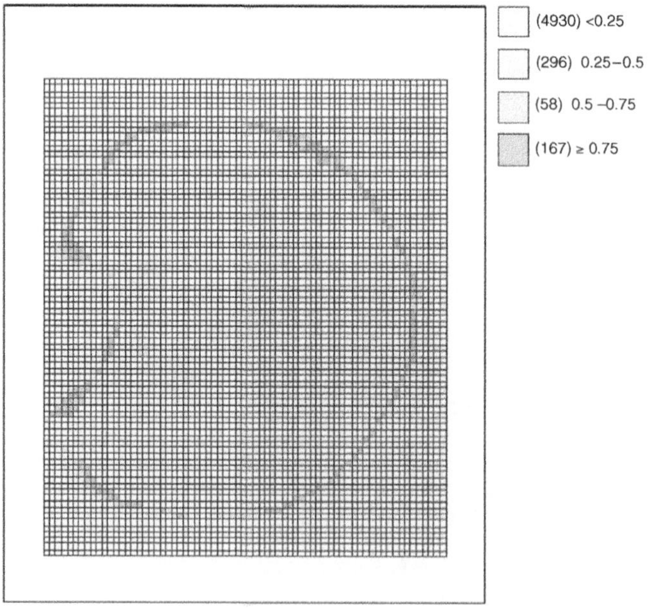

Figure 16.16 Finger-tapping experiment: posterior average field estimate of p_{jk} for the mixture model (model 4).

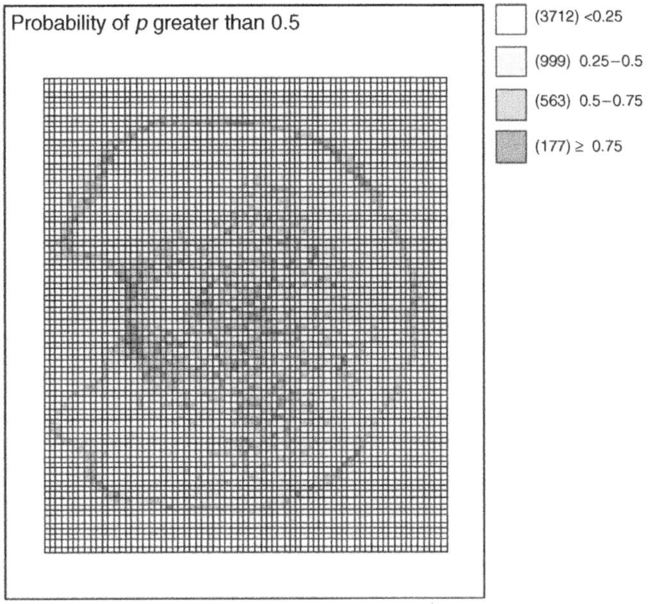

Figure 16.17 Finger-tapping experiment: posterior exceedence probability of $p_{jk} > 0.5$ for the extended mixture model (model 5).

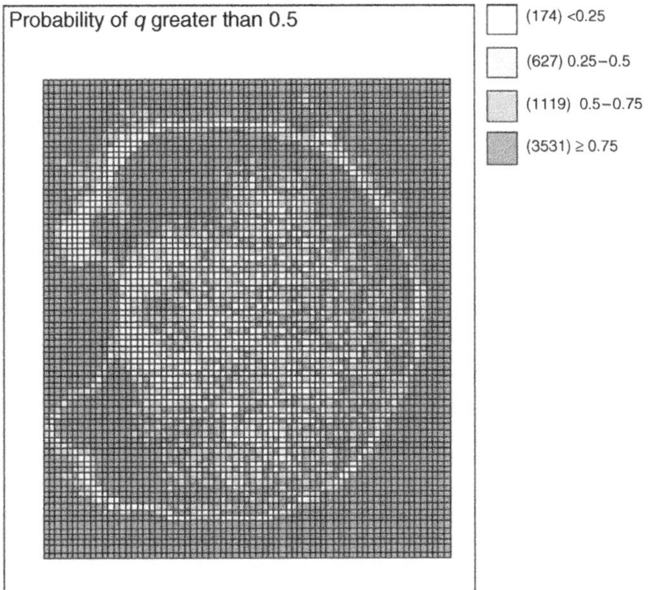

Figure 16.18 Finger-tapping experiment: posterior exceedence probability of $q_{jk} > 0.5$ for the extended mixture model (model 5).

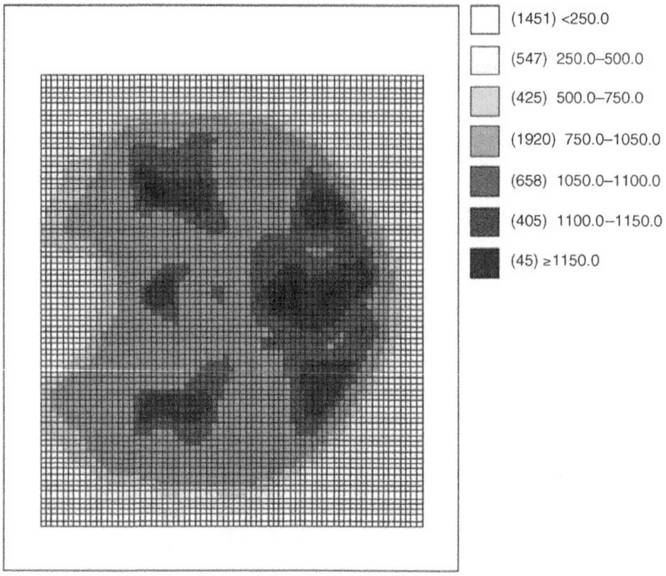

Figure 16.19 Finger-tapping experiment: posterior average of the smoothed mean field, μ_{ijk} for the extended mixture model (model 5).

More sophisticated Bayesian models have recently been proposed based on mixtures (Xu *et al.* 2009; Zhang *et al.* 2010). Alternative approaches to Bayesian spatial modeling have also been suggested based on exchangeable assumptions (Bowman *et al.* 2008) and predefined regions in connectivity applications (Derado *et al.* 2010).

Functional connectivity is a major area of concern in neuroimaging (Lange 2003). This concerns the connection or correlation between areas of the brain. Hence, correlation of activity level is a focus, but this may not be spatially defined as some areas may signal synchronously because of functional dependence but may be separated by some distance. Clearly lagged temporal effects could play a major role in the complexity of connectivity. It is beyond the scope of this chapter to further examine this topic, although we will examine some related areas in the next sections. Regions of Interest (ROIs) are areas of the brain that are of specific interest in connection with functional behavior. In the next sections, we will briefly examine modeling approaches associated with these regions. For further information about functional connectivity, the interested reader is referred to Lange (2003), Stanberry *et al.* (2008), and more generally to Lazar (2008).

16.3.1.2 Temporal models

Figure 16.20 displays time series of BOLD values for a set of four adjacent voxels.

A range of models can be considered for time series, similar to those found for longitudinal studies (see Chapter 15). Unlike longitudinal studies, however, these series are likely to be spatially correlated especially if the voxels are close neighbors. Of course, greater separation will reduce such correlation, but functional connectivity could also mean that distant voxels are correlated due to functional connections.

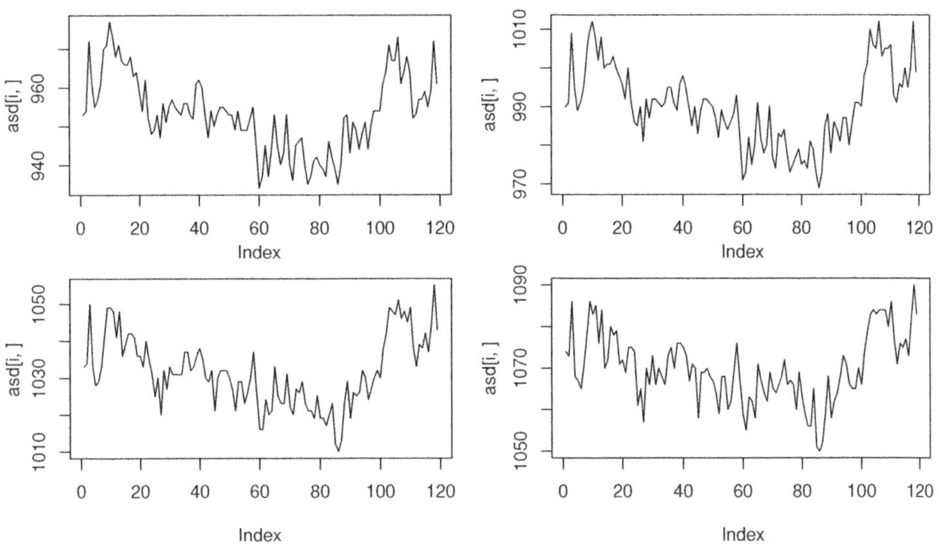

Figure 16.20 Finger-tapping experiment: multiple plot of four adjacent voxel time series for the finger data (slice = 20).

For the set of four voxel time series, we have considered a model that can capture much of the variation as follows. Let y_{ijk} denote the BOLD response at the ith time point and j–kth voxel and assume an autoregressive dependence model as follows:

$$
\begin{aligned}
y_{ijk} &\sim \mathrm{N}(\mu_{ijk}, \sigma^2); \quad \mu_{ijk} = \alpha_0 + c_{jk} + g_{ijk},\\
\alpha_0 &\sim \mathrm{N}(0, \sigma_0^2),\\
g_{ijk} &\sim \mathrm{N}(\rho g_{i-1,jk}, \sigma_g^2),\\
c_{jk} &\sim \mathrm{N}(c_T, \sigma_c^2); \; c_T \sim \mathrm{N}(0, \sigma_{ct}^2),\\
\sigma_* &\sim \mathrm{U}(0, c), \; \rho \sim \mathrm{Beta}(1, 1).
\end{aligned}
$$

The parameters α_0 and c_{jk} represent overall and series specific intercepts, whereas the temporal correlation is modeled via an AR(1) (autoregressive model with lag 1) model on g_{ijk}. The temporal correlation parameter is ρ. For the example in Figure 16.20, we show the posterior average estimates (and standard deviations) in Table 16.3.

Hence, for this model we can see that the AR(1) model is virtually a random walk with common correlation close to $\rho \approx 1.0$. The series specific components range from 126.7 to 130.7 with common mean 133.90. More sophisticated models could be envisaged which allow for more complex temporal and spatial dependence. However, the latter leads into space–time (ST) analysis.

16.3.1.3 Spatio-temporal models

Sequences of images can be analyzed via space–time (ST) models. ROIs are often the focus when ST models are to be examined, and so a spatial subset of the image is used. There is a

Table 16.3 Four voxel time series: posterior mean estimates of parameters in a model.

Parameter	Estimate	SD
α_0	772.1	14.44
c_1	126.7	23.68
c_2	128.4	23.39
c_3	133.1	23.36
c_4	130.7	22.98
c_T	133.9	28.20
ρ	0.997	0.002

growing literature on the Bayesian analysis of ST image sequences (see Woolrich *et al.* 2004; Gossl *et al.* 2001; Quiros *et al.* 2010; Derado *et al.* 2010). Here, we do not intend to provide an exhaustive review of this area. Instead, we note that some modeling principles which can be applied within disease mapping can also be considered relevant to image analysis. Denote the BOLD value for the j-kth voxel at the ith time as y_{ijk}. One approach to modeling assumes that we can consider a mixed model where we have spatial (S), temporal (T) and ST components. We can think of S and T as main effects and ST as interaction. Define the model for a sequence of images, excluding fixed effects, as

$$y_{ijk} \sim \text{N}(\mu_{ijk}, \sigma_y^2),$$
$$\mu_{ijk} = \alpha_0 + S + T + ST,$$

where

$$S = v_{jk} + u_{jk},$$
$$T = g_i + h_i,$$
$$ST = \psi_{ijk}.$$

Hence a parsimonious description of the space-time behavior can have temporal structure (uncorrelated or correlated) via $g_i \sim \text{N}(0, \sigma_g^2)$ and $h_i \sim \text{N}(\rho h_{i-1}, \sigma_h^2)$ and spatial structure (uncorrelated or correlated) via $v_{jk} \sim \text{N}(0, \sigma_v^2)$ and $u_{jk} \sim \text{CAR}(\gamma, \tau_u)$ and interaction defined by $\psi_{ijk} \sim \text{N}(0, \sigma_\psi^2)$. In this model, we regard interaction as a kind of residual after having fitted the main S and T components. Many issues arise in definitions of neighborhoods: once the temporal domain is admitted to the spatial analysis then neighborhoods can (1) extend back in time and (2) dynamically change with time, and dependencies could be defined based on flow dynamics or gradients of flow. Hence, much complexity could be included within these extended models. A recent example of this kind of modeling can be found in Quiros *et al.* (2010). We do not pursue this here.

As one can imagine, there is much potential for the development of Bayesian methods applied in imaging, not only from the point of view of models for the image itself, but also when individuals are grouped into treatment and then treatments are monitored over time. Hence, ultimately we could have a longitudinal-ST treatment group analysis of images. Many of the issues related to these extensions are as yet unexplored.

16.3.2 A note on software

Bayesian fMRI analysis is hindered by the large data arrays that must be processed. Because of this computationally intensive MCMC has not been used to any great extent until recently. Hence, it is common for analyses to be performed either on purpose written platforms: Matlab is commonly used as is the Matlab-based statistical parameter mapping (SPM) package. Purpose written code is often found also.

FMRIB software library (FSL) is also available for some analyses. The R package does have some functionality for Bayesian imaging. Namely, the package `AnalyseFMRI` is useful for handling ANALYSE and NIFTI format image files and does provide some limited Bayesian capabilities (e.g. the mixture model of Hartvig and Jensen 2000).

WinBUGS would be an ideal platform but for the fact that the array sizes are very large and posterior sampling is slow. The basic spatial convolution model discussed above fitted to a single fMRI slice (5451 voxels) took 564 seconds for 10 000 updates on a standard Dell Latitude 830 running WinBUGS 1.4.3 under Windows XP.

17

Final chapter

17.1 What this book covered

In the first eleven chapters (Part I and II), we have reviewed Bayesian methodology: its philosophy, the language, the computational machinery, and their implementation for statistical modeling. To this end, a great variety of examples were used: cross-sectional studies, longitudinal studies, elementary spatial epidemiological studies and some basic controlled clinical trials. In addition, some elementary examples were taken of growth curve modeling, diagnostic testing research and bioinformatics. The application areas were taken from dietary research, rheumatology, stroke research, oral health research, animal research, diabetic research and oncology. In the subsequent five chapters (Part III), we have gone in more depth into the application of Bayesian methods in bioassay, measurement error and misclassification, disease mapping and image analysis, survival models and longitudinal studies.

This noted, the Bayesian approach has seen an explosion of new developments in basically every area of medical research. Hence, what this book covers both from a theoretical as well as applied perspective is a core of topics more fundamental to an understanding of the Bayesian approach to Biostatistics. Additional Bayesian developments and topics not addressed in detail here are briefly reviewed with key references for further reading.

17.2 Additional Bayesian developments

Methodological developments may be inspired by a particular class of applications. Other developments are more driven by theoretical considerations and cover basically every application area. We review both kinds of developments, but we have no ambition to be comprehensive.

17.2.1 Medical decision making

Medical decision making aims at rationalizing and improving the decision making process in health care, as well as improving patient outcomes as a consequence. The Bayesian approach is particularly appealing here since optimal decision making often needs a variety of sources

Bayesian Biostatistics, First Edition. Emmanuel Lesaffre and Andrew B. Lawson.

to choose an action and not all of that information may be quantified in data. Parmigiani (2002) treats modeling in medical decision making from a Bayesian perspective. The covered topics are: individual prediction as seen in Section 1.3.2, simulation models that generate synthetic individual-based data of hypothetical cohorts to evaluate the cost effectiveness of, say, cancer-screening programs using Bayesian decision making approaches, quality of life research and meta-analyses. Spiegelhalter *et al.* (2004) deal with similar applications but focus more on clinical trial methodologies.

We have omitted the treatment of meta-analyses, an important source for medical decision making. Note, however, that a Bayesian meta-analysis is only a Bayesian hierarchical model whereby level-2 observations are obtained from individual studies, most often RCTs. For a tutorial on meta-analyses including Bayesian approaches; see Arends *et al.* (2008) and references therein.

Another source for decision making are diagnostic tests. When a gold standard is available, but too costly or too time consuming then an imperfect test needs to be used in practice. Diagnostic testing deals with the evaluation of imperfect measurement devices. The performance of the imperfect device can be expressed by sensitivity and specificity in the presence of a gold standard, otherwise it is evaluated with agreement tests such as the kappa statistic. The Bayesian approach in combination with the MCMC machinery, can compute better these performance measures in some nonstandard situations, such as in a multilevel context (see Section 13.2.3) or when prior information needs to be imputed; see Broemeling (2007) for a general Bayesian treatment of this subject.

17.2.2 Clinical trials

About 20 years ago, O'Quigley *et al.* (1990) introduced the Bayesian approach into phase I studies. But beyond dose-finding applications, the incorporation of Bayesian methods in clinical trials evolved only slow especially in phase III trials. This was illustrated in Chapter 5. Bayesian methods are, though, well integrated in the evaluation of medical devices. There are FDA websites containing guidelines for the evaluation of medical devices using a Bayesian approach:

http://www.accessdata.fda.gov/cdrh_docs/pdf/P970033b.pdf

http://www.accessdata.fda.gov/cdrh_docs/pdf/P970015b.pdf

http://www.fda.gov/MedicalDevices/DeviceRegulationandGuidance/GuidanceDocuments/ucm106757.htm

http://www.accessdata.fda.gov/cdrh_docs/pdf/P980048b.pdf

The resistance to using Bayesian methodology in phase II and phase III trials may slowly disappear with the advent of adaptive trials. Loosely spoken, adaptive trials allow for much more freedom in trial designs. For instance, one of the ambitions of adaptive designs is to make the transition between phase II and phase III smoother and quicker. This area has seen a lot of developments in the frequentist literature. Lately, this area of research has also attracted the Bayesian world; see Berry *et al.* (2011) for a general review of the Bayesian adaptive methods for clinical trials.

17.2.3 Bayesian networks

A Bayesian network is another term for a directed acyclic graphical model. Recall that Directed Acyclic Graphs (DAGs) are the basis for WinBUGS. From Chapter 5 we know that a DAG is a probabilistic graphical model that represents a set of random variables and their conditional dependencies. For example, a Bayesian network could represent the probabilistic relationships between diseases and symptoms. Given symptoms, the network can be used to compute the probabilities of the presence of various diseases. Thus, a Bayesian network can be used to learn about causal relationships, and hence may help in understanding about a problem domain and to predict the consequences of intervention. More background on this topic can be found in Neal (1996), Borgelt and Kruse (2002), Korb and Nicholson (2004) and Williamson (2005).

17.2.4 Bioinformatics

The analysis of high-throughput genetic data has seen a tremendous evolution in the last decade. In Chapter 11, we have applied some Bayesian variable selection techniques to gene expression data. The fact that in genetic studies, a large number of genes need to be explored, stimulated the development of fast variable selection techniques. But this is just one of the statistical techniques that has seen an impetus due to genetic studies. We refer to Do *et al.* (2006), Sorensen and Gianola (2002), Mallick *et al.* (2009) and Dey *et al.* (2011) for an in-depth treatment of the Bayesian methods in bioinformatics.

17.2.5 Missing data

Many, if not all, studies are plagued with missing data. In general, a proper analysis of data in the presence of missing data is not straightforward. In Chapter 15, we have briefly outlined the basic issues in dealing with missingness applied to longitudinal studies and we have seen some analyses that take missing values and dropout into account. However, there is a large variety of possible approaches which deal with missing data some of which may be preferable above the ones we have used. In addition, it might be necessary to perform sensitivity analyses, varying the assumptions about the missing-data process. In Daniels and Hogan (2008) several Bayesian modeling approaches that deal with missing data are treated. The Bayesian approach is well suited for performing sensitivity analyses, since it allows the inclusion of all kinds of prior information into the estimation process. For yet another source of Bayesian methods for missing data, see Tan *et al.* 2010.

17.2.6 Mixture models

Mixture modeling is an important but advanced area in statistics, both from theoretical as from computational point of view. It covers, for instance, cluster analysis and change-point modeling. The approach of reversible jump MCMC, treated in Chapter 6, is one of the Bayesian approaches to deal with mixture distributions. So to some extent, we have covered mixture models in this book, but our treatment was not in-depth. For instance, we ignored the well-known problem of 'label-switching' in MCMC computations. An example of this problem is seen in Example VII.7 where there was ambiguity in the definition of prevalence, sensitivity and specificity. For a general overview of how to deal with this problem, we refer to Jasra *et al.* (2005). The standard reference to mixture modeling is McLachlan and Peel (2000) or Böhning (2003), although the focus in these books is on the frequentist approach. In a Bayesian context, there is the book on classification by Denison *et al.* (2002).

17.2.7 Nonparametric Bayesian methods

All approaches that we have dealt with in this book are parametric. But because the Bayesian approach, together with the MCMC approach and the Bayesian software, offers a flexible tool to fit a great variety of parametric models of increasing complexity we may not immediately have experienced this as a limitation. Nevertheless, a class of Bayesian approaches offers an even greater flexibility, called *nonparametric Bayesian methods*. They constitute a rapidly evolving class of Bayesian methods that provides a richer and potentially more realistic class of models. The term 'nonparametric' should not mislead. This class of Bayesian methods is still parametric, but the number of parameters grows with the sample size. A nonparametric Bayesian model is in fact a probability model on an infinite-dimensional space. This approach allows the statistical model to be specified in a flexible manner and its different components, such as the random effects distribution, the link function, etc. are estimated from the data. However, the mathematical background of this approach is quite evolved and is, therefore, beyond the scope of this textbook. Interested readers may consult the special issue of *Statistical Modelling, Volume 8, Number 1, 2008* or the more technical sources by Ghosh and Ramamoorthi (2003) and Hjort *et al.* (2010). Another possibility is to watch the two videos featuring an introduction by Peter Orbanz at http://videolectures.net/mlss09uk_orbanz_fnbm/.

17.3 Alternative reading

There are numerous books on Bayesian methods. Some of them were already referred to in earlier chapters. But for the interested reader, here is a list of some additional books:

- The book of Marin and Robert (2007) gives an overview of the computational procedures in Bayesian methods applied to a variety of statistical models, such as generalized linear models (GLIM), capture–recapture experiments, mixture models, dynamic models and image analysis. Mathematical and statistical background is provided but is limited to the essential facts. R programs are provided.
- In an impressive series of books (Congdon 2003, 2006, 2007, 2010), the author describes an enormous amount of statistical modeling applications and provides WinBUGS code for their analyses.
- For those who need a more elementary book than this one, or for those who wish to recommend biomedical researchers to grasp the concepts of Bayesian methods, here is a list of references: Moyé (2008) for a general elementary introduction into Bayesian methods in biostatistics, McCarthy (2007) for an introduction of Bayesian methods in ecology, King *et al.* (2009) for a more advanced text in that area, Taroni *et al.* (2010) for an introduction of Bayesian methods in forensic science and Colosimo and del Castillo (2006) for Bayesian process control and surveillance-related topics.

Appendix

Distributions

A.1 Introduction

We review in this appendix the most common distributions used in parametric Bayesian methods. For the univariate distributions, we provide a graphical representation. For some distributions, such as the inverse gamma, we show on the same graph also the better known gamma distribution with the same parameter values. Further, we provide the commands in R, WinBUGS, JAGS and the SAS procedure MCMC to invoke the distributions. A symbol '-' indicates that the distribution does not exist in the software.

In most of the cases, the command in WinBUGS is the same as for JAGS, but sometimes they differ. JAGS also offers a few extra distributions, namely the F-distribution, the noncentral χ^2-distribution, the beta-binomial distribution and the noncentral hypergeometric distribution. For these distributions, we basically refer to the JAGS manual. SAS also offers extra distributions. For instance, the exponential version of a variety of distributions is available, such as the exponential gamma distribution which is the distribution of $\log(\theta)$ when θ has a gamma distribution; see the SAS manual on the procedure MCMC.

For various distributions, there exists two versions: one parameterized in scale and one in rate=1/scale. We chose one, the other one can be deduced by replacing in the expression everywhere scale in 1/rate or vice versa. In the calls to the functions, the inverse of the parameter `param` is indicated by `iparam`. Finally, JAGS and SAS have aliases for several distributions to avoid confusion with other statistical software; see the respective software manuals for more details.

Bayesian Biostatistics, First Edition. Emmanuel Lesaffre and Andrew B. Lawson.

A.2 Continuous univariate distributions

Table A.1 Beta distribution: Beta(α, β).

Model	Examples
$p(\theta) = \dfrac{1}{B(\alpha, \beta)}\, \theta^{\alpha-1}(1-\theta)^{\beta-1}$ with $B(\alpha, \beta) = \dfrac{\Gamma(\alpha)\Gamma(\beta)}{\Gamma(\alpha+\beta)}$ `Condition:` $\alpha > 0, \beta > 0$ `Range:` [0,1] `Parameters:` α, β: shape	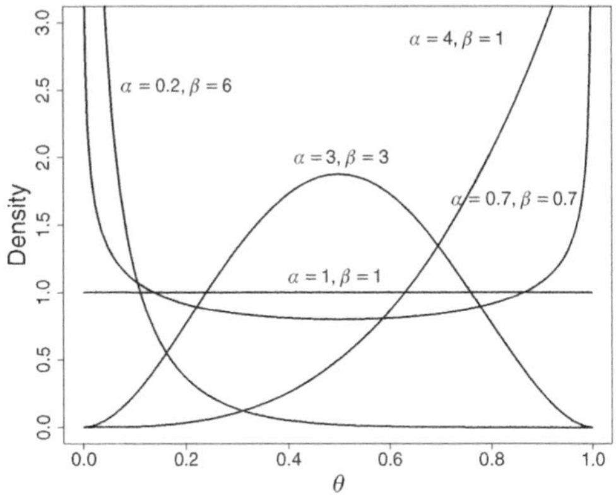

Moments		Program commands	
`Mean:`	$\dfrac{\alpha}{(\alpha+\beta)}$	`R:`	`dbeta(theta,alpha,beta)`
`Mode:`	$\dfrac{\alpha-1}{(\alpha+\beta-2)}$	`WB/JAGS:`	`theta ~ dbeta(alpha,beta)`
`Variance:`	$\dfrac{\alpha\beta}{(\alpha+\beta)^2(\alpha+\beta+1)}$	`SAS:`	`theta ~ beta(alpha,beta)`

Table A.2 Cauchy distribution: Cauchy(μ, σ).

Model	Examples
$$p(\theta) = \frac{1}{\pi}\left(\frac{\sigma}{\sigma^2 + (\theta - \mu)^2}\right)$$ `Condition:` $\sigma > 0$ `Range:` $(-\infty, \infty)$ `Parameters:` μ location, σ: scale	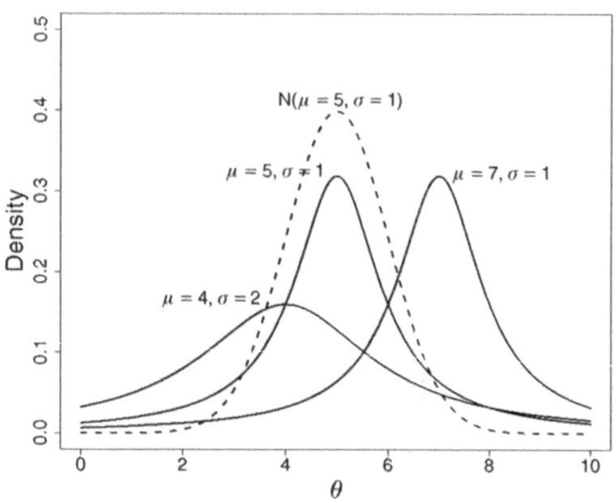

Moments		Program commands	
`Mean:`	-	`R:`	`dcauchy(theta,mu,sigma)`
`Mode:`	μ	`WB/JAGS:`	-
`Variance:`	-	`SAS:`	`theta ~ cauchy(mu,sigma)`

Note:
Cauchy distribution is a special case of location-scale t-distribution:
Cauchy$(\mu, \sigma) = t_1(\mu, \sigma)$.

Table A.3 Chi-squared distribution: $\chi^2(\nu)$.

Model	Examples
$p(\theta) = \frac{1}{\Gamma(\nu/2)2^{\nu/2}}\theta^{(\nu/2)-1}\mathrm{e}^{-\theta/2}$ `Condition:` $\nu > 0$ `Range:` $\nu = 2 : [0, \infty)$ otherwise : $(0, \infty)$ `Parameters:` ν: degrees of freedom	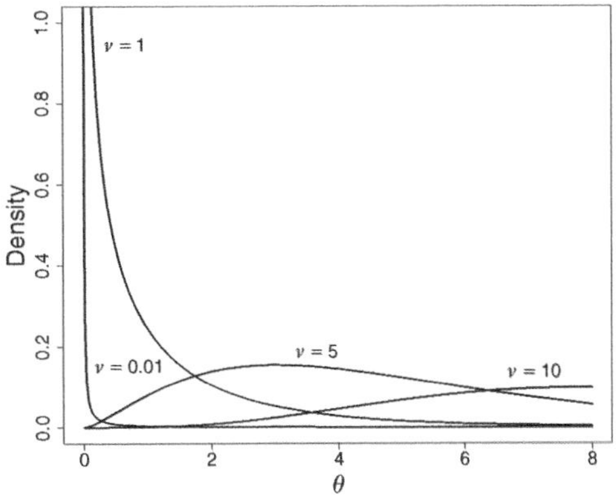

Moments		Program commands	
`Mean:`	ν	`R:`	`dchisq(theta,nu)`
`Mode:`	$\nu - 2$ $(\nu \geq 2)$, otherwise –	`WB/JAGS:`	`theta ~ dchisqr(nu)`
`Variance:`	2ν	`SAS:`	`theta ~ chisq(nu)`

Note:
Chi-squared is a special case of a gamma distribution:
$\chi^2(\nu) = \text{Gamma}(\alpha = \nu/2, \beta = 1/2)$ (rate).

JAGS offers a noncentral χ^2-distribution:
'theta ~ dnchisqr(nu,delta)', $\delta > 0$ noncentrality parameter.

JAGS offers an F-distribution (ratio of two independent χ^2s):
'theta ~ df(nu1, nu2)', with nu1, nu2 = dfs of numerator and denominator, respectively.

Table A.4 Exponential distribution: $\exp(\lambda)$.

Model	Examples
$p(\theta) = \lambda e^{-\lambda\theta}$ `Condition:` $\lambda > 0$ `Range:` $[0, \infty)$ `Parameters:` λ: rate	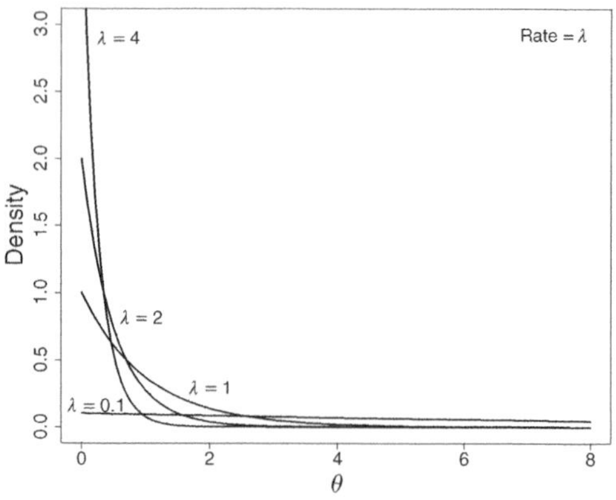

Moments		Program commands	
`Rate:`	λ		
`Mean:`	$\frac{1}{\lambda}$	`R:`	`dexp(theta,lambda)`
`Mode:`	0	`WB/JAGS:`	`theta ~ dexp(lambda)`
`Variance:`	$\frac{1}{\lambda^2}$	`SAS:`	`theta ~ expon(iscale=lambda)`
		`(scale)`	`theta ~ expon(scale=ilambda)`

Note:
Exponential is special case of gamma distribution:
$\exp(\lambda)$= Gamma($\alpha = 1, \lambda$).

Table A.5 Gamma distribution: Gamma(α, β).

Model	Examples
$p(\theta) = \dfrac{\beta^{\alpha}}{\Gamma(\alpha)}\,\theta^{(\alpha-1)}\,\mathrm{e}^{-\beta\theta}$ `Condition:` $\alpha > 0, \beta > 0$ `Range:` $\alpha = 1 : (0, \infty)$ otherwise : $[0, \infty)$ `Parameters:` α: shape, β: rate	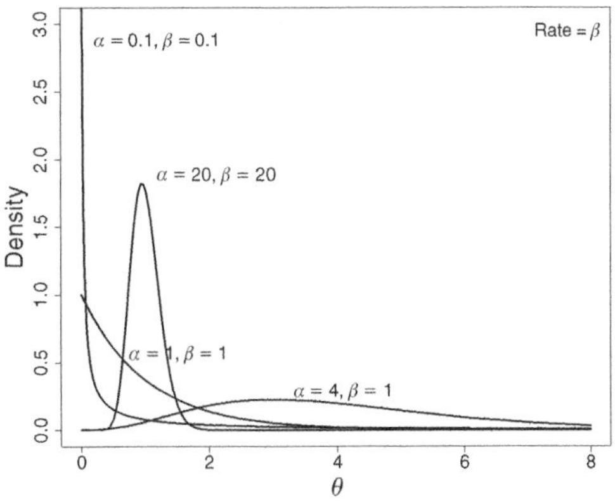

Moments		Program commands	
`Rate:`	β		
`Mean:`	$\dfrac{\alpha}{\beta}$	`R:`	`dgamma(theta,alpha,rate=beta)`
		`(scale)`	`dgamma(theta,alpha,scale=ibeta)`
`Mode:`	$\dfrac{\alpha-1}{\beta}$ $(\alpha \geq 1)$	`WB/JAGS:`	`theta ~ dgamma(alpha,beta)`
`Variance:`	$\dfrac{\alpha}{\beta^2}$	`SAS:`	`theta ~ gamma(alpha,iscale=beta)`
		`(scale)`	`theta ~ gamma(alpha,scale=ibeta)`

Note:
WB and JAGS offer a generalized gamma distribution *GenGamma*:
$\theta \sim \text{GenGamma}(\alpha, \beta^*, \lambda) \Leftrightarrow \theta^{1/\lambda} \sim \text{Gamma}(\alpha, \beta)$, with $\beta^* = \beta^{1/\lambda}$.
WB/JAGS command: 'theta ~ dgen.gamma(alpha, beta, lambda)'.

Table A.6 Inverse chi-squared distribution: Inv $-\ \chi^2(\nu)$.

Model	Examples
$p(\theta) = \dfrac{1}{\Gamma(\nu/2)2^{\nu/2}} \theta^{-(\nu/2+1)} \mathrm{e}^{-1/(2\theta)}$ `Condition:` $\nu > 0$ `Range:` $(0, \infty)$ `Parameters:` ν: degrees of freedom	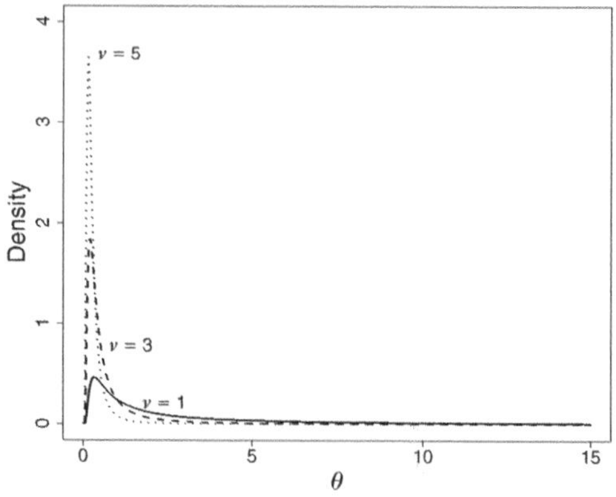

Moments			Program commands	
`Mean:`	$\dfrac{1}{\nu - 2}$	$(\nu > 2)$	`R:`	`dchisq(1/theta,nu)/theta^2`
`Mode:`	$\dfrac{1}{\nu + 2}$		`WB/JAGS:`	`theta <- 1/itheta;` `itheta ~ dchisqr(nu)`
`Variance:`	$\dfrac{2}{(\nu - 2)^2(\nu - 4)}$	$(\nu > 4)$	`SAS:`	`theta ~ ichisq(nu)`

Note:
Inverse χ^2 is a special case of the inverse gamma-distribution: (rate).
Inv $-\ \chi^2(\nu) = \mathrm{IG}(\alpha = \nu/2, \beta = 1/2)$ (rate).
Inverse χ^2 is a special case of the scaled inverse χ^2-distribution with $\nu\, s^2 = 1$.

Table A.7 Inverse gamma distribution: $\mathrm{IG}(\alpha, \beta)$.

Model	Examples
$p(\theta) = \dfrac{1}{\beta^{\alpha}\Gamma(\alpha)}\theta^{-(\alpha+1)}\,\mathrm{e}^{-\beta/\theta}$ `Condition:` $\alpha > 0, \beta > 0$ `Range:` $(0, \infty)$ `Parameters:` α: shape, β: rate	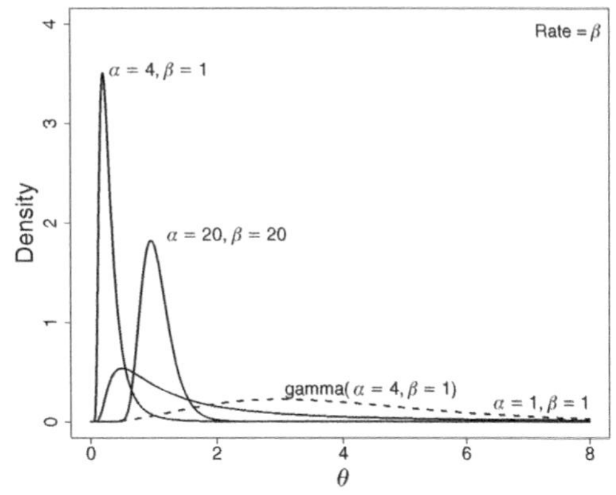

Moments		Program commands	
`Rate:`	β		
`Mean:`	$\dfrac{\beta}{(\alpha-1)}$	`R:`	`dgamma(1/theta,alpha,rate=beta)/ theta^2`
		`(scale)`	`dgamma(1/theta,alpha,scale=beta)/ theta^2`
`Mode:`	$\dfrac{\beta}{(\alpha+1)}$	`WB/JAGS:`	`theta <- 1/itheta;`
			`itheta ~ dgamma(alpha,beta)`
`Variance:`	$\dfrac{\beta^2}{(\alpha-1)^2(\alpha-2)}$	`SAS:`	`theta ~ igamma(alpha,iscale=beta)`
		`(scale)`	`theta ~ igamma(alpha,scale=ibeta)`

Note:
$\theta \sim \mathrm{IG}(\alpha, \beta) \Leftrightarrow 1/\theta \sim \mathrm{Gamma}(\alpha, \beta)$.

Table A.8 Laplace distribution: Laplace(μ, σ).

Model	Examples
$p(\theta) = \frac{1}{2\sigma}\,\mathrm{e}^{-(\theta-\mu)/\sigma}$ Condition: $\sigma > 0$ Range: $(-\infty, \infty)$ Parameters: μ: location, σ: scale	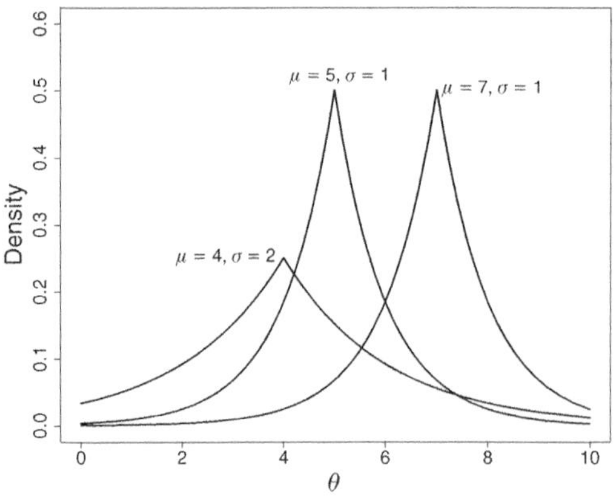

Moments		Program commands		
Scale:	σ			
Mean:	μ	R:	dlaplace(theta,mu,sigma)	
Mode:	μ	WB/JAGS:	-	
		(rate)	theta ~	ddexp(isigma)
Variance:	$2\sigma^2$	SAS:	theta ~	laplace(mu,scale=sigma)
		(rate)	theta ~	laplace(mu,iscale=isigma)

Note:
Laplace distribution is also called *double exponential distribution*.
R function dlaplace is available from R package 'VGAM'.

Table A.9 Logistic distribution: Logistic(μ, σ).

Model	Examples
$$p(\theta) = \exp\left(-\frac{\theta-\mu}{\sigma}\right)\left[\sigma \exp\left(-\frac{\theta-\mu}{\sigma}\right)\right]^2$$ `Condition:` $\sigma > 0$ `Range:` $(-\infty, \infty)$ `Parameters:` μ: location, σ: scale	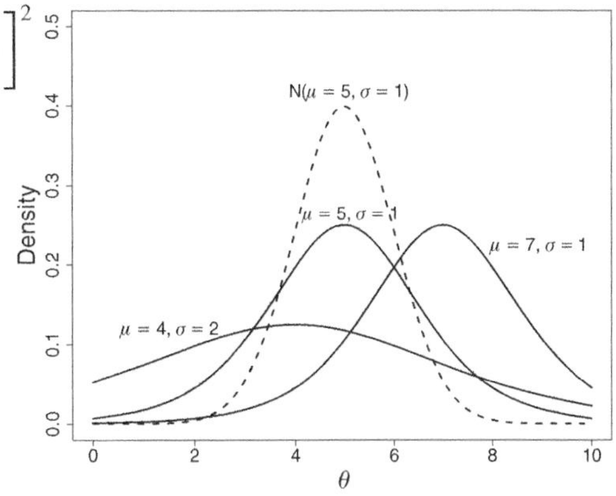

Moments		Program commands	
`Mean:`	μ	`R:`	`dlogis(theta,mu,sigma)`
`Mode:`	μ	`WB/JAGS:`	`theta ~ dlogis(mu,isigma) (rate)`
`Variance:`	$\frac{\pi^2\sigma^2}{3}$	`SAS:`	`theta ~ logistic(mu,sigma)`

Table A.10 Lognormal distribution: $\mathrm{LN}(\mu, \sigma^2)$.

Model	Examples
$p(\theta) = \frac{1}{\theta\sigma\sqrt{2\pi}} \exp\left(-\frac{(\log(\theta)-\mu)^2}{2\sigma^2}\right)$ `Condition:` $\sigma > 0$ `Range:` $(0, \infty)$ `Parameters:` μ: location, σ: scale	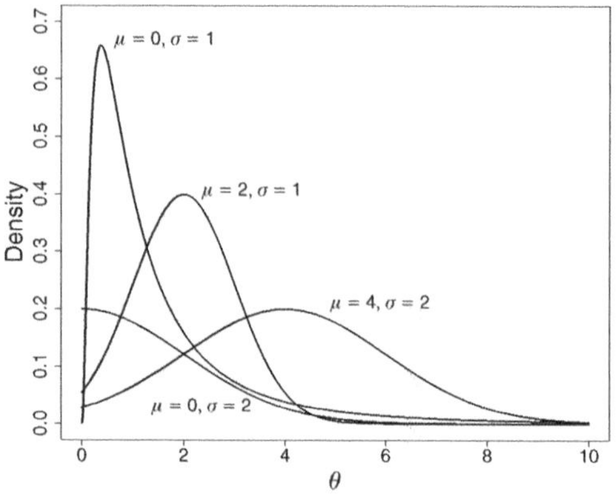

Moments		Program commands	
`Mean:`	$\exp(\mu + \sigma^2)$	`R:`	`dlnorm(theta,mu,sigma)`
`Mode:`	$\exp(\mu - \sigma^2)$	`WB/JAGS:`	`theta~dlnorm(mu,isigma2)`
`Variance:`			

$\exp(2(\mu + \sigma^2)) - \exp(2\mu + \sigma^2)$		`SAS:`	`theta~lognormal(mu,sd=sigma)`
			`theta~lognormal(mu,var=sigma2)`
			`theta~lognormal(mu,prec=isigma2)`

Table A.11 Normal distribution: $\mathrm{N}(\mu, \sigma^2)$.

Model	Examples
$$p(\theta) = \frac{1}{\sigma\sqrt{2\pi}} \exp\left(-\frac{(\theta-\mu)^2}{2\sigma^2}\right)$$ `Condition:` $\sigma > 0$ `Range:` $(-\infty, \infty)$ `Parameters:` μ: location, σ: scale	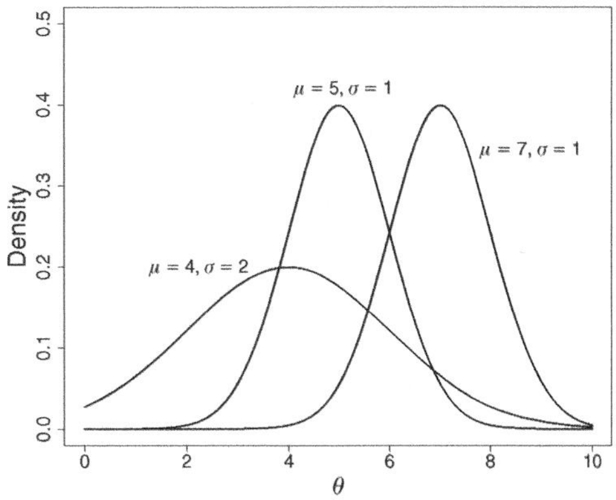

Moments		Program commands	
`Mean:`	μ	`R:`	`dnorm(theta,mu,sigma)`
`Mode:`	μ	`WB/JAGS:`	`theta ~ dnorm(mu,isigma2)`
`Variance:`	σ^2	`SAS:`	`theta ~ normal(mu,sd=sigma)`
			`theta ~ normal(mu,var=sigma2)`
			`theta ~ normal(mu,prec=isigma2)`

Table A.12 Location-scale t-distribution: $t_\nu(\mu, \sigma)$.

Model

$$p(\theta) = \frac{\Gamma\left(\frac{\nu+1}{2}\right)}{\Gamma\left(\frac{\nu}{2}\right)\sigma\sqrt{\nu\pi}}\left(1+\frac{(\theta-\mu)^2}{\nu\sigma^2}\right)^{-\frac{\nu+1}{2}}$$

Condition: $\sigma > 0, \nu > 0$
Range: $(-\infty, \infty)$
Parameters:
μ: location, σ: scale
ν: degrees of freedom

Examples

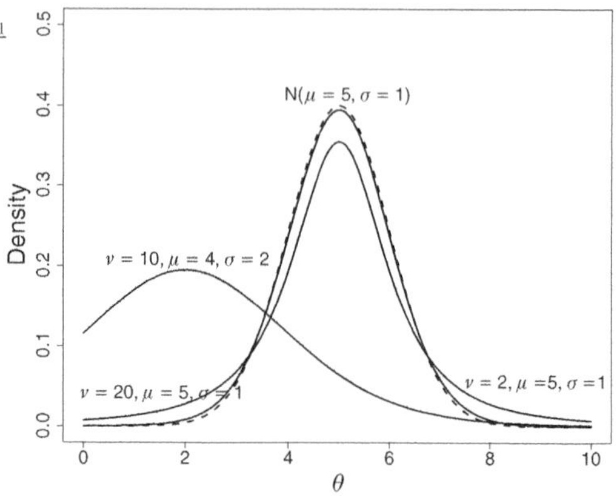

Moments		Program commands	
Mean:	μ (if $\nu > 1$)	R:	dt(nu,(theta-mu)/sigma)/sigma
Mode:	μ	WB/JAGS:	theta ~ dt(mu,isigma2,nu)
Variance:	$\frac{\nu}{\nu-2}\sigma^2$ (if $\nu > 2$)	SAS:	theta ~ t(mu,sd=sigma,nu)
			theta ~ t(mu,var=sigma2,nu)
			theta ~ t(mu,prec=isigma2,nu)

Table A.13 Pareto distribution: Pareto(α, β).

Model	Examples
$p(\theta) = \frac{\alpha}{\beta}\left(\frac{\beta}{\theta}\right)^{\alpha+1}$ `Condition:` $\alpha > 0, \beta > 0$ `Range:` (β, ∞) `Parameters:` α: shape, β: location	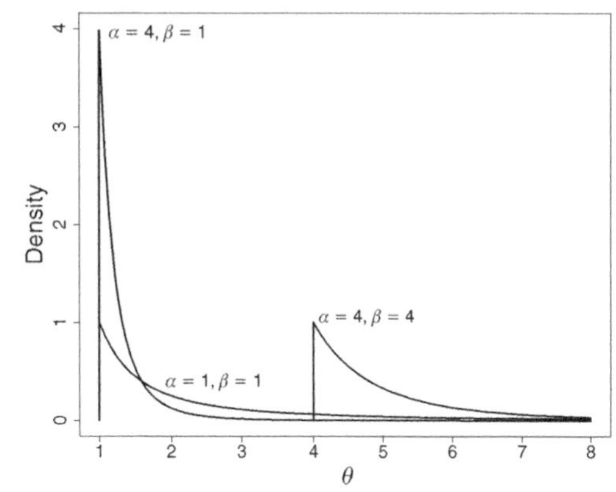

Moments			Program commands	
`Mean:`	$\frac{\alpha\beta}{\alpha - 1}$	(if $\alpha > 1$)	`R:`	`dpareto(theta,beta,alpha)`
`Mode:`	β		`WB/JAGS:`	`theta~dpareto(alpha,beta)`
`Variance:`	$\frac{\alpha\beta^2}{(\alpha - 1)^2(\alpha - 2)}$	(if $\alpha > 2$)	`SAS:`	`theta~pareto(alpha,beta)`

Note:
R function dpareto is available from R package 'VGAM'.

Table A.14 Scaled inverse chi-squared density: $\text{Inv}-\chi^2(\nu, s^2)$.

Model	Examples
$p(\theta) = \frac{(\nu/2)^{\nu/2}}{\Gamma(\nu/2)} s^{\nu} \theta^{-(\nu/2+1)} e^{-\nu s^2/(2\theta)}$ `Condition:` $\nu > 0, s > 0$ `Range:` $(0, \infty)$ `Parameters:` ν: degrees of freedom, s^2: scale	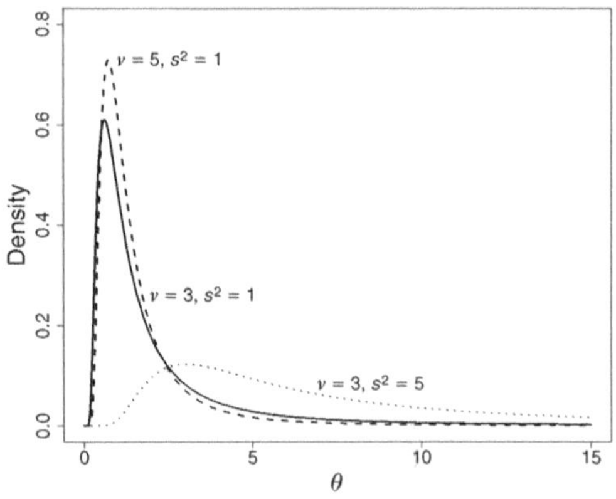

Moments		Program commands	
`Mean:`	$\frac{\nu}{\nu-2} s^2 \quad (\nu > 2)$	`R:`	`dchisq(nu*s^2/theta,nu)`
`Mode:`	$\frac{\nu}{\nu+2} s^2$	`WB/JAGS:`	`theta <- nu*s^2/itheta;` `itheta ~ dchisqr(nu)`
`Variance:`	$\frac{2\nu^2}{(\nu-2)^2(\nu-4)} s^4 \quad (\nu > 4)$	`SAS:`	`theta ~ sichisq(nu,s)`

Note:
Scaled inverse chi-squared is a special case of the inverse gamma distribution:
$\text{Inv}-\chi^2(\nu, s^2) = \text{IG}(\alpha = \nu/2, \beta = \nu\, s^2/2)$ (rate).

Table A.15 Weibull distribution: Weibull(α, β).

Model	Examples
$p(\theta) = \frac{\alpha}{\beta}\left(\frac{\theta}{\beta}\right)^{(\alpha-1)} \exp\left(-(\theta/\beta)^{\alpha}\right)$ `Condition:` $\alpha > 0, \beta > 0$ `Range:` $\alpha = 1 : [0, \infty)$ otherwise: $(0, \infty)$ `Parameters:` α: shape, β: scale	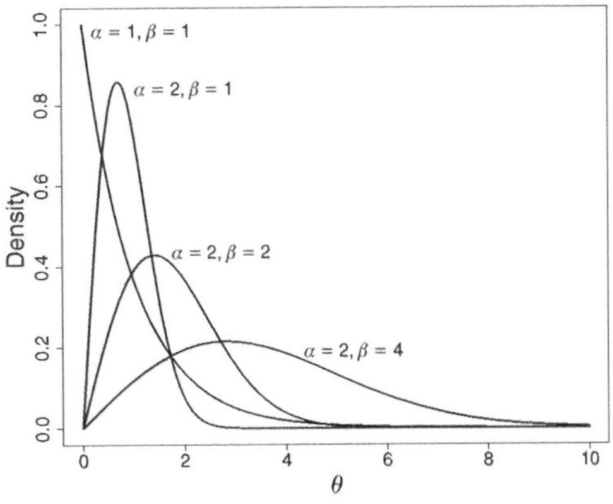

Moments	Program commands	
`Mean:` $\beta\Gamma(1 + 1/\alpha)$	`R:`	`dweibull(theta,alpha,beta)`
`Mode:` $\beta(1 - 1/\alpha)^{1/\alpha}$ (if $\alpha > 1$)	`WB/JAGS:`	`theta ~ dweib(alpha,ibeta)`
`Variance:` $\beta^2\left[\Gamma(1 + 2/\alpha) - \Gamma^2(1 + 2/\alpha)\right]$	`SAS:`	`theta ~ weibull(0,alpha,beta)`

Note:
SAS: more general Weibull distribution with additional $\mu > 0 =$ lower limit of range: 'weibull(mu,alpha,beta)', with θ/β in Weibull distribution replaced by $(\theta - \mu)/\beta$.

Table A.16 Uniform distribution: $U(\alpha, \beta)$.

Model	Examples
$p(\theta) = \dfrac{1}{\beta - \alpha}$ `Condition:` $\beta > \alpha$ `Range:` $[\alpha, \beta]$ `Parameters:` α: lower limit, β: upper limit	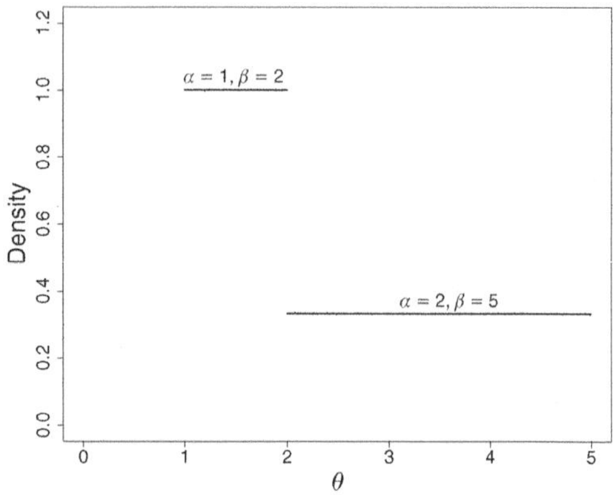

Moments		Program commands	
`Mean:`	$\dfrac{\alpha + \beta}{2}$	`R:`	`dunif(theta,alpha,beta)`
`Mode:`	–	`WB/JAGS:`	`theta ~ dunif(alpha,beta)`
`Variance:`	$\dfrac{(\beta - \alpha)^2}{12}$	`SAS:`	`theta ~ uniform(alpha,beta)`

Note:
Uniform is a special case of the beta distribution: U(0, 1) = Beta(1, 1).

A.3 Discrete univariate distributions

Table A.17 Binomial distribution: $\mathrm{Bin}(n, \pi)$.

Model	Examples

$p(\theta) = \binom{n}{\theta} \pi^{\theta} (1-\pi)^{n-\theta}$
`Conditions:`
$n = 0, 1, 2, \ldots$
$0 \leq \pi \leq 1$
`Range:` $\theta \in \{0, 1, \ldots, n\}$
`Parameters:`
n: sample size
π: probability of success
	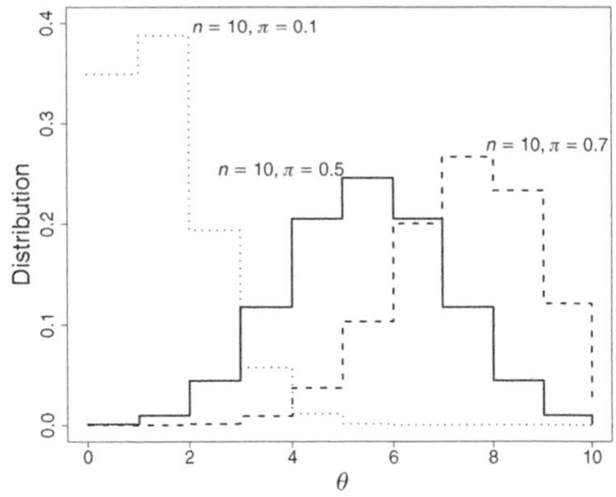

Moments		Program commands	
`Mean:`	$n\pi$	`R:`	`dbinom(theta,n,pi)`
`Mode:`	$\lfloor (n+1)\pi \rfloor$	`WB/JAGS:`	`theta ~ dbin(pi,n)`
`Variance:`	$n\pi(1-\pi)$	`SAS:`	`theta ~ binomial(n,pi)`

Note:
$\lfloor (n+1)\pi \rfloor$ = greatest integer in value.
Special case: *Bernoulli distribution* = $\mathrm{Bern}(\pi) = \mathrm{Bin}(1, \pi)$.
Commands Bernoulli dist: R: dbern(pi), WB: dbern(pi), SAS: binary(pi).

Table A.18 Categorical distribution: Cat(π).

Model	Examples

$p(\theta) = \pi_\theta$
 	
`Conditions:`
$\pi_\theta > 0, \sum \pi_\theta = 1$
`Range:` $\theta \in \{0, 1, \ldots, n\}$
`Parameters:`
π_θ: class probabilities
	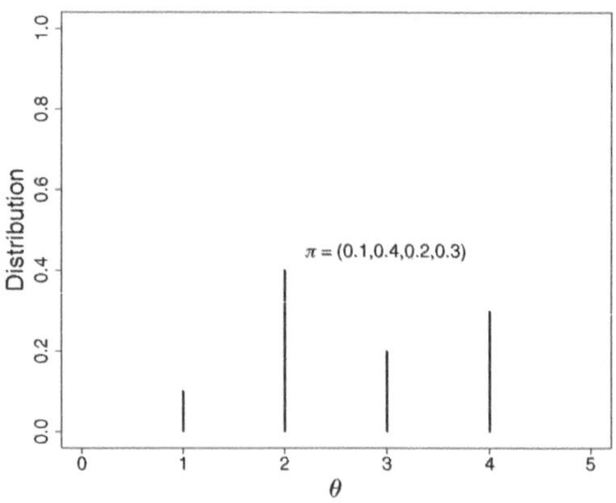

Moments		Program commands	
`Mean:`	–	`R:`	`dmultinom(theta,size=1,pi)`
`Mode:`	–	`WB/JAGS:`	`theta ~ dcat(pi)`
`Variance:`	–	`SAS:`	`theta ~ multinom(pi)`

Note:
Categorical is a special case of the multinomial distribution with $n = 1$.
JAGS only requires that π_θ is positive, they must not add up to 1.

Table A.19 Negative binomial distribution: NB(n, π).

Model	Examples

$p(\theta) = \binom{\theta + n - 1}{\theta} \pi^n (1-\pi)^\theta$
 	
`Conditions:`
$n = 0, 1, 2, \ldots$
$0 \le \pi \le 1$
`Range:` $\theta \in \{0, 1, \ldots, n\}$
`Parameters:`
n: number of successes
π: probability of success
	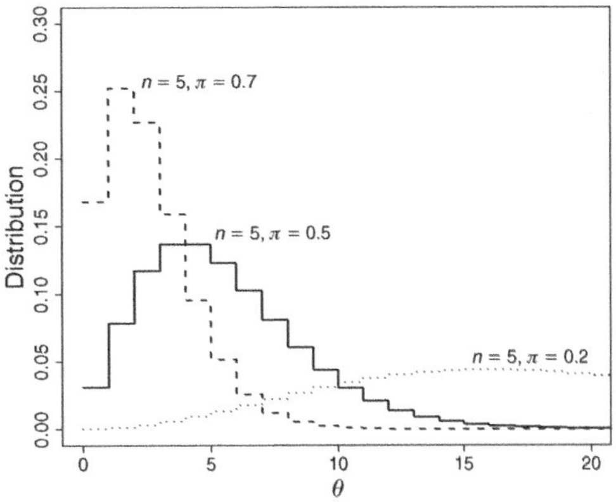

Moments		Program commands	
`Mean:`	$\mathrm{round}\left(\frac{n(1-\pi)}{\pi}\right)$	`R:`	`dnbinom(theta,n,pi)`
`Mode:`	$\mathrm{round}\left(\frac{(n-1)(1-\pi)}{\pi}\right)$	`WB/JAGS:`	`theta ~ dnbinom(pi,n)`
`Variance:`	$\frac{n(1-\pi)}{\pi^2}$	`SAS:`	`theta ~ negbin(n,pi)`

Note:
Special case: *Geometric distribution*: geom(p) = NB$(1, \pi)$.
We have seen alternative parameterizations of the negative binomial distribution in the book:
Expression (3.15): $\pi = \beta/(1+\beta)$ and $n = \alpha$ a real value.
Expression (6.19): $\pi = 1/(1+\kappa\lambda)$ and $n = 1/\kappa$ a real value.

Table A.20 Poisson distribution: Poisson(λ).

Model	Examples
$p(\theta) = \frac{\lambda^\theta}{\theta!} \exp(-\lambda)$ `Condition:` $\lambda \geq 0$ `Range:` $\theta \in \{0, 1, \ldots, \infty\}$ `Parameters:` λ: average number of counts	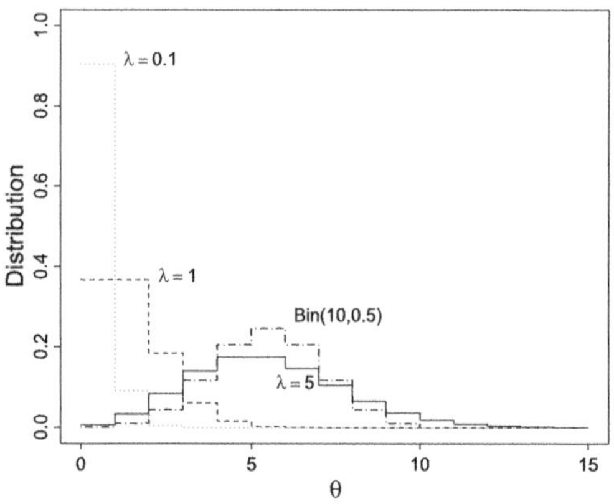

Moments		Program commands	
`Mean:`	λ	`R:`	`dpois(theta,lambda)`
`Mode:`	round(λ)	`WB/JAGS:`	`theta ~ dpois(lambda)`
`Variance:`	λ	`SAS:`	`theta ~ poisson(lambda)`

A.4 Multivariate distributions

Table A.21 Dirichlet distribution: Dirichlet($\boldsymbol{\alpha}$).

Model	Program commands
$p(\boldsymbol{\theta}) = \dfrac{\Gamma\left(\sum_{j=1}^{J}\alpha_j\right)}{\prod_{j=1}^{J}\Gamma(\alpha_j)}\prod_{j=1}^{J}\theta_j^{\alpha_j-1}$	`R: ddirichlet(vtheta,valpha)`
`Condition:` $\alpha_j > 0\ (j = 1, \ldots, J)$	`WB/JAGS: vtheta[] ~ ddirich (valpha[])`
`Range:` $\theta_j > 0,\ \sum_{j=1}^{J}\theta_j = 1$	`SAS: vtheta ~ dirich(valpha)`
`Parameters:` α_j: probabilities	
Moments	
`Mean:` $\alpha_j/\sum_{j=1}^{J}\alpha_j$	`Mode:` $(\alpha_j - 1)/\sum_{j=1}^{J}\alpha_j$
`Variances:` $\dfrac{\alpha_j\left(\sum_m\alpha_m - \alpha_j\right)}{\left(\sum_m\alpha_m\right)^2\left(\sum_m\alpha_m - \alpha_j\right)}$	`Covariances:` $-\dfrac{\alpha_j\alpha_k}{\left(\sum_m\alpha_m\right)^2\left(\sum_m\alpha_m + 1\right)}$

Table A.22 Inverse Wishart distribution: IW(R, k).

Model	Program commands
$p(\Sigma) = c\det(\mathrm{R})^{k/2}\det(\Sigma)^{-(k+p+1)/2}$ $\exp\left[-\frac{1}{2}\mathrm{tr}\,(\Sigma^{-1}\mathrm{R})\right]$	`R: diwish(Sigma, k, Rinv)` (Rinv $= \mathrm{R}^{-1}$ in MCMCpack)
with $c^{-1} = 2^{kp/2}\pi^{p(p-1)/4}\prod_{j=1}^{p}\Gamma\left(\dfrac{k+1-j}{2}\right)$	
`Condition:` R pos definite, $k > 0$ `Range:` Σ symmetric	`WB/JAGS: –` `SAS: Sigma ~ iwishart(k,R)`
`Parameters:` k: degrees of freedom & R: inverse of cov matrix	
Moments	
`Mean:` $\mathrm{R}/(k - p - 1)$ (if $k > p + 1$)	`Mode:` $\mathrm{R}/(k + p + 1)$

Table A.23 Multinomial distribution: Mult(n, $\boldsymbol{\pi}$).

Model	Program commands
$p(\boldsymbol{\theta}) = \frac{n!}{\theta_1!\theta_2!\ldots\theta_k!}\prod_{j=1}^{k}\pi_j^{\theta_j}$,	R: `dmultinom(theta,size=n,prob=vpi)`
`Condition:` $\sum_{j=1}^{k}\pi_j = 1$	WB/JAGS: `vtheta[] ~ dmulti(pi[],n)`
`Range:` $\theta_j \in \{0,\ldots,n\}$ with $\sum_{j=1}^{k}\theta_j = n$	SAS: `vtheta ~ multinom(vpi)`
`Parameters:` π_j: probabilities	
Moments	
`Mean:` $n\cdot\boldsymbol{\pi}$	
`Variances:` $n\pi_j(1-\pi_j)$	`Covariances:` $-n\pi_j\pi_k$

Table A.24 Multivariate normal distribution: $N_p(\boldsymbol{\mu}, \Sigma)$.

Model	Program commands
$p(\boldsymbol{\theta}) = \frac{1}{(2\pi)^{p/2}\det(\Sigma)^{1/2}} \times \exp\left[-\frac{1}{2}(\boldsymbol{\theta}-\boldsymbol{\mu})^T\Sigma^{-1}(\boldsymbol{\theta}-\boldsymbol{\mu})\right]$	R: `mvrnorm(vtheta,vmu,S)` (MASS)
`Condition:` Σ positive definite	WB/JAGS: `vtheta[] ~ dmnorm(vmu[],S[,])`
`Range:` $-\infty < \theta_j < \infty$	SAS: `vtheta ~ mvn(vmu,S)`
`Parameters:` $\boldsymbol{\mu}$: mean vector & Σ: $p \times p$ covariance matrix	
Moments	
`Mean:` $\boldsymbol{\mu}$	`Mode:` $\boldsymbol{\mu}$
`Variances:` Σ_{jj}	`Covariances:` Σ_{jk}

Table A.25 Multivariate t-distribution: $T_\nu(\boldsymbol{\mu}, \Sigma)$.

Model	Program commands
$p(\boldsymbol{\theta}) = c\det(\Sigma)^{-1/2}$ $\times\left[1+\frac{1}{\nu}(\boldsymbol{\theta}-\boldsymbol{\mu})^T\Sigma^{-1}(\boldsymbol{\theta}-\boldsymbol{\mu})\right]^{-(\nu+p)/2}$ with $c = \frac{\Gamma[(\nu+p)/2]}{\Gamma(\nu/2)(k\pi)^{p/2}}$	`R: -`
`Condition:` Σ positive definite, $\nu > 0$ `Range:` $-\infty < \theta_j < \infty$	`WB/JAGS: vtheta[] ~ dmt(vmu[],S[,],nu)` `SAS: -`
`Parameters:` $\boldsymbol{\mu}$: mean vector; Σ: $p \times p$ covariance matrix; ν: degrees of freedom	
Moments	
`Mean:` $\boldsymbol{\mu}$ (if $\nu > 1$)	`Mode:` $\boldsymbol{\mu}$
`Variances:` $\frac{\nu}{\nu-2}\Sigma_{jj}$ (if $\nu > 2$)	`Covariances:` $\frac{\nu}{\nu-2}\Sigma_{jk}$ (if $\nu > 2$)

Table A.26 Wishart distribution: Wishart(R, k).

Model	Program commands
$p(\Sigma) = c\det(\mathrm{R})^{-k/2}\det(\Sigma)^{(k-p-1)/2}$ $\times\exp\left[-\frac{1}{2}\mathrm{tr}\,(\mathrm{R}^{-1}\Sigma)\right]$ with $c^{-1} = 2^{kp/2}\pi^{p(p-1)/4}$ $\prod_{j=1}^{p}\Gamma\left(\frac{k+1-j}{2}\right)$	`R: dwish(Sigma, k, Rinv)` (Rinv = R^{-1} in MCMCpack)
`Condition:` R pos definite, $k > 0$ `Range:` Σ symmetric	`WB/JAGS: Sigma[,] ~ dwish(R[,],k)` `SAS: -`
`Parameters:` k: degrees of freedom & R: covariance matrix	
Moments	
`Mean:` kR	`Mode:` $(k-p-1)$R (if $k > p+1$)
`Variances:` $\mathrm{Var}(\Sigma_{ij}) = k(r_{ij}^2 + r_{ii}r_{jj})$	`Covariances:` $\mathrm{Cov}(\Sigma_{ij}, \Sigma_{kl}) = k(r_{ik}r_{jl} + r_{il}r_{jk})$

Note:
WinBUGS uses an alternative expression of the Wishart distribution: in the above expression R is replaced by R^{-1} and hence represents a covariance matrix in WinBUGS.

References

Abellan J, Richardson S and Best N 2008 Use of space-time models to investigate the stability of patterns of disease. *Environmental Health Perspectives* **116**, 1111–1118.

Abraham B and Box G 1978 Linear models and spurious observations. *Journal of the Royal Statistical Society: Series C (Applied Statistics)* **27**, 131–138.

Adler S 1981 Over-relaxation methods for the Monte Carlo evaluation of the partition function for multiquadratic actions. *Physical Review D* **23**, 2901–2904.

Agresti A 1990 *Categorical Data Analysis*. John Wiley & Sons, New York.

Agresti A and Min Y 2005 Frequentist performance of Bayesian confidence intervals for comparing proportions in 2×2 contingency tables. *Biometrics* **61**, 515–523.

Aitchison J 1964 Bayesian tolerance intervals. *Journal of the Royal Statistical Society: Series B* **26**, 161–175.

Aitchison J 1966 Expected-cover and linear utility tolerance intervals. *Journal of the Royal Statistical Society: Series B* **28**, 57–62.

Aitkin M 2010 *Statistical Inference: An Integrated Bayesian/Likelihood Approach*. Chapman and Hall/CRC Press, Boca Raton.

Akaike H 1974 A new look at the statistical model identification. *IEEE Transactions on Automatic Control* **19**, 716–723.

Albert A and Anderson J 1984 On the existence of maximum likelihood estimates in logistic regression models. *Biometrika* **71**, 1–19.

Albert J 1988 Computational methods using a Bayesian hierarchical generalized linear model. *Journal of the American Statistical Association* **83**, 1037–1044.

Albert J 1999 Criticism of a hierarchical model using Bayes factors. *Statistics in Medicine* **18**, 287–305.

Albert J and Chib S 1993 Bayesian analysis of binary and polychotomous response data. *Journal of the American Statistical Association* **88**, 669–679.

Albert J and Chib S 1995 Bayesian residual analysis for binary response regression models. *Biometrika* **82**, 747–759.

Alves C, Luime J, van Zeben D, Huisman A, Weel A, Barendregt P and Hazes J 2011 Diagnostic performance of the ACR/EULAR 2010 criteria for rheumatoid arthritis and two diagnostic algorithms in an early arthritis clinic (REACH). *Annals of Rheumatology Diseases* **70**, 1645–1647.

Anderson D and Burnham K 1999 Understanding information criteria for selection among capture–recapture or ring recovery models. *Bird Study* **46**, S14–S21.

Bayesian Biostatistics, First Edition. Emmanuel Lesaffre and Andrew B. Lawson.

Ando T 2007 Bayesian predictive information criterion for the evaluation of hierarchical Bayesian and empirical Bayes models. *Biometrika* **94**, 443–458.

Ando T 2010 *Bayesian Model Selection and Statistical Modeling*. Chapman and Hall/CRC, Boca Raton.

Andrews D and Mallows C 1974 Scale mixtures of normal distributions. *Journal of the Royal Statistical Society: Series B* **36**, 99–102.

Andrews R, Berger J and Smith A 1993 Bayesian estimation of fuel economy potential due to technology improvements. In: *Case Studies in Bayesian Statistics*, vol. 1 (C. Gatsonis *et al.*, eds.). Springer-Verlag, New York, pp. 1–77.

Arellano-Valle RB, Bolfarine H and Lachos VH 2007 Bayesian inference for skew-normal linear mixed models. *Journal of Applied Statistics* **34**, 663–682.

Arends L, Hamza T, Van Houwelingen J, Heijenbrok-kal, Hunink M and Stijnen T 2008 Multivariate random effects meta-analysis of ROC curves. *Medical Decision Making* **28**, 621–638.

Arnold B, Castillo E and Sarabia J 2001 Conditionally specified distributions: An introduction. *Statistical Science* **16**, 249–274.

Ashby D, Hutton J and McGee M 1993 Simple Bayesian analyses for case-control studies in cancer epidemiology. *The Statistician* **42**, 385–397.

Baddeley A and M. van Lieshout 1993 Stochastic geometry models in high-level vision. In: *Statistics and Images* (Mardia K, ed.). Carfax, Abingdon, pp. 233–258.

Bae K and Mallick B 2004 Gene selection using a two-level hierarchical Bayesian model. *Bioinformatics* **20**, 3423–3430.

Banerjee A and Bhattacharyya G 1979 Bayesian results for the Inverse Gaussian distribution with an application. *Technometrics* **21**, 247–251.

Banerjee S and Carlin B 2003 Semiparametric spatio-temporal frailty modeling. *Environmetrics* **14**, 523–535.

Banerjee S, Carlin B and Gelfand A 2004 *Hierarchical Modeling and Analysis for Spatial Data*. CRC Press, London.

Banerjee S, Gelfand A, Finley A and Sang H 2008 Gaussian predictive process models for large spatial data sets. *Journal of the Royal Statistical Society: Series B* **70**, 825–848.

Banuro F 1999 *Relative Risks for Disease Mapping: A New Approach Using a Spatial Mixture Model*. Doctoral Thesis: Catholic University of Leuven.

Barbieri M and Berger J 2004 Optimal predictive model selection. *Annals of Statistics* **32**, 870–897.

Barlow RE, Bartholomew D, Bremner JM and Brunk HD 1972 *Statistical Inference Under Order Restrictions: The Theory and Application of Isotonic Regression*. John Wiley & Sons, New York.

Barone P, Sebastiani G and Stander J 2002 Over-relaxation methods and coupled Markov chains for Monte Caarlo simulation. *Statistics and Computing* **12**, 17–26.

Bartlett M 1957 A comment on D.V. Lindley's statistical paradox. *Biometrika* **44**, 533–534.

Bastos L and Gamerman D 2006 Dynamical survival models with spatial frailty. *Lifetime Data Analysis* **12**, 441–460.

Bedrick E, Christensen R and Johnson W 1996 A new perspective on priors for generalized linear models. *Journal of the American Statistical Association* **91**, 1450–1460.

Bennett J, Racine-Poon A and Wakefield J 1996 Markov Chain Monte Carlo in Practice. *MCMC for Nonlinear Hierarchical Models* (WR Gilks, S Richardson, and D Spiegelhalter, eds.). CRC Press, London.

Berger J 2006 The case for objective Bayesian analysis. *Bayesian Analysis* **1**, 285–402.

Berger J and Pericchi L 2001 *Objective Bayesian Methods for Model Selection: Introduction and Comparison*, vol. 38. IMS Lectures Notes – Monograph Series.

Berger J and Sellke T 1987 Testing a point null hypothesis: The irreconcilability of p values and evidence. *Journal of the American Statistical Association* **82**, 112–122.

Berger J and Wolpert R 1984 *The Likelihood Principle*. Lecture Notes – Monograph Series, Vol 6, Institute of Mathematical Statistics.

Berkvens D, Speybroeck N, Praet N, Adel A and Lesaffre E 2006 Estimating disease prevalence in a Bayesian framework using probabilistic constraints. *Epidemiology* **17**, 145–153.

Bernardinelli L, Clayton D, Pascutto C, Montomoli C, Ghislandi M and Songini M 1995 Bayesian analysis of space-time variation in disease risk. *Statistics in Medicine* **14**, 2433–2443.

Bernardo J 1979 Reference posterior distributions for Bayesian inference (with discussion). *Journal of the Royal Statistical Society: Series B* **41**, 113–147.

Bernardo J and Smith A 1994 *Bayesian Theory*. John Wiley & Sons, Chichester.

Berry S, Carlin B, Lee J and Müller P 2011 *Bayesian Adaptive Methods for Clinical Trials*. Chapman and Hall/CRC, Boca Raton.

Besag J 1974 Spatial interaction and the statistical analysis of lattice systems. *Journal of the Royal Statistical Society: Series B* **36**, 192–236.

Besag J 1977 Some methods of statistical analyisis for spatial data. *Bulletin of the International Statistical Institute* **47**, 77–92.

Besag J 1986 On the statistical analysis of dirty pictures. *Journal of the Royal Statistical Society: Series B* **48**, 259–302.

Besag J and Green PJ 1993 Spatial statistics and Bayesian computation. *Journal of the Royal Statistical Society: Series B* **55**, 25–37.

Besag J, York J and Mollié A 1991 Bayesian image restoration with two applications in spatial statistics. *Annals of the Institute of Statistical Mathematics* **43**, 1–59.

Bickel P and Doksum K 1981 An analysis of transformations revisited. *Journal of the American Statistical Association* **76**, 296–311.

Biggeri A, Braga M and Marchi M 1993 Empirical Bayes interval estimates: An application to geographical epidemiology. *Journal of Italian Statistical Society* **3**, 251–267.

Bliss C 1935 The calculation of the dosage mortality curve. *Annals of Applied Biology* **22**, 134–167.

Böhning D 2003 *Computer-Assisted Analysis of Mixtures and Applications: Meta-Analysis, Disease Mapping and Others*. Chapman and Hall/CRC Press, Boca Raton.

Boonen S, Lesaffre E, Aerssens J, Pelemans W, Dequeker J and Bouillon R 1996 Deficiency of the growth hormone-insulin-like growth factor-i axis potentially involved in age-related alteration of body composition. *Gerontology* **42**, 330–338.

Borgelt C and Kruse R 2002 *Graphical Models: Methods for Data Analysis and Mining*. John Wiley & Sons, New York.

Bottolo L and Richardson S 2010 Evolutionary stochastic search for Bayesian model exploration. *Bayesian Analysis* **5**, 583–618.

Bowman FD, Caffo B, Bassett S and Kilts C 2008 A Bayesian hierarchical framework for spatial modeling of fMRI data. *NeuroImage* **35**, 146–156.

Box G 1980 Sampling and Bayes' inference in scientific modelling and robustness (with discussion). *Journal of the Royal Statistical Society: Series A* **143**, 383–430.

Box G and Cox D 1964 An analysis of transformations (with discussion). *Journal of the Royal Statistical Society: Series B* **26**, 211–252.

Box G and Tiao G 1968 A Bayesian approach to some outlier problems. *Biometrika* **55**, 119–129.

Box G and Tiao G 1973 *Bayesian Inference in Statistical Analysis*. Addison-Wesley, Reading, MA. Reprinted by Wiley in 1992 in the Wiley Classics Library Edition.

Box G and Tidwell P 1962 Transformation of the independent variables. *Technometrics* **4**, 531–550.

Bradlow E and Zaslavsky A 1997 Case influence analysis in Bayesian inference. *Journal of Computational and Graphical Statistics* **6**, 314–331.

Breslow N 1984 Extra-Poisson variation in log-linear models. *Journal of the Royal Statistical Society: Series C (Applied Statistics)* **33**, 38–44.

Broemeling L 2007 *Bayesian Biostatistics and Diagnostic Medicine*. Chapman and Hall/CRC, Boca Raton.

Brooks S 1998 Quantitative convergence assessment for Markov Chain Monte Carlo via cusums. *Statistics and Computing* **8**, 267–274.

Brooks S and Gelman A 1998 General methods for monitoring convergence of iterative simulation. *Journal of Computational and Graphical Statistics* **7**, 434–455.

Brooks S and Giudici P 2000 MCMC convergence assessment via two-way ANOVA. *Journal of Computational and Graphical Statistics* **9**, 266–285.

Brooks S and Roberts G 1998 Convergence assessment techniques for Markov Chain Monte Carlo. *Statistics and Computing* **8**, 319–335.

Brooks S and Roberts G 1999 On quantile estimation and Markov Chain Monte Carlo. *Biometrika* **86**, 710–717.

Brophy J and Joseph L 1995 Placing trials in context using Bayesian analysis. GUSTO revisited by reverend Bayes. *JAMA* **273**, 871–875.

Browne W and Draper D 2006 A comparison of Bayesian and likelihood-based methods for fitting multilevel models. *Bayesian Analysis* **1**, 473–514.

Buonaccorsi J 2010 *Measurement Error: Models, Methods and Applications*. Springer, Boca Raton.

Burnham K and Anderson D 2002 *Model Selection and Multimodel Inference: A Practical Information-Theoretic Approach* (2nd edition). Springer, New York.

Carlin B and Chib S 1995 Bayesian model choice via Markov Chain Monte Carlo methods. *Journal of the Royal Statistical Society: Series B* **57**, 473–484.

Carlin B and Hodges J 1999 Hierarchical proportional hazards regression models for highly stratified data. *Biometrics* **55**, 1162–1170.

Carlin B and Louis T 2009 *Bayes and Empirical Bayes Methods for Data Analysis*. Chapman and Hall/CRC Press, Boca Raton.

Carroll R, Ruppert D, Stefanski L and Crainiceanu C 2006 *Measurement Error in Nonlinear Models* (2nd edition). Chapman and Hall/CRC Press, Boca Raton.

Carstairs V 1981 Small area analysis and health service research. *Community Medicine* **3**, 131–139.

Casella G and Berger R 1987 Reconciling Bayesian and frequentist evidence in the one-sided testing problem. *Journal of the American Statistical Association* **82**, 106–111.

Casella G and George E 1992 Explaining the Gibbs sampler. *The American Statistician* **46**, 167–174.

Castelloe J and Zimmerman D 2002 Convergence assessment for Reversible Jump MCMC samplers. *Technical Report 313*.

Celeux G, Forbes F, Robert C and Titterington D 2006 Deviance information criteria for missing data models. *Bayesian Analysis* **1**, 651–705.

Chaloner K 1996 Elicitation of prior distributions. In: *Bayesian Biostatistics* (DA Berry and DK Stangl, eds.). Marcel Dekker, New York, pp. 141–156.

Chaloner K and Brant R 1988 A Bayesian approach to outlier detection and residual analysis. *Biometrika* **75**, 651–659.

Chaloner K, Church T, Louis T and Matts J 1993 Graphical elicitation of a prior distribution for a clinical trial. *The Statistician* **42**, 341–353.

Chen MH and Deely J 1996 Bayesian analysis for a constrained linear multiple regression problem for predicting the new crop of apples. *Journal of Agricultural, Biological, and Environmental Statistics* **1**, 467–489.

Chen MH and Ibrahim J 2003 Conjugate priors for generalized linear models. *Statistica Sinica* **13**, 461–476.

Chen MH and Shao QM 1999 Monte Carlo estimation of Bayesian credible intervals and HPD intervals. *Journal of Computational and Graphical Statistics* **8**, 69–92.

Chen MH, Ibrahim J and Shao Q 2000 Power prior distributions for generalized linear models. *Journal of Statistical Planning and Inference* **84**, 121–137.

Chen MH, Ibrahim J and Yiannoutsous C 1999 Prior elicitation, variable selection and Bayesian computation for logistic regression models. *Journal of the Royal Statistical Society: Series B* **61**, 223–242.

Chen X, Wang Z and McKeown M 2011 A Bayesian Lasso via reversible-jump MCMC. *Signal Processing* **91**, 1920–1932.

Chib S and Carlin B 1999 On MCMC sampling in hierarchical longitudinal models. *Statistics and Computing* **9**, 17–26.

Chib S and Greenberg E 1995 Understanding the Metropolis-Hastings algorithm. *The American Statistician* **49**, 327–335.

Chipman H 1996 Bayesian variable selection with related predictors. *The Canadian Journal of Statistics* **24**, 17–36.

Chipman HA, George EI and McCulloch RE 2010 BART: Bayesian additive regression trees. *Annals of Applied Statistics* **4**, 266–298.

Chipman H, George E, McCulloch R, Clyde M, Foster D and Stine R 2001 *Model Selection*, vol. 38. IMS Lecture Notes – Monograph Series, Beachwood OH: Institute of Mathematical Statistics.

Claeskens G and Hjort N 2008 *Model Selection and Model Averaging*. Cambridge University Press, Cambridge.

Clayton D 1994 Some approaches to the analysis of recurrent event data. *Statistical Methods in Medical Research* **3**, 244–262.

Clements J 2000 The mouse lymphoma assay. *Mutation Research* **455**, 97–110.

Clogg C, Rubin D, Schenker N, Schultz B and Weidman L 1991 Multiple imputation of industry and occupation codes in census public-use samples using Baysian logistic regression. *Journal of the American Statistical Association* **86**, 68–78.

Clyde M and George E 2004 Model uncertainty. *Statistical Science* **19**, 81–94.

(Colosimo B and del Castillo E eds.) 2006 *Bayesian Process Monitoring, Control and Optimization*. Chapman and Hall/CRC Press, Boca Raton, pp. 81–94.

Congdon P 2003 *Applied Bayesian Modelling*. John Wiley & Sons, New York.

Congdon P 2006 *Bayesian Models for Categorical Data*. John Wiley & Sons, New York.

Congdon P 2007 *Bayesian Statistical Modelling*. John Wiley & Sons, New York.

Congdon P 2010 *Applied Bayesian Hierarchical Methods*. Chapman and Hall/CRC, Boca Raton.

Cook R 1977 Detection of influential observations in linear regression. *Technometrics* **19**, 15–18.

Cook R and Lawless J 2007 *The Statistical Analysis of Recurrent Events*. Springer, New York.

Cook R and Weisberg S 1982 *Residuals and Influence in Regression*. Chapman and Hall, New York.

Cordani L and Wechsler S 2006 Teaching independence and exchangeability. *Proceedings of ICOTS-7*, July 2–6, 2006, Salvador, Brazil, pp. 1–5.

Cornfield J 1966 Sequential trials, sequential analysis and the likelihood principle. *The American Statistician* **April**, 18–23.

Cornfield J 1967 Bayes theorem. *Review of the International Statistical Institute* **35**, 34–49.

Cowles M and Carlin B 1996 Markov Chain Monte Carlo convergence diagnostics: A comparative review. *Journal of the American Statistical Association* **91**, 883–904.

Cox D 1972 Regression models and life-tables (with discussion). *Journal of the Royal Statistical Society: Series B* **34**, 187–220.

Cox D 1999 Discussion of 'Some statistical heresies'. *The Statistician* **48**, 30.

Crainiceanu C, Ruppert D and Wand M 2004 Spatially adaptive Bayesian P-splines with heteroscedastic errors. *Paper 61*. Johns Hopkins University, Department of Biostatistics Working Papers.

Crainiceanu C, Ruppert D and Wand M 2005 Bayesian analysis for penalized spline regression using WinBUGS. *Journal of Statistical Software* **14**, 1–24.

Crowne D and Marlowe D 1960 A new scale of social desirability independent of psychopathology. *Journal of Consulting Psychology* **24**, 349–354.

Cui Y, Hodges J, Kong X and Carlin B 2010 Partitioning degrees of freedom in hierarchical models and other richly parameterized models. *Technometrics* **52**, 124–136.

Dalal S and Hall W 1983 Approximating priors by mixtures of natural conjugate priors. *Journal of the Royal Statistical Society: Series B* **45**, 278–286.

Daniels M and Hogan J 2008 *Missing Data in Longitudinal Studies. Strategies for Bayesian Modeling and Sensitivity Analysis*. Chapman and Hall/CRC, Boca Raton.

Daniels M and Pourahmadi M 2002 Bayesian analysis of covariance matrices and dynamic models for longitudinal data. *Biometrika* **89**, 553–566.

Davidian M and Giltinan D 2003 Nonlinear models for repeated measurements data: An overview and update. *Journal of Agricultural, Biological, and Environmental Statistics* **8**, 387–419.

Dawid A 2002 Discussion of Bayesian measures of model complexity and fit (DJ Spiegelhalter, NG Best, BP Carlin, and A van der Linde, 2002). *Journal of the Royal Statistical Society: Series B* **64**, 624–625.

De Backer M, De Keyser P, De Vroey C and Lesaffre E 1996 A 12-week treatment for dermatophyte toe onycholysis: terbinafine 250 mg/day vs. itraconazole 200 mg/day – a double-blind comparative trial. *British Journal of Dermatology* **134**, 16–17.

de Boor C 1978 *A Practical Guide to Splines*. Springer, Berlin.

de Finetti B 1937 Foresight: Its logical laws, its subjective sources. In: *Studies in Subjective Probability* (HE Kyburg and HE Smokler, eds.). John Wiley & Sons, New York, pp. 55–187.

de Finetti B 1974 *Theory of Probability (two volumes)*. John Wiley & Sons, New York.

de Leeuw J, Hornik K and Mair P 2009 Isotone optimization in R: Pool-adjacent-violators (PAVA) and active set methods. *Journal of Statistical Software* **32**, 1–24.

Dellaportas P, Forster J and Ntzoufras I 2002 On Bayesian model and variable selection using MCMC. *Statistics and Computing* **12**, 27–36.

Dempster A, Laird N and Rubin D 1977 Maximum likelihood from incomplete data via the EM algorithm. *Journal of the Royal Statistical Society: Series B* **39**, 1–38.

Den Hond E, De Schryver M, Muylaert A, Lesaffre E and Kesteloot H 1994 The Inter regional Belgian Bank Employee Nutrition Study (IBBENS). *European Journal of Clinical Nutrition* **48**, 106–117.

Denison D, Holmes C, Mallick B and Smith A 2002 *Bayesian Methods for Nonlinear Classification and Regression*. John Wiley & Sons, New York.

Derado G, Bowman FD and Kilts C 2010 Modeling the spatial and temporal dependence in fMRI data. *Biometrics* **66**, 949–957.

Dey D, Gelfand A, Swartz T and Vlachos P 1998 A simulation-intensive approach for checking hierarchical models. *Test* **79**, 325–346.

Dey D, Ghosh S and Mallick B (eds.) 2000 *Generalized Linear Models: A Bayesian Perspective*. Marcel Dekker, Inc., New York.

Dey D, Ghosh S and Mallick B (eds.) 2011 *Bayesian Modeling in Bioinformatics*. Chapman and Hall/CRC, Boca Raton.

Diaconis P and Ylvisaker D 1985 Quantifying prior opinion. In: *Bayesian Statistics* (JM Bernardo *et al.*, eds.). North Holland, Amsterdam, vol. 2, pp. 133–156.

Diggle P 1990 *Time Series. A Biostatistical Introduction*. Oxford Science Publications, Oxford.

Do KA, Müller P and Vannucci M (eds.) 2006 *Bayesian Inference for Gene Expression and Proteomics*. Cambridge University Press, Cambridge.

Donnan G, Davis S and Chambers B 1996 Streptokinase for acute ischaemic stroke with relationship to time administration. *Journal of the American Medical Association* **276**, 961–966.

Dorny P, Phiri I, Vercruysse J, Gabriel S, Willingham A, Brandt J, Victor B, Speybroeck N and Berkvens D 2004 A Bayesian approach for estimating values for prevalence and diagnostic test characteristics of porcine cysticercosis. *International Journal for Parasitology* **34**, 569–576.

Doss H 1994 Markov chains for exploring posterior distributions. *The Annals of Statistics* **22**, 1728–1734.

Draper D 1999 Comment in: Bayesian model averaging: A tutorial. *Statistical Science* **14**, 405–409.

Draper D, Hodges J, Mallows C and Pregibon D 1993 Exchangeability and data analysis. *Journal of the Royal Statistical Society: Series A* **156**, 9–37.

Dryden I and Mardia K 1997 *The Statistical Analysis of Shape*. John Wiley & Sons, New York.

Dunson D and Herring A 2005 Bayesian model selection and averaging in additive and proportional hazards models. *Lifetime Data Analysis* **11**, 213–232.

Edwards A 1972 *Likelihood*. Cambridge University Press, Cambridge.

Edwards A 1997 What did Fisher mean by 'inverse probability' in 1912–1922? *Statistical Science* **3**, 177–184.

Efron B, Hastie T, Johnstone I and Tibshirani R 2004 Least angle regression. *The Annals of Statistics* **32**, 407–451.

Eilers P and Marx B 1996 Flexible smoothing with B-splines and penalties. *Statistical Science* **11**, 89–121.

Elliott P, Wakefield J, Best N and Briggs D (eds.) 2000 *Spatial Epidemiology: Methods and Applications*. Oxford University Press, London.

Epifani I, MacEachern S and Peruggia M 2008 Case-deletion importance sampling estimators: Central limit theorems and related results. *Electronic Journal of Statistics* **2**, 774–806.

Fearn T 1975 A Bayesian approach to growth curves. *Biometrika* **62**, 89–100.

Fernandez C, Ley E and Steel M 2001 Benchmark priors for Bayesian model averaging. *Journal of Econometrics* **100**, 381–427.

Fisher L and van Belle G 1993 Biostatistics. *A Methodology for the Health Sciences*. John Wiley & Sons, New York.

Fisher L, Dixon D, Herson J, Frankowski R, Hearon M and Pearce K 1990 Intention to treat in clinical trials. In: *Statistical Issues in Drug Research and Development* (K Pearce *et al.*, eds.). Marcel Dekker, New York, pp. 331–350.

Fisher R 1922 On the mathematical foundations of theoretical statistics. *Philosophical Transaction of the Royal Statistical Society A* **222**, 309–368.

Fisher R 1925 *Statistical Methods for Research Workers*. Oliver and Boyd, Edinburgh.

Fisher R 1935 *The Design of Experiments*. Oliver and Boyd, Edinburgh.

Fisher R 1959 *Statistical Methods and Scientific Inference* (2nd edition, revised). Oliver and Boyd, Edinburgh.

Fisher R 1993 Social desirability bias and the validity of indirect questioning. *The Journal of Consumer Research* **20**, 303–315.

Forster M 2000 Key concepts in model selection: performance and generalizability. *Journal of Mathematical Psychology* **44**, 205–231.

Fouskakis D, Ntzoufras I and Draper D 2009 Population-based reversible jump Markov Chain Monte Carlo methods for Bayesian variable selection and evaluation under cost limit restrictions. *Journal of the Royal Statistical Society: Series C (Applied Statistics)* **45**(58), 311–354.

Friston K, Ashburner J, Kiebel S, Nichols T and Penny W (eds.) 2007 *Statistical Parameter Mapping: The analysis of Functional Brain Images*. Academic Press, New York.

Gamerman D 1997 Sampling from the posterior distribution in generalized linear mixed models. *Statistics and Computing* **7**, 57–68.

Gangnon R 2006 Impact of prior choice on local Bayes factors for cluster detection. *Statistics in Medicine* **25**, 883–895.

Garcia-Zattera M, Mutsvari T, Jara A, Declerck D and Lesaffre E 2010 Correcting for misclassification for a monotone disease process with an application in dental research. *Statistics in Medicine* **29**, 3103–3117.

Geisser S 1980 Discussion of Sampling and Bayes' inference in scientific modelling and robustness (Box, 1980). *Journal of the Royal Statistical Society: Series A* **143**, 416–417.

Geisser S 1985 On the prediction of observables: A selective update. In: *Bayesian Statistics 2* (JM Bernardo *et al.*, eds.). North Holland, Amsterdam, pp. 203–230.

Geisser S and Eddy W 1979 A predictive approach to model selection. *Journal of the American Statistical Association* **74**, 153–160.

Gelfand A and Dey D 1994 Bayesian model choice: Asymptotics and exact calculations. *Journal of the Royal Statistical Society: Series B* **56**, 501–514.

Gelfand A and Ghosh S 1998 Model choice: A minimum posterior predictive loss approach. *Biometrika* **85**, 1–11.

Gelfand A and Kuo L 1991 Nonparametric Bayesian bioassay including ordered polytomous response. *Biometrika* **78**, 657–666.

Gelfand A and Sahu S 1999 Identifiability, improper priors, and Gibbs sampling for generalized linear models. *Journal of the American Statistical Association* **94**, 247–253.

Gelfand A and Smith A 1990 Sampling-based approaches to calculating marginal densities. *Journal of the American Statistical Association* **85**, 398–409.

Gelfand A, Carlin B and Smith A 1992 Hierarchical Bayesian analysis of change point problems. *Journal of the Royal Statistical Society: Series C (Applied Statistics)* **41**, 389–405.

Gelfand A, Hills S, Racine-Poon A and Smith A 1990 Illustration of Bayesian inference in normal data models using Gibbs sampling. *Journal of the American Statistical Association* **85**, 972–985.

Gelfand A, Sahu S and Carlin B 1995 Efficient parametrisations for normal linear mixed models. *Biometrika* **82**, 479–488.

Gelfand A, Sahu S and Carlin B 1996 Efficient parametrisations for generalized linear mixed models. In: *Bayesian Analysis 5* (JM Bernardo *et al.*, eds). Clarendon Press, Oxford, pp. 165–180.

Gelman A 2003 A Bayesian formulation of exploratory data analysis and goodness-of-fit testing. *International Statistical Review* **71**, 369–382.

Gelman A 2004 Exploratory data analysis for complex models. *Journal of Computational and Graphical Statistics* **13**, 755–779.

Gelman A 2006 Prior distributions for variance parameters in hierarchical models. *Bayesian Analysis* **1**, 515–533.

Gelman A and Meng XL 1996 Model checking and model improvement In: *Markov Chain Monte Carlo in Practice* (WR Gilks, S Richardson and DJ Spiegelhalter, eds), pp. 189–201. Chapman and Hall, London.

Gelman A and Rubin D 1992 Inference from iterative simulation using multiple sequences. *Statistical Science* **7**, 457–511.

Gelman A and Rubin D 1995 Avoiding model selection in Bayesian social research. Discussion of 'Bayesian model selection in social research,' by A Raftery. *Sociological Methodology* **25**, 165–173.

Gelman A, Carlin J, Stern H and Rubin D 2004 *Bayesian Data Analysis* (2nd edition). Chapman and Hall/CRC, Boca Raton.

Gelman A, Jakulin A, Pittau MG and Su YS 2008 A weakly informative default prior distribution for logistic and other regression models. *The Annals of Applied Statistics* **2**, 1360–1383.

Gelman A, Meng X and Stern H 1996 Posterior predictive assessment of model fitness via realized discrepancies. *Statistica Sinica* **6**, 733–807.

Gelman A, van Dyk AA, Huang Z and Boscardin JW 2008 Using redundant parameters to fit hierarchical models. *Journal of Computational and Graphical Statistics* **17**, 95–122.

Gelman A, Van Mechelen I, Verbeke G, Heitjan D and Meulders M 2005 Multiple imputation for model checking: completed-data plots with missing and latent data. *Biometrics* **61**, 74–85.

Geman S and Geman D 1984 Stochastic relaxation, Gibbs distributions, and the Bayesian restoration of images. *IEEE Transactions on Pattern Analysis and Machine Intelligence* **6**, 721–741.

Gentle J 1998 *Random Number Generation and Monte Carlo Methods*. Springer, New York.

George E 2000 The variable selection problem. *Journal of the American Statistical Association* **95**, 1304–1308.

George E and Foster D 2000 Calibration and empirical Bayes variable selection. *Biometrika* **87**, 731–747.

George E and McCulloch R 1993 Variable selection via Gibbs sampling. *Journal of the American Statistical Association* **88**(423), 881–889.

George E and McCulloch R 1997 Approaches for Bayesian variable selection. *Statistica Sinica* **7**, 339–373.

George E, McCulloch R and Tsay R 1996 Two approaches to Bayesian model selection with applications. In: *Bayesian Analysis and Environmetrics* (DA Berry, KM Chaloner and JK Geweke, eds.). John Wiley and Sons, New York, pp. 339–347.

Geuskens G, Hazes J, Barendregt P and Burdorf A 2008 Work and sick leave among patients with early inflammatory joint conditions. *Arthritis Rheumatology* **59**, 1458–1466.

Geweke J 1989 Bayesian inference in econometric models using Monte Carlo integration. *Econometrica* **57**, 1317–1339.

Geweke J 1992 Evaluating the accuracy of sampling-based approaches to the calculation of posterior moments. In: *Bayesian Statistics 4* (JM Bernardo *et al.*, eds.). Clarendon Press, Oxford, pp. 169–193.

Geyer C 1992 Practical Markov Chain Monte Carlo. *Statistical Science* **7**, 473–511.

Ghosh J and Ramamoorthi R 2003 *Bayesian Nonparametrics*. Springer, New York.

Ghosh M, Natarajan K, Stroud T and Carlin B 1998 Generalized linear models for small-area estimation. *Journal of the American Statistical Association* **93**, 273–282.

Ghosh S 2007 Adaptive elastic net: An improvement of elastic net to achieve oracle properties, pp. 1–26 *(http://www.math.iupui.edu/research/preprint/2007/pr07-01.pdf)*.

Gilks W and Wild P 1992 Adaptive rejection sampling for Gibbs sampling. *Journal of the Royal Statistical Society: Series C (Applied Statistics)* **41**, 337–348.

Gilks W, Richardson S and Spiegelhalter D 1996 *Markov Chain Monte Carlo in Practice*. Chapman and Hall, London.

Gilks W, Thomas A and Spiegelhalter D 1994 A language and program for complex Bayesian modelling. *The Statistician* **43**, 169–177.

Gilks, W.R. BN and Tan K 1995 Adaptive rejection Metropolis sampling. *Journal of the Royal Statistical Society: Series C (Applied Statistics)* **44**, 455–472.

Good I 1978 A. Alleged objectivity: a threat to the human spirit?. *International Statistical Review* **46**, 65–66.

Good I 1982 46556 varieties of Bayesians (letter). *The American Statistician* **25**, 62–63.

Goodman S 1993 P values, hypothesis tests, and likelihood: Implications for epidemiology of a neglected historical debate. *American Journal of Epidemiology* **137**(5), 485–500.

Goodman S 1999a Toward evidence-based medical statistics. 1: The *p*-value fallacy. *Annals Internal Medicine* **130**, 995–1004.

Goodman S 1999b Toward evidence-based medical statistics. 2: The Bayes factor. *Annals Internal Medicine* **130**, 1005–1013.

Gössl C and Küchenhoff H 2001 Bayesian analysis of logistic regression with an unknown change point and covariate measurement error. *Statistics in Medicine* **20**, 3109–3121.

Gössl C, Auer D and Fahrmeir L 2001 Bayesian spatio-temporal infernce in functional magnetic resonance imaging. *Biometrics* **57**, 554–562.

Gottardo R and Raftery A 2009 Bayesian robust transformation and variable selection: a unified approach. *The Canadian Journal of Statistics* **37**, 361–380.

Gramacy R and Pantaleoy E 2010 Shrinkage regression for multivariate inference with missing data, and an application to portfolio balancing. *Bayesian Analysis* **5**, 237–262.

Gravendeel A, Kouwenhoven M, Gevaert O, De Rooi J, Stubbs A, Duijm E, Daemen A, Bleeker F, Bralten B, Kloosterhof N, De Moor B, Eilers P, van der Spek P, Kros J, Sillevis Smitt P, van den Bent M and French P 2009 Intrinsic gene expression profiles of gliomas are a better predictor of survival than histology. *Cancer Research* **69**, 9065–9072.

Green MJ, Medley GF and Browne WJ 2009 Use of posterior predictive assessments to evaluate model fit in multilevel logistic regression. http://dx.doi.org/10.1051/vetres/2009013

Green P 1990 Bayesian reconstructions from emission tomography data using a modified EM algorithm. *IEEE Transactions on Medical Imaging* **9**, 84–93.

Green P 1995 Reversible jump Markov chain Monte Carlo computation and Bayesian model determination. *Biometrika* **82**, 711–732.

Green P and Han X 1990 Metropolis methods, Gaussian proposals and antithetic variables In: *Stochastic Models, Statistical Methods and Algortihms in Image Analysis*, vol. 74 (P Barone, A Frigessi and M Picconi, eds.). Springer-Verlag, Berlin, pp. 142–164.

Green P and Silverman B 1994 *Nonparametric Regression and Generalized Linear Models. A Roughness Penalty Approach*. Chapman and Hall, London.

Greenland S 2001 Putting background information about relative risks into conjugate prior distributions. *Biometrics* **57**, 663–670.

Greenland S 2003 Generalized conjugate priors for Bayesian analysis of risk and survival regressions. *Biometrics* **59**, 92–99.

Greenland S 2007 Prior data for non-normal priors. *Statistics in Medicine* **26**, 3578–3590.

Greenland S and Christensen R 2001 Data augmentation priors for Bayesian and semi-Bayesian analyses of conditional-logistic and proportional hazards regression. *Statistics in Medicine* **20**, 2421–2428.

Guerrero V and Johnson R 1982 Use of the Box-Cox transformation with binary response models. *Biometrika* **69**, 309–314.

Guo X and Carlin B 2004 Separate and joint modeling of longitudinal and event time data using standard computer packages. *The American Statistician* **58**, 1–9.

Gupta R and Richards DSP 2001 The history of the Dirichlet and Liouville distributions. *International Statistical Review* **69**, 433–446.

Gurrin L, Scurrah K and Hazelton M 2005 Tutorial in biostatistics: spline smoothing with linear mixed models. *Statistics in Medicine* **24**, 3361–3381.

Gustafson P 1998a Flexible Bayesian modelling for survival data. *Lifetime Data Analysis* **4**, 281–299.

Gustafson P 1998b A guided walk Metropolis algorithm. *Statistics and Computing* **8**, 357–364.

Gustafson P 2004 *Measurement Error and Misclassification in Statistics and Epidemiology*. Chapman and Hall/CRC Press, Boca Raton.

Gustafson P 2009 What are the limits of posterior distributions arising from nonidentified models, and why should we care? *Journal of the American Statistical Association* **104**, 1682–1695.

Guttman I 1967 The use of the concept of a future observation in goodness-of-fit problems. *Journal of the Royal Statistical Society: Series B* **29**, 83–100.

Guttman I and Peña D 1993 A Bayesian look at diagnostics in the univariate linear model. *Statistica Sinica* **3**, 367–390.

Hacke W, Kaste M, Bluhmki E, Brozman M, Dávalos A and al. 2008 Thrombolysis with Alteplase 3 to 4.5 hours after acute ischemic stroke. *New England Journal of Medicine* **13**, 1317–1329.

Hacke W, Kaste M, Fieschi C, Toni D, Lesaffre E, von Kummer R, Boysen R, Bluhmki E, Höxter G, Mahagne M and Hennerici M 1995 Intravenous thrombolysis with recombinant tissue plasminogen activator for acute hemispheric stroke. The European Cooperative Acute Stroke Study (ECASS). *Journal of the American Medical Association* **274**, 1017–1025.

Hacke W, Kaste M, Fieschi C, von Kummer R, Davalos T, Meier D, Larrue V, Bluhmki E, Davis S, Donnan G, Schneider D, Diez-Tejedor E and Trouillas P 1998 Randomised double-blind placebo-controlled trial of thrombolytic therapy with intravenous alteplase in acute ischaemic stroke (ECASS II). *The Lancet* **352**, 1245–1251.

Hald A 2007 *A History of Parametric Statistical Inference from Bernoulli to Fisher*, 1713–1935. Springer, New York.

Hans C 2009 Bayesian lasso regression. *Biometrika* **96**, 835–845.

Hans C, Dobra A and West M 2007 Shotgun stochastic search for 'large p' regression. *Journal of the American Statistical Association* **102**, 507–516.

Hansen M, Møller J and Tøgersen F 2002 Bayesian contour detection in a time series of ultrasound images through dynamic deformable template models. *Biostatistics* **3**, 213–228.

Hartvig N and Jensen J 2000 Spatial mixture modelling of fMRI data. *Human Brain Mapping* **11**, 233–248.

Harville D 1974 Bayesian inference for variance components using only error contrasts. *Biometrika* **61**, 383–385.

Hastie D and Green P 2012 Model choice using Reversible Jump Markov Chain Monte Carlo. *Statistica Neerlandica* **66**, accepted for publication.

Hastie T and Tibshirani R 1986 Generalized additive models. *Statistical Science* **1**, 297–318.

Hastie T, Tibshirani R and Friedman J 2009 *The Elements of Statistical Learning. Data Mining, Inference and Prediction*. New York, Springer.

Hastings W 1970 Monte Carlo sampling methods using Markov chains and their applications. *Biometrika* **57**, 97–109.

Hedeker D and Gibbons R 1994 A random-effects ordinal regression for multilevel analysis. *Biometrics* **50**, 933–944.

Heidelberger P and Welch P 1983 Simulation run length control in the presence of an initial transient. *Operations Research* **31**, 1109–1144.

Held L 2004 Simultaneous posterior probability statements from Monte Carlo output. *Journal of Computational and Graphical Statistics* **13**, 20–35.

Held L 2010 A nomogram for P values. *BMC Medical Research Methodology*. **10**:21. doi:10.1186/1471-2288-10-21.

Henderson R, Shimakura S and Gorst D 2002 Modeling spatial variation in leukaemia survival data. *Journal of the American Statistical Association* **97**, 965–972.

Higdon D 2002 Space and space-time modeling using process convolutions In: *Quantitative Methods for Current Environmental Issues* (C Anderson, V Barnett, P Chatwin, A, El-Shaarawi, eds.). Springer, London, pp. 37–54.

Hill B 1965 Inference about variance components in the one-way model. *Journal of the American Statistical Association* **60**, 806–825.

Hill B 1996 Discussion of Posterior predictive assessment of model fitness via realized discrepancies (Gelman, Meng and Stern, 1996). *Statistica Sinica* **6**, 767–773.

Hills S and Smith A 1992 Parametrization issues in Bayesian inference. In: Bayesian Analysis, vol. 4. (JM Bernardo, J Berger, AP Dawid and AFM Smith, eds.) Oxford University Press, Oxford, pp. 227–246.

Hitchcock D 2003 A history of the Metropolis-Hastings algorithm. *The American Statistician* **57**, 254–257.

Hjort NL, Holmes C, Müller P and Walker S (eds.) 2010 *Bayesian Nonparametrics*. Cambridge University Press, London.

Hobert J and Casella G 1996 The effect of improper priors on Gibbs sampling in hierarchical linear mixed models. *Journal of the American Statistical Association* **91**, 1461–1473.

Hodges J 1998 Some algebra and geometry for hierarchical models, applied to diagnostics. *Journal of the Royal Statistical Society: Series B* **60**, 497–536.

Hodges J and Sargent D 2001 Counting degrees of freedom in hierarchical models and other richly-parametrised models. *Biometrika* **88**, 367–379.

Hoeting J, Madigan D, Raftery A and Volinsky C 1999a Bayesian model averaging: A tutorial (with discussion). *Statistical Science* **14**, 382–417.

Hoeting J, Madigan D, Raftery A and Volinsky C 1999b Rejoinder: Bayesian model averaging: A tutorial. *Statistical Science* **14**, 412–417.

Hoeting J, Raftery A and Madigan D 1996 A method for simultaneous variable selection and outlier detection. *Journal of Computational Statistics* **22**, 251–271.

Hoeting J, Raftery A and Madigan D 2002 Bayesian variable and transformation selection in linear regression. *Journal of Computational and Graphical Statistics* **11**, 429–467.

Holzer M, Müllner M, Sterz F, Robak O and Kliegel A 2006 Efficacy and safety of endovascular cooling after cardiac arrest: Cohort study and Bayesian approach. *Stroke* **37**, 1792–1797.

Hossain M and Lawson A 2006 Cluster detection diagnostics for small area health data: With reference to evaluation of local likelihood models. *Statistics in Medicine* **25**, 771–786.

Howard J 1998 The 2× 2 table: A discussion from a Bayesian viewpoint. *Statistical Science* **13**, 351–367.

Hubbard R and Bayarri M 2003 Confusion over measures of evidence (p's) versus errors (α's) in classical statistical testing. *The American Statistician* **57**(3), 171–182.

Ibrahim J and Chen MH 2000 Power prior distributions for regression models. *Statistical Science* **15**, 46–60.

Ibrahim J and Laud P 1991 On Bayesian analysis of generalized linear models using Jeffrey's prior. *Journal of the American Statistical Association* **86**, 981–986.

Ibrahim J, Chen M and Sinha D 2000 *Bayesian Survival Analysis*. Springer, New York.

Ibrahim J, Chen MH and Sinha D 2003 On optimality properties of the power prior. *Journal of the American Statistical Association* **98**, 204–213.

Ibrahim J, Chu H and Chen L 2001 Basic concepts and methods for joint models of longitudinal and survival data. *Journal of Clinical Oncology* **28**, 2796–2801.

Ibrahim J, Ryan L and Chen MH 1998 Using historical controls to adjust for covariates in trend tests for binary data. *Journal of the American Statistical Association* **93**, 1282–1293.

Ioannidus J 2005 Why most published research findings are false. *PLoS Medicine* (www.plosmedicine.org) **2**, 696–701.

Ishawaran H and James L 2004 Computational methods for multiplicative intensity models using weighted gamma processes: Proportional hazards, marked point processes, and panel count data. *Journal of the American Statistical Association* **99**, 175–190.

Ishwaran H and Rao J 2003 Detecting differentially expressed genes in microarrays using Bayesian model selection. *Journal of the American Statistical Association* **98**, 438–455.

Ishwaran H and Rao J 2005 Spike and slab variable selection: Frequentist and Bayesian strategies. *The Annals of Statistics* **33**, 730–773.

Jasra A, Holmes C and Stephens D 2005 Markov Chain Monte Carlo Methods and the label switching problem in Bayesian mixture modeling. *Statistical Science* **20**, 50–67.

Jasra A, Stephens D and Holmes C 2007a On population-based simulation for static inference. *Statistics and Computing* **17**, 263–279.

Jasra A, Stephens D and Holmes C 2007b Population-based reversible Jump Markov Chain Monte Carlo. *Biometrika* **94**, 787–807.

Jeffreys H 1946 An invariant form for the prior probability in estimation problems. *Proceedings of the Royal Statistical Society: Series A* **186**, 453–461.

Jeffreys H 1961 *Theory of Probability* (3rd edition). Oxford University Press, Oxford.

Jennison C and Turnbull B 2000 *Group Sequential Methods with Applications to Clinical Trials*. Chapman and Hall/CRC, Boca Raton.

Johnson S, Tomlinson G, Hawker G, Granton J and Feldman B 2010 Methods to elicit beliefs for Bayesian priors: A systematic review. *Journal of Clinical Epidemiology* **63**, 355–369.

Johnson W and Geisser S 1983 A predictive view of the detection and characterization of influential observations in regression analysis. *Journal of the American Statistical Association* **78**, 137–144.

Jones G and Hobert J 2001 Honest exploration of intractable probability distributions via Markov Chain Monte Carlo. *Statistical Science* **16**, 312–334.

Joseph L, Gyorkos T and Coupal L 1995 Bayesian estimation of disease prevalence and the parameters of diagnostic tests in the absence of a gold standard. *American Journal of Epidemiology* **141**, 263–272.

Kadane J and Lazar N 2004 Methods and criteria for model selection. *Journal of the American Statistical Association* **99**, 279–290.

Kadane J and Wolfson L 1996 Priors for the design and analysis of clinical trials. In: *Bayesian Biostatistics* (DA Berry and DK Stangl, eds.). Marcel Dekker, New York, pp. 157–184.

Kadane J and Wolfson L 1997 Experiences in elicitation. *The Statistician* **46**, 1–17.

Kadane J, Dickey J, Winkler R, Smith W and Peters S 1980 Interactive elicitation of opinion for a normal linear model. *Journal of the American Statistical Association* **75**, 845–854.

Kahn H and Marshall A 1953 Methods of reducing sample size in Monte Carlo computations. *Journal of the Operations Research Society of America* **1**, 263–278.

Kahn M and Raftery A 1996 Discharge rates of Medicare stroke patients to skilled nursing facilities: Bayesian logistic regression with unobserved heterogeneity. *Journal of the American Statistical Association* **91**, 29–41.

Kaldor J, Day N, Clarke E and Van Leeuwen F 1990 Leukemia following Hodgkin's disease. *New England Journal of Medicine* **322**, 7–13.

Kass R and Raftery A 1995 Bayes factors. *Journal of the American Statistical Association* **90**, 773–795.

Kass R and Wasserman L 1996 The selection of prior distributions by formal rules. *Journal of the American Statistical Association* **91**, 1343–1370.

Kass R, Carlin B, Gelman A and Neal R 1998 Markov Chain Monte Carlo in practice: A roundtable discussion. *The American Statistician* **52**, 93–100.

Kass R, Tierney L and Kadane J 1989 Approximate methods for assessing influence and sensitivity in Bayesian analysis. *Biometrika* **76**, 663–674.

Kiiveri H 2003 A Bayesian approach to variable selection when the number of variables is very large. *Lecture Notes-Monograph Series. Statistics and Science: A Festschrift for Terry Speed* **40**, 127–143.

Kim B and Margolin B 1999 Statistical methods for the Ames Salmonella assay: A review. *Mutation Research: Reviews in Mutation Research* **436**, 113–122.

Kim JI, Lawson A, McDermott S and Aelion C 2010 Bayesian spatial modeling of disease risk in relation to multivariate environmental risk fields. *Statistics in Medicine* **29**, 142–157.

King R, Morgan B, Gimenez O and Brooks S 2009 *Bayesian Analysis for Population Ecology*. Chapman and Hall/CRC Press, Boca Raton.

Kipnis V, Carroll R, Freedman L and Li L 1999 A new dietary measurement error model and its application to the estimation of relative risk: Application to four validation studies. *American Journal of Epidemiology* **150**, 642–651.

Kipnis V, Midthune D, Freedman L, Bingham S, Schatzkin A, Subar A and Carroll R 2001 Empirical evidence of correlated biases in dietary assessment instruments and its implications. *American Journal of Epidemiology* **153**, 394–403.

Kipnis V, Subar A, Midthune D, Freedman L, Ballard-Barbash L, Troiano R, Bingham S, Schoeller D, Schatzkin A and Carroll R 2003 The structure of dietary measurement error: Results of the OPEN biomarker study. *American Journal of Epidemiology* **158**, 14–21.

Kirkland DJ (eds.) 2008 *Statistical Evaluation of Mutagenicity test Data*. Cambridge University Press, New York.

Kirkpatrick S, Gelatt CD and Vecchi MP 1983 Optimization by simulated annealing. *Science* **220**, 671–680.

Kloek T and van Dijk H 1978 Bayesian estimates of equation system parameters: An application of integration by Monte Carlo. *Econometrica* **46**, 1–20.

Komárek A and Lesaffre E 2008 Bayesian accelerated failure time model with multivariate doubly-interval-censored data and flexible distributional assumptions. *Journal of the American Statistical Association* **103**, 523–533.

Komárek A, Lesaffre E and Hilton J 2005 Accelerated failure time model for arbitrarily censored data with smoothed error distribution. *Journal of Computational and Graphical Statistics* **14**, 726–745.

Kooperberg C, Stone C and Truong Y 1995 Hazard regression. *Journal of the American Statistical Association* **90**, 78–94.

Korb K and Nicholson A 2004 *Bayesian Artificial Intelligence*. Chapman and Hall/CRC, Boca Raton.

Krause R, Anand V, Gruemer HD and Willke T 1975 The impact of laboratory error on the normal range: A Bayesian model. *Clinical Chemistry* **21**, 321–324.

Krewski D, Leroux BG, Bleuer S and Broekhoven L 1993 Modeling the Ames Salmonella/Microsome Assay. *Biometrics* **49**, 499–510.

Krishna A, Bondell H and Ghosh S 2009 Bayesian variable selection using an adaptive powered correlation prior. *Journal of the Statistical Planning and Inference* **139**, 2665–2674.

Krishnamoorthy K and Mathew T 2009 *Statistical Tolerance Regions*. John Wiley & Sons, New York.

Kuha J 2004 AIC and BIC: Comparisons of assumptions and performance. *Sociological Methods and Research* **33**, 188–229.

Kulldorff M and Nagarwalla N 1995 Spatial disease clusters:Detection and inference. *Statistics in Medicine* **14**, 799–810.

Kunsch H 1987 Intrinsic autoregressions and related models on the two-dimensional lattice. *Biometrika* **74**, 517–524.

Kuo L and Mallick B 1998 Variable selection for regression models. *The Indian Journal of Statistics: Series B* **60**, 65–81.

Kwon D, Landi M, Vannucci M, Issaq H, Prieto D and Pfeiffer R 2011 An efficient stochastic search for Bayesian variable selection with high-dimensional correlated predictors. *Computational Statistics and Data Analysis* **55**, 2807–2818.

Kyung M, Gill J, Ghosh J and Casella G 2010 Penalized regression, standard errors, and Bayesian Lassos. *Bayesian Analysis* **5**, 369–412.

Lambert P 2006 A comment on the article of Browne and Draper. *Bayesian Analysis* **1**, 543–546.

Lang S and Brezger A 2004 Bayesian P-splines. *Journal of Computational and Graphical Statistics* **13**, 183–212.

Lange KL, Little R and Taylor J 1989 Robust statistical modeling using the t-distribution. *Journal of the American Statistical Association* **84**, 881–896.

Lange N 2003 What can modern statistics offer imaging neuroscience? *Statistical Methods in Medical Research* **12**, 447–469.

Lange N, Carlin B and Gelfand A 1992 Hierarchical Bayes models for the progression of HIV infection using longitudinal CD4+ counts (with discussion). *Journal of the American Statistical Association* **87**, 615–632.

Laud P and Ibrahim J 1995 Predictive model selection. *Journal of the Royal Statistical Society: Series B* **57**, 247–262.

Lawson A 2006 *Statistical Methods in Spatial Epidemiology* (2nd edition). John Wiley & Sons, New York.

Lawson A 2009 *Bayesian Disease Mapping: Hierarchical Modeling in Spatial Epidemiology*. Chapmand and Hall/CRC, New York.

Lawson A and Banerjee S 2010 Bayesian spatial analysis. In: *Handbook of Spatial Analysis* (S Fotheringham and P Rogerson, eds.). Sage, New York, Chapter 9.

Lawson A and Clark A 1999 Markov chain Monte Carlo methods for clustering in case event and count data in spatial epidemiology. In: *Statistics and Epidemiology: Environment and Clinical Trials* (ME Halloran and D Berry, eds.). Springer-Verlag, New York, pp. 193–218.

Lawson A and Denison D 2002 Spatial cluster modelling: An overview. In: *Spatial Cluster Modelling* (AB Lawson and D Denison, eds.). CRC Press, New York, Chapter 1, pp. 1–19.

Lawson A and Song H-R 2010 Semiparametric space-time survival modeling of chronic wasting disease in deer. *Environmental and Ecological Statistics* **17**, 559–571.

Lawson A, Browne W and Vidal Rodeiro C 2003 *Disease Mapping with WinBUGS and MLwiN, v2.10*. John Wiley & Sons, New York.

Lazar N 2008 *The Statistical Analysis of Functional fMRI Data*. Springer, New York.

Lee K, Sha N, Dougherty E, Vannucci M and Mallick B 2003 Gene selection: A Bayesian variable selection approach. *Bioinformatics* **19**, 90–97.

Lee Y, Nelder J and Pawitan Y 2006 *Generalized Linear Models with Random Effects. Unified Analysis via H-Likelihood*. Chapman and Hall/CRC, Boca Raton.

Leng C, Tran M and Nott D 2009 Bayesian adaptive Lasso. *Technical Report*: *http://arxiv.org/abs/1009.2300*, pp. 1–18.

Lesaffre E and Albert A 1989 Partial separation in logistic discrimination. *Journal of the Royal Statistical Society: Series B* **51**, 109–116.

Lesaffre E and Kaufmann H 1992 Existence and uniqueness of the maximum likelihood estimator for a multivariate probit model. *Journal of the American Statistical Association* **87**, 805–811.

Lesaffre E and Marx B 1993 Collinearity in generalized linear regression. *Communications in Statistics, Theory and Methods* **22**, 1933–1952.

Lesaffre E and Spiessens B 2001 On the effect of the number of quadrature points in a logistic random-effects model: An example. *Journal of the Royal Statistical Society: Series C (Applied Statistics)* **50**, 325–335.

Lesaffre E and Willems J 1988 Measuring the certainty of a decision rule with applications in electrocardiography. *Methods of Information in Medicine* **27**, 155–160.

Lesaffre E, Asafa M and Verbeke G 1999 Assessing the goodness-of-fit of the Laird and Ware model – An example: The Jimma Infant Survival Differential Longitudinal Study. *Statistics in Medicine* **18**, 835–854.

Lesaffre E, Küchenhoff H, Mwalili S and Declerck D 2009 On the estimation of the misclassification table for finite count data with an application in caries research. *Statistical Modelling* **9**, 99–118.

Lesaffre E, Mwalili S and Declerck D 2004 Analysis of caries experience taking inter-observer bias and variability into account. *Journal of Dental Research* **83**, 951–955.

Li B, Lingsma H, Steyerberg E and Lesaffre E 2011 Logistic random effects regression models: A comparison of statistical packages for binary and ordinal outcomes. *BMC Medical Research Methodology* **11**: 77. doi:10.1186/1471-2288-11-77.

Li Q and Lin N 2010 The Bayesian Elastic Net. *Bayesian Analysis* **5**, 151–170.

Liang F and Wong WH 2000 Evolutionary Monte Carlo: Applications to Cp model sampling and change point problems. *Statistica Sinica* **45**, 311–354.

Liang F, Paulo R, Molina G, Clyde M and Berger J 2008 Mixtures of *g*-priors for Bayesian variable selection. *Journal of the American Statistical Association* **103**, 410–423.

Liang K and Zeger S 1986 Longitudinal data analysis using generalized linear models. *Biometrika* **73**, 13–22.

Liese A, Schulz M, Moore C and Mayer-Davis E 2004 Dietary patterns, insulin sensitivity and adiposity in the multi-ethnic Insulin Resistance Atherosclerosis Study population. *British Journal of Nutrition* **92**, 973–84.

Lin T and Dayton CM 1997 Model selection information criterion criteria for non-nested latent class models. *Journal of Educational and Behavioral Statistics* **22**, 249–264.

Lindley D 1957 A statistical paradox. *Biometrika* **44**, 187–192.

Lindley D 1971 The estimation of many parameters. *Foundations of Statistical Inference* (VP Godambe and DA Sprott, eds.), pp. 435–455, Toronto: Holt, Rinehart and Winston.

Lindley D 2006 *Understanding Uncertainty*. John Wiley & Sons, New York.

Lindley D and Smith A 1972 Bayes estimates for the linear model (with discussion). *Journal of the Royal Statistical Society: Series B* **34**, 14–46.

Lindstrom M and Bates D 1990 Nonlinear mixed effects models for repeated measures data. *Biometrics* **46**, 673–687.

Little R and Rubin D 2002 *Statistical Analysis with Missing Data* (2nd edition). John Wiley & Sons, New York.

Liu C and Wu Y 1999 Parameter expansion for data augmentation. *Journal of the American Statistical Association* **94**, 1264–1274.

Liu C, Rubin D and Wu Y 1998 Parameter expansion to accelerate EM: The PX-EM algorithm. *Biometrika* **85**, 755–770.

Liu J and Hodges J 2003 Posterior bimodality in the balanced one-way random effects model. *Journal of the Royal Statistical Society: Series B* **65**, 247–255.

Lu H, Hodges J and Carlin B 2007 Measuring the complexity of generalized linear hierarchical models. *The Canadian Journal of Statistics* **35**, 69–87.

Lunn D, Best N and Whittaker J 2009a Generic reversible jump MCMC using graphical models. *Statistics and Computing* **19**, 395–408.

Lunn D, Spiegelhalter D, Thomas A and Best N 2009b The BUGS project: evolution, critique and future directions. *Statistics in Medicine* **25**, 3049–3067.

Madigan D, York J and Allard D 1995 Bayesian graphical models for discrete data. *International Statistical Review* **63**, 215–232.

Mallick B, Gold D and Balandandaythapani V 2009 *Bayesian Analysis of Gene Expression Data*. John Wiley & Sons, New York.

Mansourian M, Kazemnejad A, Kazemi I, Zayeri F and Soheilian M 2012 Bayesian analysis of longitudinal ordered data with flexible random effects using McMC: Application to diabetec macular Edema data. *Journal of Applied Statistics* **39**, 1087–1100.

Margolin B, Kim B and Risko K 1989 The Ames Salmonelle/Microsome Mutagenicity Assay: Issues of Inference and Validation. *Journal of the American Statistical Association* **84**, 651–661.

Marin JM and Robert C 2007 *Bayesian Core: A Practical Approach to Computational Bayesian Statistics*. Springer, New York.

Marshall E and Spiegelhalter D 2007 Identifying outliers in Bayesian hierarchical models: A simulation-based approach. *Bayesian Analysis* **2**, 409–444.

Mc Grayne S 2011 *The Theory That Would Not Die. How Bayes' Rule Cracked the Enigma Code, Hunted Down Russian Submarines & Emerged Triumphant from Two Centuries of Controversy*. Yale University Press, New Haven and London.

McCarthy M 2007 *Bayesian Methods for Ecology*. Cambridge University Press, Cambridge.

McCullagh P and Nelder J 1989 *Generalized Linear Models* (2nd edition). Chapman and Hall, London.

McLachlan G and Peel D 2000 *Finite Mixture Models*. John Wiley & Sons, New York.

Meng X 1994 Posterior predictive p-values. *The Annals of Statistics* **22**, 1142–1160.

Mengersen K, Knight S and Robert C 1999 MCMC: How do we know when to stop? *Proceedings of the 52nd Bulletin of the International Statistical Institute. Book 1*, Helsinki, Finland.

Metropolis N, Rosenbluth A, Rosenbluth M, Teller A and Teller E 1953 Equations of state calculations by fast computing machines. *Journal of Chemical Physics* **21**, 1087–1092.

Meyn S and Tweedie R 1993 *Markov Chains and Stochastic Stability*. Springer-Verlag, London.

Millar R 2009 Comparison of hierarchical Bayesian models for overdispersed count data using DIC and Bayes' factors. *Biometrics* **65**, 962–969.

Millar R and Stewart W 2007 Assessment of locally influential observations in Bayesian models. *Bayesian Analysis* **2**, 365–384.

Miller A 2002 *Subset Selection in Regression*. Chapman and Hall/CRC Press, Boca Raton.

Mitchell T and Beauchamp J 1988 Bayesian variable selection in linear regression. *Journal of the American Statistical Association* **83**(404), 1023–1032.

Möhner M, Stabenow R and Eisinger B 1994 *Atlas der Krebsinzidenz in der DDR 1961–1989*. Berlin: Ullstein Mosby.

Molenberghs G and Verbeke G 2005 *Models for Discrete Longitudinal Data*. Springer, New York.

Molina R and Ripley B 1989 Using spatial models as priors in astronomical image analysis. *Journal of Applied Statistics* **16**, 193–206.

Mollié A 1999 Bayesian and empirical Bayes approaches to disease mapping. In: *Disease Mapping and Risk Assessment for Public Health* (A Lawson, and A Biggeri, D Boehning, E Lesaffre, J-F Viel and R Bertollini, eds.). John Wiley & Sons, Chichester, Chapter 2, pp. 15–29.

Moore M, Honma M and Clements Jea 2003 Mouse lymphoma thymidine kinase gene mutation assay: International workshop on genotoxicity tests workgroup report – Plymouth, UK 2002. *Mutation Research* **540**, 127–140.

Moreau T, O'Quigley J and Mesbah M 1985 A global goodness-of-fit statistic for the proportional hazards model. *Journal of the Royal Statistical Society: Series C (Applied Statistics)* **34**, 212–218.

Mortelmans K and Zeiger E 2000 The Ames Salmonella/microsome mutagenicity assay. *Mutation Research* **455**, 29–60.

Moyé L 2008 *Elementary Bayesian Biostatistics*. Chapman and Hall/CRC, Boca Raton.

Mutsvari T, Lesaffre E, Garcia-Zattera M, Diya L and Declerck D 2010 Factors that influence data quality in caries experience screening: A multi-level modeling approach. *Caries Research* **44**, 438–444.

Mwalili S, Lesaffre E and Declerck D 2005 A Bayesian ordinal logistic regression model to correct for inter-observer measurement error in a geographical oral health study. *Journal of the Royal Statistical Society: Series C (Applied Statistics)* **54**, 77–93.

Mwalili S, Lesaffre E and Declerck D 2008 The zero-inflated negative binomial regression model with correction for misclassification: An example in caries research. *Statistical Methods in Medical Research* **17**, 123–139.

Myers R 1998 *Classical and Modern Regression Analysis with Applications*. PWS-Kent Publishing Company.

Natarajan R and Kass R 2000 Reference Bayesian methods for generalized linear mixed models. *Journal of the American Statistical Association* **95**, 227–237.

Naylor J and Smith A 1982 Applications of a method for the efficient computation of posterior distributions. *Journal of the Royal Statistical Society: Series C (Applied Statistics)* **31**, 214–225.

Neal R 1995 Suppressing random walks in Markov chain Monte Carlo using ordered overrelaxation. *Technical Report 9508 (http://www/statslab.cam.ac.uk/mcmc/)*.

Neal R 1996 *Bayesian Learning for Neural Networks*. Springer, New York.

Neuhaus J 1999 Bias and efficiency loss due to misclassified responses in binary regression. *Biometrika* **86**, 843–855.

Newton M and Raftery A 1994 Approximate Bayesian inference with the weighted likelihood bootstrap. *Journal of the Royal Statistical Society: Series B* **56**, 3–48.

Neyman J and Pearson E 1928a On the use and interpretation of certain test criteria for purposes of statistical inference. Part I. *Biometrika* **20A**, 175–240.

Neyman J and Pearson E 1928b On the use and interpretation of certain test criteria for purposes of statistical inference. Part II. *Biometrika* **20A**, 263–294.

Neyman J and Pearson E 1933 On the problem of the most efficient tests of statistical hypotheses. *Philosophical Transactions of the Royal Society of London, Seriesi A* **231**, 289–337.

Niinima A and Oja H 1999 Multivariate median. In: *Encyclopedia of Statistical Sciences*, vol. 3 (S Kotz, CB Read and D Banks, eds.). John Wiley & Sons, New York.

Ntzoufras I 2009 *Bayesian Modeling Using WinBUGS*. John Wiley & Sons, New York.

Ntzoufras I, Dellaportas P and Forster J 2003 Bayesian variable and link determination for generalized linear models. *Journal of Statistical Planning and Inference* **111**, 165–180.

O'Hagan A 1998 Eliciting expert beliefs in substantial practical applications. *The Statistician* **47**, 21–35.

O'Hagan A and Forster J 2004 Bayesian Inference. In: *Bayesian Inference in the series Kendall's Advanced Theory of Statistics*, vol. 2B. Arnold, London.

O'Hagan A and Leonhard T 1976 Bayes estimation subject to uncertainty about parameter constraints. *Biometrika* **63**, 201–202.

O'Hagan A, Buck C, Daneshkrah A, Eiser J, Garthwaite P, Jenkinson D, Oakly J and Rakow T 2006 *Uncertain Judgments: Eliciting Expert's Probabilities*. John Wiley & Sons, New York.

O'Hagan T 2006 Bayes Factors. *Significance* **3**, 184–186.

O'Hara R and Sillanpää 2009 A review of Bayesian variable selection methods: What, how and which. *Bayesian Analysis* **4**, 85–118.

O'Quigley J, Pepe M and Fisher L 1990 Continual reassessment method: A practical design for phase I clinical trials in cancer. *Biometrics* **46**, 33–48.

Park T and Casella G 2008 The Bayesian Lasso. *Journal of the American Statistical Association* **103**, 681–686.

Parmigiani G 2002 *Modeling in Medical Decision Making: A Bayesian Approach.* John Wiley & Sons, New York.

Pawitan Y 2001 *In All Likelihood: Statistical Modelling and Influence Using Likelihood.* Oxford Science Publications, New York.

Peruggia M 1997 On the variability of case-deletion importance sampling weights in the Bayesian linear model. *Journal of the American Statistical Association* **92**, 199–207.

Peruggia M 2007 Bayesian model diagnostics based on artificial autoregressive errors. *Bayesian Analysis* **2**, 817–842.

Peskun P 1973 Optimum Monte-Carlo sampling using Markov chains. *Biometrika* **60**, 607–612.

Pettit L and Smith A 1985 Outliers and influential observations in linear models. In: *Bayesian Statistics 2* (JM Bernardo *et al.*, eds.). North Holland, Amsterdam, pp. 473–494.

Pettitt L 1990 The conditional predictive ordinate for the normal distribution. *Journal of the Royal Statistical Society: Series B* **52**, 175–184.

Pham-Gia T 2004 Bayesian Inference. In: *Handbook of Beta Distribution and Its Applications* (A Gupta and S Nadarajah, eds.). Marcel Dekker, New York, pp. 361–422.

Piegorsch W and Bailer J 2005 *Analyzing Environmental Data.* John Wiley & Sons, New York.

Pikkuhookana P and Silanpää M 2009 Correcting for relatedness in Bayesian models for genomic data association analysis. *Heredity* **103**, 223–237.

Plummer M 2008 Penalized loss functions for Bayesian model comparison. *Biostatistics* **9**, 523–539.

Popper KR 1959 *Logic of Scientific Discovery.* Hutchinson, London.

Potthoff R and Roy S 1964 A generalized multivariate analysis of variance model useful especially for growth curve problems. *Biometrika* **5**, 313–326.

Pourahmadi M and Daniels M 2002 Dynamic conditionally linear mixed models for longitudinal data. *Biometrics* **58**, 225–231.

Pregibon D 1981 Logistic regression diagnostics. *The Annals of Statistics* **9**, 705–724.

Press J 2003 *Subjective and Objective Bayesian Statistics. Principles, Models and Applications.* John Wiley & Sons, New York.

Press S and Tanur J 2001 *The Subjectivity of Scientists and the Bayesian Approach.* John Wiley & Sons, New York.

Quiros A, Diez RM and Gamerman D 2010 Bayesian spatiotemporal model of fMRI data. *NeuroImage* **40**, 442–456.

Raftery A 1995 Bayesian model selection in social research. *Sociological Methodology* **25**, 111–163.

Raftery A 1996 Approximate Bayes factors and accounting for model uncertainty in generalized linear models. *Biometrika* **83**, 251–266.

Raftery A 1999 Bayes factors and BIC. *Sociological Methods & Research* **27**, 411–427.

Raftery A and Akman V 1986 Bayesian analysis of a Poisson process with a change-point. *Biometrika* **73**, 85–89.

Raftery A and Lewis S 1992 How many iterations in the Gibbs sampler? In: *Bayesian Statistics 4* (JM Bernardo *et al.*, eds.). Clarendon Press, London, pp. 765–776.

Raftery A and Madigan D 1994 Model selection and accounting for model uncertainty in graphical models using Occam's window. *Journal of the American Statistical Association* **89**, 1535–1546.

Raftery A, Madigan D and Hoeting J 1997 Bayesian model averaging for linear regression models. *Journal of the American Statistical Association* **92**, 179–191.

Raftery A, Madigan D and Volinsky C 1996 Accounting for model uncertainty in survival analysis improves predictive performance (with discussion). In: *Bayesian Statistics 5* (JM Bernardo *et al.*, eds.). Oxford Science Publications, Oxford, pp. 323–349.

Ramgopal P, Laud P and Smith A 1993 Nonparametric Bayesian bioassay with prior constraints on the shape of the potency curve. *Biometrika* **80**, 489–498.

Rao C 1973 *Linear Statistical Inference and Applications*. John Wiley & Sons, New York.

Rasbash J, Steele F, Browne W and Goldstein H 2009 *A Users Guide to MLwiN, v2.10*. Centre for Multilevel Modelling, University of Bristol.

Richardson S 2002 Discussion of Bayesian measures of model complexity and fit (DJ Spiegelhalter, NC Best, BP Carlin and A van der Linde, 2002). *Journal of the Royal Statistical Society: Series B* **64**, 626–627.

Richardson S, Thomson A, Best N and Elliott P 2004 Interpreting posterior relative risk estimates in disease mapping studies. *Environmental Health Perspectives* **112**, 1016–1025.

Ripley B 1987 *Stochastic Simulation*. John Wiley & Sons, New York.

Ripley B 1988 *Statistical Inference for Spatial Processes*. Cambridge University Press, Cambridge.

Robert C and Casella G 2004 *Monte Carlo Statistical Methods*. Springer Texts in Statistics, New York.

Robert C and Titterington D 2002 Discussion of Bayesian measures of model complexity and fit (DJ Spiegelhalter, NG Best, BP Carlin and A van der Linde, 2002). *Journal of the Royal Statistical Society: Series B* **64**, 621–622.

Roberts G and Sahu S 1997 Updating schemes, correlation structures, blocking and parametrization for the Gibbs sampler. *Journal of the Royal Statistical Society: Series B* **59**, 291–317.

Roberts G, Gelman A and Gilks W 1997 Weak convergence and optimal scaling of random walk Metropolis algorithms. *Annals Applied Probability* **7**, 110–120.

Robins J, van der Vaart A and Ventura V 2000 The asymptotic distribution of p-values in composite null models. *Journal of the American Statistical Association* **95**, 1143–1172.

Rockova V, Lesaffre E, Luime J and Löwenberg B 2012 Hierarchical Bayesian formulations for selecting variables in regression models. *Statistics in Medicine (accepted)*. DOI: 10.1002/sim.4439.

Ross S 2000 *Introduction to Probability Models* (7th edition). Academic Press, San Diego.

Rosset S and Zhu J 2004 Corrected proof of the results of 'a prediction error property of the lasso estimator and its generalization' by Huang (2003). *Australian and New Zealand Journal of Statistics* **46**, 505–510.

Rowe D 2003 *Multivariate Bayesian Statistics*. Chapman and Hall/CRC Press, London.

Royall R 1997 *Statistical Evidence: A Likelihood Paradigm*. Chapman and Hall, London.

Royston P and Altman D 1994 Regression using fractional polynomials of continuous covariates: Parsimonious modelling. *Journal of the Royal Statistical Society: Series C (Applied Statistics)* **43**, 429–467.

Rubin D 1984 Bayesian justifiable and relevant frequency calculations for the applied statistician. *The Annals of Statistics* **12**, 1151–1172.

Rubin D 1988 Using the SIR algorithm to simulate posterior distributions. In: *Bayesian Statistics 3* (JM Bernardo *et al*., eds.). Clarendon Press, Oxford, pp. 395–402.

Rue H and Held L 2005 *Gaussian Markov Random Fields: Theory and Applications*. Chapman and Hall/CRC Press, New York.

Rue H, Martino S and Chopin N 2009 Approximate Bayesian inference for latent Gaussian models by using integrated nested Laplace approximations (with discussion). *Journal of the Royal Statistical Society: Series B* **71**, 319–392.

Ruppert D, Wand M and Carroll R 2003 *Semiparametric Regression*. Cambridge University Press, Cambridge.

Sabanés Bové D and Held L 2011a Bayesian fractional polynomials. *Statistics and Computing* **21**, 309–324.

Sabanés Bové D and Held L 2011b Hyper-*g*-priors for generalized linear models. *Bayesian Analysis* **6**, 387–410.

Schabenberger O and Gotway C 2004 *Statistical Methods for Spatial Data Analysis.* Chapman and Hall/CRC Press, Boca Raton.

Scheipl F 2011 spikeSlabGAM: Bayesian variable selection, model choice and regularization for generalized additive mixed models in R. *Journal of Statistical Software* **43**, 1–24.

Schwarz G 1978 Estimating the dimension of a model. *Annals of Statistics* **6**, 461–464.

Scott J and Berger J 2010 Bayes and empirical-Bayes multiplicity adjustment in the variable selection problem. *The Annals of Statistics* **38**, 2587–2619.

Seber G and Wild C 1989 *Nonlinear Regression*. John Wiley & Sons, New York.

Sellke T, Bayarri M and Berger J 2001 Calculation of p values for testing precise null hypotheses. *The American Statistician* **55**, 62–71.

Seltzer M 1993 Sensitivity analysis for fixed effects in the hierarchical model: A Gibbs sampling approach. *Journal of Educational and Behaviorial Statistics* **18**, 207–235.

Seltzer M, Wong W and Bryk A 1996 Bayesian analysis in applications of hierarchical models: Issues and methods. *Journal of Educational and Behaviorial Statistics* **21**, 131–167.

Serruys P, de Feyter P, Macaya C, Kokott N, Puel J, Vrolix M, Branzi A, Bertolami M, Jackson G, Strauss B and Meier B 2002 Fluvastatin for prevention of cardiac events following successful first percutaneous coronary intervention. A randomised controlled trial. *Journal of the American Medical Association* **287**, 3215–3222.

Sha N, Vannucci M, Tadesse M, Brown P, Dragoni I, Davies N, Roberts T, Contestabile A, Salmon M, Buckley C and Falciani F 2004 Bayesian variable selection in multinomial probit models to identify molecular signatures of disease stage. *Biometrics* **60**, 812–819.

Shapiro S and Francia R 1972 An approximate analysis of variance test for normality. *Journal of the American Statistical Association* **67**, 215–216.

Sharef E, Strawderman R, Ruppert D, Cowen M and Halasyamani L 2010 Bayesian adaptive B-spline estimation in proportional hazards frailty models. *Electronic Journal of Statistics* **4**, 606–642.

Sinharay S and Stern H 2003 Posterior predictive model checking in hierarchical models. *Journal of Statistical Planning and Inference* **111**, 209–221.

Smith A 1973a Bayes estimates in one-way and two-way models. *Biometrika* **60**, 319–329.

Smith A 1973b A general Bayesian linear model. *Journal of the Royal Statistical Society: Series B* **35**, 67–75.

Smith A and Gelfand A 1992 Bayesian statistics without tears: A sampling-resampling perspective. *The American Statistician* **46**, 84–88.

Smith M and Kohn R 1996 Nonparametric regression using Bayesian variable selection. *Journal of Econometrics* **75**, 317–343.

Song HR, Lawson A and Nitcheva D 2010 Bayesian hierarchical models of dietary assessment via food frequency. *Canadian Journal of Statistics* **38**, 506–516.

Sorensen D and Gianola D 2002 *Likelihood, Bayesian, and MCMC Methods in Quantitative Genetics.* Springer, New York.

Spiegelhalter D, Abrams K and Myles J 2004 *Bayesian Approaches to Clinical Trials and Health-Care Evaluation.* John Wiley & Sons, New York.

Spiegelhalter D, Best N, Carlin B and van der Linde A 2002 Bayesian measures of model complexity and fit (with discussion). *Journal of the Royal Statistical Society: Series B* **64**, 583–639.

Spiegelhalter, DJ, Freedman L and Myles J 1994 Bayesian approaches to randomised trials. *Journal of the Royal Statistical Society: Series A* **57**, 357–387.

Stanberry L, Murua A and Cordes D 2008 Functional connectivity mapping using the ferromagnetic Potts spin model. *Human Brain Mapping* **29**, 422–440.

Steinbakk G and Storvik G 2009 Posterior predictive p-values in Bayesian hierarchical models. *Scandinavian Journal of Statistics* **36**, 320–336.

Stern H and Sinharay S 2005 Bayesian model checking and model diagnostics. *Handbook of Statistics* **25**, 171–192.

Sturtz S, Ligges U and Gelman A 2005 R2WinBUGS: A package for running WinBUGS from R. *Journal of Statistical Software* **12**, 1–16.

Sun D, Speckman P and Tsutakawa R 2000 Random Effects in Generalized Linear Mixed models (GLMMs). In: *Generalized Linear Models: A Bayesian Perspective* (DK Dey, SK Ghosh and BK Mallick, eds.). Marcel Dekker, Inc., New York, pp. 23–39.

Sun D, Tsutakowa R and He Z 2001 Propriety of posteriors with improper priors in hierarchical linear mixed models. *Statistica Sinica* **11**, 77–95.

Swartz M and Shete S 2007 The null distribution of stochastic search gene suggestion: a Bayesian approach to gene mapping. *BMC Proceedings* **1**(S113), 1–5.

Swartz M, Kimmel M, Mueller P and Amos C 2006 Stochastic search gene suggestion: A Bayesian hierarchical model for gene mapping. *Biometrics* **62**, 495–503.

Tadesse M, Sha N and Vannucci M 2005 Bayesian variable selection in clustering high-dimensional data. *Journal of the American Statistical Association* **100**, 602–617.

Tan SB, Chung YF, Tai BC, Cheung YB and Machin D 2003 Bayesian approaches to randomised trials. *Controlled Clinical Trials* **24**, 110–121.

Tan T, Tian GL and Ng KW 2010 *Bayesian Missing Data Problems. EM, Data Augmentation and Noniterative Computation*. Chapman and Hall/CRC, Boca Raton.

Tanner M 1993 *Tools for Statistical Inference* (2nd edition). Springer Series in Statistics, Springer-Verlag, New York.

Tanner M 1996 *Tools for Statistical Inference* (3rd edition). Springer Series in Statistics, Springer-Verlag, New York.

Tanner M and Wong W 1987 The calculation of posterior distributions by data augmentation (with discussion). *Journal of the American Statistical Association* **82**, 528–550.

Tarone R 1982 The use of historical control information in testing for a trend in Poisson means. *Biometrics* **38**, 457–462.

Taroni F, Bozza S, Biedermann A, Garbolino P and Aitkin C 2010 *Data Analysis in Forensic Science: A Bayesian Decision Perspective*. John Wiley & Sons, New York.

Tennant R, Margolin B, Shelby M, Zeigler E, Haseman J, Spalding J, Caspary W, Resnick M, Stasiewicz S, Andersob B and Minor R 1987 Prediction of chemical carcinogenicity in rodents from in vitro genetic toxicity assays. *Science* **236**(4804), 933–941.

Thall P and Vail S 1990 Some covariance models for longitudinal count data with overdispersion. *Biometrics* **46**, 657–671.

The GUSTO Investigators 1993 An international randomized trial comparing four thrombolytic strategies for acute myocardial infarction. *New England Journal of Medicine* **329**, 673–682.

The Scandinavian Simvastatin Survival Study Group 1994 Randomized trial of cholesterol lowering in 4444 patients with coronary heart disease: The Scandinavian Simvastatin Survival Study (4S). *The Lancet* **344**, 1383–1389.

Tiao G and Tan W 1965 Bayesian analysis of random-effect models in the analysis of variance. I.: Posterior distribution of variance components. *Biometrika* **52**, 37–53.

Tibshirani R 1996 Regression shrinkage and selection via the Lasso. *Journal of the Royal Statistical Society: Series B* **58**, 267–288.

Tibshirani R, Saunders M, Rosset S, Zhu J and Knight K 2005 Sparsity and smoothness via the fused Lasso. *Journal of the Royal Statistical Society: Series B* **67**, 91–108.

Tierney L 1994 Markov chains for exploring posterior distributions (with discussion). *Annals of Statistics* **22**, 1701–1762.

Topal B, Van de Moortel M, Fieuws S, Vanbeckevoort D, Van Steenbergen W, Aerts R and Penninckx F 2003 The value of magnetic resonance cholangiocreatography in predicting common bile duct stones in patients with gallstone disease. *British Journal of Surgery* **90**, 42–47.

Tsiatis A, Gruttola V and Wulfsohn M 1995 Modeling the relationship of survival to longitudinal data measured with error. Applications to survival and CD4 counts in patients with AIDS. *Journal of the American Statistical Association* **90**, 27–37.

Ugarte M, Goicoa T, Ibanez B and Militano A 2009 Evaluating the performance of spatio-temporal Bayesian models in disease mapping. *Environmetrics* **20**, 647–665. DOI: 10.1002/env.969.

Vaida F and Blanchard S 2005 Conditional Akaike information for mixed-effects models. *Biometrika* **92**, 351–370.

van Dyk D and Meng X 2001 The art of data augmentation (with discussion). *Journal of Computational and Graphical Statistics* **10**, 1–111.

Van Houwelingen J and Le Cessie S 1992 Ridge estimators in logistic regression. *Journal of the Royal Statistical Society: Series C (Applied Statistics)* **41**, 191–201.

van Weel V, Toes R, Seghers L, Deckers M, de Vries M, Eilers P, Sipkens J, Schepers A, Eefting D, van Hinsbergh V, van Bockel J and Quax P 2007 Natural killer cells and $CD4^+$ T-cells modulate collateral artery development. *Artheriosclerosis, Thrombosis, and Vascular Biology* **27**, 2310–2318.

Vanobbergen J, Martens L and Declerck D 2001 Caries prevalence in Belgian children: A review. *International Journal of Paediatric Dentistry* **11**, 164–170.

Vanobbergen J, Martens L, Lesaffre E and Declerck D 2000 The Signal-Tandmobiel® project – a longitudinal intervention health promotion study in Flanders (Belgium): Baseline and first year results. *European Journal of Paediatric Dentistry* **2**, 87–96.

Verbeke G and Lesaffre E 1996 A linear mixed-effects model with heterogeneity in the random-effects population. *Journal of the American Statistical Association* **91**, 217–221.

Verbeke G and Molenberghs G 2000 *Linear Mixed Models for Longitudinal Data*. Springer, New York.

Vines S, Giks W and Wild P 1996 Fitting Bayesian multiple random effects models. *Statistics and Computing* **6**, 337–346.

Waagepetersen R and Sorensen D 2001 A tutorial on reversible jump MCMC with a view toward applications in QTL-mapping. *International Statistical Review* **69**, 49–61.

Wakefield J 2004 A critique of statistical aspects of ecological studies in spatial epidemiology. *Environmental and Ecological Statistics* **11**, 31–54.

Wakefield J and Morris S 2001 The Bayesian modeling of disease risk in relation to a point source. *Journal of the American Statistical Association* **96**, 77–91.

Wakefield J and Shaddick G 2006 Health-exposure modeling and the ecological fallacy. *Biostatistics* **7**, 438–455.

Ward E 2008 A review and comparison of four commonly used Bayesian and maximum likelihood model selection tools. *Ecological Modelling* **211**, 1–10.

Weinberg C 2001 It's time to rehabilitate the *P*-value. *Epidemiology* **12**, 288–290.

Weiss R 1996 An approach to Bayesian sensitivity analysis. *Journal of the Royal Statistical Society: Series B* **58**, 739–750.

West M 2000 Bayesian factor regression models in the large p small n paradigm. In: *Bayesian Statistics 7* (JM Bernardo *et al.*, eds.). Oxford University Press, Oxford, pp. 733–742.

Wheeler D, Hickson D and Waller L 2010 Assessing local model adequacy in Bayesian hierarchical models using the partitioned deviance information criterion. *Computational Statistics and Data Analysis* **54**, 1657–1671.

Wilks W and Roberts G 1996 Strategies from improving MCMC. In: *Markov Chain Monte Carlo in Practice* (WR Gilks, S Richardson and DJ Spiegelhalter, eds.). Chapman and Hall, London, pp. 89–113.

Wilks W, Wang C, Yvonnet B and Coursager P 1993 Random-effects models for longitudinal data using Gibbs sampling. *Biometrics* **49**, 441–453.

Williamson J 2005 *Bayesian Nets and Causality*. Oxford University Press, Oxford.

Winkler G 2006 *Image Analysis, Random Fields and Markov Chain Monte Carlo Methods* (2nd edition). Springer, New York.

Woolrich M, Jenkinson M, Brady J and Smith S 2004 Fully Bayesian spatio-temporal modeling of fMRI data. *IEEE Transactions on Medical Imaging* **2**, 213–231.

Wulfsohn M and Tsiatis A 1997 A joint model for survival and longitudinal data measured with error. *Biometrics* **53**, 330–339.

Xu L, Johnson T, Nichols T and Nee D 2009 Modeling inter-subject variability in fMRI activation location: A Bayesian hierarchical spatial model. *Biometrics* **65**, 1041–1051.

Yang AJ and Song XY 2010 Bayesian variable selection for disease classification using gene expression data. *Bioinformatics* **26**, 215–222.

Yi N, Yandell B, Churchill G, Allison D, Eisen E and Pomp D 2005 Bayesian model selection for genomic-wide epistatic quantitative trait loci analysis. *Genetics* **170**, 1333–1344.

Yuan M and Lin Y 2006 Model selection and estimation in regression with grouped variables. *Journal of the Royal Statistical Society: Series B* **68**, 49–67.

Zellner A 1975 Bayesian analysis of regression error terms. *Journal of the American Statistical Association* **70**, 138–144.

Zellner A 1986 On assessing prior distributions and Bayesian regression analysis with *g*-prior distributions. In: *Bayesian Inference and Decision Techniques: Essays in Honor of Bruno de Finetti* (PK Goel and A Zellner, eds.). North Holland, Amsterdam, pp. 223–243.

Zhang J and Lawson AB 2011 Accelerated failure time spatial model and its application to prostate cancer. *Journal of Applied Statistics* **38**(3), 591–603.

Zhang X, Johnson T, Little R and Cao Y 2010 Longitudinal image analysis of tumour-healthy brain change in contrast uptake induced by radiation. *Journal of the Royal Statistical Society: Series C (Applied Statistics)* **59**, 821–838.

Zhao P and Yu B 2006 On model selection consistency of Lasso. *Journal of Machine Learning Research* **7**, 2541–2563.

Zhu L and Carlin B 2000 Comparing hierarchical models for spatio-temporally misaligned data using the deviance information criterion. *Statistics in Medicine* **19**, 2265–2278.

Zou H 2006 The adaptive Lasso and its oracle properties. *Journal of the American Statistical Association* **101**, 1418–1429.

Zou H and Hastie T 2005 Regularization and variable selection via the Elastic Net. *Journal of the Royal Statistical Society: Series B* **67**, 301–320.

Index

Printed and bound by CPI Group (UK) Ltd, Croydon, CR0 4YY

26/04/2023

03214205-0002